Essentials of Obstetrics and Gynecology

Essentials of Obstetrics and Gynecology

Edited by **Larry Stone**

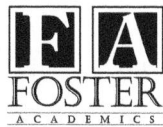

FA
FOSTER
ACADEMICS

New Jersey

Published by Foster Academics,
61 Van Reypen Street,
Jersey City, NJ 07306, USA
www.fosteracademics.com

Essentials of Obstetrics and Gynecology
Edited by Larry Stone

International Standard Book Number: 978-1-63242-462-4 (Hardback)

The publisher's policy is to use permanent paper from mills that operate a sustainable forestry policy. Furthermore, the publisher ensures that the text paper and cover boards used have met acceptable environmental accreditation standards.

Trademark Notice: Registered trademark of products or corporate names are used only for explanation and identification without intent to infringe.

Printed in the United States of America.

Contents

Preface

Obstetrics and gynecology is that branch of medical science which is concerned with the health of a women's reproductive organs like vagina, uterus, ovaries, etc. It covers the study of childbirth, pregnancy and also post-natal care. It also includes some sub-specialties like maternal-fetal medicine, reproductive endocrinology, infertility, menopausal and geriatric gynecology, etc. This book elucidates the concepts and innovative models around prospective developments with respect to this field. It will outline the concepts and core areas of this subject to provide comprehensive insights to the readers. From theories to research to practical applications, case studies from all across the globe, related to all contemporary topics of relevance to obstetrics and gynecology have been included in this text. Students, researchers, experts, gynecologists and all associated with this discipline will benefit alike from this book.

This book unites the global concepts and researches in an organized manner for a comprehensive understanding of the subject. It is a ripe text for all researchers, students, scientists or anyone else who is interested in acquiring a better knowledge of this dynamic field.

I extend my sincere thanks to the contributors for such eloquent research chapters. Finally, I thank my family for being a source of support and help.

Editor

Alternate Sequential Suture Tightening: A Novel Technique for Uncontrolled Postpartum Hemorrhage

Sharda Brata Ghosh[1] and Y. M. Mala[2]

[1]*Saudi German Hospital, Dubai, UAE*
[2]*Department of Obstetrics & Gynaecology, Lok Nayak Hospital, Maulana Azad Medical College, Delhi 110002, India*

Correspondence should be addressed to Sharda Brata Ghosh; shardabg2005@gmail.com

Academic Editor: Gian Carlo Di Renzo

Objective. The most commonly described technique of modified B-Lynch suture may not be suitable for all the patients presenting with flabby, atonic uterus. *Study Design*. A retrospective analysis of twelve patients with uncontrolled postpartum haemorrhage, who underwent this procedure from March 2007 to September 2012, was conducted. In this novel technique, sutures are passed in the lower uterine segment and are tightened alternately to control uterine bleeding. *Results*. Average duration of the procedure was 4 minutes (range 2–7 minutes). Average blood loss was 1625 mL (range 1300–1900 mL). Eleven patients (91.66%) were seen to have a successful outcome with only this technique. No patient required hysterectomy and one patient (8.33%) required additional bilateral internal iliac artery ligation. All the patients had a minimum follow-up of 2 yrs and none of them reported any infertility problems. *Conclusion*. This technique is simple, quick, and effective. There was no adverse effect on the fertility potential for the observed 2 years; however, a long-term follow-up is required to comment on its actual rate. This technique cannot replace the standard modified B-Lynch technique for uncontrolled postpartum haemorrhage but can be used for unresponsive, flabby, and atonic uterus.

1. Introduction

Postpartum haemorrhage remains one of the leading causes of maternal morbidity and mortality [1]. In developed countries, it accounts for 0.1% of maternal deaths [2] and is responsible for approximately yearly deaths of around 125,000 women all over the world [3]. For more than a decade, modified B-Lynch suture has been the standard technique for managing uncontrolled postpartum haemorrhage [4–6], but, in some patients, it does not have a successful outcome. In developing countries, this may lead to emergency hysterectomy or maternal mortality due to inadequate medical facilities. In order to avoid or reduce the rate of such avoidable complications, we have tried to modify the original technique of modified B-Lynch suture and present our results as seen in the operated patients of uncontrolled PPH.

2. Material and Methods

A retrospective study was conducted on all the women who were diagnosed with postpartum haemorrhage from March 2007 up to September 2012. The data was analyzed regarding total number and mode of deliveries, number of cases of postpartum haemorrhage, their complications, and duration of hospital stay. Blood loss was estimated based on the swab count (one small 10×10 cm fully saturated swab: around 60 mL of blood loss; one large 45×45 cm fully saturated swab: around 350 mL blood loss). Patients having PPH after vaginal delivery and PPH without uterine atony were excluded from the study.

This technique was described and developed by the corresponding author. It was used as a secondary procedure in the first patient following a failed modified B-Lynch suture and then as a primary procedure in the other eleven patients (Table 1). Primary indication in these 11 patients was persistent atonic uterus which did not respond to other conservative measures including uterotonics (I/V oxytocin, ergometrine, carboprost, and misoprostol) and uterine massage. Uterotonic treatment included bolus dose of 5 units of the oxytocin followed by infusion of 20 units of oxytocin; 0.2 mg of ergometrine was given and repeated 2-3 times;

TABLE 1: Showing diagnoses, treatment, complications, blood loss, and hospital stay.

Age of patient (yrs)	Diagnosis	Preop Hb (gm%)	Technique	O	Estimated blood loss (mL)	Postop Hb (gm%)	Number of units of blood transfusion	Hospital stay (days)	Complications
29	G2P1L1 37 wks with fetal distress	8.4	**Failed MBLS;** ASTS	S	1400	8.9	2	10	Fever for 3 days
24.5	Primi. with 40 weeks with thick meconium in early labor	7.8	Failed MT ASTS	S	1900	8.3	3	8	—
35	G5P4L4 with 36 wks with APH (PP IIb)	9.7	Failed MT ASTS	S	1600	9.2	1	16	—
33	G3A2 with 41 weeks with PROM	9.4	Failed MT ASTS	S	1800	9.3	2	10	—
29	G3A2 with 41 weeks with CPD	8.9	Failed MT ASTS	S	1500	9.6	2	8	Superficial infection
31	G3A2 with 37 wks with gestational HTN with failed induction	10.1	Failed MT ASTS	S	1900	9.2	1	8	—
26	G2A1 with thick meconium in early labor	8.7	Failed MT ASTS	S	1800	9.4	2	8	—
36	G5A2P2L2 with 36 wks with previous 2 LSCS	9.8	Failed MT ASTS	S	1600	9.4	1	10	Fever for 3 days
37.5	G7AOP6L3 with 38 wks with placenta previa with APH	7.6	A failed MT STS	S	1700	9.3	4 with 10 units of FFP	8	
28.5	G3A1P1L1 with 39 wks with prolonged LPV with failed induction	12.2	Failed MT ASTS	S	1400	11.3		16	
30	G4A1P2L1 with 37 wks with previous 2 LSCS	8	Failed MT ASTS	S	1300	9.7		10	
27	G2P1L1 with 39	9.8	Failed MT ASTS	S	1600	9.4	1	8	Superficial infection

O: outcome; S: successful; EBL: estimated blood loss; MBLS: modified B-Lynch suture; ASTS: Alternate Sequential Suture Tightening; APH: antipartum hemorrhage; MT: medical treatment; PP: placenta previa; PROM: prelabor rupture of membrane; CPD: cephalopelvic disproportion; LPV: leaking per vagina; FFP: fresh frozen plasma; LSCS: lower segment cesarean section.

250 micrograms of carboprost was given by intramyometrial route and was repeated 2-3 times; 1000 micrograms of the misoprostol was given rectally. All the patients were discharged after a minimum of 8 days of hospital stay and were followed up regularly.

3. Alternate Sequential Suture Tightening (ASST) Technique

3.1. Position and Technique. After induction of anaesthesia, patient is positioned, cleaned, and draped for lower segment caesarean section. After delivery of the baby, if atonic PPH is observed, medical management (as described in Section 2) and uterine massage are started. If patient does not respond to this treatment, then resuscitation is started along with the arrangement and transfusion of adequate blood and blood products. If medical treatment fails then the uterus is exteriorized and bimanual compression is applied to assess the feasibility of the Alternate Sequential Suture Tightening (modified B-Lynch) technique. Two number 2 Vicryl sutures preferably on straight needles are mounted. First needle (right side) is inserted into the uterus above (1-2 cm) the bladder reflection and 1-2 cm medial to the lateral edge of lower uterine segment and 1–3 cm below the lower uterine incision. Then needle from this point of insertion into the anterior wall is taken out from the posterior wall at the same level. Then both free ends of the sutures are tied by a knot (double throw) at the fundus of the uterus. Then the knot is held by artery forceps. Similarly, another suture is applied and tied over the fundus and is held with artery forceps on the left side. Then artery forceps on the right side are opened and the suture is tightened further and again forceps are held at further tightened point. Now similar procedure is repeated on the left side. Such alternative sequential tightening of both sutures is repeated 3-4 times till the uterus is completely compressed and bleeding is controlled. Both sutures can be tightened up to around 3–5 cm of their extra length from the initial level of tightening by this Alternate Sequential Suture Tightening technique. Finally, one square knot is applied on both sides to lock the sutures. Now incision line is observed for any bleeding; if there is no bleeding, uterus is closed in the regular manner.

3.2. Postoperative Management. All the patients were monitored for hypovolemia and contracted uterus. Vulval examination was done to detect any vaginal bleeding. All the patients were discharged after a minimum of 8 days of hospital stay. Patients were followed up regularly at 1.5, 3, 6, 12, and 24 months after the index procedure.

4. Results

A total of 199 patients had atonic postpartum haemorrhage of which 174 patients developed it after vaginal deliveries and 25 patients after caesarean sections. Out of the 25, thirteen patients responded to uterotonics with uterine massage; the remaining twelve patients did not respond and hence were managed by this technique. Average duration of the procedure was 4 minutes (range 2–7 minutes). Average blood loss was 1625 mL (range 1300–1900 mL). Average duration of hospital stay was 10 days (range 8–16 days).

Eleven patients (91.66%) were seen to have a successful outcome with this technique alone. No patient required hysterectomy and one patient (8.33%) required additional bilateral internal iliac artery ligation. Two patients had postoperative fever for 3 days while two had mild superficial infection, all of whom recovered well with conservative treatment. All the patients had minimum follow-up of 2 yrs and none of them reported any infertility problems.

5. Discussion

Postpartum haemorrhage is a potentially life threatening complication associated with foetal delivery [1]. It may occur after vaginal delivery (4%) or caesarean section (6%) [7, 8]. It is usually unpredictable and remains a challenge for obstetricians worldwide. In the developing world, due to factors such as high prevalence of high risk pregnant women, nonavailability of blood products and/or of operation theatre/intensive care unit back-up may further complicate the situation. Risk factors for PPH include anemia, uncontrolled hypertension, multigravida mothers, multiple pregnancies, coagulopathy, previously scared uterus, prolonged labor, and instrumental delivery [2, 7, 8]. Some common underlying causes include uterine atony, retained conception product, abnormal placental implantation, uterogenital trauma, and undetected coagulopathies [9].

The most important step in the management of PPH is to identify the underlying cause and correct the same [4]. Most of the cases of PPH can be controlled by traditional treatment modalities like uterotonic agents, uterine massage, and balloon tamponade [4]. Uncontrolled PPH is usually managed by different uterine suture techniques (B-Lynch, modified B-Lynch, and square suture) or with stepwise devascularization surgical procedures. These techniques have reported variable outcomes and many of the patients finally require emergency hysterectomy [4, 5, 10, 11].

B-Lynch suture was first described and was shown to be the most effective suture technique for managing uncontrolled postpartum haemorrhage due to atonic uterus. But it requires expertise and reopening of the uterus. As a result, a lot of complications (partial necrosis or sloughing of the uterine wall, cervical stenosis, and hematometra) have been reported in literature [12]. Hayman et al. [5] have performed a modified original B-Lynch suture independently. They did not reopen the uterine cavity and used number 2 Vicryl or Dexon suture to control the bleeding. Sutures are taken on long straight needle to transfix the uterus from front to back, just above the reflection of the bladder, and are then tied at the fundus of the uterus. Since then, modified suture has become one of the most popular and standard treatments for managing uncontrolled postpartum haemorrhage [5, 6, 13].

This technique is also used to control massive uterine bleeding due to abnormal placental implantations, midtrimester abortion, and patients with coagulation disorders [5, 12, 13]. A number of suture materials like Dexon (polyglycolic acid), Vicryl (polyglactin 910), PDS (polydioxanone), Prolene (monofilament polypropylene), and nylon

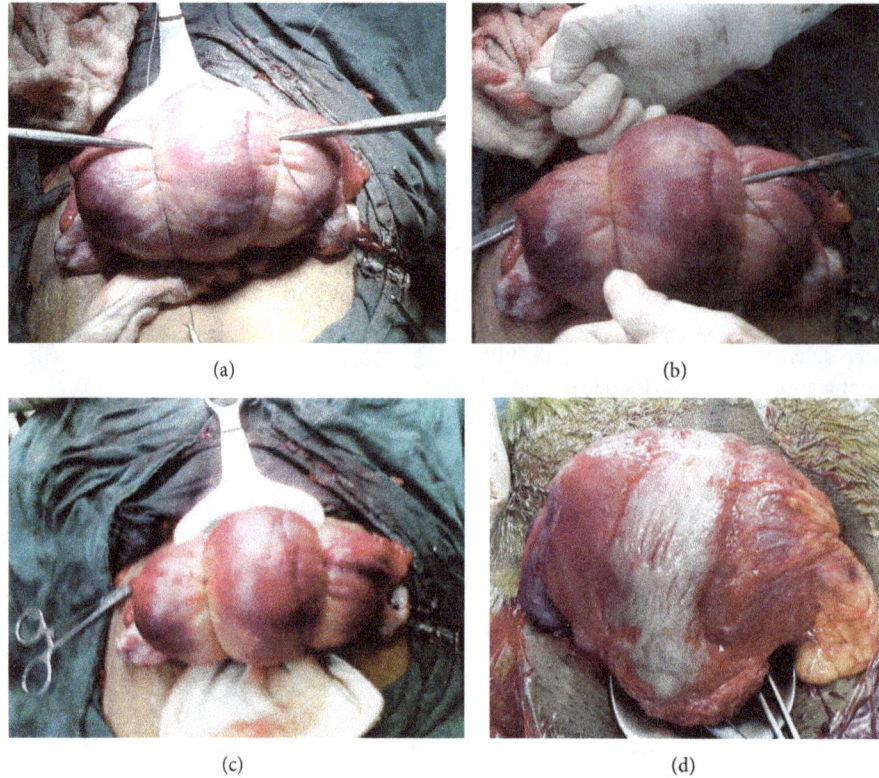

FIGURE 1: (a) Clinical photograph showing the first level of double tie knot being held with two artery forceps. (b) Clinical photograph showing artery forceps holding the tightened knot on Lt side and the Rt side which is being further tightened (with reduction in the size of uterus). (c) Clinical photograph showing both knots after final tightening of both sutures with marked reduction in the size of uterus. (d) Clinical photograph showing the uterus at 1.5 yrs follow-up during second cesarean section.

have been used for applying these sutures [14, 15]. Many centers use a specially designed Monocryl (poliglecaprone 25, Ethicon) monofilament suture with a 60% tensile strength at 7 days, 0% at 21 days, and complete absorption at 90–120 days [14, 15]. Kaoiean [16] reported successful outcome of B-Lynch suture in 23 patients out of total 24 patients. One patient did not respond and was managed by emergency hysterectomy. Xiao and Zhang reported successful outcome in a patient with PPH managed with combination of B-Lynch and modified Cho suture [17]. Marasinghe et al. [18] did a prospective observational study to evaluate the performance of a modified anchored B-Lynch suture for postpartum atonic uterus in 17 women. They reported successful outcomes in 13 patients (76%) while 4 patients (24%) required emergency postpartum hysterectomy. Kayem et al. [19] did a prospective population based study to assess maternal outcomes after application of uterine compression suture and to characterize the risk factors for obstetric hysterectomy. Two hundred eleven women were managed with a uterine compression suture to control postpartum haemorrhage. The overall rate of failure, leading to hysterectomy, was 25%. However, there were no significant differences in failure rates among B-Lynch sutures, modified B-Lynch sutures, and other suture techniques. They reported that women were more likely to have a hysterectomy if they were aged 35 years or older, were multiparous, had a vaginal delivery, or had a delay between 2 and 6 hours from delivery to uterine suture compression.

So, a single or combination of these suture techniques has produced variable results in different published studies. In many patients, uterus may remain flabby which may lead to emergency hysterectomy or maternal mortality due to inadequate medical facilities. Such difficult situations forced us to incorporate some changes in the modified B-Lynch technique.

This modified technique (Alternate Sequential Suture Tightening) was used as a secondary procedure in the first patient for failed modified B-Lynch suture and then as a primary procedure in the other eleven patients. We believe that uterus remained flabby in some cases, because it could not be compressed fully by the standard modified B-Lynch suture technique. But when we used this technique, uterus could be compressed more effectively and bleeding could be controlled. We used number 2 Vicryl sutures in all of our patients due to unavailability of the Monocryl (poliglecaprone 25, Ethicon) suture. Two number 2 Vicryl sutures, preferably on straight needles, were used in this technique. The first needle (right side) is inserted into the uterus above (1-2 cm) bladder reflection, 1-2 cm medial to the lateral edge of lower uterine segment, and 1–3 cm below the lower uterine incision. Then needle from this point of insertion into the anterior wall is taken out from the posterior wall at the same level. Then both free ends of the sutures are tied by a knot (double throw) at the fundus of the uterus. Then the knot is held by artery forceps (Figure 1). Similarly, another suture is applied and tied over the fundus and is held with artery forceps on the left side. Then artery forceps on the right side are opened and the suture is tightened further and again forceps are held at further tightened point. Now similar procedure is repeated on the left side. Such alternative sequential tightening of both sutures is repeated 3-4 times till the uterus is completely compressed and bleeding is controlled. Finally, one square knot is applied on both sides to lock the sutures.

Almost 75–100% successful outcomes have been reported with modified B-Lynch suture in published literature [18, 19]. But, in our study, eleven patients (91.66%) had successful outcome with our technique only. No patient required hysterectomy and only one patient (8.33%) required additional bilateral internal artery ligation. All the patients had minimum follow-up of 2 yrs and none of them reported any infertility problems. Weakness of this study includes retrospective nature, lack of control, and short follow-up.

This technique is simple, quick, and effective (91.66% successful outcome). There was no adverse effect on the fertility potential for the observed 2 years; however, a long term follow-up is required to comment on its actual rate. This technique cannot replace the standard B-Lynch [20] or modified B-Lynch technique for uncontrolled postpartum haemorrhage but can be used for unresponsive, flabby, and atonic uterus.

Disclosure

Part of this paper has been presented in Arab Health Gynae Conference (2012).

Conflict of Interests

There is no conflict of interests.

Authors' Contribution

It is certified that both authors have contributed to this paper; work is original.

References

[1] G. Lewis and The Confidential Enquiry into Maternal and Child Health (CEMACH), Eds., *Saving Mothers' Lives: Reviewing Maternal Deaths to Make Motherhood Safer—2003-2005. The Seventh Report on the Confidential Enquiries into Maternal Deaths in the United Kingdom*, The Confidential Enquiry into Maternal and Child Health (CEMACH), London, UK, 2007.

[2] V. D. Tsu, "Postpartum haemorrhage in Zimbabwe: a risk factor analysis," *British Journal of Obstetrics & Gynaecology*, vol. 100, no. 4, pp. 327–333, 1993.

[3] J. Drife, "Management of primary postpartum haemorrhage," *British Journal of Obstetrics and Gynaecology*, vol. 104, no. 3, pp. 275–277, 1997.

[4] A. B. Weisbrod, F. R. Sheppard, M. R. Chernofsky et al., "Emergent management of postpartum hemorrhage for the general and acute care surgeon," *World Journal of Emergency Surgery*, vol. 4, no. 1, article 43, 2009.

[5] R. G. Hayman, S. Arulkumaran, and P. J. Steer, "Uterine compression sutures: surgical management of postpartum hemorrhage," *Obstetrics and Gynecology*, vol. 99, no. 3, pp. 502–506, 2002.

[6] E. El-Hamamy and C. B-Lynch, "A worldwide review of the uses of the uterine compression suture techniques as alternative to hysterectomy in the management of severe post-partum haemorrhage," *Journal of Obstetrics and Gynaecology*, vol. 25, no. 2, pp. 143–149, 2005.

[7] C. A. Combs, E. L. Murphy, and R. K. Laros Jr., "Factors associated with postpartum hemorrhage with vaginal birth," *Obstetrics & Gynecology*, vol. 77, no. 1, pp. 69–76, 1991.

[8] W. Prasertcharoensuk, U. Swadpanich, and P. Lumbiganon, "Accuracy of the blood loss estimation in the third stage of labor," *International Journal of Gynecology & Obstetrics*, vol. 71, no. 1, pp. 69–70, 2000.

[9] M. Moore, J. P. Morales, T. Sabharwal, E. Oteng-Ntim, and G. O'Sullivan, "Selective arterial embolisation: a first line measure for obstetric haemorrhage?" *International Journal of Obstetric Anesthesia*, vol. 17, no. 1, pp. 70–73, 2008.

[10] C. B-Lynch, A. Coker, A. H. Lawal, J. Abu, and M. J. Cowen, "The B-Lynch surgical technique for the control of massive postpartum haemorrhage: an alternative to hysterectomy? Five cases reported," *British Journal of Obstetrics and Gynaecology*, vol. 104, no. 3, pp. 372–375, 1997.

[11] J. H. Cho, H. S. Jun, and C. N. Lee, "Hemostatic suturing technique for uterine bleeding during cesarean delivery," *Obstetrics & Gynecology*, vol. 96, no. 1, pp. 129–131, 2000.

[12] V. B. Ghodake, S. N. Pandit, and S. M. Umbardand, "Role of modified B-lynch suture in modern day management of atonic postpartum haemorrhage," *Bombay Hospital Journal*, vol. 50, no. 2, pp. 205–211, 2008.

[13] K. Hillaby, J. Ablett, and L. Cardozo, "Successful use of the B-Lynch brace suture in early pregnancy," *Journal of Obstetrics and Gynaecology*, vol. 24, no. 7, pp. 841–842, 2004.

[14] N. Price and C. B-Lynch, "Technical description of the B-Lynch brace suture for treatment of massive postpartum hemorrhage and review of published cases," *International Journal of Fertility and Women's Medicine*, vol. 50, no. 4, pp. 148–163, 2005.

[15] E. Koh, K. Devendra, and L. K. Tan, "B-Lynch suture for the treatment of uterine atony," *Singapore Medical Journal*, vol. 50, no. 7, pp. 693–697, 2009.

[16] S. Kaoiean, "Successful use of the B-Lynch uterine compression suture in treating intractable postpartum hemorrhage after cesarean delivery in Rajavithi Hospital," *Journal of the Medical Association of Thailand*, vol. 96, no. 11, pp. 1408–1415, 2013.

[17] J. P. Xiao and B. Zhang, "Combination of B-Lynch and modified Cho sutures for postpartum hemorrhage caused by low-lying placenta and placenta accreta," *Clinical and Experimental Obstetrics and Gynecology*, vol. 38, no. 3, pp. 274–275, 2011.

[18] J. P. Marasinghe, G. Condous, H. R. Seneviratne, and U. Marasinghe, "Modified anchored B-Lynch uterine compression suture for post partum bleeding with uterine atony," *Acta Obstetricia et Gynecologica Scandinavica*, vol. 90, no. 3, pp. 280–283, 2011.

[19] G. Kayem, J. J. Kurinczuk, Z. Alfirevic, P. Spark, P. Brocklehurst, and M. Knight, "Uterine compression sutures for the management of severe postpartum hemorrhage," *Obstetrics & Gynecology*, vol. 117, no. 1, pp. 14–20, 2011.

[20] F. C. A. Reynders, L. Senten, W. Tjalma, and Y. Jacque-myn, "Postpartum hemorrhage: practical approach to a life-threatening complication," *Clinical and Experimental Obstetrics and Gynecology*, vol. 33, no. 2, pp. 81–84, 2006.

A Case-Control Study on Intimate Partner Violence during Pregnancy and Low Birth Weight, Southeast Ethiopia

Habtamu Demelash,[1] Dabere Nigatu,[2] and Ketema Gashaw[2]

[1]*Department of Public Health, College of Medicine and Health Sciences, Madawalabu University, Goba, Bale, Ethiopia*
[2]*Department of Nursing, College of Medicine and Health Sciences, Madawalabu University, Goba, Bale, Ethiopia*

Correspondence should be addressed to Habtamu Demelash; hab2396@yahoo.com

Academic Editor: Curt W. Burger

Introduction. Violence against women has serious consequences for their reproductive and sexual health including birth outcomes. In Ethiopia, though the average parity of pregnant women is much higher than in other African countries, the link between intimate partner violence with low birth weight is unknown. *Objective.* The aim of this study was to examine the association between intimate partner violence and low birth weight among pregnant women. *Method.* Hospital based case-control study was conducted among 387 mothers (129 cases and 258 controls). Anthropometric measurements were taken both from mothers and their live births. The association between intimate partner violence and birth weight was computed through bivariable and multivariable logistic regression analyses and statistical significance was declared at $P < 0.05$. *Result.* Out of 387 interviewed mothers, 100 (25.8%) had experienced intimate partner violence during their index pregnancy period. Relatively more mothers of low birth weight infants were abused (48%) compared with controls (16.4%). Those mothers who suffered acts of any type of intimate partner violence during pregnancy were three times more likely to have a newborn with low birth weight (95% CI; (1.57 to 7.18)). The association between overall intimate partner violence and LBW was adjusted for potential confounder variables. *Conclusion.* This research result gives insight for health professional about the importance of screening for intimate partner violence during pregnancy. Health care providers should consider violence in their practice and try to identify women at risk.

1. Introduction

The World Health Organization (WHO) defines violence against women as "the range of sexually, psychologically, and physically coercive acts used against women by current or former male intimate partners" [1]. It is related to violence of any kind that is likely to result in harm or suffering of women whether it occurs in private or in public [2].

Domestic violence is one of the most common forms of violence against women. It is the violence perpetrated by persons who have or had a relationship of kinship or affection with the woman and generally refers to the current or former male intimate partner [1, 2]. Intimate partner violence against women is a major worldwide epidemic which has been found in practically all societies [3]. According to WHO 2013 report, 1 in 3 women throughout the world will experience physical and/or sexual violence by a partner

or sexual violence by a nonpartner [1]. Pregnancy may be a time of unique vulnerability to intimate partner violence (IPV) victimization because of changes in women's physical, social, emotional, and economic needs during pregnancy [1, 2, 4]. International studies suggested that 1–25% of pregnant women are exposed to physical violence by intimate partners during pregnancy [5].

Violence against women has serious consequences for their reproductive and sexual health including birth outcomes [6–8]. Violence during pregnancy has been associated with low birth weight, a major cause of infant death in the developing world [3], because stress due to violence raises cortisol levels leading to constriction of the blood vessels, limiting blood flow to the uterus [4].

A systematic review and meta-analysis study revealed that women who reported physical, sexual, or emotional abuse during pregnancy were more likely than nonabused women to give birth to a baby with low birth weight (LBW) [5]. The association between physical violence and LBW remained significant even after adjustment for parity, socioeconomic status, mother's age, and smoking habits [6].

But research linking intimate partner violence during pregnancy to LBW has not been conclusive and was mainly cross-sectional studies. Consequently, how much LBW is attributable to intimate partner violence during pregnancy remained unknown. Most of the research was also conducted in developed countries. In Ethiopia, the average parity of pregnant women is much higher than that in other African countries and no study has been conducted to link intimate partner violence with low birth weight [7]. Thus, we sought to investigate the effects of intimate partner violence during pregnancy period on birth weight of the babies born to women at the four governmental hospitals in Bale Zone, Oromia regional state, Ethiopia.

2. Method

2.1. Study Setting and Population. A hospital-based case-control study design was conducted in Bale Zone, Southeast Ethiopia, from April 1 to August 30, 2013. This study was conducted at the four government hospitals: Goba, Robe, Delomena, and Ginir. All mothers who gave live births in the study hospitals were eligible for this study. Cases were mothers who gave live births of weight less than 2500 g and controls were mothers who gave live births of weight 2500 g and above. All mothers selected as cases and controls were mothers with singleton and full term births. Additionally, mothers who had serious illness, hypertension, and/or diabetes mellitus were excluded from the study. Seven cases and respective controls' data were excluded because of missing data making the response rate 94%.

For each case there were two controls. Following each case two consecutive controls were included in the study until the required sample sizes were satisfied.

Since the cases (LBW) were rare, all eligible cases fulfilling the inclusion criteria in each hospital were included in the study until the required sample sizes were satisfied within the study period.

2.2. Data Collection Procedures. The data were collected by face-to-face interview method using structured and pretested questionnaire. The questionnaire was adopted from the Ethiopian Demographic and Health Survey (EDHS) and Behavioral Surveillance Survey (BSS). It consists of sociodemographic, obstetric, and experiences-of-violence related questions. The same interviewer was used to interview the mother for a case and the respective two consecutive controls. The weight of the newborns was measured within 15 minutes after birth using a balanced Seca scale. Maternal height was measured against a wall height scale to the nearest centimeter. Maternal weight was also measured by beam balance to the nearest kilogram and body mass index (BMI) was subsequently calculated.

The interview and anthropometric measurements were obtained by eight (two in each study hospital) trained midwives and nurses who were working in labor ward.

2.3. Data Analysis. The data were analyzed using SPSS for Windows version 20.0 (IBM SPSS Statistics, IBM Corp., New York). Bivariable logistic regression analyses were done to evaluate the association of low birth weight with each construct of intimate partner violence (IPV) (physical violence, psychological violence, and sexual violence) and overall IPV. Multivariable logistic regression analysis was used to control for potential confounding variables. A multivariable analysis was based on multiple logistic regression models. Two multivariable logistic regression models were constructed: one is to see the interaction of the three constructs of IPV, socioeconomic factors, and other maternal factors with the dependent variable low birth weight while the other model is constructed to see the interaction of overall IPV, socioeconomic factors, and other maternal factors with low birth weight. Furthermore, the relationship between the socioeconomic factors (residence, maternal education, maternal occupational status, family monthly income level, and husband's educational and occupational status) and intimate partner violence was evaluated by logistic regression analysis. In order to evaluate the strength of association, both crude and adjusted odds ratios with 95% confidence interval were calculated for exposure to intimate partner violence, socioeconomic factors, and other maternal factors in relation to LBW. Statistical significance was defined as $P < 0.05$.

2.4. Operational Definition

2.4.1. Emotional/Psychological Violence. Emotional/psychological violence is defined as being humiliated, insulted, intimidated, or threatened and/or controlling behaviors by a partner.

2.4.2. Physical Violence. Physical violence is defined as being slapped or having something thrown at her that could hurt her, being pushed or shoved, being hit with a fist or something else that could hurt, being kicked, dragged, or beaten up, being choked or burnt on purpose, and/or being threatened with, or actually having, a gun, a knife, or another weapon used on her by an intimate partner.

2.4.3. Sexual Violence. Sexual violence is defined as being physically forced to have sexual intercourse when she did not want to, having sexual intercourse because she was afraid of what her partner might do, and/or being forced to do something sexual that she found humiliating or degrading to her by an intimate partner.

2.4.4. Overall Intimate Partner Violence. Overall intimate partner violence is defined as follows: those mothers who experienced any act of intimate partner violence whether they encounter physical, psychological, or sexual violence during the index pregnancy period.

3. Results

In this study, from a total of 408 mothers that we planned to interview, 387 mothers (mothers of 129 cases and 258 controls) completed the interview which made the response rate of 94% for both cases and controls. Fifty-one percent of mothers of LBW babies and 69.4% of mothers of normal birth weight (NBW) babies were in the age range of 21–35 years. The predominant religion was found to be Islam, 66.7% of mothers of cases and 53.9% of mothers of controls. Related to occupational status the majority, 69.8%, of LBW mothers and 45.3% of NBW mothers were housewives. The significant number, 45.7%, of mothers of low birth weight babies was illiterate compared to 15.5% of mothers of normal birth weight babies. Concerning monthly family income among the study population, relatively high percentage of mothers with low birth weight babies, 24.6%, had less than 500 ETB monthly income compared to mothers with normal birth weight babies, 7.8%.

Fifty percent of mothers with LBW babies spaced between present and past pregnancy more than two years compared to 75% of mothers with NBW babies. Almost eighty-eight percent of mothers of cases and 95.3% of mothers of controls weighed more than 50 kg. Measurements of maternal height showed that 84.5% of mothers of cases and 93.8% of mothers of controls were greater than 150 cm tall. Forty-eight percent of mothers of cases and 24.8% of mothers of controls were residing in rural part of the study area. Almost all, 93%, of the study participants were currently married (Table 1).

A total of 387 mothers were interviewed about their experience of any violence during their current pregnancy period. Of them, 100 (25.8%) experienced some violence by their intimate partners during their index pregnancy period. Relatively more mothers of low birth weight infants were abused, 59 (48%), compared with controls, 41 (16.4%). Thirty percent of the mothers of LBW infants had been sexually abused by their partners during their current pregnancy, compared with 7.3% of mothers of the controls. Around forty-one percent of mothers of cases and 10% of mothers of controls had been abused physically by their intimate partners. In addition to physical and sexual violence, 38% of mothers of cases had been psychologically abused by their intimate partners, compared to 11.6% of mothers of controls. Overall, proportionally more mothers in the cases group reported experiences of abuse than in the controls group.

More than half, 54 (14%), of the mothers faced a type of intimate partner violence: the most frequent was being slapped or punched on the face. Seven (1.8%) of the mothers experienced a type of violence less frequent which was not being allowed to enter home or being locked in. Besides the above violence, 46 (11.9%) of the mothers had their contact with friends/family members limited, 44 (11.4%) of the mothers have been criticized by partners for what they were doing, 21 (5.4%) of the mothers were verbally abused by partners somewhere, and 9 (2.3%) of the mothers were threatened with some harmful objects.

Multivariable logistic regression analyses were performed to control confounding variables and to identify the strength of association with significant explanatory variables. In the logistic regression analysis, mothers with no formal education were more likely to encounter physical violence than mothers with advanced educational status (OR = 2.74; 95% CI = 1.38 to 5.47), and housewife mothers were more likely to be physically violated by their partner than employed

Table 1: Distribution of mothers by sociodemographic characteristics in Bale Zone, Oromia regional state, August 2013.

Variables	LBW		NBW		Total	
	Number	%	Number	%	Number	%
Age group (years)						
<20	52	40.3	56	21.7	108	28.0
21–35	66	51.2	179	69.4	245	63.3
>35	11	8.5	23	8.9	34	8.7
Weight group (kg)						
<50	16	12.4	12	4.7	28	7.2
>50	113	87.6	246	95.3	359	92.8
Height (Cm)						
≤150	20	15.5	16	6.2	36	9.3
>150	109	84.5	242	93.8	351	90.7
Religion						
Muslim	86	66.7	139	53.9	225	58.1
Orthodox	38	29.5	100	38.8	138	35.7
Protestant	5	3.9	14	5.4	19	4.9
Catholic	0	0	5	1.9	5	1.3
Ethnicity						
Oromo	103	79.8	183	70.9	186	73.9
Amhara	14	10.9	64	24.8	78	20.2
Others	12	9.3	11	1.3	23	5.9
Marital status						
Married	116	89.9	243	94.2	359	92.7
Others	13	10.1	15	5.8	28	7.3
Residence						
Urban	67	51.9	194	75.2	261	67.4
Rural	62	48.1	64	24.8	126	32.6
Head of household						
Male	117	90.7	233	90.3	350	90.4
Female	12	9.3	25	9.7	37	9.6
Maternal occupation						
Employed	10	7.8	40	15.5	50	12.9
Housewife	90	69.8	117	45.3	207	53.4
Farmer	8	6.2	31	12.0	39	10.0
Merchant	12	9.3	63	24.4	75	19.3
Daily laborer	9	7.0	7	2.7	16	4.3
Monthly income (ETB)						
≤500	31	24.6	20	7.8	51	13.3
501–1000	40	31.7	49	19.1	89	23.2
1001–1500	15	11.9	39	15.2	54	14.1
>1500	40	31.7	149	58	189	49.3
Maternal education						
Illiterate	59	45.7	40	15.5	99	25.6
Read and write only	2	1.6	5	1.9	7	1.8
Primary (1–8)	49	38.0	109	42.2	158	40.8
Secondary (9–12)	14	10.9	81	31.4	95	24.5
Tertiary	5	3.9	23	8.9	28	7.2

mothers (OR = 2.859; 95% CI = 1.073 to 7.616). Similarly, mothers living in a family with monthly income less than

TABLE 2: Sexual, physical, and psychological and all intimate violence during pregnancy and the risk of delivering a low birth weight infant among mothers in Bale Zone, Oromia regional state, August 2013.

Violence	LBW	NBW	COR [95% CI]	P value	AOR* [95% CI]	P value
			Sexual violence			
Yes	38	16	5.4 [2.92, 10.08]	<0.001	1.5 [0.43, 5.54]	0.513
No	84	228	1		1	
			Physical violence			
Yes	50	25	6.2 [3.56, 10.66]	<0.001	8.5 [3.36, 21.73]	<0.001
No	73	225	1		1	
			Psychological violence			
Yes	47	29	4.7 [2.77, 8.01]	<0.001	1.03 [0.29, 3.75]	0.957
No	76	221	1		1	
			Over all types of violence			
Yes	59	41	4.7 [2.89, 7.65]	<0.001	3.4 [1.57, 7.18]	0.002
No	64	209	1		1	

*Adjusted for birth interval, maternal height, BMI, maternal weight, antenatal care follow-up, and khat chewing status of the mother.

500 ETB (OR = 3.35; 95% CI = 1.58 to 7.13) or in the range of 1001–1500 ETB (OR = 2.83; 95% CI = 1.37 to 5.83) were at a higher risk of physical violence compared to mothers living in a family with monthly income greater than 1500 ETB. Psychological violence also significantly increased with residence and family income level. Mothers residing in rural area and with lower income level were associated with increased psychological violence. The relationship between exposure to any type of intimate partner violence and LBW was evaluated after adjusting for residence, maternal education, maternal occupational status, husband's educational and occupational status, family monthly income, maternal body mass index (BMI), antenatal care, and khat chewing and alcohol drinking status of mothers. Therefore, the multivariable logistic regression model indicated that those mothers who suffered acts of any type of intimate partner violence during pregnancy were three times more likely to have a newborn with low birth weight (95% CI: 1.57 to 7.18) (Table 2).

Similarly, the association was examined for subcategories of intimate partner violence (sexual, physical, and psychological) (Table 2). Physical violence during pregnancy was consistently associated with a significant increase in LBW. A slightly higher proportion of mothers of low birth weight infants reported having been abused sexually and psychologically compared with controls, but the difference was not statistically significant.

4. Discussion

In this study, 26% of the mothers had experienced intimate partner violence during their index pregnancy period. This result is consistent with other study in Nicaragua where 27% of the mothers had been abused by their intimate partners during their pregnancy [6]. But it is less than the study result in South Carolina where 35% reported intimate partner violence before and during index pregnancy period [7]. The difference might be due to differences in community awareness of violence during pregnancy. This study revealed that relatively more mothers of low birth weight infants were abused compared with controls. This result is supported by other similar studies in which slightly more mothers of low birth weight babies faced intimate partner violence than mothers with normal birth weight babies [2, 5, 6].

Although some studies have found that abuse during pregnancy increases the risk of LBW [1, 4, 7] other studies did not find a significant association [6, 9, 10]. This discrepancy might be due to differences in study populations, sample size, study design, measurements of violence, analytic approaches, and handling of potentially confounding variables.

In our study mothers who suffered from any type of intimate partner violence during pregnancy were more likely to have a newborn with low birth weight. This result is supported by results from hospital-based case-control study in León, Nicaragua, which found that, after adjusting for other known risk factors of low birth weight, partner violence against pregnant women increased the risk of low birth weight by a factor of three [11]. It has also been demonstrated through a systematic review and meta-analyses that the risk of violence during pregnancy increases for both low birth weight and preterm birth [5, 7, 12].

In our study we tried to analyze the association of birth weight for subgroups of intimate partner violence (sexual, physical, and psychological). As a result, physical violence during pregnancy was consistently associated with a significant increase in LBW. This finding is in line with other similar studies where physical violence by intimate partners during pregnancy period was independently associated with low birth weight [4, 6, 13, 14]. While a slightly higher proportion of mothers of low birth weight infants reported having been abused sexually and psychologically compared with controls, the difference was not statistically significant. Other studies demonstrate that statistically significant associations were not seen for those reporting only sexual or only psychological violence during pregnancy [4, 15, 16]. Further, a history of physical intimate partner violence exposure was found to be associated with low infant birth weight in the recent study in South Africa. But neither sexual nor psychological violence exposure yielded significant associations with low birth weight in this study [17].

5. Conclusion

The results of the present study indicate that there is an independent effect of overall and physical violence during pregnancy on the birth weight of the offspring. But neither sexual nor psychological violence exposure yielded significant associations with low birth weight in our study.

Health service providers should be aware of the impact of intimate violence on pregnant women and on their newborns and try to identify women at risk using the knowledge of maternal characteristics statistically associated with violence in pregnancy.

Longitudinal studies would also be valuable in addressing the causal mechanisms between intimate violence and low birth weight.

Ethical Approval

Ethical clearance letter was obtained from the Institutional Research Ethics Review Committee of Research and Community Services Directorate Office of Madawalabu University. Permission letters were secured from Bale Zone Health Bureau and from the four respective hospitals. Additionally, all the information obtained from each study participant was kept confidential throughout the process of this study.

Consent

Verbal consent was obtained from each mother prior to interview.

Conflict of Interests

All authors declare that they have no competing interests.

Authors' Contribution

Dabere Nigatu designed the study, participated in the process of data collection, performed data clerking and data analysis, interpreted the result, and drafted and critically reviewed the paper. Habtamu Demelash participated in the development of the study design as well as developing the questionnaire. He contributed in drafting and writing of the paper, supervised the data collection process, interpreted the result, and reviewed the paper. Ketema Gashaw contributed to the development of the overall study concept and design of the study and drafted and reviewed the paper. All authors read and approved the final paper.

Acknowledgments

The authors would like to acknowledge Madawalabu University for giving them an opportunity to work on identified thematic areas and the financial grants. They would like to thank the medical directors of the four hospitals (Delomena, Goba, Ginir, and Robe) and respective supervisors for their cooperation and assistance during data collection. Finally, they would like to forward their gratitude to the study participants and data collectors for their great contribution for the completion of this study.

References

[1] WHO, *Global and Regional Estimates of Violence against Women: Prevalence and Health Effects of Intimate Partner Violence and Non-Partner Sexual Violence*, World Health Organization, Geneva, Switzerland, 2013.

[2] D. K. Kaye, F. M. Mirembe, G. Bantebya, A. Johansson, and A. M. Ekstrom, "Domestic violence during pregnancy and risk of low birthweight and maternal complications: a prospective cohort study at Mulago hospital, Uganda," *Tropical Medicine and International Health*, vol. 11, no. 10, pp. 1576–1584, 2006.

[3] E. V. Cardoza, *Partner violence during pregnancy, psychosocial factors and child outcomes in Nicaragua [Ph.D. thesis]*, 2005.

[4] M. A. A. Nunes, S. Camey, C. P. Ferri, P. Manzolli, C. N. Manenti, and M. I. Schmidt, "Violence during pregnancy and newborn outcomes: a cohort study in a disadvantaged population in Brazil," *The European Journal of Public Health*, vol. 21, no. 1, pp. 92–97, 2010.

[5] E. Valladares, M. Ellsberg, R. Peña, U. Högberg, and L. Å. Persson, "Physical partner abuse during pregnancy: a risk factor for low birth weight in Nicaragua," *Obstetrics & Gynecology*, vol. 100, no. 4, pp. 700–705, 2002.

[6] H. Grimstad, B. Schei, B. Backe, and G. Jacobsen, "Physical abuse and low birthweight: a case-control study," *British Journal of Obstetrics and Gynaecology*, vol. 104, no. 11, pp. 1281–1287, 1997.

[7] WHO, *Multi-Country Study on Women's Health and Domestic Violence against Women Initial Results on Prevalence, Health Outcomes and Women's Responses*, WHO, 2005.

[8] M. L. Urquia, P. J. O'Campo, M. I. Heaman, P. A. Janssen, and K. R. Thiessen, "Experiences of violence before and during pregnancy and adverse pregnancy outcomes: an analysis of the Canadian Maternity Experiences Survey," *BMC Pregnancy and Childbirth*, vol. 11, article 42, 2011.

[9] N. Zareen, N. Majid, S. Naqvi, S. Saboohi, and H. Fatima, "Effect of domestic violence on pregnancy outcome," *Journal of the College of Physicians and Surgeons Pakistan*, vol. 19, no. 5, pp. 291–296, 2009.

[10] J. Campbell, S. Torres, J. Ryan et al., "Physical and nonphysical partner abuse and other risk factors for low birth weight among full term and preterm babies: a multiethnic case-control study," *American Journal of Epidemiology*, vol. 150, no. 7, pp. 714–726, 1999.

[11] K. Åsling-Monemi, R. Peña, M. C. Ellsberg, and L. Å. Persson, "Violence against women increases the risk of infant and child mortality: a case-referent study in Nicaragua," *Bulletin of the World Health Organization*, vol. 81, no. 1, pp. 10–18, 2003.

[12] C. C. Murphy, B. Schei, T. L. Myhr, and J. Du Mont, "Abuse: a risk factor for low birth weight? A systematic review and meta-analysis," *Canadian Medical Association Journal*, vol. 164, no. 11, pp. 1567–1572, 2001.

[13] V. E. C. Cokkinides, L. Ann, M. Sanderson, C. Addy, and L. Bethea, "Physical violence during pregnancy: maternal complications and birth outcomes," *CRVAW Faculty Journal Articles*, vol. 93, no. 5, pp. 661–666, 1999, Paper 133.

[14] J. Ntaganira, A. S. Muula, F. Masaisa, F. Dusabeyezu, S. Siziya, and E. Rudatsikira, "Intimate partner violence among pregnant women in Rwanda," *BMC Women's Health*, vol. 8, article 17, 2008.

[15] M. Mercedes, "Intimate partner violence against women during pregnancy: a critical reading from a gender perspective," *Revista Colombiana de Enfermería*, vol. 10, no. 10, pp. 64–77, 2015.

[16] F. Abdollahi, F. R. Abhari, M. A. Delavar, and J. Y. Charati, "Physical violence against pregnant women by an intimate partner, and adverse pregnancy outcomes in Mazandaran Province, Iran," *Journal of Family and Community Medicine*, vol. 22, no. 1, pp. 13–18, 2015.

[17] N. Koen, G. E. Wyatt, J. K. Williams et al., "Intimate partner violence: associations with low infant birthweight in a South African birth cohort," *Metabolic Brain Disease*, vol. 29, no. 2, pp. 281–299, 2014.

3

Comparison of Perinatal Outcome of Preterm Births Starting in Primary Care versus Secondary Care in Netherlands: A Retrospective Analysis of Nationwide Collected Data

A. J. van der Ven,[1] **J. M. Schaaf,**[1,2] **M. A. van Os,**[3] **C. J. M. de Groot,**[3] **M. C. Haak,**[4] **E. Pajkrt,**[1] **and B. W. J. Mol**[5]

[1]*Department of Obstetrics and Gynaecology, Academic Medical Center, P.O. Box 22700, 1100 DE Amsterdam, Netherlands*
[2]*Department of Medical Informatics, Academic Medical Center, Amsterdam, Netherlands*
[3]*Department of Obstetrics and Gynaecology, VU University Medical Center, Amsterdam, Netherlands*
[4]*Department of Obstetrics and Gynaecology, Leiden University Medical Center, Leiden, Netherlands*
[5]*School of Paediatrics and Reproductive Health, University of Adelaide, SA 5000, Australia*

Correspondence should be addressed to A. J. van der Ven; a.j.vanderven@amc.uva.nl

Academic Editor: Curt W. Burger

Introduction. In Netherlands, the obstetric care system is divided into primary and secondary care by risk level of the pregnancy. We assessed the incidence of preterm birth according to level of care and the association between level of care at time of labor onset and delivery and adverse perinatal outcome. *Methods*. Singleton pregnancies recorded in Netherlands Perinatal Registry between 1999 and 2007, with spontaneous birth between 25^{+0} and 36^{+6} weeks, were included. Three groups were compared: (1) labor onset and delivery in primary care; (2) labor onset in primary care and delivery in secondary care; (3) labor onset and delivery in secondary care. Multivariable logistic regression analyses were performed to calculate the risk of perinatal mortality and Apgar score ≤4. *Results*. Of all preterm deliveries, 42% had labor onset and 7.9% had also delivery in primary care. Women with labor onset between 34^{+0} and 36^{+6} weeks who were referred before delivery to secondary care had the lowest risk of perinatal mortality (aOR 0.49 (0.30–0.79)). Risk of perinatal mortality (aOR 1.65; 95% CI 1.20–2.27) and low Apgar score (aOR 1.95; 95% CI 1.53–2.48) were significantly increased in preterm home delivery. *Conclusion*. Referral before delivery is associated with improved perinatal outcome in the occurrence of preterm labor onset in primary care.

1. Introduction

Spontaneous preterm birth (PTB), defined by the World Health Organization as birth before 37 completed weeks of gestation, is one of the main causes of perinatal death in the developed countries [1]. PTB has multifactorial causes and a heterogeneous outcome [2–7]. For surviving preterm neonates, there may be significant health consequences with lasting disabilities, including respiratory problems, hearing and vision impairment, cerebral palsy, and mental retardation [2, 3].

In 2008, the EURO-PERISTAT study showed that perinatal mortality in Netherlands was relatively high when compared to other European countries [8]. The pathways leading to this are not completely clear and under investigation [9–11].

It has been suggested that PTB (<28 weeks) is a major cause of the low ranking of Netherlands in the EURO-PERISTAT study [12], although the incidence of PTB in Netherlands is comparable with the rest of Europe [13]. Among singleton pregnancies, the incidence of preterm deliveries is 6.0% and of very preterm deliveries, that is, before 32 completed weeks, 0.9% [10].

The Dutch obstetric care system is different from most other developed countries, since the level of care is organised according to the presence or absence of risk factors in medical and/or obstetrical history. However, it is not known if levels of care at labor onset and at time of delivery are determining factors in the pathway to adverse perinatal outcome.

The Dutch obstetric care system is structured as follows. Pregnant women without risk factors are under surveillance by primary obstetric care providers (midwives and in rural areas a few general practitioners who provide primary obstetric care (GPs)). Women with an a priori high risk profile, due to their medical or obstetrical history, receive secondary care from the beginning of pregnancy. If complications occur during pregnancy, women will be referred to secondary care during pregnancy. As risk factors can arise at any time, risk-selection remains a continuous process during pregnancy and delivery. Indications for primary and secondary care have been formulated by consensus between primary and secondary care providers in the so-called "List of Obstetric Indications" (LOI) [14] and all professionals involved in pregnancy care are bound to follow these guidelines. In the LOI, the policy regarding PTB is set as follows.

(i) Preterm labor defined as preterm rupture of membranes and/or preterm contractions before 37 completed weeks of gestation is of its nature an indication for referral to secondary care.

(ii) Women with previous PTB before 33 completed weeks have an indication for secondary care from the beginning of prenatal care until 37 weeks.

(iii) Women with previous PTB after 33 completed weeks can be cared for in primary care.

Women attending primary care will visit their midwife or GP on a regular consulting basis at the practice premises, which is in most cases within a twenty-minute drive of their home. In case of predefined changes in their normal pregnancy process, they will contact their primary care giver. Subsequently, the pregnant woman will be invited for an extra check or the care provider will visit her at home to assess the changes in order to distinguish between normal and abnormal changes and to assess if referral to secondary care is mandatory. This takes time and may sometimes be the cause of delay when referral to secondary care is indicated because of impending preterm delivery. In case of precipitous PTB, the midwife or GP will evaluate whether there is sufficient time for transport to hospital or if not will accept PTB at home. Thus in case of rapidly progressing spontaneous PTB there is always a risk of an unintended home delivery.

In contrast, patients in secondary care will contact their attending obstetricians by phone in case of signs of imminent PTB. After triage, they will be advised to come straight to hospital, thereby reducing delay and consequently reducing the risk of an unexpected home delivery. However, precipitous preterm labor may also occur in secondary care patients. In case of insufficient time to reach the hospital, the obstetrician will request the nearest midwife on call to assist the pregnant woman with her delivery at home.

Unfortunately, unintended home delivery is not registered as such in Netherlands Perinatal Registry.

To gain insight in the incidence of PTB and if levels of care at labor onset and at time of delivery are determining factors in the pathway to adverse perinatal outcome, we aimed to conduct an exploratory study.

2. Methods

2.1. Dataset. This study was performed in a nationwide retrospective cohort using Netherlands Perinatal Registry (PRN). The PRN consists of population-based data containing information on pregnancies, deliveries, and (re)admissions until 28 days after birth. The PRN database is obtained by a validated linkage of 3 different registries: the midwifery registry (LVR1), the obstetrics registry (LVR2), and the neonatology registry (LNR) of hospital admissions of newborns [15]. The coverage of the PRN is about 96% of all deliveries in Netherlands. All data contained in PRN are voluntarily recorded by the caregiver during prenatal care, delivery, and perinatal period. The data are sent annually to the national registry office, where a number of range and consistency checks are conducted [16].

2.2. Inclusion and Exclusion Criteria. For this study, all singleton spontaneous PTBs between 1 January, 1999, and 31 December, 2007, were selected. PTB was defined as birth before 37 completed weeks of gestation (before 259 days). Spontaneous onset of birth was considered in case of spontaneous contractions or spontaneous rupture of membranes. Women with iatrogenic PTB as a consequence of induction of labor or an elective Caesarean section were not included. Gestational age data were predominantly based on the date of the last menstrual period and/or the crown-rump length (CRL). We excluded all pregnancies of women who delivered before gestational age (GA) of 25^{+0} as this was the threshold for fully active perinatal treatment during the study period.

In this study, we focused solely on spontaneous PTB (with or without pPROM). Pregnancies with an unknown gestational age or resulting in antenatal intrauterine fetal death or the birth of a child weighing less than 500 grams were excluded from this study. Antenatal intrauterine fetal death is registered as such in the PRN. In the calculation of perinatal mortality, all fetuses with a positive heart rate at the start of the delivery, confirmed by auscultation or any sign of life observed after birth, were included.

Moreover, we excluded all fetuses with congenital abnormalities as well as all cases with an unknown obstetric care provider.

2.3. Definition of Determinant. The primary variable of interest was the level of care in which labor and/or delivery took place. We defined three categories: (1) onset of labor and delivery in primary care, (2) onset of labor in primary care and delivery in secondary care (intrapartum referral), and (3) onset of labor and delivery in secondary care.

2.4. Definition of Outcome Measures. The primary outcome measure was perinatal mortality, defined as intrapartum or

TABLE 1: Study population.

	N	%		
Total births in Netherlands 1999–2007			1,633,636	
Included births at gestational age of 25^{+0}–36^{+6}			123,388	7.6%
Exclusion of the total births between 25^{+0} and 36^{+6} wks	N	%		
Multiple pregnancies	30,041	24.4%		
Congenital anomalies	6,367	6.8%		
Antenatal death	3,400	4%		
Induction of labor and primary Caesarean section	31,039	37%		
Unknown level of care at onset of labor and delivery	144	0%		
	70,991		70,991	
Study population			52,397	3.2%

neonatal mortality in the first week of life. The secondary outcome measure was an Apgar score less than or equal to 4 after 5 minutes as criterion for diagnosing perinatal asphyxia.

2.5. Statistics. Baseline characteristics of the three patient groups under investigation were assessed. We analysed maternal age, parity, maternal ethnicity (European white versus other), socioeconomic status, and living in a deprived neighbourhood (yes or no, based on four-digit zip codes and a public list of deprived neighbourhoods issued by the Dutch government) according to both outcome measures. To analyse the association between variables and spontaneous PTB related perinatal mortality and low Apgar score, we performed univariable logistic regression analysis. Subsequently, multivariable regression analysis was performed to obtain adjusted odds ratios (aOR). We calculated the incidence of our outcome measures for each individual year to investigate trends over time. Data were analyzed using SAS statistical software package version 9.2 (SAS Institute Inc., NC, USA).

3. Results

Between 1999 and 2007, there were 52,397 births that met our inclusion criteria (Table 1).

Table 2 shows the baseline characteristics of the study population. In total, 22,121 (42%) of all spontaneous singleton PTBs had labor onset in primary care.

Of those, 4,134 (7.9%) were subsequently also delivered in primary care (Figure 1).

The proportion of perinatal death and Apgar score less than or equal to 4 are also presented in Table 2.

There were no major differences in baseline characteristics between cases with onset in primary care and those with onset in secondary care, making the two groups comparable at the onset of delivery. The median gestational age at delivery was 36^{+2} weeks in the group with onset and delivery in primary care versus, respectively, 35^{+6} in the group with onset in primary care and delivery in secondary care and 35^{+3} in the group with onset and delivery in secondary care (P value < 0.0001). Of all PTBs, 20.9% (10,957/52,397) occurred before a GA of 34^{0} weeks.

Table 3 shows the rates and odds ratios for Apgar score less than or equal to 4 and perinatal mortality after

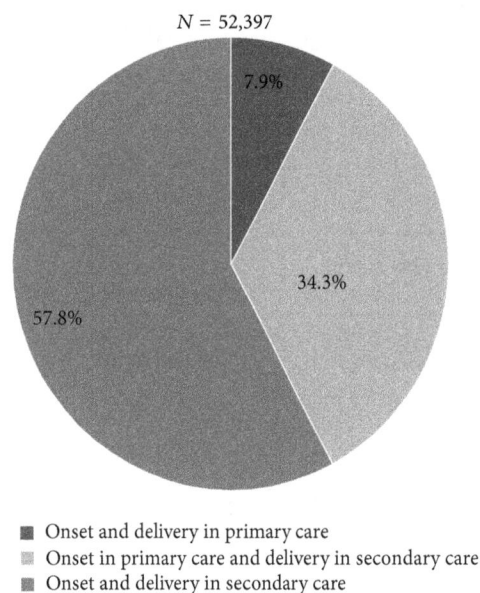

N = 52,397

7.9%

34.3%

57.8%

■ Onset and delivery in primary care
▨ Onset in primary care and delivery in secondary care
■ Onset and delivery in secondary care

FIGURE 1: Study population (PTB 25^{+0}–36^{+6}) divided by level of care at onset and delivery.

adjustment for maternal age, parity, ethnicity, socioeconomic status, fetal sex, and gestational age.

After adjustment, nulliparous women had the lowest risk of perinatal mortality and Apgar score less than or equal to 4. Both risk of perinatal mortality and risk of low Apgar score were decreased if women were referred before delivery to a secondary care setting. However, the risk was significantly increased if onset of labor and delivery took place in primary care.

A subgroup analysis was performed for late PTBs, that is, between 34^{+0} and 36^{+6} weeks of gestation. Table 4 shows the baseline characteristics of this group.

Of the total group of PTBs with onset in primary care, 86% (19,001/22,121) were late preterm compared to 74% (22,439/30,272) being late preterm with onset in secondary care. Within the group of PTBs with onset and delivery in primary care, almost 60% took place between GA of 36^{+0} and 36^{+6} weeks (Figure 2(a)).

TABLE 2: Baseline characteristics and outcome of 52,397 women with preterm delivery (GA 25^{+0}–36^{+6}).

Population 1999–2007	Total N/%	Onset and delivery Primary care	Onset in prim. care Delivery in sec. care	Onset and delivery Secondary care
Total GA 25^0–36^6 minus exclusions n (%)	52397 (100)	4134 (7.9)	17987 (34.3)	30279 (57.8)
Maternal age				
<25 years, n (%)	7573 (14.5)	603 (14.6)	2858 (15.9)	4112 (13.6)
25–29 years, n (%)	16662 (31.8)	1311 (31.7)	6499 (36.1)	8852 (29.2)
30–34 years, n (%)	19432 (37.1)	1568 (37.9)	6521 (36.3)	11343 (37.5)
≥35 years, n (%)	8730 (16.7)	652 (15.8)	2109 (11.7)	5969 (19.7)
Parity				
0, n (%)	31115 (59.4)	2365 (57.2)	12386 (68.9)	16364 (54.1)
1, n (%)	14407 (27.5)	1193 (28.9)	4047 (22.5)	9167 (30.3)
2+, n (%)	6875 (13.1)	576 (13.9)	1554 (8.6)	4745 (15.7)
Ethnicity				
European white, n (%)	43898 (83.8)	3377 (81.7)	15381 (85.5)	25140 (83.0)
Socioeconomic status				
High, n (%)	11976 (22.9)	929 (22.5)	4119 (22.9)	6928 (22.9)
Medium, n (%)	26080 (49.8)	2099 (50.8)	9184 (51.0)	14797 (48.9)
Low, n (%)	14341 (27.4)	1106 (26.8)	4784 (26.0)	8551 (28.2)
Deprived neighborhood				
Yes, n (%)	3730 (7.1)	276 (6.7)	1129 (6.3)	2325 (7.9)
Fetal sex				
Male fetal sex, n (%)	29686 (56.7)	2337 (56.5)	10295 (57.2)	17054 (56.7)
Apgar score ≤4 after 5 min				
Apgar ≤4, n (%)	805 (1.5)	94 (2.3)	158 (0.9)	553 (1.8)
Perinatal death				
Perinatal death, n (%)	575 (1.10)	58 (1.4)	99 (0.6)	418 (1.4)

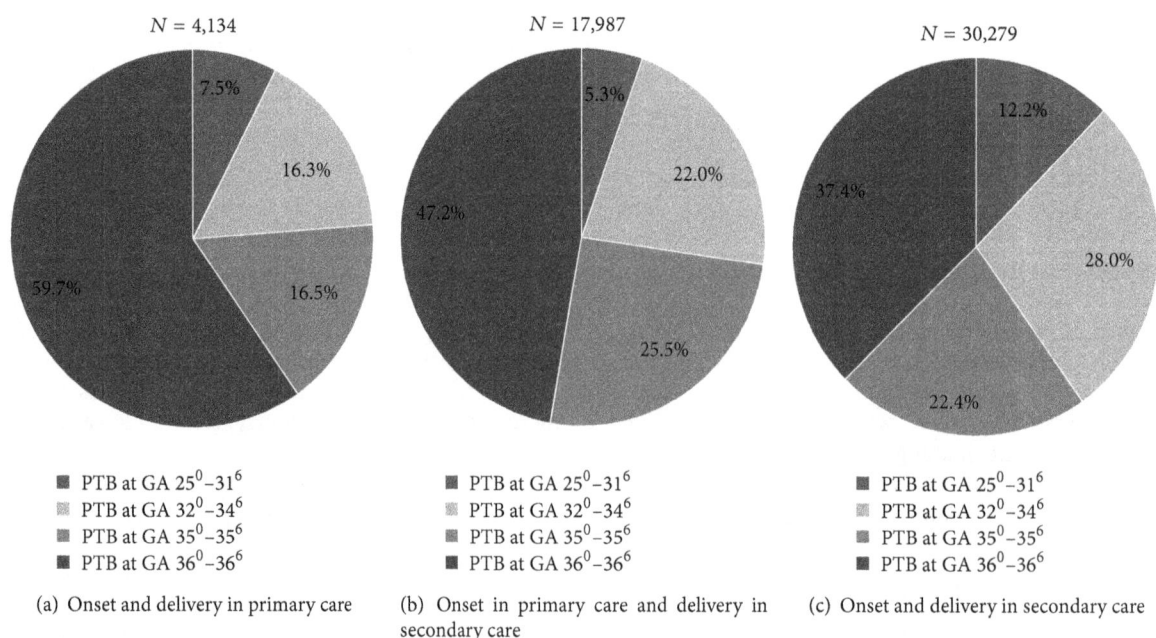

(a) Onset and delivery in primary care

(b) Onset in primary care and delivery in secondary care

(c) Onset and delivery in secondary care

FIGURE 2: All preterm births (N = 52,397) per level of care divided by gestational age (GA).

TABLE 3: Unadjusted and adjusted* odds ratios (OR) for 5-minute Apgar score ≤4 and perinatal mortality (GA 25^{+0}–36^{+6}).

Characteristics GA 25^{+0}–36^{+6} N 52397	Apgar score ≤4 after 5 minutes			Mortality intrapartum and ≤7 dgn postpartum		
	N (%)	Unadjusted OR (95% CI)	Adjusted OR (95% CI)	N (%)	Unadjusted OR (95% CI)	Adjusted OR (95% CI)
Parturition	805 (1.54)			575 (1.1)		
Onset and delivery in primary care	94 (0.18)	1.25 (1.00–1.56)	1.95 (1.53–2.48)	58 (0.11)	1.02 (0.77–1.34)	1.65 (1.20–2.27)
Onset primary and delivery in sec. care	158 (0.3)	0.48 (0.40–0.57)	0.89 (0.74–1.08)	99 (0.19)	0.40 (0.32–0.49)	0.86 (0.67–1.09)
Onset and delivery in secondary care	553 (1.06)	Reference	Reference	418 (0.8)	Reference	Reference
Maternal age						
<25 years		1.38 (1.11–1.70)	1.11 (0.88–1.40)		1.44 (1.12–1.86)	1.14 (0.85–1.52)
25–29 years		Reference	Reference		Reference	Reference
30–34 years		1.08 (0.90–1.29)	1.02 (0.85–1.27)		1.13 (0.92–1.40)	1.06 (0.84–1.34)
≥35 years		1.40 (1.14–1.72)	1.10 (0.88–1.38)		1.50 (1.18–1.91)	1.08 (0.81–1.42)
Parity						
0		0.78 (0.66–0.92)	0.74 (0.62–0.88)		0.80 (0.66–0.97)	0.74 (0.60–0.93)
1		Reference	Reference		Reference	Reference
2+		1.46 (1.2–1.8)	1.19 (0.95–1.48)		1.46 (1.2–1.8)	1.43 (1.10–1.87)
Ethnicity						
European white		Reference	Reference		Reference	Reference
Non-European white		1.36 (1.14–1.61)	0.88 (0.72–1.07)		1.27 (1.03–1.56)	0.69 (0.53–0.89)
Socioeconomic status						
High		Reference	Reference		Reference	Reference
Medium		1.11 (0.92–1.33)	1.07 (0.88–1.38)		1.04 (0.84–1.28)	0.98 (0.77–1.24)
Low		1.29 (1.05–1.57)	1.09 (0.87–1.35)		1.15 (0.91–1.46)	0.95 (0.73–1.25)
Fetal sex						
Female		Reference	Reference		Reference	Reference
Male		0.94 (0.81–1.08)	0.89 (0.77–1.04)		0.95 (0.81–1.12)	

*Adjusted for onset and location of delivery, maternal age, parity before study delivery, ethnicity, socioeconomic status, fetal sex, and gestational age.

TABLE 4: Baseline characteristics and outcome of 41,440 women with late preterm delivery (GA 34^{+0}–36^{+6}).

Population 1999–2007	Total N/%	Onset and delivery Primary care	Onset in prim. care Delivery in sec. care	Onset and delivery Secondary care
Total GA 34^0–36^6 minus exclusions n (%)	41440 (100)	3494 (8.4)	15507 (37.4)	22439 (54.2)
Maternal age				
<25 years, n (%)	5799 (14.0)	484 (13.9)	2393 (15.4)	2922 (13.0)
25–29 years, n (%)	13278 (32.0)	1117 (32.0)	5629 (36.3)	6532 (32.0)
30–34 years, n (%)	15496 (37.4)	1332 (38.1)	5654 (36.5)	8510 (37.9)
≥35 years, n (%)	6867 (16.6)	561 (16.1)	1831 (11.8)	4475 (19.9)
Parity				
0, n (%)	24453 (59.0)	1936 (55.4)	10527 (67.9)	11990 (53.4)
1, n (%)	11651 (28.1)	1065 (30.5)	3595 (23.2)	6991 (31.3)
2+, n (%)	5336 (12.9)	493 (14.1)	1385 (8.9)	3458 (15.4)
Ethnicity				
European white, n (%)	34881 (84.2)	2871 (82.2)	13252 (85.5)	18758 (83.6)
Socioeconomic status				
High, n (%)	9572 (23.1)	784 (22.4)	3575 (23.05)	5213 (23.2)
Medium, n (%)	20736 (50.0)	1789 (51.2)	7956 (51.3)	10991 (49.0)
Low, n (%)	11132 (26.9)	921 (26.4)	3976 (25.6)	6235 (27.8)
Deprived neighborhood				
Yes, n (%)	2853 (6.9)	225 (6.4)	968 (6.2)	1660 (7.4)
Fetal sex				
Male fetal sex, n (%)	23143 (55.9)	1965 (56.3)	8807 (56.8)	12371 (55.1)
Apgar score ≤4 after 5 min				
Apgar ≤4, n (%)	243 (0.6)	35 (1.0)	61 (0.4)	147 (0.7)
Perinatal death				
Perinatal death, n (%)	123 (0.3)	18 (0.5)	22 (0.1)	83 (0.4)

Table 5 shows the adjusted odds ratios in the subgroup of late PTBs (GA 34^{+0}–36^{+6}).

Women with preterm onset of labor between 34^{+0} and 36^{+6} weeks, who were referred before delivery to secondary care, had the lowest risk of low Apgar score (aOR 0.72 (0.53–0.98)) and perinatal mortality (aOR 0.49 (0.30–0.79)). The risk for a 5-minute Apgar score less than or equal to 4 was significantly increased for women with onset and delivery in primary care comparing to onset and delivery in secondary care. The increased risk on perinatal mortality for women with onset and delivery in primary care reached the border of significance (aOR 1.61 (0.96–2.21)). In the subgroup of late PTBs, multiparous women (≥2) had the highest risk on perinatal mortality (aOR 2.14 (1.31–3.51)).

3.1. Trends. Figure 3(a) shows the trends over the years 1999–2007 in incidence of the total of all births according to the type of supervision at the time of onset of labor and delivery. Figure 3(b) shows the trends in incidence of preterm births according to level of care.

The incidence of PTBs in a primary care setting has steadily decreased. In 1999, 38.4% of all deliveries took place under supervision of a midwife or GP; in 2007, this rate declined to 33%, indicating a relative decrease of 14%. However, of all PTBs in 1999, 13,2% had onset and delivery in primary care compared to 4.7% in 2007, a relative decrease of 64%. Although the overall share of primary care in the birthrate has declined over the years, the reduction in PTBs is stronger. Subsequently, the number of PTBs in a secondary care setting increased from 53.5% to 63.6% (a relative increase of 19%) while referrals from primary to secondary care during preterm labor showed a relative decrease of 5%.

4. Discussion

4.1. Principal Findings. Our study shows that the risk of adverse perinatal outcome after spontaneous PTB was lowest for women with labor onset in primary care who were referred to a secondary care setting before delivery. The risk of perinatal mortality and the risk of low Apgar score after 5 minutes were significantly increased for those women with both labor onset and delivery in primary care compared to women with labor onset and delivery in a secondary care setting.

Of all spontaneous singleton PTBs, 42.2% (Figure 1(a)) had labor onset in primary care and 7.9% of these births

TABLE 5: Unadjusted and adjusted* odds ratios (OR) for 5-minute Apgar score ≤4 and perinatal mortality (GA 34^{+0}–36^{+6}).

Characteristics GA 34^{+0}–36^{+6} N 41440	Apgar score ≤4 after 5 minutes			Mortality intrapartum and ≤7 dgn postpartum		
	N (%)	Unadjusted OR (95% CI)	Adjusted OR (95% CI)	N (%)	Unadjusted OR (95% CI)	Adjusted OR (95% CI)
Parturition	243 (0.59)			123 (0.30)		
Onset and delivery in primary care	35 (0.08)	1.54 (1.06–2.22)	1.75 (1.20–2.55)	18 (0.04)	1.40 (0.84–2.33)	1.61 (0.96–2.21)
Onset primary and delivery in secondary care	61 (0.15)	0.60 (0.44–0.81)	0.72 (0.53–0.98)	22 (0.05)	0.38 (0.24–0.61)	0.49 (0.30–0.79)
Onset and delivery in secondary care	147 (0.35)	Reference	Reference	83 (0.2)	Reference	Reference
Maternal age						
<25 years		0.98 (0.63–1.51)	0.92 (0.59–1.44)		1.11 (0.62–1.99)	1.14 (0.63–2.06)
25–29 years		Reference	Reference		Reference	Reference
30–34 years		1.24 (0.91–1.69)	1.9 (0.86–1.61)		1.18 (0.76–1.48)	1.05 (0.67–1.63)
≥35 years		1.37 (0.94–1.98)	1.13 (0.77–1.67)		1.27 (0.75–2.15)	0.88 (0.51–1.53)
Parity						
0		0.72 (0.54–0.96)	0.78 (0.58–1.05)		0.78 (0.51–1.20)	0.82 (0.53–1.27)
1		Reference	Reference		Reference	Reference
2+		1.39 (0.97–2.00)	1.30 (0.90–1.90)		2.13 (1.32–3.44)	2.14 (1.31–3.51)
Ethnicity						
European white		Reference	Reference		Reference	Reference
Non-European white		1.21 (0.88–1.68)	1.03 (0.73–1.47)		0.97 (0.60–1.59)	0.72 (0.43–1.21)
Socioeconomic status						
High		Reference	Reference		Reference	Reference
Medium		1.24 (0.88–1.75)	1.24 (0.88–1.75)		1.15 (0.72–1.85)	1.10 (0.68–1.77)
Low		1.47 (1.02–2.13)	1.39 (0.94–2.04)		1.40 (0.84–2.33)	1.22 (0.72–2.08)
Fetal sex						
Female		Reference	Reference		Reference	Reference
Male		0.91 (0.77–1.17)	0.89 (0.69–1.15)		0.89 (0.62–1.26)	0.86 (0.60–1.22)
Gestational age						
34^0–34^6		1.87 (1.35–2.57)	2.14 (1.55–2.96)		2.00 (1.27–3.17)	2.38 (1.491–3.78)
35^0–35^6		1.51 (1.13–2.02)	1.68 (1.25–2.25)		1.82 (1.21–2.73)	2.06 (1.37–3.11)
36^0–36^6		Reference	Reference		Reference	Reference

*Adjusted for onset and location of delivery, maternal age, parity before study delivery, ethnicity, socioeconomic status, fetal sex, and gestational age.

(a) Total births per year divided by level of care

(b) Total *preterm* births per year divided by level of care

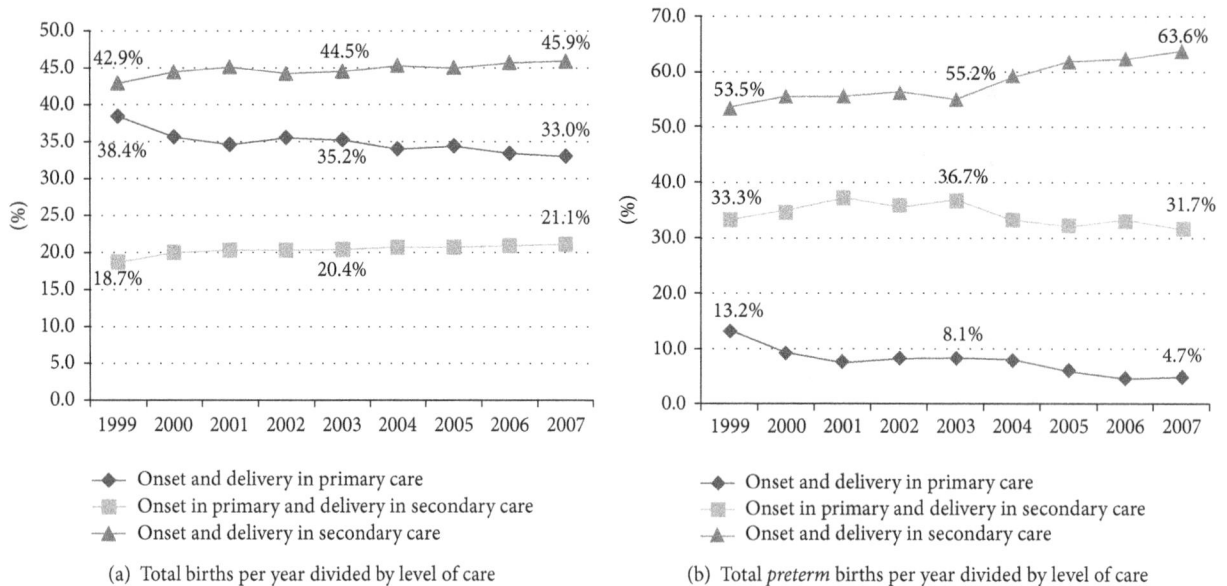

FIGURE 3: Trends over 1999–2007.

subsequently ended in primary care. Of all PTBs in primary care, 85% were late preterm (34^{+0}–36^{+6} weeks) and almost 60% between 36^{+0} and 36^{+6} weeks (Figure 2(a)).

4.2. Strengths and Weaknesses. Our study was based on data of a large population-based national perinatal registry. Most professionals in obstetrical care contribute to the PRN and it thus comprises approximately 96% of all pregnancy and birth characteristics in Netherlands. The 4% of missing birth data are due to 1-2% nonreporting general practitioners and 2-3% nonreporting midwives.

The Dutch obstetrical system has received a great deal of attention over the last few years, both nationally and internationally, mainly because of its relatively high perinatal mortality compared to other developed countries and the possible contribution of our obstetric care system with distinct differentiation between primary and secondary care. As far as we know, this is the first study that examines the incidence of PTB according to level of care in which the share of both levels in perinatal mortality and low Apgar score is studied.

The method of pregnancy dating can influence the incidence of PTB [17–19]. In the last decade, the vast majority of women in Netherlands received an early pregnancy ultrasound to confirm or change the gestational age that was based on date of last menstrual period. Since this strategy did not change during the study period, the effect of miscalculated gestational age on the studied outcome of PTB should be marginal.

During the study period, approximately 83% [20] of all pregnant women received primary care at the onset of pregnancy. We assume that the majority of the remaining 17% of women had a high risk profile according to the LOI guidelines (e.g., diabetes, hypertension, multiple pregnancies, previous Caesarean section, and chronic disease) at the onset

of the pregnancy, including a history of PTB before 33 completed weeks. During pregnancy, changing level of care is not uncommon and can go both ways, but overall this generally results in more referrals from primary to secondary care than vice versa. Consequently, at the onset of labor, 39.5% of all pregnant women are under obstetrician-led care. Some of those women may have risk factors related to a higher risk of (indicated) preterm labor or risk factors that may affect neonatal outcome. In our study, we evaluated the difference in perinatal outcome in spontaneous PTB according to the level of care at the onset of delivery and at delivery. We excluded induced PTBs in this study but did not adjust for risk factors in medical or obstetrical history nor for pregnancy related complications and this may have influenced our neonatal data. If we compare our three groups, it is evident that (initially low risk) pregnancies with onset and preterm delivery in primary care had the worst outcome. In the crude analysis, the group with onset in primary care and preterm delivery in secondary care had the best outcome. This concerns all low risk pregnancies with a referral to secondary care before delivery, in case of spontaneous PTB. However, after adjusting (Tables 3 and 4), there was no significant difference between this group and the group with onset and delivery in secondary care. This is remarkable because the latest group concerns women who are at increased risk as a result of their medical or obstetric history. If we had adjusted for risk factors, the results would probably be even more in favour of the group with onset and delivery in secondary care. Comparing neonatal outcome based on setting at onset of delivery implies comparing outcome in low and high risk patients, without correction for risk factors. However, we do not feel this would undermine our results; namely, healthy low risk women with PTB cared for in primary care do not have better perinatal outcome than women at increased risk as a result of a number of unspecified conditions cared for in secondary care. On the contrary, the adjusted risk outcomes are worse if PTB occurs in primary care setting although referral before delivery affects the results positively.

We suggested that precipitous PTB could be one of the reasons why delivery ended at home by midwifery-led care. It may take some time for the midwife to travel to the pregnant woman for further examination after the first call and it is possible that there is not enough time for hospital referral. Nonetheless, a precipitous (preterm) birth can also occur in secondary care. If the obstetrician suspects a precipitous (preterm) birth at the first call while the patient is still at home, there are two options: firstly, to send an ambulance for emergency transport to the hospital and secondly, to alert the nearest midwife with the request to assist the woman at home. In that case, the birth is registered as a primary care birth. The probability that there is no medical assistance available at the time of birth is very rare but occurs incidentally. Unfortunately this is not registered consequently.

4.3. Relation to Other Studies. In our study, we found lower odds of perinatal mortality in case of PTB for ethnicity other than European white and the odds of a 5-minute Apgar score less than or equal to 4 reached the border of significance. This is entirely consistent with the study of Schaaf et al. [21]. They concluded that although African and South Asian women had an increased risk of PTB, they had a decreased risk of adverse neonatal outcome after PTB. Mediterranean women had a decreased risk of PTB when compared to European white women but also a significant decreased risk of subsequent adverse neonatal outcome.

Several studies have compared the outcome associated with planned home births and planned hospital births in low risk women [22, 23]. Planned home birth was associated with less medical interventions, but the interpretation of perinatal outcome differed in these studies [24, 25]. Evers et al. [26] have also investigated the incidence of perinatal mortality and morbidity in low risk term pregnancies supervised by a midwife and compared those to high risk pregnancies in secondary care. Their study suggested that the Dutch system of risk selection, which is based on two independent and separately working obstetric care levels, is not as effective as it should be. However, as the authors themselves stated in a reply on comments on their study, a causal association between the results and the obstetric care system cannot be shown because of limitations of the chosen study design. The authors indicated that little is known regarding delay in primary as well as in secondary care after referral and/or during transport. Also, essential information could be lost during referral causing inadequate treatment in the hospital. It is not known to what extent these factors have contributed to adverse outcomes.

de Jonge et al. [14] compared perinatal mortality and morbidity between planned home and hospital births in low risk pregnancies in Netherlands. This study did not show an increased risk for adverse outcome in planned home birth in the Dutch obstetric care system with well-trained midwives and good referral and transportation system.

Comparability of our results with the results of these studies and others [22–25] on perinatal outcome according to

the intended place of birth is limited because PTB in primary care is not planned as such. Preterm onset of labor is an indication for referral to a secondary care setting because of the risks of PTB for the neonate. None of the studies compared the outcome of PTB under primary care versus secondary care. However, our study does show that the Dutch obstetric care system is well organized, since the group of low risk women with onset in primary care and PTB in secondary care had the best neonatal outcome as expected.

The number of women with onset of labor in primary care decreased from 60.5% in 1999 to 54.3% in 2007 [20], a relative decrease of 10.3%. Meanwhile, the incidence of spontaneous singleton PTB between 25^{+0} and 37^{+0} weeks with onset and delivery in primary care decreased during the study period from 13.2% to 4.7%, resulting in an absolute decrease of 7.5% and a relative decrease of 64%. These data indicate that referral by primary care providers in case of (imminent) PTB has markedly improved.

The epidemiology of PTBs and trends in the last decade are well investigated [4–7, 9]. In Netherlands, the risk on adverse outcome in preterm singleton pregnancies decreased significantly during the study period from 8.0% to 7.7% [8]. The reduction was mainly due to a decrease of two types of PTB: first of all the decrease of spontaneous PTB with or without preterm prelabor rupture of membranes (pPROM) from 3.6% to 3.1% and secondly a decrease in PTB within gestational age of 34–36 weeks from 4.6% to 4.2%.

During our study period, there was a relative decrease of PTBs with onset and delivery in primary care of 64% (13.2% of all PTBs in 1999 versus 4.7% in 2007). Both abovementioned trends are partly responsible for this decrease because PTBs in primary care setting are always spontaneous PTBs and 85% of them occur between 34^{+0} and 36^{+6} weeks. Another contributor is the overall decreasing share of primary care in birth assistance. However, all these factors do not explain the 64% relative decrease as we mentioned before. We can only welcome the decline, given the poorer outcome of PTBs in primary care setting.

Even so, the Dutch perinatal mortality declined steadily over the years 2000–2006, according to the study of Ravelli et al. [10]. These dates indicate that the decrease in perinatal mortality risk was most prominent among births with congenital anomalies (45% decline), among term births (25% decline) and among PTBs with 32.0–36.6 weeks' gestation (30% decline).

This positively influenced the primary outcome of our study.

4.4. Meaning of the Results and Proposal for Future Research. Our study shows that the risk of perinatal mortality and Apgar score less than or equal to 4 after spontaneous PTB is higher if birth takes place in primary care. In late PTB, the risk of low Apgar score is still higher than for births in a secondary care setting. Because of its impact on perinatal outcome and costs, reducing PTB is a worldwide challenge in obstetrics and a topic of research [27–30].

One of the most important aspects of midwifery care in Netherlands is risk selection. Midwives in Netherlands are independent practitioners, qualified to provide full maternity care to all women whose pregnancy and childbirth are uncomplicated. When risk factors occur in pregnancy or during birth, women are referred to a secondary care setting.

In case of imminent PTB, referral to an obstetrician is indicated according to the Dutch guidelines. Nevertheless, there are factors that may hamper referral before delivery to a hospital for delivery.

Firstly, patient related factors: we hypothesize that pregnant women may be insufficiently aware of the signs associated with the onset of labor and when to contact the obstetric caregiver or did not understand the advice of her obstetric caregiver, maybe due to a language barrier. In these cases, it is useful to examine in which way pregnant women, especially nulliparous, could be informed to raise the awareness.

Secondly, obstetric care related factors: the obstetric caregiver did not think of imminent PTB with the specified complaints or did not respond adequately enough or underestimated the problem and was subsequently confronted with a preterm parturition. In case of late PTB, there might be acceptation of the parturition by the obstetric caregiver, but it is not known to what extent this occurs.

Thirdly, unforeseeable circumstances: the fastness of the delivery left no time for referral to the hospital and transportation of the woman in labor was not a safe option anymore.

Ravelli et al. [31] investigated the impact of travel time, from home to hospital during delivery, on neonatal outcome in Netherlands. They concluded that there is a significant association between a travel time of 20 minutes or longer and adverse outcomes.

Considering all conceivable reasons for preterm delivery in a primary care setting, it is of major importance that both midwives and pregnant women are aware of the risk outcome of (late) spontaneous PTB.

A risk assessment to predict PTB in low risk women without any symptoms would be very valuable but a good risk selection tool is not available yet. Despite all research, the clinical applicability of the previously developed prediction models is still limited [27, 32, 33]. Therefore, the focus should be on increasing awareness in patients and midwives of potential signals of impending PTB and of the risks of (late) PTB in primary care setting.

5. Conclusion

Our study shows that the risk of adverse perinatal outcome was significantly increased after spontaneous preterm birth for healthy women with low risk singleton pregnancies with labor onset and delivery in primary care. For women with labor onset in primary care who were referred to a secondary care setting before delivery, the adjusted risk of adverse perinatal outcome is comparable to those with onset and delivery in secondary care setting. We recommend improving the awareness of both the complaints and, above all, the risks associated with preterm labor of primary obstetric care providers as well as of the pregnant women in order to achieve an increasing referral before delivery to secondary care, because this improves perinatal outcome after preterm onset of labor.

Conflict of Interests

The authors declare that there is no conflict of interests regarding the publication of this paper.

Acknowledgments

The authors would like to thank all Dutch midwives, obstetricians, neonatologists, and other perinatal healthcare providers for the registration of perinatal information. They would also like to thank the Foundation of the Netherlands Perinatal Registry (http://www.perinatreg.nl/) for permission to use and analyze the registry data (no. 11.46). This study was funded by ZonMw, the Dutch Organization for Health Research and Development, Grant no. 50–50110-96-530.

References

[1] G. J. Bonsel, E. Birnie, S. Denktas, J. Poeran, and E. Steegers, *Lijnen in de Perinatale Sterfte, Signalementstudie Zwangerschap en Geboorte*, Erasmus MC, Rotterdam, The Netherlands, 2010.

[2] E. M. Boyle, G. Poulsen, D. J. Field et al., "Effects of gestational age at birth on health outcomes at 3 and 5 years of age: population based cohort study," *The British Medical Journal*, vol. 344, no. 7848, article e896, 2012.

[3] D. Moster, R. T. Lie, and T. Markestad, "Long-term medical and social consequences of preterm birth," *The New England Journal of Medicine*, vol. 359, no. 3, pp. 262–273, 2008.

[4] J. J. Henderson, O. A. McWilliam, J. P. Newnham, and C. E. Pennell, "Preterm birth aetiology 2004–2008. Maternal factors associated with three phenotypes: spontaneous preterm labour, preterm pre-labour rupture of membranes and medically indicated preterm birth," *The Journal of Maternal-Fetal & Neonatal Medicine*, vol. 25, no. 6, pp. 642–647, 2012.

[5] R. L. Goldenberg, J. F. Culhane, J. D. Iams, and R. Romero, "Epidemiology and causes of preterm birth," *The Lancet*, vol. 371, no. 9606, pp. 75–84, 2008.

[6] EURO-PERISTAT Project in Collaboration with SCPE E&E, "European perinatal health report. Percent of preterm live births in 2004 and difference between 2010 and 2004," http://www.europeristat.com/reports/european-perinatal-health-report-2010.html.

[7] H. Blencowe, S. Cousens, M. Z. Oestergaard et al., "National, regional, and worldwide estimates of preterm birth rates in the year 2010 with time trends since 1990 for selected countries: a systematic analysis and implications," *The Lancet*, vol. 379, no. 9832, pp. 2162–2172, 2012.

[8] A. D. Mohangoo, S. E. Buitendijk, C. W. P. M. Hukkelhouen et al., "Higher perinatal mortality in the Netherlands than in other European countries: the Peristat-II study," *Nederlands Tijdschrift voor Geneeskunde*, vol. 152, no. 50, pp. 2718–2727, 2008.

[9] J. P. de Graaf, A. C. J. Ravelli, G. H. A. Visser et al., "Increased adverse perinatal outcome of hospital delivery at night," *BJOG: An International Journal of Obstetrics & Gynaecology*, vol. 117, no. 9, pp. 1098–1107, 2010.

[10] A. C. J. Ravelli, M. Tromp, M. van Huis et al., "Decreasing perinatal mortality in the Netherlands, 2000–2006: a record linkage study," *Journal of Epidemiology and Community Health*, vol. 63, no. 9, pp. 761–765, 2009.

[11] M. Tromp, M. Eskes, J. B. Reitsma et al., "Regional perinatal mortality differences in the Netherlands; care is the question," *BMC Public Health*, vol. 9, article 102, 2009.

[12] A. de Jonge, R. Baron, M. Westerneng, J. Twisk, and E. K. Hutton, "Perinatal mortality rate in the Netherlands compared to other European countries: a secondary analysis of Euro-PERISTAT data," *Midwifery*, vol. 29, no. 8, pp. 1011–1018, 2013.

[13] J. M. Schaaf, B. W. J. Mol, A. Abu-Hanna, and A. C. J. Ravelli, "Trends in preterm birth: singleton and multiple pregnancies in the Netherlands, 2000–2007," *BJOG: An International Journal of Obstetrics & Gynaecology*, vol. 118, no. 10, pp. 1196–1204, 2011.

[14] *Verloskundig Vademecum*, College van Zorgverzekeringen, Diemen, The Netherlands, 2003.

[15] N. Méray, J. B. Reitsma, A. C. J. Ravelli, and G. J. Bonsel, "Probabilistic record linkage is a valid and transparent tool to combine databases without a patient identification number," *Journal of Clinical Epidemiology*, vol. 60, no. 9, pp. 883.e1–883.e11, 2007.

[16] M. Tromp, A. C. J. Ravelli, N. Méray, J. B. Reitsma, and G. J. Bonsel, "An efficient validation method of probabilistic record linkage including readmissions and twins," *Methods of Information in Medicine*, vol. 47, no. 4, pp. 356–363, 2008.

[17] C. S. Hoffman, L. C. Messer, P. Mendola, D. A. Savitz, A. H. Herring, and K. E. Hartmann, "Comparison of gestational age at birth based on last menstrual period and ultrasound during the first trimester," *Paediatric and Perinatal Epidemiology*, vol. 22, no. 6, pp. 587–596, 2008.

[18] D. A. Savitz, J. W. Terry Jr., N. Dole, J. M. Thorp Jr., A. M. Siega-Riz, and A. H. Herring, "Comparison of pregnancy dating by last menstrual period, ultrasound scanning, and their combination," *The American Journal of Obstetrics & Gynecology*, vol. 187, no. 6, pp. 1660–1666, 2002.

[19] H. Yang, M. S. Kramer, R. W. Platt et al., "How does early ultrasound scan estimation of gestational age lead to higher rates of preterm birth?" *The American Journal of Obstetrics & Gynecology*, vol. 186, no. 3, pp. 433–437, 2002.

[20] The Netherlands Perinatal Registry, *10 Years Perinatal Registration Broadly Outlined, 2011Stichting Perinatale Registratie Nederland. Grote Lijnen 10 jaar Perinatale Registratie Nederland*, Stichting Perinatale Registratie Nederland, Utrecht, The Netherlands, 2011, http://www.perinat.nluploads/174/146/Perinatale_Registratie_Nederland_Grote_Lijnen_1999-2012_2.pdf.

[21] J. M. Schaaf, B.-W. J. Mol, A. Abu-Hanna, and A. C. J. Ravelli, "Ethnic disparities in the risk of adverse neonatal outcome after spontaneous preterm birth," *Acta Obstetricia et Gynecologica Scandinavica*, vol. 91, no. 12, pp. 1402–1408, 2012.

[22] J. van der Kooy, J. Poeran, J. P. de Graaf et al., "Planned home compared with planned hospital births in the netherlands: intrapartum and early neonatal death in low-risk pregnancies," *Obstetrics & Gynecology*, vol. 118, no. 5, pp. 1037–1046, 2011.

[23] E. K. Hutton, A. H. Reitsma, and K. Kaufman, "Outcomes associated with planned home and planned hospital births in low-risk women attended by midwives in Ontario, Canada, 2003–2006: a retrospective cohort study," *Birth*, vol. 36, no. 3, pp. 180–189, 2009.

[24] P. A. Janssen, L. Saxell, L. A. Page, M. C. Klein, R. M. Liston, and S. K. Lee, "Outcomes of planned home birth with registered midwife versus planned hospital birth with midwife or physician," *Canadian Medical Association Journal*, vol. 181, no. 6-7, pp. 377–383, 2009.

[25] J. R. Wax, F. L. Lucas, M. Lamont, M. G. Pinette, A. Cartin, and J. Blackstone, "Maternal and newborn outcomes in planned home birth vs planned hospital births: a metaanalysis," *The American Journal of Obstetrics & Gynecology*, vol. 203, no. 3, pp. 243–248, 2010.

[26] A. C. Evers, H. A. Brouwers, C. W. Hukkelhoven et al., "Perinatal mortality and severe morbidity in low and high risk term pregnancies in the Netherlands: prospective cohort study," *The British Medical Journal*, vol. 341, no. 7780, Article ID c5639, 2010.

[27] M. W. Davey, I. Watson, J. A. Rayner, and S. Rowland, "Risk scoring systems for predicting preterm birth with the aim of reducing associated adverse outcomes," *Cochrane Database of Systematic Reviews*, no. 11, Article ID CD004902, 2011.

[28] J. E. Norman, A. Shennan, P. Bennett et al., "Trial protocol OPPTIMUM—does progesterone prophylaxis for the prevention of preterm labour improve outcome?" *BMC Pregnancy and Childbirth*, vol. 12, no. 1, article 79, 2012.

[29] M. A. van Os, J. A. van der Ven, C. E. Kleinrouweler et al., "Preventing preterm birth with progesterone: costs and effects of screening low risk women with a singleton pregnancy for short cervical length, the Triple P study," *BMC Pregnancy and Childbirth*, vol. 11, article 77, 2011.

[30] H. Honest, C. A. Forbes, K. H. Durée et al., "Screening to prevent spontaneous preterm birth: systematic reviews of accuracy and effectiveness literature with economic modelling," *Health Technology Assessment*, vol. 13, no. 43, 2009.

[31] A. C. J. Ravelli, K. J. Jager, M. H. de Groot et al., "Travel time from home to hospital and adverse perinatal outcomes in women at term in the Netherlands," *BJOG: An International Journal of Obstetrics & Gynaecology*, vol. 118, no. 4, pp. 457–465, 2011.

[32] J. M. Schaaf, A. C. J. Ravelli, B. W. J. Mol, and A. Abu-Hanna, "Development of a prognostic model for predicting spontaneous singleton preterm birth," *European Journal of Obstetrics & Gynecology and Reproductive Biology*, vol. 164, no. 2, pp. 150–155, 2012.

[33] K. A. Lee, M. H. Chang, M.-H. Park et al., "A model for prediction of spontaneous preterm birth in asymptomatic women," *Journal of Women's Health*, vol. 20, no. 12, pp. 1825–1831, 2011.

4

Risk Factors for Preterm Birth among HIV-Infected Tanzanian Women: A Prospective Study

Rachel M. Zack,[1] **Jenna Golan,**[2] **Said Aboud,**[3] **Gernard Msamanga,**[4] **Donna Spiegelman,**[1,2,5] **and Wafaie Fawzi**[1,2,6]

[1] *Department of Epidemiology, Harvard School of Public Health, 1633 Tremont Street, Boston, MA 02115, USA*
[2] *Department of Nutrition, Harvard School of Public Health, Boston, MA, USA*
[3] *Department of Microbiology and Immunology, Muhimbili University of Health and Allied Sciences, Dar es Salaam, Tanzania*
[4] *Department of Community Health, Muhimbili University of Health and Allied Sciences, Dar es Salaam, Tanzania*
[5] *Department of Biostatistics, Harvard School of Public Health, Boston, MA, USA*
[6] *Department of Global Health and Population, Harvard School of Public Health, Boston, MA, USA*

Correspondence should be addressed to Rachel M. Zack; rmzack@gmail.com

Academic Editor: Everett Magann

Premature delivery, a significant cause of child mortality and morbidity worldwide, is particularly prevalent in the developing world. As HIV is highly prevalent in much of sub-Saharan Africa, it is important to determine risk factors for prematurity among HIV-positive pregnancies. The aims of this study were to identify risk factors of preterm (<37 weeks) and very preterm (<34 weeks) birth among a cohort of 927 HIV positive women living in Dar es Salaam, Tanzania, who enrolled in the Tanzania Vitamin and HIV Infection Trial between 1995 and 1997. Multivariable relative risk regression models were used to determine the association of potential maternal risk factors with premature and very premature delivery. High rates of preterm (24%) and very preterm birth (9%) were found. Risk factors (adjusted RR (95% CI)) for preterm birth were mother <20 years (1.46 (1.10, 1.95)), maternal illiteracy (1.54 (1.10, 2.16)), malaria (1.42 (1.11, 1.81)), *Entamoeba coli* (1.49 (1.04, 2.15)), no or low pregnancy weight gain, and HIV disease stage ≥2 (1.41 (1.12, 1.50)). Interventions to reduce pregnancies in women under 20, prevent and treat malaria, reduce *Entamoeba coli* infection, and promote weight gain in pregnant women may have a protective effect on prematurity.

1. Introduction

Preterm delivery is recognized as a significant cause of child mortality and morbidity worldwide. Preterm birth is the leading cause of neonatal mortality [1]. It is estimated that preterm birth is the direct cause of 29% of deaths in children under 28 days and 11% of deaths in children under 5 years [1–3].

Prematurity disproportionately affects newborns in resource-constrained countries, where it is both more common and more often leads to adverse health outcomes. A systematic review from 2010 reports that 7.5% and 11.9% of births in developed countries and in Africa, respectively, were preterm [4]. In Tanzania, 11% of births are premature

and prematurity is the second leading cause of neonatal death [5]. In a study of hospitalized neonates in Tanzania, the neonatal mortality rate for preterm infants was twice as high as that for full-term infants, 26% versus 13% [6].

Expending extra resources on additional medical care for pregnant women with risk factors for prematurity could reduce the incidence of prematurity. Not only would this have immediate benefits, such as reducing neonatal mortality, but it could also reduce the risk of chronic disease due to preterm delivery throughout the life course [7, 8]. This could substantially lower long-term health expenditures.

The prevalence of HIV infection among Tanzanian women is estimated to be 6.6% [9]. Given the significant proportion of pregnant women who are HIV-infected in some regions of the world, it is important to determine not only the risk factors for prematurity among the general population but also risk factors for prematurity among HIV-infected women, because such factors could be distinct from those in HIV uninfected women.

As the 2015 deadline of the Millennium Development Goals (MDGs) draws near, it is clear that MDG 4, the goal of reducing the under-five child mortality rate by two-thirds between 1990 and 2015, cannot be reached unless efforts are drastically increased [10]. While under-five mortality is declining in many countries, neonatal mortality still lags behind. Since preterm birth is responsible for 11% of under-five child mortality worldwide, knowledge of risk factors for prematurity may help the global community to reach MDG 4 [11]. This paper aims to contribute to the evidence base needed for a reduction in premature delivery by finding determinants of preterm and very preterm birth through the analysis of a cohort of 927 HIV-infected Tanzanian women. We examined potential risk factors for preterm delivery, many of which were previously found to be associated with preterm delivery in healthy populations.

2. Methods

2.1. Study Population and Design. Study participants were enrolled in a trial of vitamin supplements on pregnancy outcomes and HIV disease progression. Participants were HIV-infected pregnant women living in Dar es Salaam, Tanzania. Women were recruited from four prenatal clinics. They were enrolled in the study between April 1995 and July 1997. Inclusion criteria included 12 to 27 weeks gestation, intention to continue residing in Dar es Salaam for at least one year following delivery, World Health Organization (WHO) HIV disease stages 1–3, and informed consent to be randomized to a treatment regimen. The study has previously been described in further detail [12–15].

Of 1078 women enrolled in the trial, 949 had a live birth with known gestational age at delivery. For the prematurity analyses, we excluded 22 additional women because of missing data on key potential risk factors for preterm birth including age, maternal literacy, maternal malaria, HIV disease stage, hypertension status, height, or at least two measures of weight during pregnancy. None of the women reported smoking during pregnancy. This resulted in a sample of 927 pregnant women.

Consistent with the Tanzanian Ministry of Health's standard of prenatal care at the time of the study, study participants were provided with anemia and malaria prophylaxis during pregnancy. During pregnancy, all study participants received daily doses of 400 mg of ferrous sulfate and 5 mg of folic acid for anemia prophylaxis and weekly doses of 500 mg of chloroquine phosphate for malaria prophylaxis. Study participants were treated for hypertension and syphilis during pregnancy if found to have either disease. Study participants did not receive antiretrovirals (ARVs), as they were not available in Tanzania at the time of the study.

The trial was approved by the Research and Publications Committee of Muhimbili University of Health and Allied Sciences, the ethics committee of the Tanzania Ministry of Health's National AIDS Control Program, and the Institutional Review Board of the Harvard School of Public Health.

2.2. Measurements. Premature was defined as birth at fewer than 37 weeks of gestation and very premature was defined as fewer than 34 weeks of gestation. Gestational age was based on last menstrual period (LMP), which was self-reported by the participant at both screening and enrollment. Fundal height was measured as the distance, in centimeters, from the top of the pubic bone to the top of the uterus by trained doctors during the screening visit.

Anthropometric measurements, genital swabs, and blood, urine, and stool samples were collected at enrollment. These specimens were used to diagnose malaria, sexually transmitted infections (STIs), and parasitic infections and to measure micronutrient levels, hemoglobin concentration, HIV viral load, and CD4 cell count. By design, vitamin A, vitamin E, viral load, parasitic infections, and STIs were only measured in a subsample of study participants.

The following STIs were tested for at enrollment: trichomoniasis, gonorrhea, syphilis, and vaginal candidiasis. Syphilis was diagnosed as active if syphilis antibodies from sera were found to be present by both the Venereal Disease Research Laboratory (VDRL; Murex Diagnostic, Dartford, United Kingdom) and *Treponema pallidum* haemagglutination (TPHA; Fijurebio, Tokyo, Japan) tests. Gonorrhea was diagnosed based on a culture of the genital swab to detect *Neisseria gonorrhea* and *Trichomonas vaginalis* was diagnosed based upon wet mounts that were prepared and examined using microscopy. Vaginal candidiasis was diagnosed clinically by physician exam.

The following intestinal parasitic infections were tested for at enrollment: *Ascaris lumbricoides, Cryptosporidium parvum, Entamoeba coli, Entamoeba histolytica, Enterobius, Giardia lamblia,* hookworm, isospora, microsporidia, *Strongyloides stercoralis, Taenia,* and *Trichuris trichiura*. Stool samples were examined macroscopically for the previously mentioned worms and microscopically using saline and iodine wet mount and the formalin-ether concentration technique for larvae, ova, and cysts.

Malaria was diagnosed by use of thick-smear blood films stained with Giemsa. Vitamin A deficiency was defined as plasma vitamin A <20 μg/dL. Low vitamin E levels were defined as plasma vitamin E <9.7 μmol/L. CD4 cell counts were dichotomized by <200 cell/mm^3. We categorized hemoglobin levels according to three cutpoints: 7.0, 8.5, and 11.0 g/L. The WHO defines anemia in pregnancy as a hemoglobin concentration below 11 g/dL [16]. Prehypertension was defined as systolic blood pressure (SBP) $\geq$120 or diastolic blood pressure (DBP) $\geq$80 and hypertension was defined as SBP $\geq$140 or DBP $\geq$90 [17]. Selenium and mid-upper arm circumference (MUAC) were categorized by quartile. WHO HIV disease stage was dichotomized (stage < 2 versus stage $\geq$ 2) because of the limited number of women with HIV stage >2.

Trained research nurses interviewed study participants at enrollment. Maternal age and relationship status were self-reported. Maternal age at conception was estimated by subtracting gestational age at enrollment from maternal age at enrollment. Having a partner was defined as self-report of being married or cohabiting.

2.3. Statistical Analyses. Prematurity status, the outcome variable, was determined based on self-reported LMP. In order to validate the quality of LMP as a measure of gestational age we performed a supplemental analysis where we calculated the Spearman correlation between gestational ages based on LMP and fundal height.

Risk factors measured at enrollment that we examined were mother's age at conception, having no partner, being illiterate, mid-upper arm circumference (MUAC), height, vitamin A, vitamin E, selenium, hemoglobin, malaria, parasitic infections, STIs, HIV disease stage ≥ 2, CD4 cell count, and viral load. Whether or not the pregnancy resulted in twins and weight change during pregnancy were also included as exposures. Although the Tanzania Vitamin and HIV Infection Trial found that multivitamins reduced the risk of very preterm delivery [12], we did not adjust for assigned vitamin regimen because vitamin regimen was randomized and thus did not confound the relationships between the risk factors we examined and preterm delivery.

Weight change during pregnancy was calculated for each individual by using linear regression to regress weight on week of gestation [18–20]. Weight change was then categorized into three groups: no gain (≤0 grams per week), gain below the 25th percentile, and gain at or above the 25th percentile.

Missing indicators were created for each of the parasitic infections, each of the STIs, viral load, CD4 count, vitamin A deficiency, vitamin E, selenium, hemoglobin, and MUAC [21].

Unadjusted and adjusted relative risk regression models were run to calculate relative risks (RRs) and 95% confidence intervals (CIs) [22]. Log-binomial regression was used for all unadjusted regressions. Poisson was used for the adjusted regressions because the adjusted log-binomial regressions did not converge. Each regression was run twice, once with preterm versus full term as the dependent variable and again with very preterm versus full term as the dependent variable. Deliveries of ≥34–<37 weeks were excluded from the very preterm versus full term analysis. Explanatory variables were included in the adjusted models if the P-value in the unadjusted model was less than 0.2 [23]. Wald tests for trend were calculated for categorical variables by taking the median value of each category and setting missing values to the overall median. Wald tests were calculated for dichotomous and continuous variables.

We calculated a Spearman correlation coefficient comparing gestational age as measured by LMP and fundal height on 1077 women. The analysis included data on all trial participants with a known LMP and fundal height at the screening visit, excluding only one woman who was missing data on LMP.

A P value of ≤0.05 was considered to be statistically significant. All statistical analyses were performed using SAS software 9.3 (SAS Institute, Inc., http://www.sas.com, Cary, North Carolina).

3. Results

The median gestational age at enrollment was 21 weeks (IQR 18–23). The median gestational age at delivery was 39 weeks (IQR 37–41). Seventy-six percent of deliveries were full-term, 24% were premature and 9% were very premature. The characteristics of the cohort are shown in Table 1.

The results of unadjusted and adjusted relative risk regressions assessing the relationships of maternal factors and the risk for preterm versus full-term deliveries are shown in Table 2. After adjustment, maternal age less than 20 years (RR, 1.46; 95% CI, 1.10–1.95), maternal illiteracy (RR, 1.54; 95% CI, 1.10–2.61), low weight gain during pregnancy (P for trend = 0.006), malaria (RR, 1.42; 95% CI, 1.11–1.81), *Entamoeba coli* infection (RR, 1.49; 95% CI, 1.04–2.15), and HIV disease stage ≥ 2 (RR, 1.41; 95% CI, 1.12–1.79), and prehypertension or hypertension (RR, 1.26; 95% CI, 1.00–1.59) were significantly and independently associated with increased risk of preterm delivery. After adjustment, vitamin A deficiency, *Entamoeba histolytica* infection, and carrying twins were all associated with an increased risk of preterm delivery with borderline significance.

The results of unadjusted and adjusted relative risk regressions comparing maternal factors for very preterm versus full-term deliveries are presented in Table 3. Maternal age less than 20 years (RR, 1.91; 95% CI, 1.21–3.03), small MUAC (P for trend = 0.03), low weight gain during pregnancy (P for trend = 0.0005), malaria (RR, 1.81; 95% CI, 1.19–2.76), *Entamoeba coli* infection (RR, 2.38; 95% CI, 1.38–4.09), and *Entamoeba histolytica* infection (RR, 2.62; 95% CI, 1.09–6.28), and HIV disease stage ≥ 2 (RR, 1.68; 95% CI, 1.11–2.53) were significantly and independently associated with increased risk of preterm delivery. Maternal illiteracy was associated with increased risk of very preterm delivery with borderline significance.

For the analysis, we dichotomized maternal age with a cutpoint at 20 years. We chose not to include an age group for older mothers because analyses showed that the risk of prematurity in mothers aged 30 and older was not significantly greater than the risk of prematurity in mothers aged 20 to 30 (data not shown).

There may be concern that gestational age based on self-reported LMP is potentially unreliable. However, we found a correlation of 0.78 (95% CI, 0.76–0.80) between gestational age at screening based on LMP and fundal height, suggesting that, for this population, self-reported LMP can be used as a reasonable measure of gestational age.

4. Discussion

4.1. Main Findings. Our study found that HIV disease stage ≥ 2, no or low weight gain during pregnancy, *Entamoeba coli*, malaria, and maternal age less than 20 years were significantly associated with risk of preterm and very preterm

Table 1: Study population characteristics, $N = 927^{a}$.

Characteristic	N (%) or median [IQR]
Preterm births (<37 wks)	227 (24%)
Very preterm births (<34 wks)	87 (9%)
Gestational age at enrollment (weeks)	21 [18, 23]
Gestational age at birth (weeks)	39 [37, 41]
Sociodemographic	
Maternal age at conception (years)	25 [22, 29]
<20	96 (10%)
No partner	103 (11%)
Illiterate	70 (8%)
Nutrition and Anthropometric	
Plasma vitamin A (μg/dL)	23.4 [17.9, 30.2]
<20	246 (34%)
Plasma vitamin E (μmol/L)	9.6 [8.0, 11.4]
<9.7	368 (51%)
Selenium (mg/mL)	0.12 [0.11, 0.14]
<0.11	218 (26.49%)
0.11-0.12	148 (17.98%)
0.12–0.14	250 (30.38%)
≥0.14	207 (25.15%)
Hemoglobin (g/dL)	9.5 [8.4, 10.5]
<7.0	59 (6%)
7.0–8.4	188 (21%)
8.5–10.9	508 (56%)
≥11.0	112 (12%)
Mid-upper arm circumference (cm)	25.0 [23.5, 27.5]
≤23.5	225 (26%)
23.6–25.0	203 (24%)
25.1–27.5	220 (26%)
>27.5	203 (24%)
Weight gain (g per week)	255 [116, 380]
≤0	112 (12%)
1–119	126 (14%)
≥120	689 (74%)
Height (cm)	156 [152, 160]
<150	90 (10%)
Infections	
Malaria	176 (19%)
Hookworm	92 (12%)
Entamoeba coli	69 (9%)
Ascaris lumbricoides	43 (6%)
Cryptosporidium parvum	34 (4%)
Entamoeba histolytica	15 (2%)
Strongyloides stercoralis	14 (2%)
Trichuris trichiura	9 (1%)
Giardia lamblia	4 (1%)
Enterobius	0 (0%)
Isospora	0 (0%)
Microsporidia	0 (0%)
Taenia	0 (0%)

Table 1: Continued.

Characteristic	N (%) or median [IQR]
Trichomoniasis	232 (25%)
Syphilis	44 (6%)
Vaginal candidiasis	41 (6%)
Gonorrhea	9 (1%)
HIV/AIDS	
WHO HIV disease stage ≥ 2	189 (20%)
CD4 count (cells/mm^3)	402 [275, 530]
<200	112 (13%)
Viral load (copies/mL)	47819 [11626, 146135]
≥50,000	193 (50%)
Other clinical variables	
Twins	22 (2%)
Diastolic blood pressure (mmHg)	70 [60, 70]
Systolic blood pressure (mmHg)	110 [100, 110]
Prehypertension or hypertension^b	259 (28%)

AIQR: interquartile range.
^{a}Not all numbers add up to 927 due to missing data.
^{b}Systolic blood pressure > 120 mmHg or diastolic blood pressure > 80 mmHg.

delivery. Illiteracy and pre-hypertension/hypertension were associated with preterm delivery; however, the relationship of illiteracy with very preterm was only borderline significant and pre-hypertension/hypertension was not associated with very preterm delivery. *Entamoeba histolytica*, an intestinal parasitic infection, and MUAC were associated with very preterm delivery but not preterm delivery.

4.2. Strengths and Limitations. Although there have been several studies on risk factors for premature delivery, this study is unique in that it is based upon a large sample of HIV-infected, ART-naïve pregnant women in sub-Saharan Africa. However, there are some potential limitations to our study and analyses. Many of the potential risk factors we examined were only measured at enrollment and not throughout the pregnancy. Additional useful information would have been obtained if lab samples had been taking throughout participants' pregnancies, since this would have provided more complete data on parasitic infections, STIs, HIV disease progression, and nutritional status throughout pregnancy.

The potential lack of reliability of using LMP to estimate gestational age is a limitation to our study, although this approach is used frequently, both clinically and for research, in sub-Saharan Africa given the expense and lack of access to ultrasound machines. We expect that the definition of prematurity will be misclassified in a random way with respect to various strata of a particular risk factor in our analyses. Thus, we expect that our findings are biased towards the null because nondifferential exposure of a binary outcome will bias the results towards the null [24]. We found gestational age based on fundal height and LMP to be highly correlated. However, ultrasound, not fundal height measurements is the gold standard for measuring gestational age. Fundal height is thought to be accurate to 1-3 weeks. A future study

TABLE 2: Risk factors for preterm birth (<37 weeks versus ≥37 weeks), $N = 927$.

Characteristic	Unadjusted		Adjusted[a]	
	RR [95% CI]	P value	RR [95% CI]	P value
Sociodemographic				
Age < 20 at conception	1.58 [1.18, 2.11]	0.002	1.47 [1.10, 1.97]	0.01
No partner	1.17 [0.84, 1.63]	0.35		
Illiterate	1.58 [1.14, 2.20]	0.006	1.53 [1.09, 2.15]	0.01
Nutrition				
Plasma vitamin A < 20 (μg/dL)	1.24 [1.19, 1.96]	0.0008	1.25 [0.97, 1.62]	0.08
Plasma vitamin E < 9.7 (μmol/L)	0.88 [0.69, 1.13]	0.31		
Selenium (mg/mL)		0.12		0.16
<0.11	1.37 [0.97, 1.96]		1.40 [0.98, 2.00]	
0.11-0.12	1.15 [0.77, 1.73]		1.11 [0.74, 1.65]	
0.12–0.14	1.39 [0.98, 1.95]		1.48 [1.05, 2.08]	
≥0.14	Reference		Reference	
Hemoglobin (g/dL)		0.11		0.90
<7.0	1.29 [0.83, 2.01]		0.98 [0.64, 1.52]	
7.0–8.4	1.05 [0.74, 1.49]		0.90 [0.63, 1.28]	
8.5–10.9	0.82 [0.60, 1.11]		0.78 [0.58, 1.07]	
≥11.0	Reference		Reference	
Mid-upper arm circumference (cm)		0.19		0.23
≤23.5	1.29 [0.92, 1.81]		1.32 [0.93, 1.87]	
23.6–25.0	0.95 [0.66, 1.39]		0.91 [0.63, 1.33]	
25.1–27.5	1.11 [0.78, 1.58]		1.07 [0.75, 1.53]	
>27.5	Reference		Reference	
Weight gain (g per week)		<0.0001		0.006
≤0	1.95 [1.51, 2.53]		1.60 [1.20, 2.14]	
1–120	1.18 [0.85, 1.65]		1.12 [0.81, 1.57]	
≥120	Reference		Reference	
Height < 150 cm	0.95 [0.64, 1.40]	0.79		
Infections				
Malaria	1.53 [1.20, 1.96]	0.0006	1.41 [1.10, 1.81]	0.006
Hookworm	1.30 [0.92, 1.84]	0.13	1.19 [0.83, 1.70]	0.34
Entamoeba coli	1.49 [1.04, 2.14]	0.03	1.49 [1.04, 2.15]	0.03
Ascaris lumbricoides	1.21 [0.73, 1.99]	0.46		
Cryptosporidium parvum	0.88 [0.45, 1.72]	0.70		
Entamoeba histolytica	1.73 [0.92, 3.27]	0.09	1.79 [0.99, 3.26]	0.06
Strongyloides stercoralis	1.23 [0.53, 2.84]	0.63		
Trichuris trichiura	1.44 [0.56, 3.65]	0.45		
Trichomoniasis	1.18 [0.92, 1.52]	0.19	1.13 [0.88, 1.45]	0.35
Syphilis	1.28 [0.80, 2.05]	0.31		
Vaginal candidiasis	1.10 [0.66, 1.85]	0.72		
Gonorrhea	1.83 [0.88, 3.85]	0.11	1.68 [0.84, 3.35]	0.14
HIV/AIDS				
WHO HIV disease stage ≥ 2	1.60 [1.26, 2.03]	0.0001	1.40 [1.11, 1.78]	0.005
CD4 count < 200 cells/mm^3	0.92 [0.64, 1.32]	0.65		
Viral load ≥ 50,000 copies/mL	1.02 [0.74, 1.42]	0.89		
Other clinical variables				
Twins	1.50 [0.85, 2.64]	0.16	1.85 [0.94, 3.66]	0.07
Prehypertension or hypertension[b]	1.25 [0.98, 1.58]	0.07	1.27 [1.01, 1.60]	0.04

ARR: risk ratio; CI: confidence interval.

[a]Adjusted for age < 20 years, literacy, plasma vitamin A < 20 μg/dL, selenium, mid-upper arm circumference, weight gain, malaria, hookworm, *Entamoeba coli*, *Entamoeba histolytica*, trichomoniasis, gonorrhea, WHO HIV disease stage ≥ 2, twins, and prehypertension or hypertension.

[b]Systolic blood pressure >120 mmHg or diastolic blood pressure >80 mmHg.

TABLE 3: Risk factors for very preterm birth (<34 weeks versus ≥37 weeks), $N = 787$.

Characteristic	Unadjusted		Adjusted[a]	
	RR [95% CI]	P value	RR [95% CI]	P value
Sociodemographic				
Age < 20 at conception	2.21 [1.37, 3.55]	0.001	1.94 [1.22, 3.06]	0.005
No partner	1.20 [0.66, 2.16]	0.55		
Illiterate	1.93 [1.09, 3.41]	0.02	1.66 [0.91, 3.02]	0.10
Nutrition				
Plasma vitamin A < 20 (μg/dL)	1.89 [1.24, 2.87]	0.003	1.38 [0.89, 2.13]	0.15
Plasma vitamin E < 9.7 (μmol/L)	0.86 [0.57, 1.32]	0.50		
Selenium (mg/mL)	0.003 [<0.01, 58]	0.24		
<0.11	1.64 [0.87, 3.09]			
0.11-0.12	1.13 [0.53, 2.40]			
0.12–0.14	1.82 [1.00, 3.32]			
≥0.14	Reference			
Hemoglobin (g/dL)		0.45		
<7.0	0.72 [0.43, 1.23]			
7.0–8.4	0.72 [0.43, 1.23]			
8.5–10.9	1.12 [0.63, 2.01]			
≥11.0	Reference			
Mid-upper arm circumference (cm)		0.03		0.03
≤23.5	1.90 [0.99, 3.67]		2.07 [1.03, 4.16]	
23.6–25.0	1.50 [0.75, 3.00]		1.50 [0.74, 3.06]	
25.1–27.5	1.10 [0.52, 2.32]		1.03 [0.49, 2.20]	
>27.5	Reference		Reference	
Weight gain (g per week)		<0.0001		0.0005
≤0	3.21 [2.06, 5.00]		2.32 [1.36, 3.96]	
1–120	1.78 [1.05, 3.03]		1.85 [1.05, 3.25]	
≥120	Reference		Reference	
Height < 150 cm	0.93 [0.47, 1.86]	0.84		
Infections				
Malaria	2.03 [1.34, 3.07]	0.0009	1.87 [1.20, 2.89]	0.005
Hookworm	1.18 [0.61, 2.27]	0.63		
Entamoeba coli	2.34 [1.36, 4.02]	0.002	2.38 [1.38, 4.09]	0.002
Ascaris lumbricoides	1.34 [0.58, 3.13]	0.49		
Cryptosporidium parvum	0.64 [0.17, 2.50]	0.53		
Entamoeba histolytica	2.44 [0.89, 6.66]	0.08	2.62 [1.09, 6.28]	0.03
Strongyloides stercoralis	0.86 [0.13, 5.65]	0.88		
Trichuris trichiura	No data			
Trichomoniasis	1.30 [0.84, 1.99]	0.24		
Syphilis	1.34 [0.58, 3.13]	0.49		
Vaginal candidiasis	0.82 [0.27, 2.45]	0.72		
Gonorrhea	2.61 [0.80, 8.57]	0.11	2.72 [0.86, 8.58]	0.09
HIV/AIDS				
WHO HIV disease stage ≥ 2	2.09 [1.39, 3.14]	0.0004	1.67 [1.11, 2.51]	0.01
CD4 count < 200 cells/mm^3	0.72 [0.36, 1.45]	0.36		
Viral load ≥ 50,000 copies/mL	0.79 [0.46, 1.36]	0.40		
Other clinical variables				
Twins	2.06 [0.85, 5.00]	0.11	1.86 [0.68, 5.07]	0.22
Prehypertension or hypertension[b]	1.16 [0.76, 1.79]	0.49	1.22 [0.81, 1.85]	0.33

ARR: risk ratio; CI: confidence interval.

[a] Adjusted for age < 20 years, literacy, plasma vitamin A < 20 μg/dL, mid-upper arm circumference, weight gain, malaria, *Entamoeba coli*, *Entamoeba histolytica*, gonorrhea, WHO HIV disease stage ≥ 2, twins, and prehypertension or hypertension.

[b] Systolic blood pressure > 120 mmHg or diastolic blood pressure > 80 mmHg.

comparing gestational age based on LMP versus ultrasound in a developing country context, where recall of LMP may be especially inaccurate, could provide further information on the reliability of gestational age based on self-reported LMP.

Our study took place before zidovudine (AZT) and other ARVs were in use in Tanzania, allowing us to identify risk factors for prematurity among children born to ARV-naive HIV-positive women. The use of highly active antiretroviral therapy (HAART), but not AZT monotherapy, during pregnancy has been shown to increase the risk of preterm delivery [25]. In 2012, only 71% of HIV-infected pregnant women in Tanzania were receiving ARVs for prevention of mother-to-child transmission (PMTCT) [26]. This indicates that in Tanzania the risk factors we have found for preterm delivery in HIV-infected women are directly relevant for 29% of the pregnancies in HIV-infected women. A review of PMTCT coverage in 108 countries between 2007 and 2009 found that only 35% of HIV-infected pregnant women received PMCTC [27]. The WHO estimates that in 21 priority countries in sub-Saharan Africa in 2012, only 64% of HIV-infected pregnant women received any ARVs for PMCTC [28]. Among these 21 countries, PMCTC coverage ranged from 13% in the Democratic Republic of the Congo to >95% in both Botswana and Zambia [28].

Furthermore, the WHO guidelines recommend that low-income countries choose from one of three options (A, B, or B+) for PMTCT. The guidelines suggest that all patients with a CD4 count of <350 cells/mm^3 begin HAART and that pregnant women with CD4 counts >350 cells/mm^3 be provided with either option A, B, or B+. Option A is the provision of AZT monotherapy beginning at no sooner than 14 weeks gestation. Option B is the provision of HAART beginning at no sooner than 14 weeks gestation. Option B+ is the provision of HAART as soon as HIV infection is diagnosed. While some countries have adopted option B or B+ for prevention of mother-to-child transmission of HIV, several countries have opted to adopt Option A of the WHO guidelines whereby women receive HAART only if they are advanced in their disease. For example, Kenya has adopted a combination of options A and B, in which health centers adopt option A if they do not have the capacity to adopt option B [29]. In these settings, a majority of pregnant women are in early stages of disease and are thus not initiated on triple ARVs, and for whom our findings are applied.

4.3. Interpretation. Preterm delivery and very preterm delivery were analyzed as separate outcomes for two reasons. First, because very preterm delivery leads to more severe health outcomes than preterm delivery, identification of differing risk factors would make possible the targeting of available resources toward very preterm delivery prevention. However, we found that risk factors for very preterm and preterm deliveries were similar. Our results suggest that the same interventions can be used to reduce both preterm and very preterm deliveries. Furthermore, analyzing preterm and very preterm deliveries separately provided a sensitivity analysis. The regression analysis of very preterm deliveries excluded

deliveries between 34 and 37 weeks, reducing misclassification bias that may be associated with gestational age assessment.

Because very preterm deliveries are a subset of preterm deliveries, they have a smaller sample size, resulting in larger standard errors and P values, and wider confidence intervals. Many of the point estimates are larger in the very preterm regression. This may be because there is less misclassification bias due to incorrectly estimated gestational age. Deliveries with a reported gestational age of less than 34 weeks were more likely to be correctly classified as preterm than those with a reported gestational age of less than 37 weeks.

The rate of prematurity that we observed, 24%, is higher than that found in other HIV-infected populations. A study of 1626 HIV-positive Nigerian women from 2004–2010 found a preterm delivery rate of 11.1% [30]. This may partially be due to improvements in nutrition and maternal health from 1995–1997 to 2004–2010. A study in the United States in the early 1990's found that 19% of infants born to HIV-infected mothers were premature [31]. This difference is likely due, in part, to better healthcare in the US.

We found lack of weight gain during pregnancy to be associated with preterm and very preterm delivery. Weight gain is a marker of maternal nutritional status, and thus no or low weight gain during pregnancy could be a marker of inadequate nutrition during pregnancy. However, this finding may be due to reverse causality, as it is unknown whether lack of weight gain caused the premature delivery or the premature delivery led to less time for gestational weight gain.

We found that HIV disease stage ≥ 2 at enrollment increased the risk of prematurity. However, we did not find any further association between prematurity and either CD4 cell count or viral load. A study in South Africa found no effect of HIV-infection in ART-naïve women on prematurity [32]. However, a previous study in China did report an effect of CD4 count and viral load on prematurity [33].

We found younger maternal age, but not older maternal age, to be a risk factor for preterm birth. Women younger than 20 years were more likely to deliver preterm compared to women 20 years and older. However, women 30 years of age and older were not found to be at a higher risk of premature delivery compared to women aged 20–30. The result that young mothers are at an increased risk for premature delivery has also been found in studies in other sub-Saharan African countries such as Cameroon [34], but not Zimbabwe [35]. The result that older maternal age is not associated with premature delivery was also found in a Turkish study that found adolescent pregnancy to be a weak risk factor for prematurity but did not find maternal age of 39 and older to increase the risk of prematurity [36]. However, a study in the US found women aged 30–34 and aged 35 and older to be at an increased risk for premature delivery compared to women aged 25–29 [37].

5. Conclusion

As the preventable and treatable major killers of children such as malaria, diarrheal disease, and respiratory disease are increasingly managed, with the presumption that mortality from these causes will decrease, the proportion of child mortality due to premature birth will increase. In order to further reduce needless child deaths, it will be important to reduce the modifiable determinants of preterm birth so as to increase the percentage of children that are born full-term. Interventions to promote nutritional status and to slow HIV disease progression are likely to be critical for reducing the risk of prematurity.

Ethical Approval

The study was approved by the Research and Publications Committee of Muhimbili University of Health and Allied Sciences, the ethics committee of the Tanzania Ministry of Health's National AIDS Control Program, and the Institutional Review Board of the Harvard School of Public Health (no. 10399).

Conflict of Interests

The authors declare that there is no conflict of interests regarding the publication of this paper.

Authors' Contribution

Wafaie Fawzi proposed the study question and edited the paper. Said Aboud contributed to study design and data collection and edited the paper. Donna Spiegelman edited the paper and provided statistical advice. Gernard Msamanga contributed to study design and execution of the fieldwork and edited the paper. Rachel M. Zack conducted the analyses, interpreted the results, and wrote the paper along with Jenna Golan.

Funding

The Trial of Vitamins study was sponsored by the National Institute of Child Health and Human Development (NICHD R01 32257) and the Fogarty International Center (NIH D43 TW00004). RMZ was supported in part by an NIH T32 training grant (CA 09001).

Acknowledgments

The authors would like to thank James Okuma and Ellen Hertzmark who helped them access and analyze the data. They would also like to thank everyone who conducted the study and the women who participated in it.

References

[1] J. E. Lawn, S. Cousens, and J. Zupan, "4 Million neonatal deaths: when? Where? Why?" *The Lancet*, vol. 365, no. 9462, pp. 891–900, 2005.

[2] C. Mathers, G. Stevens, and M. Mascarenhas, *Global Health Risks: Mortality and Burden of Disease Attributable to Selected Major Risks*, World Health Organization, 2009.

[3] R. Lozano, M. Naghavi, K. Foreman et al., "Global and regional mortality from 235 causes of death for 20 age groups in 1990 and 2010: a systematic analysis for the Global Burden of Disease Study 2010," *The Lancet*, vol. 380, no. 9859, pp. 2095–2128, 2012.

[4] S. Beck, D. Wojdyla, L. Say et al., "The worldwide incidence of preterm birth: a systematic review of maternal mortality and morbidity," *Bulletin of the World Health Organization*, vol. 88, no. 1, pp. 31–38, 2010.

[5] K. Manji, "Situation analysis of newborn health in Tanzania: current situation, existing plans and strategic next steps for newborn health," 2009.

[6] C. Klingenberg, R. Olomi, M. Oneko, N. Sam, and N. Langeland, "Neonatal morbidity and mortality in a Tanzanian tertiary care referral hospital," *Annals of Tropical Paediatrics*, vol. 23, no. 4, pp. 293–299, 2003.

[7] L. K. Rogers and M. Velten, "Maternal inflammation, growth retardation, and preterm birth: insights into adult cardiovascular disease," *Life Sciences*, vol. 89, no. 13-14, pp. 417–421, 2011.

[8] G. Filler, A. Yasin, P. Kesarwani, A. X. Garg, R. Lindsay, and A. P. Sharma, "Big mother or small baby: which predicts hypertension?" *Journal of Clinical Hypertension*, vol. 13, no. 1, pp. 35–41, 2011.

[9] Tanzania Commission for AIDS (TACAIDS), Zanzaibar AIDS Commission (ZAC), National Burea of Statistics (NBS), Office of the Chief Government Statistiian (OCGS), and Macro International, "Tanzania HIV/AIDS and Malaria Indicator Survey 2007-2008," 2008.

[10] R. Lozano, H. Wang, K. J. Foreman et al., "Progress towards Millennium Development Goals 4 and 5 on maternal and child mortality: an updated systematic analysis," *The Lancet*, vol. 378, no. 9797, pp. 1139–1165, 2011.

[11] C. Mathers, G. Stevens, and M. Mascarenhas, "Global Health Risks: mortality and burden of disease attributable to selected major risks," Tech. Rep., WHO, 2009.

[12] W. W. Fawzi, G. I. Msamanga, D. Spiegelman et al., "Randomised trial of effects of vitamin supplements on pregnancy outcomes and T cell counts in HIV-1-infected women in Tanzania," *The Lancet*, vol. 351, no. 9114, pp. 1477–1482, 1998.

[13] W. W. Fawzi, G. I. Msamanga, D. Spiegelman et al., "A randomized trial of multivitamin supplements and HIV disease progression and mortality," *The New England Journal of Medicine*, vol. 351, no. 1, pp. 23–32, 2004.

[14] W. W. Fawzi, G. I. Msamanga, D. Hunter et al., "Randomized trial of vitamin supplements in relation to transmission of HIV-1 through breastfeeding and early child mortality," *AIDS*, vol. 16, no. 14, pp. 1935–1944, 2002.

[15] W. W. Fawzi, G. Msamanga, D. Hunter et al., "Randomized trial of vitamin supplements in relation to vertical transmission of HIV-1 in Tanzania," *Journal of Acquired Immune Deficiency Syndromes*, vol. 23, no. 3, pp. 246–254, 2000.

[16] B. de Benoist, E. McLean, I. Egli, and M. Cogswell, *Worldwide Prevalence of Anaemia 1993–2005: WHO Global Database on Anaemia*, WHO, Geneva, Switzerland, 2008.

[17] X. Guo, X. Zhang, L. Guo et al., "Association between pre-hypertension and cardiovascular outcomes: a systematic review and meta-analysis of prospective studies," *Current Hypertension Reports*, vol. 15, pp. 703–716, 2013.

[18] E. Villamor, G. Msamanga, D. Spiegelman et al., "Effect of multivitamin and vitamin A supplements on weight gain during pregnancy among HIV-1-infected women," *The American Journal of Clinical Nutrition*, vol. 76, no. 5, pp. 1082–1090, 2002.

[19] E. Villamor, M. L. Dreyfuss, A. Baylín, G. Msamanga, and W. W. Fawzi, "Weight loss during pregnancy is associated with adverse pregnancy outcomes among HIV-1 infected women," *Journal of Nutrition*, vol. 134, no. 6, pp. 1424–1431, 2004.

[20] E. Villamor, E. Saathoff, G. Msamanga, M. E. O'Brien, K. Manji, and W. W. Fawzi, "Wasting during pregnancy increases the risk of mother-to-child HIV-1 transmission," *Journal of Acquired Immune Deficiency Syndromes*, vol. 38, no. 5, pp. 622–626, 2005.

[21] O. S. Miettinen, *Theoretical Epidemiology: Principles of Occurrence Research in Medicine*, Delmar, 1985.

[22] D. Spiegelman and E. Hertzmark, "Easy SAS calculations for risk or prevalence ratios and differences," *The American Journal of Epidemiology*, vol. 162, no. 3, pp. 199–200, 2005.

[23] G. Maldonado and S. Greenland, "Simulation study of confounder-selection strategies," *The American Journal of Epidemiology*, vol. 138, no. 11, pp. 923–936, 1993.

[24] K. J. Rothman, S. Greenland, and T. L. Lash, *Modern Epidemiology*, Lippincott Williams & Wilkins, 2008.

[25] F. Martin and G. P. Taylor, "The safety of highly active antiretroviral therapy for the HIV-positive pregnant mother and her baby: is "the more the merrier"?" *Journal of Antimicrobial Chemotherapy*, vol. 64, no. 5, pp. 895–900, 2009.

[26] F. Mrisho, "Country Progress Reporting 2012".

[27] W. Y. N. Man, H. Worth, A. Kelly, D. P. Wilson, and P. Siba, "Is endemic political corruption hampering provision of ART and PMTCT in developing countries?" *Journal of the International AIDS Society*, vol. 17, Article ID 18568, 2014.

[28] WHO, UNICEF, and UNAIDS, "Global update on HIV treatment 2013: results, impact and opportunities," WHO Report in Partnership with UNICEF and UNAIDS, 2013.

[29] E. du Plessis, S. Y. Shaw, M. Gichuhi et al., "Prevention of mother-to-child transmission of HIV in Kenya: challenges to implementation," *BMC Health Services Research*, vol. 14, article S10, 2014.

[30] O. C. Ezechi, A. N. David, C. V. Gab-Okafor et al., "Incidence of and socio-biologic risk factors for spontaneous preterm birth in HIV positive Nigerian women," *BMC Pregnancy and Childbirth*, vol. 12, article 93, 2012.

[31] R. Martin, P. Boyer, H. Hammill et al., "Incidence of premature birth and neonatal respiratory disease in infants of HIV-positive mothers," *Journal of Pediatrics*, vol. 131, no. 6, pp. 851–856, 1997.

[32] J. Ndirangu, M.-L. Newell, R. M. Bland, and C. Thorne, "Maternal HIV infection associated with small-for-gestational age infants but not preterm births: evidence from rural South Africa," *Human Reproduction*, vol. 27, no. 6, pp. 1846–1856, 2012.

[33] L. Yu, W.-Y. Li, R. Y. Chen et al., "Pregnancy outcomes and risk factors for low birth weight and preterm delivery among HIV-infected pregnant women in Guangxi, China," *Chinese Medical Journal*, vol. 125, no. 3, pp. 403–409, 2012.

[34] E. J. Kongnyuy, P. N. Nana, N. Fomulu, S. C. Wiysonge, L. Kouam, and A. S. Doh, "Adverse perinatal outcomes of adolescent pregnancies in cameroon," *Maternal and Child Health Journal*, vol. 12, no. 2, pp. 149–154, 2008.

[35] S. A. Feresu, S. D. Harlow, and G. B. Woelk, "Risk factors for prematurity at Harare Maternity Hospital, Zimbabwe," *International Journal of Epidemiology*, vol. 33, no. 6, pp. 1194–1201, 2004.

[36] U. Kuyumcuoglu, A. I. Guzel, and Y. Çelik, "Comparison of the risk factors for adverse perinatal outcomes in adolescent age pregnancies and advanced age pregnancies," *Ginekologia Polska*, vol. 83, no. 1, pp. 33–37, 2012.

[37] M. M. Hillemeier, C. S. Weisman, G. A. Chase, and A.-M. Dyer, "Individual and community predictors of preterm birth and low birthweight along the rural-urban continuum in central Pennsylvania," *Journal of Rural Health*, vol. 23, no. 1, pp. 42–48, 2007.

5

Correlation of Endometrial Glycodelin Expression and Pregnancy Outcome in Cases with Polycystic Ovary Syndrome Treated with Clomiphene Citrate Plus Metformin: A Controlled Study

Selda Uysal,[1] **Ahmet Zeki Isik,**[2] **Serenat Eris,**[3] **Seyran Yigit,**[4] **Yakup Yalcin,**[5] **and Pelin Ozun Ozbay**[6]

[1]*Gynecology and Obstetrics Department, Ataturk Training and Research Hospital, Basin Sitesi, Yesilyurt, 35360 İzmir, Turkey*
[2]*Gynecology and Obstetrics Department, Izmir University Hospital, 35360 İzmir, Turkey*
[3]*Gynecology and Obstetrics Department, Isparta Obstetrics and Pediatrics Hospital, 32000 Isparta, Turkey*
[4]*Pathology Department, Ataturk Training and Research Hospital, Basin Sitesi, Yesilyurt, 35360 İzmir, Turkey*
[5]*Gynecologic Oncology Department, Suleyman Demirel University Hospital, 32000 Isparta, Turkey*
[6]*Gynecology and Obstetrics Department, Aydın Obstetrics and Pediatrics Hospital, 09100 Aydın, Turkey*

Correspondence should be addressed to Serenat Eris; serenateris@hotmail.com

Academic Editor: Curt W. Burger

Objective. The purpose of this study was to evaluate the relationship between clomiphene citrate (CC) plus metformin treatment and endometrial glycodelin expression and to then correlate this relationship with pregnancy outcomes. *Material and Methods.* A total of 30 patients diagnosed with polycystic ovary syndrome (PCOS) according to the Rotterdam criteria constituted our study group. All had been admitted to the gynecology outpatient clinic between June 1, 2011, and January 1, 2012, for infertility treatment. Our control group consisted of 20 patients admitted for routine Pap smear control. They had no history of infertility and were not using contraceptives and they were actively attempting pregnancy. Midluteal progesterone measurement and pipelle endometrial biopsies were performed with both groups. For PCOS patients, metformin treatment was initiated right after the biopsy and CC was added in the second menstrual cycle. Pipelle endometrial biopsies were repeated. Histological dating and immunohistochemistry for glycodelin were performed by a single pathologist who was blinded to the patients' clinical data. *Result(s).* The posttreatment ovulation rate in the study group was 93.3%. No pregnancies were achieved in either group when glycodelin expression was not present, even in the presence of ovulation. When glycodelin expression was high in PCOS group, the pregnancy rate was 60% and all pregnancies ended in live births. In weak expression group, however, three out of four pregnancies ended as early pregnancy losses. *Conclusion(s).* Endometrial glycodelin expression is an important predictor of pregnancy outcomes in both PCOS and fertile groups.

1. Introduction

Polycystic ovary syndrome (PCOS) is the most common cause of anovulatory infertility and occurs at a rate between 6% and 12% during the reproductive period [1–3]. This endocrinopathy, the etiology of which has not been fully elucidated, begins in the postmenarcheal period and continues until the premenopausal period [3, 4]. It is characterized by chronic anovulation and hyperandrogenemia [1–4]. In addition to anovulation-related infertility, the frequency of early pregnancy loss in PCOS is three times higher than in the normal population [2, 3]. In cases with PCOS, the rate of pregnancy loss following the clinical identification of assisted or spontaneous pregnancy is 30%–50% [1–3].

The most important feature of PCOS is compensatory hyperinsulinemic insulin resistance [1–5]. By stimulating ovarian androgen production and decreasing serum sex hormone-binding globulin (SHBG) concentrations, hyperinsulinemic insulin resistance leads to hyperandrogenism [1, 2] and anovulation [1, 2, 6–8]. With the suppression of endometrial glycodelin levels, endometrial functions are impaired, the preimplantation environment is adversely affected, and the rate of early pregnancy loss increases [1, 2].

Glycodelin is a major glycoprotein induced by progesterone and secreted from the secretory and decidual endometrium during the luteal phase [1, 2, 9, 10]. It is observed during the ovulatory cycles and facilitates implantation by inhibiting the immune response [9, 10]. The downregulation of maternal immune response against fetal alloantigenicity is achieved via the T-cells [9–11]. Glycodelin induces the apoptosis of monocytes before their differentiation into macrophages through the mitochondrial pathway, without affecting phagocytic activity. The decrease of glycodelin in the endometrium and serum is associated with growth retardation of endometrium, early pregnancy loss, and recurrent early pregnancy loss [1, 2].

Insulin-sensitizing drugs and metformin in particular not only are involved in the correction of insulin resistance but also serve to treat reproductive abnormalities [3, 4]. Biguanide metformin is the most frequently used insulin-sensitizing agent in type 2 diabetes mellitus (DM). Aside from the liver, biguanide metformin also has an effect on the skeletal muscles, the adipose tissue, the endothelium, and the ovaries. It increases ovulation, corrects the menstrual cycle, and decreases the levels of serum androgens. It achieves its reproductive effects both via insulin and through direct effects on ovarian functions. It is an effective agent for ensuring ovulation [1–4].

In PCOS, hyperinsulinemic insulin resistance decreases the concentration of circulating glycodelin [1, 2]. In nonpregnant PCOS patients, metformin increases serum glycodelin levels threefold during the luteal phase [1, 2].

The aim of our study was to demonstrate the effect of clomiphene citrate (CC) plus metformin treatment on endometrial glycodelin expression in PCOS patients and then correlate the relationship with rates of successful pregnancies and pregnancy outcomes. The effect of the intensity of endometrial glycodelin expression on pregnancy outcome was also controlled with the fertile group of women.

2. Materials and Methods

A total of 30 patients diagnosed with PCOS according to the Rotterdam criteria [12] constituted our study group. All were admitted to the gynecology outpatient clinic for fertility treatment between June 1, 2011, and January 1, 2012. Our control group consisted of 20 patients admitted for routine Pap smears. These women had no history of infertility and no contraceptive use and they were actively attempting pregnancy. Nine out of these twenty patients had previously given live births (45%). Before entering this prospective cohort study, the protocol was explained to patients and a written consent was obtained from patients agreeing to participate. Consent forms and the protocol were approved by the local ethical

committees. The physical and pelvic examination findings of these healthy patients, as well as their menstrual cycles, were normal, and none of them had a history of hormonal drug or intrauterine device (IUD) use in the previous three months. The study and control groups consisted entirely of nonsmoking patients between 20 and 40 years of age with no history of systemic or clinically active diseases. All women were naïve to clomiphene and had not undergone any significant treatment for infertility or ovulation induction earlier. Patients with hyperprolactinemia, thyroid disorder, male factor, suspected tubal factor, or endometriosis were not included in the study. There were no weight or Body Mass Index (BMI) restrictions. The complete blood-count values, follicle stimulating hormone (FSH), luteinizing hormone (LH), estradiol (E2), prolactin, thyroid stimulating hormone (TSH), total and free test, dehydroepiandrosterone sulfate (DHEA-S), 17-hydroxyprogesterone (17-OHP), luteal phase progesterone, and oral glucose tolerance test (OGTT) levels were measured during the routine clinical chemistry tests of all patients on the third day of the cycle. The BMI indices of the patients were also measured.

Following the completion of their routine tests, patients diagnosed with PCOS were administered with medroxyprogesterone acetate (MPA) 5 mg b.i.d. for six days. To perform endometrial dating, the level of progesterone was evaluated and a pipelle biopsy was taken in the period between the 21st and 24th days following the patients' menstrual bleeding. Tissue glycodelin levels were assessed in these endometrial samples.

Following biopsy, 16 patients with BMI <25 were administered metformin 500 mg b.i.d., while 14 patients with BMI >25 were given a dosage of 500 mg t.i.d. Blood biochemistry samples were obtained again following the spontaneous or induced second menstrual bleeding. Between the 5th and 9th days of the second menstrual cycle, ovulation induction was performed with clomiphene citrate under ultrasound monitoring. When the dimensions of the leading follicle reached between 18 mm and 22 mm, hCG was administered (Ovitrelle 250 μg, Merck Serono, Istanbul, Turkey). The serum progesterone level and ovulation were evaluated 9–11 days later. Pipelle biopsies were taken from 21–24 days after the beginning of the menstrual cycle. Tissue glycodelin levels were also assessed in these endometrial samples in addition to histological endometrial dating. For the study group, both pre- and posttreatment biopsies were conducted. We did not give any treatment to the control group and only one biopsy was taken of the fertile patients. All patients were followed up for three cycles. Any dose changes were made during the follow-up visits. Metformin treatment was discontinued after fetal cardiac activity observed.

2.1. Evaluation of Endometrial Biopsies. A pathologist evaluated all biopsies and confirmed that the specimens had normal endometria with no signs of pathology. Endometrial dating was performed as described in the literature [13]. Immunohistochemical analyses for glycodelin were carried out by using the horseradish peroxidase labelled streptavidin-biotin (HRP-LSAB) method. Briefly, 5 μm thick sections were

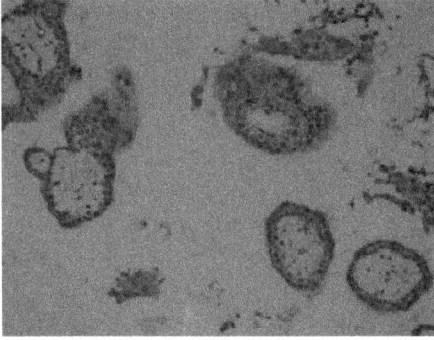

FIGURE 1: Immunohistochemical staining of glycodelin positive control in chorion villous tissue (×20).

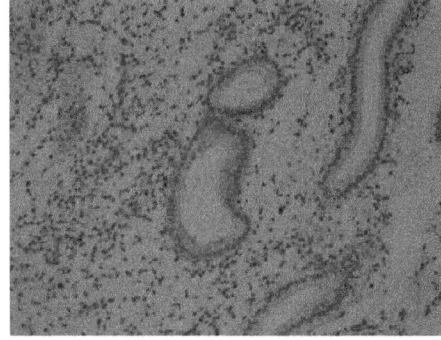

FIGURE 2: Weak glycodelin expression (×20).

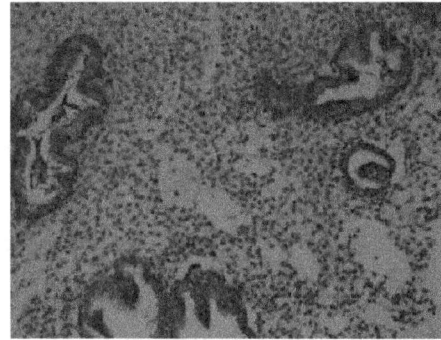

FIGURE 3: Strong glycodelin expression (×20).

cut from each paraffin block, deparaffinized, rehydrated, and subjected pre-treatment to enhance immunoreactivity, for which ethylenediaminetetraacetic acid (EDTA) 1/150 dilution was used for 25 minutes in a pretreatment procedure. Placental protein 14/glycodelin A antibody [EP870Y] (ab53289 Abcam, Cambridge, MA, USA) was used as a primary antibody 1 : 150 dilution for one hour at room temperature. The second antibody used was Horse Radish Peroxidase (DAKO, Glostrup, Denmark). Diaminobenzidine (DAB) was used as a chromogen for reaction visualization. Finally, the sections were counterstained with Mayer's hematoxylin, then dehydrated, cleared with xylene, and mounted with coverslips using a permanent mounting medium.

Cytoplasmic staining of trophoblastic cells in chorionic villous tissue was used as a positive control (Figure 1).

The antibody reacts with secretory glands and the luminal surface of normal secretory endometrium from the fifth postovulatory day. In normal proliferative endometrium, the antibody does not react with the antibody. We found no stromal staining.

For immunohistochemical analysis, all endometrial tissues were examined at low magnification (×10). For the antibody in the glandular epithelial cells, at ×20 magnification, the percentage of stained cells was determined semiquantitatively and subjectively. The immunostaining was evaluated on a scale of 0–3 points according to the percentage of cytoplasmic glandular cells that stained positively. Less than 5% of glandular cell staining was termed negative, 6–25% positivity was rated as 1 point, 26–50% positivity was rated as 2 points, and more than 50% positivity was rated as 3 points. According to the staining intensity, the immunostaining was evaluated on a scale of 1–3 points (1 point: weak; 2 points: moderate; 3 points: strongly positive). Points for the intensity staining (IS) and percentage (%S) of positive cells were added together, and an overall score (OS 0–2) was assigned. Staining was categorized into three groups based on the OS as follows: 1 point was negative expression (0 or <5% cells stained regardless of intensity); 2 points were a weak expression (OS, 1); 2 to 3 points; 3 points were a strong expression (OS, 2); 4 to 6 points; (Figures 2-3).

2.2. Statistical Analysis. Statistical analysis of the collected data was performed by using SPSS 16.0 (SPSS, Inc., Chicago,

IL, USA). Fisher's Exact Test and Pearson's chi square test were used for the statistical comparisons for categorical data between the groups. The Kruskal-Wallis H test was used for the statistical comparisons for continuous data between more than two groups and the Mann Whitney U test was used for the statistical comparisons for continuous data between the two groups. P values of <0.05 or less were considered as statistically significant.

For patients who became pregnant following the conduction of the study, the cycle in which they become pregnant, the outcome of the pregnancy, and complications were all recorded and evaluated.

3. Results

The mean age of the 30 patients in the study group was 25.6 ± 3.78, while the mean age of the 20 patients in the control group was 26.11 ± 4.21. The mean BMI values were determined to be 26.24 ± 4.91 for the study group and 24.51 ± 3.21 for the control group. The BMI values of the study group were significantly higher than the values for the control group ($P < 0.05$). When the laboratory values were evaluated, the pretreatment (predrug) LH and free testosterone values were significantly higher than the values for the control group, while the FSH and pretreatment progesterone values were significantly lower ($P < 0.05$). No significant differences were identified between the groups with respect to the other laboratory variables (Table 1). Posttreatment midluteal

TABLE 1: Mean distribution of age, BMI, and laboratory values in the study and control groups.

	Study group		Control group		P
	n	Mean ± S.D.	n	Mean ± S.D.	
Age (years)	30	25.6 ± 3.78	20	26.5 ± 4.57	0.605
Body Mass Index (kg/m^2)	30	26.24 ± 4.91	20	24.51 ± 3.21	**0.019**
FSH (mIU/mL)	30	5.74 ± 1.94	20	7.71 ± 2.64	**0.005**
LH (mIU/mL)	30	10.36 ± 8.68	20	4.6 ± 1.23	**0.025**
E2 (pg/mL)	30	68.89 ± 74.18	20	46.65 ± 17.8	0.452
Prolactin (ng/mL)	30	10.84 ± 5.06	20	14.46 ± 8.11	0.088
TSH (uIU/mL)	30	2.67 ± 1.51	20	2.41 ± 1.12	0.692
17-OHP (ng/mL)	30	1.59 ± 1.34	20	1.03 ± 0.43	0.088
DHEA-S (ug/dL)	30	247.2 ± 55.4	20	229.7 ± 87.6	0.428
Total testosterone (ng/mL)	30	49.48 ± 20.27	20	48.6 ± 24.24	0.707
Free testosterone (ng/mL)	30	7.20 ± 3.93	20	3.54 ± 1.18	**0.002**
HDL (mg/dL)	30	43.00 ± 8.73	20	51.25 ± 13.97	0.056
LDL (mg/dL)	30	117 ± 79.84	20	90.25 ± 24.12	0.153
OGTT (mg/dL) (2^h glucose concentration)	30	109.6 ± 35.56	20	110.5 ± 29.2	0.451
Progesterone (pretreatment) (ng/mL)	30	3.84 ± 4.34	20	11.98 ± 5.35	**0.001**

progesterone levels increased and a decrease was identified in the free testosterone values.

Among patients in the study group, a significant difference was identified between the pre- and posttreatment endometrial biopsy results ($P < 0.05$). There were 26 (86.7%) proliferative and 4 postovulatory (13.3%) endometria in the pretreatment period among PCOS patients (i.e., the study group); the rate of ovulation among these 30 patients reached 93.3% (28/30) following treatment. In the control group, the endometrial biopsy results in 19 out of 20 cases (95%) were postovulatory.

While no glycodelin expression was identified during the pretreatment period in the biopsy specimens of the 30 patients belonging to the study group, including the ovulatory patients, glycodelin was identified in 22 of the 28 patients (73.3%) who were classified as ovulatory during the posttreatment period. A statistically significant difference was identified between the pre- and posttreatment glycodelin levels of the study group ($P < 0.05$).

In the control group, no glycodelin was identified in 3 patients (15%) whereas glycodelin was positive in 17 patients (85%).

Spontaneous pregnancies occurred in 12 patients (60%) within the control group. All twelve were in the glycodelin positive group (12/17).

With respect to glycodelin positivity, pregnancies occurred in three out of five patients who showed weak staining positivity (60%). Nine out of 12 patients who had shown strong staining positivity (75%) also became pregnant.

In brief, 10 of 30 patients (33.3%) within the study group became pregnant. For both the study and control groups, a total of 22 patients who displayed glycodelin staining positivity became pregnant. In this group, the pregnancy rate was 45.4%. With respect to glycodelin positivity, four of the pregnancies occurred among women with positivity values of 1, while six pregnancies resulted after positivity values of 2.

TABLE 2: Pregnancy rates within the study and control groups with respect to glycodelin positivity.

	Pregnancy		No pregnancy		Total		P
	n	%	n	%	n	%	
Study group							
Glycodelin							
Negative	—	—	8	40.0	8	26.7	
1+	4	40.0	6	30.0	10	33.3	0.027
2+	6	60.0	6	30.0	12	40.0	
Control group							
Glycodelin							
Negative	—	—	3	37.5	3	15.0	
1+	3	60.0	2	40.0	5	25.0	0.030
2+	9	75.0	3	25.0	12	60.0	

Within the study and control groups, the increase in pregnancy rates following an increase in glycodelin positivity was found to be statistically significant P value for study and control groups were 0.027 and 0.030, respectively (Fisher's Exact Test, $P < 0.05$) (Table 2).

While two out of total twelve pregnancies in the control group resulted in miscarriages, ten of the pregnancies resulted in live births. With regard to the pregnancy cycles, six pregnancies occurred during the first cycle, while six other pregnancies occurred during the second and third cycles (the patients were followed for a total of three cycles).

In the study group, seven out of ten pregnancies occurred in the first cycle, while the remaining three pregnancies occurred in the second and third cycles. In addition, while three out of ten pregnancies resulted in early pregnancy loss (EPL), seven of the pregnancies resulted in live births.

When the glycodelin positivity rates were evaluated, one of the two pregnancy losses in the control group displayed

TABLE 3: Glycodelin expression and progesterone values of patients.

	Patient number (n)	Progesterone (mean ± SD)	P value
Study group			
Glycodelin			
Negative	8	13.25 ± 10.57	
Positive: 1+	10	16.9 ± 6.97	0.346
Positive: 2+	12	20.1 ± 5.16	
Control group			
Glycodelin			
Negative	3	7.85 ± 7.10	
Positive: 1+	5	12.98 ± 1.74	0.542
Positive: 2+	12	12.59 ± 5.81	

glycodelin (+) positivity, while the other had glycodelin (++) positivity. Within the study group, one of four pregnancies with glycodelin (+) positivity progressed successfully, while three resulted in early pregnancy loss. The early pregnancy loss rate was 75% in the glycodelin (+) study group.

Five out of seven of the pregnancies among the study group resulted in live and healthy births. In two of our cases, a caesarean section was performed at the 36th week due to placental abruption. No maternal and neonatal complications were observed.

When the mean progesterone values of the study group were evaluated for glycodelin positivity, no significant difference was identified between the groups (Table 3).

4. Discussion

Implantation involves the adhesion of the embryo to the decidua, its descent towards the basal membrane, and its invasion into the stroma. This process between the endometrium and the embryo is regulated by a complex system that involves the interaction of growth factors, hormones, adhesion molecules, extracellular matrices, and prostaglandins. Although assisted reproductive techniques are able to achieve fertilization rates in 70%–80% of cases, the average rate of resulting live births remains at only 35%–40%. This observation can be explained by implantation failures and deficiencies in endometrial receptivity [9].

Glycodelin is an important and promising indicator of implantation. It is involved in the processes pertaining to endometrial receptivity and implantation [9]. Low levels of glycodelin during the midcycle fertile window are conducive to fertilization, while higher glycodelin levels during the midluteal implantation window (between day 19 and day 24 during the 28-day cycle) allow for implantation to take place [14].

It has been demonstrated that the expression of glycodelin increases in the endometrium during the implantation window and late luteal phase, starting from postovulatory day five [14, 15]. Glycodelin has apoptotic [16] and antiproliferative [17] effects on T-lymphocytes, as well as immunosuppressive and inhibiting effects on natural killer (NK) lymphocytes.

It ensures implantation by protecting the embryo from the maternal immune system [3, 9]. In other words, it plays a significant role in the early interactions between the embryo and the endometrium [9].

In anovulatory cycles as well as cases with PCOS, low levels of serum and endometrial glycodelin are observed; as a result, endometrial functions are impaired and the preimplantation environment is rendered less suitable [18]. It is known that compensatory hyperinsulinemic insulin resistance has the same effect in cases with PCOS [1, 2, 19]. Thus, low levels of glycodelin can lead to implantation failures, early pregnancy losses, and recurrent pregnancy losses.

In hyperinsulinemia, signals directly and indirectly originating from the endometrial stroma are inhibited, thus contributing to low glycodelin concentrations [1, 2]. Metformin treatment is known to decrease the levels of serum insulin, glucose, and androgen while increasing serum SHBG [1, 6–8]. In another study, the concentrations of circulating glycodelin were found to have increased nearly threefold during the CC-induced postovulatory luteal phase as a result of metformin use [1].

In their study, Li et al. [20] evaluated the levels of glycodelin in the endometrial flushings of fertile subjects with normal cycles. Glycodelin levels were low during the proliferative phase and the periovulatory fertile period. However, in the early luteal phase, levels increased starting from the sixth day after the LH peak and reached their maximum during the late luteal phase. Similarly, Mylonas et al. [10] found levels increasing significantly in endometrial tissue samples during the late luteal phase. Kao et al. [21] on the other hand evaluated the genes regulating glycodelin in endometrial tissue. Glycodelin genes expressions during the secretory phase were found to be 14.6 times higher in comparison to the proliferation phase. Brown et al. found that glycodelin expression began in the endometrial glands on the 16th day of the cycle in both controlled ovarian hyperstimulation and natural cycles and increased progressively over time [22].

The goal of our study was to ensure ovulation with CC+ metformin treatment, to increase glycodelin secretion by reducing serum insulin levels with metformin treatment, and to identify the effects of this treatment on luteal phase endometrial functions and the preimplantation environment in patients with PCOS.

In our study, the pretreatment ovulation rate of the 30 patients with PCOS was 13.3%, and no glycodelin was found in their endometrial samples, including those who were identified as being ovulatory. Following CC+ metformin treatment, 28 of them (93.3%) ovulated and a glycodelin expression rate of 73.3% was obtained for 22 of the 30.

No pregnancies occurred among women in either group when glycodelin expression did not occur during ovulation. In the study group, where all patients had PCOS, the pregnancy rate was 60% and all pregnancies resulted in live births when glycodelin expression had been strong. However, among the low-expression group, three out of four pregnancies ended in early miscarriages.

Serum glycodelin concentrations are found to be low during early and recurrent pregnancy losses [1, 23]. This decrease occurs especially in the endometrium [1, 24]. Glycodelin A is secreted from the decidual endometrium and is found in the amniotic fluid. Glycodelin A protects the embryo from the maternal immune system during implantation. It is also observed in the endometrium during the entrance of the embryo into the uterine cavity [1]. Deficiencies in endometrial glycodelin production can lead to local immunological responses. Observational studies have demonstrated that insulin resistance adversely affects endometrial functions, reduces the amount of circulating glycodelin, and increases the risk of pregnancy loss [2, 23]. In comparison to normal pregnancies, a significant decrease is observed in the serum glycodelin levels of pregnant women with PCOS during the first trimester, especially during the first two months. These levels return to normal between the 9th and 11th weeks. This decrease and fluctuation in glycodelin levels are significant with regard to the early and recurrent pregnancy losses observed in PCOS. Impaired glycodelin secretion limits the ability to control the maternal immune response against the embryo; at the same time, deficiencies related to the decrease in glycodelin concentrations arise in the implantation environment [4, 14, 25].

The rate of early pregnancy loss (EPL) is three times higher in PCOS patients [2, 26, 27]. While the rate of EPL is 10%–15% within the normal population [2, 28], it is 30%–50% among women with PCOS [2].

Insulin-sensitizing agents such as metformin decrease EPL in patients with PCOS by increasing the levels of glycodelin [2, 6].

In the study of Salim et al. [28], 20 patients with recurrent EPL and 16 fertile controls were evaluated. For the EPL group, a significant decrease was identified in the glycodelin levels of the uterine flushings, which were performed on the 7th day following the LH peak.

Dalton et al. [29] compared 49 patients with recurrent EPL and 15 fertile women. In that study, glycodelin levels in the serum and uterine flushings were assessed between the 10th and 12th days of the LH peak. While no differences were identified in the serum glycodelin levels, the uterine flushing levels were very low in the recurrent EPL group. In the ensuing stages of the study, the uterine flushing glycodelin levels of cases that resulted in abortus were lower in comparison to cases resulting in live births, while no difference was identified in the serum values.

Glycodelin was also assessed in ART cycles. Westergaard et al. [30] assessed serum glycodelin levels in the pretreatment cycle and the treatment cycle in 20 patients with planned ICSI on the 2nd, 8th, 12th, 14th, 20th, 24th, and 28th days of their cycles. In comparison to the other thirteen patients who are unable to conceive, a significantly lower level of glycodelin was identified in the seven patients who became pregnant on the treatment and two pretreatment cycles while a significantly higher level of glycodelin was identified during the late luteal phase of the cycle in which they became pregnant.

Chryssikopoulos et al. [31] and Liu et al. [32] identified higher serum glycodelin values on the oocyte retrieval and embryo transfer days of the women that became pregnant.

Although glycodelin is mainly induced by progesterone, the timing of its expression is not compatible or synchronous with progesterone levels [30]. In other words, expression of glycodelin is relatively delayed from the initiation of progesterone release [14, 20].

When we evaluated the mean progesterone values of our patients according to glycodelin positivity, no significant difference was identified between the two groups. This demonstrates that progesterone values cannot be used as a clear indicator of endometrial receptivity and implantation.

One of the significant advantages of our study was the ability to directly observe glycodelin levels in the endometrium. When the serum values were evaluated, we found that glycodelin was also produced in the extrauterine tissues (i.e., bone marrow, sweat glands, breasts, and ovaries). Although insulin primarily affects endometrial glycodelin secretion, it may also affect expression in these tissues.

Our study has demonstrated that, depending on its level of expression, glycodelin is associated with pregnancy outcome. In cases with PCOS, it was observed that glycodelin expression levels, rather than progesterone, were important during the administration of CC and metformin combination. Those patients with poor or little glycodelin expression had difficulties in achieving pregnancies or experienced EPLs. This information may be helpful for patients with early pregnancy losses or those who experience recurrent implantation failure in assisted reproductive techniques. In this group of patients, new studies could be planned and performed to assess whether metformin increases expression in patients with a low level of midluteal glycodelin expression. Further studies pertaining to this subject obviously are necessary.

In conclusion, according to both the results of our study and recent literatures [1, 2, 30–32], it has been demonstrated that insulin resistance and hyperinsulinemia lead to delays in the endometrial function of women with PCOS, yet they decrease the concentration of circulating glycodelin. They also adversely affect the implantation environment and lead to infertility and early and recurrent pregnancy losses. Metformin, on the other hand, serves to increase the levels of glycodelin.

Consent

Written informed consent was obtained from patients who participated in this study.

Conflict of Interests

No conflict of interests was declared by the authors.

Authors' Contribution

Concept is done by Selda Uysal and Ahmet Zeki Isik; design is done by Selda Uysal and Ahmet Zeki Isik; supervision is done by Selda Uysal and Ahmet Zeki Isik; resource is got by Serenat Eris, Yakup Yalcin, and Pelin Ozun Ozbay; materials were brought by Selda Uysal and Serenat Eris; data collection and/or processing are done by Selda Uysal, Serenat Eris, Pelin Ozun Ozbay, and Yakup Yalcin; analysis and/or interpretation are done by Selda Uysal, Ahmet Zeki Isik, and Serenat Eris; literature search is done by Selda Uysal, Serenat Eris, and Yakup Yalcin; writing is done by Selda Uysal, Ahmet Zeki Isik, and Serenat Eris; critical reviews are done by Selda Uysal and Ahmet Zeki Isik.

References

[1] D. J. Jakubowicz, M. Seppälä, S. Jakubowicz et al., "Insulin reduction with metformin increases luteal phase serum glycodelin and insulin-like growth factor-binding protein 1 concentrations and enhances uterine vascularity and blood flow in the polycystic ovary syndrome," *The Journal of Clinical Endocrinology & Metabolism*, vol. 86, no. 3, pp. 1126–1133, 2001.

[2] D. J. Jakubowicz, P. A. Essah, M. Seppälä et al., "Reduced serum glycodelin and insulin-like growth factor-binding protein-1 in women with polycystic ovary syndrome during first trimester of pregnancy," *Journal of Clinical Endocrinology and Metabolism*, vol. 89, no. 2, pp. 833–839, 2004.

[3] J. M. Lord, I. H. K. Flight, and R. J. Norman, "Metformin in polycystic ovary syndrome: systematic review and meta-analysis," *British Medical Journal*, vol. 327, no. 7421, pp. 951–953, 2003.

[4] E. Diamanti-Kandarakis, C. D. Christakou, E. Kandaraki, and F. N. Economou, "Metformin: an old medication of new fashion: evolving new molecular mechanisms and clinical implications in polycystic ovary syndrome," *European Journal of Endocrinology*, vol. 162, no. 2, pp. 193–212, 2010.

[5] D. A. Ehrmann, J. Sturis, M. M. Byrne, T. Karrison, R. L. Rosenfield, and K. S. Polonsky, "Insulin secretory defects in polycystic ovary syndrome. Relationship to insulin sensitivity and family history of non-insulin-dependent diabetes mellitus," *The Journal of Clinical Investigation*, vol. 96, no. 1, pp. 520–527, 1995.

[6] D. J. Jakubowicz, M. J. Iuorno, S. Jakubowicz, K. A. Roberts, and J. E. Nestler, "Effects of metformin on early pregnancy loss in the polycystic ovary syndrome," *The Journal of Clinical Endocrinology & Metabolism*, vol. 87, no. 2, pp. 524–529, 2002.

[7] Thessaloniki ESHRE/ASRM-Sponsored PCOS Consensus Workshop Group, "Consensus on infertility treatment related to polycystic ovary syndrome," *Human Reproduction*, vol. 23, no. 3, pp. 462–477, 2008.

[8] M. Karaköse, E. Cakal, K. Ertan, and T. Delibaşı, "The metabolic effects of drugs used for the treatment of polycystic ovary syndrome," *Journal of the Turkish German Gynecological Association*, vol. 14, no. 3, pp. 168–173, 2013.

[9] A. Stavreus-Evers, E. Mandelin, R. Koistinen, L. Aghajnova, O. Hovatta, and M. Seppälä, "Glycodelin is present in pinopodes of receptive-phase human endometrium and is associated with down-regulation of progesterone receptor B," *Fertility and Sterility*, vol. 85, no. 6, pp. 1803–1811, 2006.

[10] I. Mylonas, U. Jeschke, C. Kunert-Keil et al., "Glycodelin A is expressed differentially in normal human endometrial tissue throughout the menstrual cycle as assessed by immunohistochemistry and in situ hybridization," *Fertility and Sterility*, vol. 86, no. 5, pp. 1488–1497, 2006.

[11] A. Alok and A. A. Karande, "The role of glycodelin as an immune-modulating agent at the feto-maternal interface," *Journal of Reproductive Immunology*, vol. 83, no. 1-2, pp. 124–127, 2009.

[12] Rotterdam ESHRE/ASRM-Sponsored PCOS Consensus Workshop Group, "Revised 2003 consensus on diagnostic criteria

[13] D. Carter, J. K. Greenson, V. E. Reuter, M. H. Stoler, and S. Mills, *Sternberg's Diagnostic Surgical Pathology*, 5th edition, 2009.

[14] M. Seppälä, H. Koistinen, R. Koistinen, P. C. N. Chiu, and W. S. B. Yeung, "Glycosylation related actions of glycodelin: gamete, cumulus cell, immune cell and clinical associations," *Human Reproduction Update*, vol. 13, no. 3, pp. 275–287, 2007.

[15] M. Seppälä, L. Riittinen, M. Julkunen et al., "Structural studies, localization in tissue and clinical aspects of human endometrial proteins," *Journal of Reproduction and Fertility. Supplement*, vol. 36, pp. 127–141, 1988.

[16] D. Mukhopadhyay, S. SundarRaj, A. Alok, and A. A. Karande, "Glycodelin A, not glycodelin S, is apoptotically active: relevance of sialic acid modification," *The Journal of Biological Chemistry*, vol. 279, no. 10, pp. 8577–8584, 2004.

[17] R. Jayachandran, C. M. Radcliffe, L. Royle et al., "Oligosaccharides modulate the apoptotic activity of glycodelin," *Glycobiology*, vol. 16, no. 11, pp. 1052–1063, 2006.

[18] M. Seppälä, H. Koistinen, R. Koistinen, L. Hautala, P. C. Chiu, and W. S. Yeung, "Glycodelin in reproductive endocrinology and hormone-related cancer," *European Journal of Endocrinology*, vol. 160, no. 2, pp. 121–133, 2009.

[19] H. Watson, D. S. Kiddy, D. Hamilton-Fairley et al., "Hypersecretion of luteinizing hormone and ovarian steroids in women with recurrent early miscarriage," *Human Reproduction*, vol. 8, no. 6, pp. 829–833, 1993.

[20] T. C. Li, E. Ling, C. Dalton, A. E. Bolton, and I. D. Cooke, "Concentration of endometrial protein PP14 in uterine flushings throughout the menstrual cycle in normal, fertile women," *British Journal of Obstetrics and Gynaecology*, vol. 100, no. 5, pp. 460–464, 1993.

[21] L. C. Kao, S. Tulac, S. Lobo et al., "Global gene profiling in human endometrium during the window of implantation," *Endocrinology*, vol. 143, no. 6, pp. 2119–2138, 2002.

[22] S. E. Brown, E. Mandelin, S. Oehninger, J. P. Toner, M. Seppala, and H. W. Jones Jr., "Endometrial glycodelin-A expression in the luteal phase of stimulated ovarian cycles," *Fertility and Sterility*, vol. 74, no. 1, pp. 130–133, 2000.

[23] M. Tulppala, M. Julkunen, A. Tiitinen, U.-H. Stenman, and M. Seppälä, "Habitual abortion is accompanied by low serum levels of placental protein 14 in the luteal phase of the fertile cycle," *Fertility and Sterility*, vol. 63, no. 4, pp. 792–795, 1995.

[24] M. Julkunen, R. Koistinen, J. Sjoberg, E. M. Rutanen, T. Wahlström, and M. Seppälä, "Secretory endometrium synthesizes placental protein 14," *Endocrinology*, vol. 118, no. 5, pp. 1782–1786, 1986.

[25] C. M. Boomsma, M. J. C. Eijkemans, E. G. Hughes, G. H. A. Visser, B. C. J. M. Fauser, and N. S. Macklon, "A meta-analysis of pregnancy outcomes in women with polycystic ovary syndrome," *Human Reproduction Update*, vol. 12, no. 6, pp. 673–683, 2006.

[26] R. H. Gray, "Subfertility and risk of spontaneous abortion," *The American Journal of Public Health*, vol. 90, no. 9, pp. 1452–1454, 2000.

[27] L. Regan, E. J. Owen, and H. S. Jacobs, "Hypersecretion of luteinising hormone, infertility, and miscarriage," *The Lancet*, vol. 336, no. 8724, pp. 1141–1144, 1990.

[28] R. Salim, J. Miel, M. Savvas, C. Lee, and D. Jurkovic, "A comparative study of glycodelin concentrations in uterine flushings in women with subseptate uteri, history of unexplained

recurrent miscarriage and healthy controls," *European Journal of Obstetrics Gynecology and Reproductive Biology*, vol. 133, no. 1, pp. 76–80, 2007.

[29] C. K. Dalton, S. M. Laird, S. E. Estdale, H. G. Saravelos, and T. C. Li, "Endometrial protein PP14 and CA-125 in recurrent miscarriage patients; Correlation with pregnancy outcome," *Human Reproduction*, vol. 13, no. 11, pp. 3197–3202, 1998.

[30] L. G. Westergaard, N. Wiberg, C. Yding Andersen et al., "Circulating concentrations of placenta protein 14 during the natural menstrual cycle in women significantly reflect endometrial receptivity to implantation and pregnancy during successive assisted reproduction cycles," *Human Reproduction*, vol. 13, no. 9, pp. 2612–2619, 1998.

[31] A. Chryssikopoulos, T. Mantzavinos, N. Kanakas, E. Karagouni, E. Dotsika, and P. A. Zourlas, "Correlation of serum and follicular fluid concentrations of placental protein 14 and CA-125 in *in vitro* fertilization-embryo transfer patients," *Fertility and Sterility*, vol. 66, no. 4, pp. 599–603, 1996.

[32] H.-M. Liu, F.-Q. Xing, and F.-L. Wu, "Glycodelin in IVF-ET cycles: its association with endometrial receptivity and impact on the outcome of pregnancy," *Nan Fang Yi Ke Da Xue Xue Bao*, vol. 26, no. 8, pp. 1227–1229, 2006.

6

Placental Oxidative Status throughout Normal Gestation in Women with Uncomplicated Pregnancies

Jayasri Basu, Bolek Bendek, Enyonam Agamasu, Carolyn M. Salafia, Aruna Mishra, Nerys Benfield, Ronak Patel, and Magdy Mikhail

Department of Obstetrics & Gynecology, Bronx Lebanon Hospital Center, 1650 Grand Concourse, Bronx, NY 10457, USA

Correspondence should be addressed to Jayasri Basu; jbasu@bronxleb.org

Academic Editor: Gian Carlo Di Renzo

The effects of gestational age on placental oxidative balance throughout gestation were investigated in women with uncomplicated pregnancies. Placental tissues were obtained from normal pregnant women who delivered at term or underwent elective pregnancy termination at 6 to 23 + 6 weeks of pregnancy. Placental tissues were analyzed for total antioxidant capacity (TAC) and lipid peroxide (malondialdehyde, MDA) levels using commercially available kits. Two hundred and one placental tissues were analyzed and the mean ± SD MDA (pmol/mg tissue) and TAC (μmol Trolox equivalent/mg tissue) levels for first, second, and third trimester groups were 277.01 ± 204.66, 202.66 ± 185.05, and 176.97 ± 141.61, $P < 0.004$ and 498.62 ± 400.74, 454.90 ± 374.44, and 912.19 ± 586.21, $P < 0.0001$ by ANOVA, respectively. Our data reflects an increased oxidative stress in the placenta in the early phase of normal pregnancy. As pregnancy progressed, placental antioxidant protective mechanisms increased and lipid peroxidation markers decreased resulting in diminution in oxidative stress. Our findings provide a biochemical support to the concept of a hypoxic environment in early pregnancy. A decrease in placental oxidative stress in the second and third trimesters appears to be a physiological phenomenon of normal pregnancy. Deviations from this physiological phenomenon may result in placental-mediated disorders.

1. Introduction

During the first trimester of pregnancy, the conceptus develops in a low oxygen environment that favors organogenesis in the embryo and angiogenesis in the placenta [1]. This low oxygen environment is created when maternal arterial blood is prevented from entering the intervillous space of the placenta by plugs of cytotrophoblast cells that invade the uterine spiral arteries. As pregnancy continues, higher concentrations of oxygen are required to support the rapid growth of the fetus and the placenta. At the end of first trimester, the maternal intraplacental circulation is fully established when cytotrophoblast cell plugs are dislodged, by an unknown mechanism and maternal blood flow to the intervillous space ensues. The normoxic environment thus created in the placenta is then maintained until term [1]. Perturbations in such an oxidative environment as pregnancy continues are suggested to play a role in the pathophysiology

of pregnancy disorders such as preeclampsia, intrauterine growth restriction, and early pregnancy loss [1].

The altered hormonal status during pregnancy results in increased accumulation of maternal fat depots and hyperlipidemia [2]. Maternal plasma triglycerols and nonesterified fatty acids are reported to correlate with fetal lipid and fetal growth, suggesting that these molecules do traverse through the placenta [3]. The abundant presence of membrane phospholipids at sites where reactive oxygen species are formed makes them easily accessible endogenous targets for lipid peroxidation [4]. The free radical chemistry of lipid peroxidation is complex. Lipid peroxidation occurs as a chain reaction initiated by free radicals, which propagates itself and can result in the formation of many equivalents of lipid peroxides. MDA is one of the several low-molecular-weight end products formed from the decomposition of certain primary and secondary lipid peroxidation products. Nevertheless, MDA is not exclusively generated through lipid peroxidation. Oxidative modification of lipid can be induced *in vitro* or could occur *in vivo* during aging [5] and certain diseased conditions [6, 7]. The host of other lipid peroxidation products include: diene hydroperoxide, cyclic peroxides, bicyclic peroxides, or epoxy alcohol [7]. Of all these products of lipid peroxidation, MDA and 4-hydroxynonenal are naturally occurring biproducts. The determination of MDA is rather fairly simple and prompt. MDA readily participates with 2-thiobarbituric acid at a low pH and an elevated temperature. The reaction product is a 1:2 MDA-TBA adduct that is red in color, which can readily be determined colorimetrically. The ease of the assay has fostered MDA determination to be the most widely employed format for monitoring lipid peroxidation in a wide array of samples.

Efforts in understanding the increased oxidative stress during pathological states of pregnancy have been the focus of many studies in recent times. For this, investigators have measured lipid peroxides and antioxidant levels either in the blood or in the placenta of women, primarily with preeclampsia, and have compared the levels to that of normal women with uncomplicated pregnancies [8–12]. However, information regarding the change in placental oxidative stress throughout pregnancy is not well-studied. The objective of the present study was to investigate the effects of gestational age on the oxidative balance throughout gestation in women with uncomplicated pregnancies. In this study, the levels of placental malondialdehyde (MDA) were determined as a marker of lipid peroxidation and reactive oxygen species (ROS). Since a large number of antioxidants are present in our body in the form of several micro and macro molecules, as well as enzymes, and these molecules function synergistically in preventing oxidative stress, hence quantitative measurement of the total antioxidant capacity (TAC) of the placenta was simultaneously measured as a marker for antioxidant defenses.

2. Materials and Methods

The investigative protocol for this study was approved by the Institutional Review Board of the Bronx Lebanon Hospital Center. A total of 201 placental tissues were obtained from either normal pregnant women who delivered at term or from women who underwent elective pregnancy termination at 6 to 23 weeks and 6 days of pregnancy. Placental tissues from women with a history of hypertension or pregnancies that were complicated by diabetes, peripheral vascular disease, chronic renal disease, multifetal gestation, or major fetal anomalies were excluded from the study.

Placental samples were collected within 10 minutes of completion of the procedure. The locations of the placental tissues obtained following elective termination of pregnancies are unknown; however, placental tissues obtained in the third trimester were taken from one of the peripheral cotyledons. Each sample was washed thoroughly in saline to remove maternal blood and was then dissected in saline to identify chorionic villi without associated decidua. Villous samples were transported to the laboratory on ice and stored at −80°C until assay. The placental tissues were analyzed for

TAC using TAC assay kit from Sigma Aldrich (St. Louis, MO, Catalog number CS0790). The principle of the assay is that, in the presence of hydrogen peroxide, metmyoglobin forms ferryl myoglobin radical which oxidizes ABTS (2,2′-azino-bis(3-ethylbenzthiazoline-6-sulfonic acid)) to produce a radical cation ABTS$^{\cdot+}$. ABTS is colorless but when ABTS$^{\cdot+}$ is produced a soluble green colored chromogen is formed that can be determined spectrophotometrically at 750 nm. Antioxidants suppress the production of the radical cation in a concentration dependent manner and the color intensity decreases proportionately. Trolox, a water soluble vitamin E analog, is used in the assay to serve as a standard or control antioxidant. The lipid peroxidation (MDA) assay kit used for the study was obtained from Abcam (Cambridge, MA, Catalog # ab118970). The principle of the MDA assay is that MDA present in the sample is reacted with thiobarbituric acid (TBA) to generate MDA-TBA adduct. The MDA-TBA adduct is then quantified spectrophotometrically. For each assay, tissue homogenate was prepared using the buffer supplied with each kit and the assays were carried out as per the manufacturers' instructions. A Tecan Infinite 200 Pro Microplate Reader was used for the assays. For MDA, the absorbance of the color was measured at 532 nm. MDA levels were expressed as pmol/mg tissue. For TAC, the absorbance was measured at 750 nm and the results were expressed as μmol Trolox equivalent/mg tissue. The intra-assay and interassay variations for both MDA and TAC were between 2–5% and 5–7%, respectively.

3. Statistical Analysis

Statistical evaluation of the data was carried out using SPSS^{R} statistical package version 22 [13]. Descriptive statistics was performed. Since the data was not normally distributed, Kruskal-Wallis test was performed to compare the differences among three trimester groups followed by Mann-Whitney U test for intergroup comparisons. Spearman's bivariate correlation was used to determine correlation between the MDA, TAC and gestational age in days and partial correlation was performed to determine the correlation between MDA and TAC after controlling for gestational age in days. A value of $P < 0.05$ was considered statistically significant.

4. Results

In the study, a total of 201 placentas were evaluated for both MDA and TAC levels. Of these, 106 placental tissues were collected from women up to 13 weeks of gestation and were grouped as first trimester; 48 placental tissues were collected from women from 13$^+$ to 23 weeks + 6 days of gestation and were grouped as second trimester; and 47 tissues were obtained from term normal placentas which were selected from deliveries of a newborn without maternal or fetal-neonatal pathologies and were grouped as third trimester.

Placental oxidative status throughout normal gestation is presented in Table 1. Placental MDA levels were the highest in the first trimester of normal pregnancy. In the second and third trimesters, placental MDA levels were progressively lower. Placental TAC levels on the other hand were found

TABLE 1: Placental MDA and TAC levels throughout normal gestation.

Groups	N	MDA (pmol/mg tissue)	TAC (μmol Trolox equivalent/mg tissue)	Age (yrs)
First trimester	106	277.01 ± 204.66	498.62 ± 400.74	26.77 ± 6.27
Second trimester	48	202.66 ± 185.05	454.90 ± 374.44	25.87 ± 6.50
Third trimester	47	176.97 ± 141.61	912.19 ± 586.21	26.83 ± 6.33

MDA: malondialdehyde; TAC: total antioxidant capacity. Data expressed as mean ± SD.
Placental MDA levels were highest in the first trimester and progressively declined thereafter, while TAC levels showed a significant increase beyond the second trimester of normal pregnancy.

TABLE 2: Comparison of placental MDA and TAC levels by trimester groups.

Groups	N	MDA Mean rank	TAC Mean rank
First trimester	106	114.39	91.44
Second trimester	48	86.81	85.52
Third trimester	47	85.30	138.37

MDA: malondialdehyde; TAC: total antioxidant capacity. Kruskal-Wallis test results.
The critical values for MDA and TAC levels were 11.895 ($P < 0.003$) and 25.665 ($P < 0.0001$), respectively.

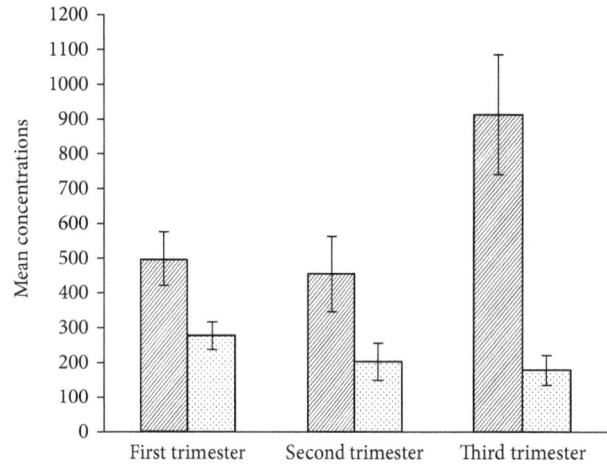

FIGURE 1: MDA: malondialdehyde; TAC: total antioxidant capacity. A box plot representating mean placental concentrations of TAC and MDA levels throughout gestation in normal pregnancy. The hatched bars represent mean placental TAC levels (μmol Trolox equivalent/mg tissue); the dotted bars represent mean placental MDA levels (pmol/mg tissue); and the error bars denote 95% CI.

to be significantly higher in the third trimesters. A bar plot and depicting the effects of gestational age on placental MDA and TAC levels by trimester is presented in Figure 1. The mean maternal age between the trimester groups as shown in Table 1 was not significantly different. Kruskal-Wallis test (Table 2) revealed significant differences in both placental MDA and TAC levels ($P < 0.003$, $P < 0.0001$, resp.), among the three trimester groups. Pairwise comparisons of MDA and TAC levels by trimester groups were performed using Mann-Whitney U test and the results are presented in Tables 3 and 4, respectively. While the placental MDA levels were noted to decrease with an increase in gestational age, the TAC levels on the other hand showed an increase. Two scatter plots depicting the MDA and TAC levels with gestational age in days are presented in Figures 2 and 3. A downward trend in MDA and an upward trend in TAC levels can be seen as pregnancy progressed. Spearman's bivariate correlation computed to determine the correlation between placental MDA and TAC levels with gestational age (GA, in days) showed a negative significant correlation between MDA and gestational age ($r = -0.191$, $P < 0.007$). TAC and gestational age were positively correlated and the correlation was significant ($r = 0.262$, $P < 0.0001$). The correlation between MDA and TAC levels was negative ($r = -0.065$, 0.362) (Table 5). Partial correlation after controlling for gestational age between TAC and MDA was not significant ($r = 0.067$, $P = 0.345$).

5. Discussion

The results of the present study demonstrate that placental MDA levels were the highest in the first trimester of normal pregnancy. Thereafter, the levels showed a gradual decline as pregnancy continued and there was a negative correlation between placental MDA levels and gestational age (Table 5). On the other hand placental TAC levels were found to be the lowest in the first and second trimester but the levels steadily increased as pregnancy progressed (Table 1 and Figure 1). Our data are in agreement with an *in vitro* study which demonstrated that the production of lipid peroxide peaked in early placental samples but, by the end of pregnancy, there was minimal lipid peroxide produced [14]. In another previously reported study, the levels of conjugated diene, a breakdown product of lipid peroxidation, in the serum was found to rise more than 45% in the second trimester over the first trimester values but by the third trimester the levels declined [15].

Since lipid peroxide levels of the placenta in our study were the highest in the first trimester while the TAC levels were the lowest, the findings provide a biochemical support of the concept of the existence of physiologic hypoxia in the placenta during the first trimester. Our findings are in agreement with other nonbiochemical studies that also reported placental hypoxia in the first trimester [1, 16–18]. Morphological studies have shown that placental hypoxia occurs in the first trimester when extravillous trophoblast plugs block the maternal spiral arteries and prevent the

TABLE 3: Pairwise comparison of placental MDA levels.

	First trimester Test Score, P value	Second trimester Test Score, P value	Third trimester Test score, P value
First trimester	—	1885.0, 0.01	1731.0, 0.003
Second trimester		—	1106.0, 0.87
Third trimester			—

MDA: malondialdehyde; the nonparametric Mann-Whitney U test was applied.
Significant differences were noted between first and second trimester ($P < 0.01$) and first and third trimester ($P < 0.003$) groups. The difference in MDA levels between second and third trimester groups was not significant.

TABLE 4: Pairwise comparison of placental TAC levels.

	First trimester Test score, P value	Second trimester Test score, P value	Third trimester Test score, P value
First trimester	—	2394.0, 0.558	1327.5, 0.0001
Second trimester		—	535.0, 0.0001
Third trimester			—

TAC: total antioxidant capacity; the nonparametric Mann-Whitney U test was applied.
Significant differences were noted between first and third trimester ($P < 0.0001$) and second and third trimester ($P < 0.0001$) groups. The difference in TAC levels between first and second trimester groups was not significant.

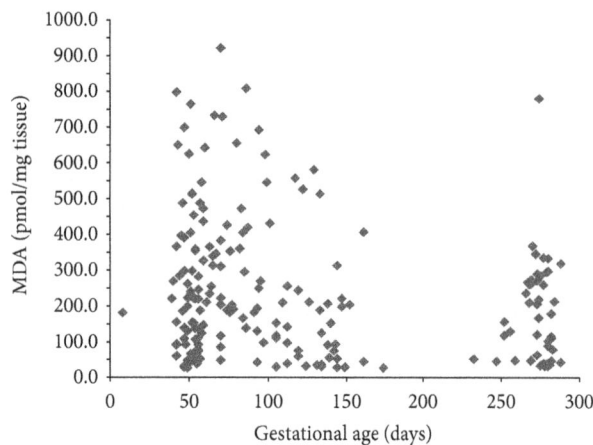

FIGURE 2: MDA: malondialdehyde. The scatter plot showing a downward trend in placental MDA levels with an increase in gestational age in days.

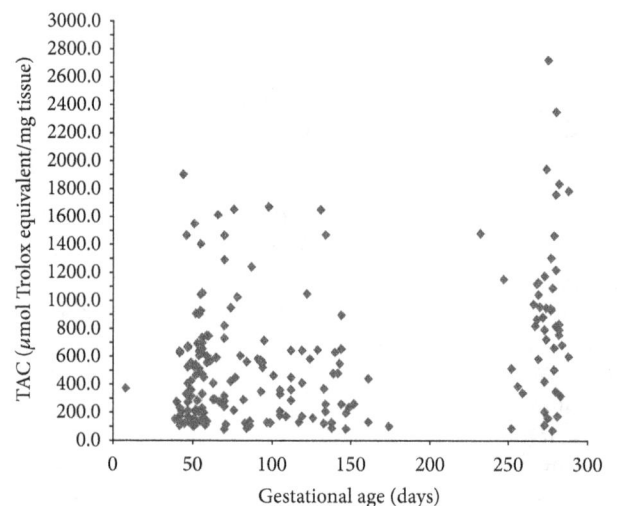

FIGURE 3: TAC: total antioxidant capacity. The scatter plot showing an upward trend in placental TAC levels with an increase in gestational age in days.

maternal blood from entering the intervillous space [16]. In normal pregnancies, Doppler studies have confirmed the absence of blood flow into the intervillous space prior to 10 weeks of gestation [17]. Additionally, direct comparison of oxygen tension between the placenta and its adjacent endometrial tissue also revealed that the partial pressure of oxygen in the placenta was significantly lower compared to that of the endometrium [18]. Investigators believe that such a hypoxic environment in the first trimester is essential for the regulation of trophoblast differentiation, embryogenesis, and/or placental development for a normal pregnancy outcome. The oxidative status of the placenta is not geographically homogenous. At high altitude, where the partial pressure of oxygen is low, placental hypoxic stress is induced that thwarts the high-altitude pregnancies more toward a preeclamptic phenotype [19].

For normal pregnancy to progress efficiently, the transition from a hypoxic to a normoxic environment is vitally important. During first trimester, antioxidant mechanisms are induced in the placenta to neutralize the excess accumulation of ROS and to trigger mechanisms that can remove or repair any damaged cells [20]. Our study shows that placental oxidative stress wanes off as normal pregnancy continues. By third trimester, a progressive increase in TAC levels was noted with a simultaneous decrease in MDA levels compared to the first trimester values (Tables 1, 3, and 4). Similar results of higher serum TAC levels in the third trimester of normal pregnancy over the first trimester values have also been previously reported [21]. Our results

TABLE 5: Correlation between MDA, TAC, and gestational age.

	MDA		TAC		GAD	
	Rho	P	Rho	P	Rho	P
MDA	1.000	—	−0.065	0.362	−0.191	0.007
TAC			1.000	—	0.262	0.0001
GAD					1.000	—

MDA: malondialdehyde; TAC: total antioxidant capacity; GAD: gestational age in days.
The nonparametric test Spearman's correlation was applied. Results show significant negative correlations between MDA and GAD and significant positive correlation between TAC and GAD. MDA and TAC levels were negatively correlated, but the correlation was not statistically significant.

indicate that by the third trimester placental antioxidant protection mechanisms become efficient enough to counteract the oxidative challenge. Failure to establish such efficient antioxidant protection may contribute to the development of preeclampsia.

Low oxygen environment favors the generation of ROS which are characterized as molecules having one or more unpaired electrons [22]. The unpaired electron gives considerable reactivity to the free radicals and their nonradical intermediates. Recent *in vitro*, cell culture, and animal model studies have confirmed that ROS can activate a variety of transcription factors and protein kinases, influence the expression of a number of genes, are involved in signal transduction pathways, and can act as subcellular messengers for certain growth factors [22–26]. Placental adaptation in response to low oxygen tension occurs early in the pregnancy and during the process ROS act as key cell signaling molecules [24–26]. The increased levels of lipid peroxide in the first trimester of pregnancy in our study could reflect a period when excessive production of ROS might have taken place (Table 1). The physiological role of ROS during early pregnancy is suggested to influence a number of functions including remodeling of the spiral arteries, angiogenesis, and proliferation of the cytotrophoblast cells. Additionally, increased ROS in the placenta in the early phase of normal pregnancy has been shown to alter cell permeability and vascular biology, stimulate cellular and matrix remodeling, and protect the fetus from intrauterine infection [24–27]. The increased production of ROS in the first trimester of normal pregnancy could induce cytotrophoblast proliferation and the expression of key developmental genes involved in embryogenesis and placental development. This increase in cytotrophoblast proliferation in the first trimester is suggested by Douglas and Haddad [28] to be a natural protective mechanism to establish a mature placenta in advance of the period of rapid fetal growth.

Our study has limitations. The short questionnaire that was approved by our Institutional Review Board for the study included collecting information on maternal age, parity, gestational age as confirmed by ultrasound, and infection status. Smoking status of the patients, though was included in the questionnaire, was, however, not strictly monitored. Moreover, information on dietary and/or vitamin intake throughout the gestational period was not included. It is noteworthy, however, that the catchment area of the Bronx

from where the pregnant women came from comprised primarily of African American (38%) and Hispanic (52%) descent. A previous study carried out on women from the same catchment area of the Bronx revealed that dietary and vitamin intakes were comparable between the pregnant and the nonpregnant groups (unpublished data).

Oxidative stress status in human placentas throughout normal pregnancy has not been well studied previously. Correlating the fetal blood oxidative status to the placenta and the placenta to the maternal systemic blood could ideally reflect the placental oxidative status and perhaps would be highly desirable. The focus of this study was in understanding the placental oxidative status throughout normal gestation. Comparative investigation of cord blood and maternal blood samples to identify any association can only be carried out in late stage of pregnancy and needs to be addressed in future studies. Our findings demonstrate that a decrease in oxidative stress with increase in gestational age may be a normal physiological phenomenon of normal pregnancy. Our data demonstrate the presence of a placental oxidative stress in the first trimester when the placental MDA levels are significantly high, with minimum protection offered by placental antioxidant system. As pregnancy progresses, the placental environment switches to a normoxic state as reflected by a gradual increase in the total antioxidant capacity of the placenta and a decrease in lipid peroxidation markers. By the third trimester, our results show that placental antioxidant mechanisms become more efficient to counteract the oxidative challenge. Deviation from this physiological balance whether caused by increased generation of ROS or decreased neutralization by antioxidants can cause placental damage and may contribute to abnormal pregnancy outcome.

Conflict of Interests

The authors declare that there is no conflict of interests regarding the publication of this paper.

Acknowledgments

The authors would like to thank the staff nurses in the Department of OB/GYN, Bronx Lebanon Hospital Center, for their support and Elaine Marchi of the Basic Research Institute, Staten Island, NY, for her contribution in the initial set up of the study.

References

[1] G. J. Burton and E. Jauniaux, "Oxidative stress," *Best Practice and Research: Clinical Obstetrics and Gynaecology*, vol. 25, no. 3, pp. 287–299, 2011.

[2] D. Mankuta, M. Elami-Suzin, A. Elhayani, and S. Vinker, "Lipid profile in consecutive pregnancies," *Lipids in Health and Disease*, vol. 9, article 58, 2010.

[3] E. Harrera and H. Ortega-Senovilla, "Lipid metabolism during pregnancy and its implications for fetal growth," *Current Pharmaceutical Biotechnology*, vol. 15, no. 1, pp. 24–31, 2014.

[4] L. L. de Zwart, J. H. N. Meerman, J. N. M. Commandeur, and N. P. E. Vermeulen, "Biomarkers of free radical damage

applications in experimental animals and in humans," *Free Radical Biology and Medicine*, vol. 26, no. 1-2, pp. 202–226, 1999.

[5] D. Harman, "Free radical theory of aging: an update—increasing the functional life span," *Annals of the New York Academy of Sciences*, vol. 1067, no. 1, pp. 10–21, 2006.

[6] D. A. Slatter, C. H. Bolton, and A. J. Bailey, "The importance of lipid-derived malondialdehyde in diabetes mellitus," *Diabetologia*, vol. 43, no. 5, pp. 550–557, 2000.

[7] A. Ayala, M. F. Muñoz, and S. Argüelles, "Lipid peroxidation: production, metabolism, and signaling mechanisms of malondialdehyde and 4-hydroxy-2-nonenal," *Oxidative Medicine and Cellular Longevity*, vol. 2014, Article ID 360438, 31 pages, 2014.

[8] R. E. Little and B. C. Gladen, "Levels of lipid peroxides in uncomplicated pregnancy: a review of the literature," *Reproductive Toxicology*, vol. 13, no. 5, pp. 347–352, 1999.

[9] M. S. Mikhail, A. Anyaegbunam, D. Garfinkel, P. R. Palan, J. Basu, and S. L. Romney, "Preeclampsia and antioxidant nutrients: decreased plasma levels of reduced ascorbic acid, α-tocopherol, and beta-carotene in women with preeclampsia," *The American Journal of Obstetrics and Gynecology*, vol. 171, no. 1, pp. 150–157, 1994.

[10] P. R. Palan, M. S. Mikhail, and S. L. Romney, "Placental and serum levels of carotenoids in preeclampsia," *Obstetrics and Gynecology*, vol. 98, no. 3, pp. 459–462, 2001.

[11] Y. Takehara, T. Yoshioka, and J. Sasaki, "Changes in the levels of lipoperoxide and antioxidant factors in human placenta during gestation," *Acta Medica Okayama*, vol. 44, no. 2, pp. 103–111, 1990.

[12] A. Agarwal, A. Aponte-Mellado, B. J. Premkumar, A. Shaman, and S. Gupta, "The effects of oxidative stress on female reproduction: a review," *Reproductive Biology and Endocrinology*, vol. 10, article 49, 2012.

[13] IBM SPSS Statistics for Windows, version 22, IBM Corporation, Armonk, NY, USA.

[14] K. Sekiba and T. Yoshioka, "Changes of lipid peroxidation and superoxide dismutase activity in the human placenta," *The American Journal of Obstetrics and Gynecology*, vol. 135, no. 3, pp. 368–371, 1979.

[15] J. Uotila, R. Tuimala, T. Aarnio, K. Pyykko, and M. Ahotupa, "Lipid peroxidation products, selenium-dependent glutathione peroxidase and vitamin E in normal pregnancy," *European Journal of Obstetrics Gynecology and Reproductive Biology*, vol. 42, no. 2, pp. 95–100, 1991.

[16] G. J. Burton, E. Jauniaux, and A. L. Watson, "Maternal arterial connections to the placental intervillous space during the first trimester of human pregnancy: the Boyd Collection revisited," *The American Journal of Obstetrics and Gynecology*, vol. 181, no. 3, pp. 718–724, 1999.

[17] L. Valentin, P. Sladkevicius, R. Laurini, H. Söderberg, and K. Marsal, "Uteroplacental and luteal circulation in normal first-trimester pregnancies: Doppler ultrasonographic and morphologic study," *The American Journal of Obstetrics and Gynecology*, vol. 174, no. 2, pp. 768–775, 1996.

[18] E. Jauniaux, A. Watson, O. Ozturk, D. Quick, and G. Burton, "In-vivo measurement of intrauterine gases and acid-base values early in human pregnancy," *Human Reproduction*, vol. 14, no. 11, pp. 2901–2904, 1999.

[19] S. K. Palmer, L. G. Moore, D. A. Young, B. Cregger, J. C. Berman, and S. Zamudio, "Altered blood pressure course during normal pregnancy and increased preeclampsia at high altitude (3100 meters) in Colorado," *The American Journal of Obstetrics and Gynecology*, vol. 180, no. 5, pp. 1161–1168, 1999.

[20] A. Mueller, C. Koebnick, H. Binder et al., "Placental defence is considered sufficient to control lipid peroxidation in pregnancy," *Medical Hypotheses*, vol. 64, no. 3, pp. 553–557, 2005.

[21] V. Toescu, S. L. Nuttall, U. Martin, M. J. Kendall, and F. Dunne, "Oxidative stress and normal pregnancy," *Clinical Endocrinology*, vol. 57, no. 5, pp. 609–613, 2002.

[22] T. Finkel, "Oxygen radicals and signaling," *Current Opinion in Cell Biology*, vol. 10, no. 2, pp. 248–253, 1998.

[23] R. G. Allen and M. Tresini, "Oxidative stress and gene regulation," *Free Radical Biology and Medicine*, vol. 28, no. 3, pp. 463–499, 2000.

[24] P. A. Dennery, "Effects of oxidative stress on embryonic development," *Birth Defects Research Part C—Embryo Today*, vol. 81, no. 3, pp. 155–162, 2007.

[25] L. Myatt, "Review: reactive oxygen and nitrogen species and functional adaptation of the placenta," *Placenta*, vol. 31, supplement A, pp. S66–S69, 2010.

[26] D. S. Charnock-Jones, P. Kaufmann, and T. M. Mayhew, "Aspects of human fetoplacental vasculogenesis and angiogenesis. I. Molecular regulation," *Placenta*, vol. 25, no. 2-3, pp. 103–113, 2004.

[27] S.-Y. Oh, T. Chu, and Y. Sadovsky, "The timing and duration of hypoxia determine gene expression patterns in cultured human trophoblasts," *Placenta*, vol. 32, no. 12, pp. 1004–1009, 2011.

[28] R. M. Douglas and G. G. Haddad, "Genetic models in applied physiology: invited review: effect of oxygen deprivation on cell cycle activity: a profile of delay and arrest," *Journal of Applied Physiology*, vol. 94, no. 5, pp. 2068–2083, 2003.

7

Factors Influencing Women's Preferences for Places to Give Birth in Addis Ababa, Ethiopia

Yibeltal Tebekaw, Yohana James Mashalla, and Gloria Thupayagale-Tshweneagae

Department of Health Studies, University of South Africa, Pretoria, South Africa

Correspondence should be addressed to Yibeltal Tebekaw; ytebekaw@gmail.com

Academic Editor: Gian Carlo Di Renzo

The main aim of this study was to examine factors determining women's preference for places to give birth in Addis Ababa, Ethiopia. A quantitative and cross-sectional community based study design was employed. Data was collected using structured questionnaire administered to 901 women aged 15–49 years through a stratified two-stage cluster sampling technique. Multinomial logistic regression model was employed to identify predictors of delivery care. More than three-fourth of slum women gave birth at public healthcare facilities compared to slightly more than half of the nonslum residents. Education, wealth quintile, the age of respondent, number of children, pregnancy intention, and cohabitation showed net effect on women's preference for places to give birth. Despite the high number of ANC attendances, still many pregnant women especially among slum residents chose to deliver at home. Most respondents delivered in public healthcare institutions despite the general doubts about the quality of services in these institutions. Future studies should examine motivating factors for continued deliveries at home and whether there is real significant difference between the quality of maternal care service offered at public and private health facilities.

1. Introduction

Assurance of healthcare for all segments of the population with special attention given to the health needs of women and children was one of the top priorities in the Ethiopian Health Policy [1]. The endorsement of MDG 5 in the HSDPs is an indication of the commitment or political will of the government towards reducing maternal mortality across the nation [2]. Yet, Ethiopia's health system is underdeveloped and underfinanced [3]. While some progress has been made in providing basic health services to poor women and their children, the progress may be uneven because many people are not reached with services [4].

Ethiopia's total health expenditure as a percentage of the gross domestic product (GDP) has remained stable at 4.3% for years. With emphasis given to publicly funded healthcare, out-of-pocket payment constitutes 42% [5]. The public health sector is the main provider of primary healthcare and serves two-thirds of the population who cannot afford private healthcare [6]. The main objective of the public sector service provision, as stated in the National Health Policy, is "*to give comprehensive and integrated primary health care services in a decentralized and equitable fashion*" [1].

Childbirth and its process are one of the most significant life events to a woman [7]. The time of birth as well as shortly thereafter is the most dangerous period in a child's life especially in the developing world [7, 8]. Hence the choice of place of delivery for a pregnant woman is an important aspect of maternal healthcare. The place of delivery is an important factor often related to the quality of care received by the mother and infant for influencing maternal and child healthcare outcomes [7]. In Addis Ababa, the capital of Ethiopia, though the private health facilities (hospitals and clinics) outnumber public clinics [9], only 20% of deliveries take place in the private sectors and 17% of mothers deliver at home [4].

This study aims to systematically explore the differences and the factors that influence women's preferences for places to give birth in Addis Ababa. It is envisaged that a clear understanding of such factors is key in building a responsive maternal healthcare system and improving health outcomes in Ethiopia.

2. Research Design and Methods

2.1. Sampling and Data Collection. Addis Ababa, the study area, is divided into 10 subcities and each subcity is further divided into several small administrative units called Kebeles. In the 2007 Ethiopia Housing and Population Census, Kebeles were further subdivided into enumeration areas (EAs). An EA is a geographic area consisting of a convenient number of dwelling units which was used as a counting unit for the census. The average number of households (HHs) per EA in urban Ethiopia is 169. The number of clusters (EAs) in Addis Ababa was about 3865 [3].

Because of the different levels of political or administrative structures and wider geographic areas, cluster sampling technique was employed for this study. The study employed a stratified, two-stage cluster design. Since Addis Ababa is entirely urban, stratification was achieved by using the subcities (10 strata). Using the 2007 Population and Housing Census data, in the first stage 30 enumeration areas (EAs) were selected independently from all the strata with probability proportional to (EA) size (PPS) of households. In the second stage, 906 households were selected with PPS of households in each EA. The systematic random sampling of the eligible households was done based on the number of households recorded during the complete listing of households in each EA during the last EDHS 2011 [3]. To minimize sampling errors that may arise due to changes in the years after the last enumeration (complete household listing), approaching the subcity and Kebele administrations as well as community members in the respective EAs was an important step in the survey process. It was necessary to be aware of and be sensitive to the various community level dynamics in the study area. Hence, the demolition of significant portions of four EAs from four strata due to the city's reconstruction process was the major change reported and verified by the first author. Three EAs were replaced by other randomly selected three adjacent EAs and remaining households of the fourth EA were completed from a section of a randomly selected adjacent EA.

In this study verbal face-to-face interview was administered using a structured questionnaire. Recall bias was taken into consideration during the development of the questionnaire. Therefore, women were asked about their most recent or last birth and the date of birth of the child was asked. Ethical clearance was obtained from the National Research Ethics Review Committee of the Ministry of Science and Technology, Ethiopia. The target population was all women of 15–49 years of age who have experienced at least one birth in the last 1–3 years before the date of data collection, December 2013–January 2014.

2.2. Description of Variables. The independent variables for this study were selected based on a modified version of the Behavioural Model of Health Services [10]. The model distinguished three sets of factors related to healthcare seeking behaviour of individuals: the predisposing, enabling, and need factors.

Under the *predisposing factors*, demographic variables such as age, number of living children, current marital status, and pregnancy intention related to last childbirth and social structure variables such as education, occupation, and ethnicity were considered at individual, household, and community levels. As regards pregnancy intention, women were asked about their recent births whether they wanted it then, wanted it later, or did not want to have any more children at all. In the analyses, the intention status of the birth was further defined as a dichotomy variable: intended for births wanted by then versus unintended for being either mistimed or unwanted by then. Women's education was defined here as the highest level of schooling attended regardless of whether the woman completed the level.

Under the *enabling factors*, individual and family resource indicator variables including housing tenure, health insurance, and wealth quintile were included. Those who visited health facility for ANC were also asked whether there was an organization or agency that either partially or fully covered their expenses and the responses were grouped as "yes" or "no." Housing tenure was categorised as the house in which the respondent lives is either owned by her or not owned by her, that is, owned versus rental. The type of residence was categorised as slum and nonslum residences based on the five indicators including access to improved water, access to improved sanitation, sufficient living area, durability of housing, and secure tenure (housing tenure) developed by United Nations Human Settlements Programme [11].

The outcome variable was *"preference for places to give birth"* which represented three choices that a woman can make: *deliver at a public healthcare facility*, *deliver at private healthcare facility*, and *deliver at home with or without professional assistance.*

2.3. Data Analysis. Data was entered using the Census and Survey Processing System (CSPro) software and was analysed for both descriptive and inferential statistics using the Statistical Package for Social Sciences (SPSS) version 16.0 [12]. Bivariate (Chi-square) tests were also applied. Multinomial logistic regression model was fitted to investigate the potential factors influencing preferred places to give birth. The base category was delivery at public healthcare institute. For this study, $P < 0.05$ was considered statistically significant at 95% confidence interval.

3. Results

In this study, the data collection response rate was 99.4%, 901 out of 906. Women were asked about their place of ANC follow-up and places of delivery during their last birth. The inquiry was about where the majority of the ANC visits occurred as there could be possibility of shifting from one place of care to another during the same pregnancy period.

3.1. Disparities by Socioeconomic and Demographic Characteristics of Respondents. More than two-thirds (69.2%) and slightly less than a quarter (24.0%) of all the study participants gave birth at public and private healthcare facilities, respectively. About 6.8% of them delivered at home. Both slum and nonslum residents accessed ANC mainly at public healthcare facilities. More than three-fourths of slum resident women gave birth at public healthcare facilities compared to slightly more than half of the nonslum residents. Higher proportion of the nonslum residents (41.7%) gave birth at private facilities compared to only 15.3% of the slum residents.

Table 1 presents the results of the association between socioeconomic, demographic, and healthcare variables and women's preferences for places to give birth. Younger age, having fewer number of children, having unintended pregnancy, and cohabitation were associated with delivery at public healthcare facilities. The educational status of women associated significantly negatively with delivery at home but positively with delivery at private healthcare facilities. The employment status of women did not show statistically significant association with preference for place of delivery. Ethnically, delivery at private healthcare facilities was more likely among the Tigraways followed by the Amharas. Women having health insurance coverage were more likely to deliver at healthcare facilities than those without. Similarly, slum residents were more than twice likely to deliver at home compared to the nonslum residents.

About 6.3% of the ANC attendees finally delivered at home. Only 1.7% of the private facility ANC clients delivered at home compared to 6.7% of the public facility clients. In terms of shifting between types of facility, 30.0% of the private facility ANC clients delivered at public healthcare facilities while 22.6% of the public facility ANC clients delivered at private facilities.

The mother's knowledge about danger signs of pregnancy showed an effect on women's preferences for place of delivery. About 94.9% of those women counselled about the danger signs of pregnancy delivered at a health facility compared to 92.1% of those who were not counselled ($P = 0.01$). About 81.7% and 72.8% of clients of private and public healthcare facilities respectively were counselled on danger signs of pregnancy during antenatal follow-up.

The reasons behind women's preference for their places of delivery were further explored. Hence, preference for public healthcare facilities was attributed to short distance (72.7% versus 36.4%; $P = 0.000$), perceived low cost service (6.1% versus 2.4%; $P = 0.037$), and experienced low cost service (16.7% versus 4.3%; $P = 0.000$). On the other hand, preference for private healthcare facilities associated positively with short waiting time (19.1% versus 8.7%; $P = 0.000$), perceived good quality of service (15.2% versus 7.6%; $P = 0.001$), experienced good quality of service (43.1% versus 20.6%; $P = 0.000$), perceived good approach of service provider (10.0% versus 5.7%; $P = 0.034$), and experienced good approach of service provider (22.9% versus 10.5%; $P = 0.000$). There was no statistically significant influence of families, friends, or husbands on women's preference for places to give birth ($P > 0.05$).

3.2. Determinants of Preferences for Places to Give Birth. In Table 2, the results of the logit model show that younger women and those with 0–2 living children were less likely to deliver at home (OR = 0.90 and OR = 0.24) compared to older women and those with three or more living children, respectively. Women who had unintended pregnancy for

their last birth and those with no formal education were 2.1 and 3.6 times more likely to deliver at home compared to those with intended pregnancy and those with secondary and above educational attainment level, respectively.

Contrary to home delivery preference, women with unintended pregnancy were less likely to deliver at private healthcare facilities. Conversely, women with intended pregnancy were 1.75 times more likely to deliver at private healthcare facilities compared to those with unintended pregnancies. Similarly, women with no formal education (OR = 0.18) or with primary education (OR = 0.33) were less likely to deliver at private healthcare facilities compared to those with secondary and above education.

The wealth class to which the household of the respondent belongs was a significant factor in predicting the preferred place of delivery. The lower the wealth quintile, the greater the likelihood of delivering at home. Women who belong to the middle class wealth quintile were 2.79 times more likely to deliver at home compared to the household with high class wealth quintile. It was also found that the odds of delivery at private healthcare facilities were low among women of low wealth quintile (OR = 0.56) compared to those in high wealth quintile.

4. Discussion

Our multinomial regression model shows that young women have lower probability of giving birth at home compared to older women. In Uganda [13] and in urban Kenya [14], young women were found to be better users of skilled professional assistance. The same is true in Nepal and India where institutional delivery was more common among young mothers compared to older ones [15, 16]. It has been argued that older women may consist of more traditional cohorts and may resist modern healthcare services [17].

We have also shown in this study that women with two or less living children were more likely to deliver at public healthcare facilities than at home compared to those with three or more living children. Our findings support results of a study from Entebbe, Uganda, which showed that primigravidae were more likely to attend government hospitals [18]. It is possible that women with three or more living children claim to be experienced and see no reason to deliver at health facilities. Alternatively, negative previous experiences may deter women from delivering at health facilities thereby exposing themselves to the complications of childbirth.

In relation to pregnancy intention we observed that women whose last pregnancy was unintended preferred delivery at home (OR = 2.11). Although the reasons for not utilising health facilities for unintended pregnancies are not very clear, it may be related to intention to conceal the delivery, lessened employment opportunities or lack of income, and delayed prenatal care [19–21].

Education is one of the key social determinants of health and healthcare. Low levels of female education [22] and lack of empowerment prevent women from seeking maternal care [23]. In the current study, women with no formal education were almost four times more likely to deliver at home compared to those with secondary and above educational

TABLE 1: Demographic variables and preferred place of delivery, Addis Ababa, January 2014.

Variables	Place of delivery		
	Home	Public facility	Private facility
Demographic variables			
Age group			
15–24	9.6**	75.1	15.3
25–29	5.8	66.9	27.3
30–49	5.8	67.7	26.5
Number of living children			
0–2	5.1**	71.7	23.2
3–6	11.7	61.7	26.6
Current marital status			
Currently married	5.5***	65.5	29.0
Cohabiting/living together	6.1	81.7	12.2
Others	15.8	72.6	11.6
Pregnancy intention			
Unintended	13.0***	74.4	12.6
Intended	4.4	67.3	28.2
Social structure variables			
Mother's educational status			
No education	19.8***	71.9	8.3
Primary education	7.4	79.5	13.1
Secondary education	2.8	65.5	31.7
Tertiary education	1.5	47.8	50.7
Mother's occupation			
Unemployed	6.9	70.9	22.3
Employed	6.8	64.1	29.1
Wealth index			
Low	6.4	77.9	15.6
Middle	6.7	72.6	20.7
High	7.2	59.3	33.4
Health insurance			
Yes	0.0**	60.9	39.1
No	4.7	71.6	23.7
Type of residence			
Slum	8.4***	76.3	15.3
Nonslum	3.8	54.5	41.7
Ethnicity			
Amhara	4.8***	68.9	26.3
Guragie	7.1	75.8	17.0
Oromo	8.0	74.1	17.8
Tigraway	1.8	54.5	43.6
Others	15.2	56.5	28.3
Healthcare variables			
Place of ANC visit			
Public facilities	6.7	70.7	22.6
Private facilities	1.7	30.0	68.3
Counselled on danger signs of pregnancy			
Yes	5.1	68.0	26.9
No	7.9	75.3	16.7

Note. **$P < 0.01$; ***$P < 0.001$.

TABLE 2: Odds ratios from multinomial logistic regression for preferences for places to give birth, Addis Ababa, January 2014.

Variables	Preferred place of delivery, AOR [95% CI]	
	Home	Private facility
Age	0.90 [0.83, 0.98]*	1.02 [0.97, 1.07]
Number of living children		
0–2	0.24 [0.10, 0.56]**	1.20 [0.71, 2.03]
3–6	1	1
Marital status		
Currently married	0.70 [0.25, 1.91]	1.33 [0.61, 2.90]
Cohabiting/living together	0.51 [0.16, 1.66]	0.80 [0.32, 2.00]
Others	1	1
Mother's pregnancy intention		
Unintended	2.11 [1.03, 4.33]*	0.57 [0.34, 0.94]*
Intended	1	1
Mother's educational status		
No education	3.56 [1.38, 9.21]**	0.18 [0.08, 0.40]***
Primary education	1.20 [0.51, 2.85]	0.33 [0.22, 0.52]***
Secondary and above	1	1
Wealth index		
Low	0.63 [0.29, 1.38]	0.56 [0.37, 0.82]**
Middle	2.79 [1.18, 6.61]*	0.61 [0.31, 1.21]
High	1	1
Type of residence		
Slum	1.32 [0.53, 3.24]	0.35 [0.24, 0.51]***
Nonslum	1	1
Religion		
Christian	1.19 [0.51, 2.78]	0.42 [0.27, 0.68]***
Muslim	1	1
High risk pregnancy		
Yes	0.89 [0.36, 2.19]	0.77 [0.48, 1.23]
No	1	1
Adequacy of ANC services		
Inadequate	1.40 [0.31, 6.36]	0.40 [0.24, 0.67]**
Adequate	1	1

Note. (*$P < 0.05$; **$P < 0.01$; ***$P < 0.001$). ANC: antenatal care, CI: confidence interval, COR: crude odds ratio, and AOR: adjusted odds ratio.

level. If they use health facilities, those with no formal education and those with primary level of education were 82% and 67% less likely to use private healthcare facilities, respectively. Similar studies show that well educated mothers are more likely to go to private hospitals seeking for maternal healthcare [18]. The findings point to the power of education in empowering women to seek maternal care and high socioeconomic opportunities both of which reduce the risks of childbirths in areas which lack professional care.

With regard to wealth status, in this study, middle class women were more likely to deliver at home compared to those in the rich wealth quintile households. Women in the low wealth quintile households were less likely to deliver at private healthcare facilities compared to those in the rich wealth quintile households. The findings concur with the report of a cross-country study which used DHS data and showed that the poorest women were over three times more likely

to report giving birth at home [24]. Further previous studies have also indicated that poor women rely more on public or governmental health services than on private healthcare facilities [25] compared to women of better living conditions. Private facilities are not affordable to the poor although the quality of services is still questionable [26].

In this study, adequacy of ANC positively correlated with giving birth at private healthcare facilities. Though there are limited sources which examined the effect of adequacy of ANC as a composite indicator, available evidences indicate that the timing of visits and number of visits as well as content of services received have significant effect on mothers' preferences for places to give birth. Studies from Bangladesh [27] and Kenya [13, 28] showed that the less the number of ANC visits is the more likely the woman is to deliver at home. Inadequate services generally prevent women from seeking care during pregnancy or childbirth [29]. Other study findings have indicated that women wishing to give birth in a health facility also make the most use of ANC services [30]. It has been suggested that each antenatal visit creates an opportunity to teach pregnant mothers how to recognize signs of pregnancy complications and how to seek for emergency obstetric care [8].

5. Conclusion

Despite the high number of ANC attendances among mothers in the study area, a notable number of pregnant women especially among slum residents still chose to deliver at home. While women's perception of the private sector in Addis Ababa is that it offers better quality services than that offered in the public facilities, still most respondents preferred to deliver in public healthcare institutions despite the general doubts about the quality of services delivered. The preferences were attributed to short distance and perceived as well as experienced low cost of care at public facilities. The observation that utilisation of health facilities was high among younger age groups compared to older women was interesting and factors that demotivate older women from utilising health facilities need to be studied further. To prevent women from reverting back to home delivery, effective communication and particularly counselling of women during ANC visits about the danger signs and complications of pregnancy and childbirth should be enhanced, and concerted effort should be made to encourage every pregnant woman to attend ANC services. Efforts should be directed at the healthcare facilities so that they should provide quality ANC services.

In interpreting this study's findings, it is advisable to consider some of the limitations of the study. The cross-sectional nature of the data does not allow making causal inferences about the relationship between delivery care and the risk factors. It is important to keep in mind that the analysed data includes information reported by mothers only from last pregnancies or childbirths. This study did not collect data about the views and practices of service providers related to quality of services. The study was also limited to the capital city and findings might not reflect the situation of the rest of the country.

Conflict of Interests

The authors declare that they have no competing interests.

Authors' Contribution

Yibeltal Tebekaw conceived of the research topic, designed the methods and materials, supervised the data collection, conducted the statistical analysis, and drafted and finalized the paper. Yohana James Mashalla and Gloria Thupayagale-Tshweneagae guided the interpretation and presentation of results and were involved in subsequent drafting and revision of the paper. All the authors have read and approved the final paper.

Acknowledgment

The authors are indebted to the University of South Africa for its financial support for data collection.

References

[1] Federal Ministry of Health, *Health Sector Strategic Plan (HSDP-III)*, Planning and Programming Department, 2005.

[2] Federal Ministry of Health, "Health sector development program IV 2010/11–2014/15," Final Draft, Federal Democratic Republic of Ethiopia, Addis Ababa, Ethiopia, 2010.

[3] Central Statistical Agency and Inner City Fund International (CSA and ICF International), *Ethiopia Demographic and Health Survey 2011*, Central Statistical Agency, Addis Ababa, Ethiopia; ICF International, Calverton, Md, USA, 2012.

[4] D. Balabanova, A. Mills, L. Conteh et al., "Good Health at Low Cost 25 years on: lessons for the future of health systems strengthening," *The Lancet*, vol. 381, no. 9883, pp. 2118–2133, 2013.

[5] Federal Ministry of Health, *National Reproductive Health Strategy 2006–2015*, Federal Ministry of Health, Addis Ababa, Ethiopia, 2006.

[6] J. B. Etowa, "Becoming a mother: the meaning of childbirth for African-Canadian women," *Contemporary Nurse*, vol. 41, no. 1, pp. 28–40, 2012.

[7] M. S. R. Murthy, P. V. Murthy, M. Hari, V. K. R. Kumar, and K. Rajasekhar, "Place of birth: why urban women still prefer home deliveries?" *Journal of Human Ecology*, vol. 21, no. 2, pp. 149–154, 2007.

[8] S. Singh, L. Remez, U. Ram, A. M. Moore, and S. Audam, *Barriers to Safe Motherhood in India*, Guttmacher Institute, New York, NY, USA, 2009.

[9] Federal Ministry of Health, *Health and Health Related Indicators 2011*, Policy Planning Directorate, Addis Ababa, Ethiopia, 2011.

[10] R. Andersen and J. F. Newman, "Societal and individual determinants of medical care utilization in the United States," *The Milbank Quarterly*, vol. 83, no. 4, pp. 1–28, 2005.

[11] United Nations Human Settlements Programme (UN-Habitat), *Urban Inequities Report: Addis Ababa. Cities and Citizens. (Series 2)*, United Nations Human Settlements Programme (UN-Habitat), 2003.

[12] L. A. Kirkpatrick and B. C. Feeney, *A Simple Guide to SPSS for Version 17.0*, Cengage Learning, Boston, Mass, USA, 2011.

[13] J. Kitui, S. Lewis, and G. Davey, "Factors influencing place of delivery for women in Kenya: an analysis of the Kenya demographic and health survey, 2008/2009," *BMC Pregnancy and Childbirth*, vol. 13, article 40, 2013.

[14] R. Ochako, J.-C. Fotso, L. Ikamari, and A. Khasakhala, "Utilization of maternal health services among young women in Kenya: insights from the Kenya Demographic and Health Survey, 2003," *BMC Pregnancy and Childbirth*, vol. 11, article 1, 2011.

[15] Y. R. Baral, K. Lyons, J. Skinner, and E. R. van Teijlingen, "Maternal health services utilisation in Nepal: progress in the new millennium?" *Health Science Journal*, vol. 6, no. 4, pp. 618–633, 2012.

[16] S. R. Mahapatro, "Utilization of maternal and child Health care services in India: does women's autonomy matter?" *The Journal of Family Welfare*, vol. 58, no. 1, pp. 22–33, 2012.

[17] S. Gabrysch and O. M. R. Campbell, "Still too far to walk: literature review of the determinants of delivery service use," *BMC Pregnancy and Childbirth*, vol. 9, article 34, 2009.

[18] C. J. Tann, M. Kizza, L. Morison et al., "Use of antenatal services and delivery care in Entebbe, Uganda: a community survey," *BMC Pregnancy and Childbirth*, vol. 7, article 23, 2007.

[19] Y. Dibaba, M. Fantahun, and M. J. Hindin, "The association of unwanted pregnancy and social support with depressive symptoms in pregnancy: evidence from rural Southwestern Ethiopia," *BMC Pregnancy and Childbirth*, vol. 13, article 135, 2013.

[20] A. Exavery, A. M. Kanté, A. Hingora, G. Mbaruku, S. Pemba, and J. F. Phillips, "How mistimed and unwanted pregnancies affect timing of antenatal care initiation in three districts in Tanzania," *BMC Pregnancy and Childbirth*, vol. 13, article 35, 2013.

[21] Y. Tebekaw, B. Aemro, and C. Teller, "Prevalence and determinants of unintended childbirth in Ethiopia," *BMC Pregnancy and Childbirth*, vol. 14, no. 1, p. 326, 2014.

[22] Q. Long, T. Zhang, L. Xu, S. Tang, and E. Hemminki, "Utilisation of maternal health care in western rural China under a new rural health insurance system (New Co-operative Medical System)," *Tropical Medicine and International Health*, vol. 15, no. 10, pp. 1210–1217, 2010.

[23] World Health Organization, *Countdown to 2015 Report*, WHO, Geneva, Switzerland, 2012, http://www.countdown2015mnch .org/documents/2012Report/2012-part-2.pdf.

[24] D. Montagu, G. Yamey, A. Visconti, A. Harding, and J. Yoong, "Where do poor women in developing countries give birth? A multi-country analysis of demographic and health survey data," *PLoS ONE*, vol. 6, no. 2, Article ID e17155, 2011.

[25] A. H. Ibnouf, H. W. van den Borne, and J. A. Maarse, "Utilization of antenatal care services by Sudanese women in their reproductive age," *Saudi Medical Journal*, vol. 28, no. 5, pp. 737–743, 2007, http://www.smj.org.sa/index.php/smj/article/view/ 5811/3585.

[26] R. Sciortino, N. Ridarineni, and B. Marjadi, "Caught between social and market considerations: a case study of Muhammadiyah charitable health services," *Reproductive Health Matters*, vol. 18, no. 36, pp. 25–34, 2010.

[27] J. Pervin, A. Moran, M. Rahman et al., "Association of antenatal care with facility delivery and perinatal survival—a population-based study in Bangladesh," *BMC Pregnancy and Childbirth*, vol. 12, article 111, 2012.

[28] African Population and Health Research Center (APHRC), "The maternal health challenge in poor urban communities in Kenya," Policy Brief 12, Health Policy of the Transitional Government of Ethiopia, Nairobi, Kenya, 2009.

[29] *Health Policy of the Transitional Government of Ethiopia*, 1993.

[30] B. Nikiéma, G. Beninguisse, and J. L. Haggerty, "Providing information on pregnancy complications during antenatal visits: unmet educational needs in sub-Saharan Africa," *Health Policy and Planning*, vol. 24, no. 5, pp. 367–376, 2009.

8

Resveratrol, Acetyl-Resveratrol, and Polydatin Exhibit Antigrowth Activity against 3D Cell Aggregates of the SKOV-3 and OVCAR-8 Ovarian Cancer Cell Lines

Simon J. Hogg,[1] Kenny Chitcholtan,[2] Wafaa Hassan,[3] Peter H. Sykes,[2] and Ashley Garrill[3]

[1]Peter MacCallum Cancer Centre, St Andrews Place, East Melbourne, Melbourne, VIC 3002, Australia
[2]Department of Obstetrics and Gynaecology, University of Otago, Christchurch, 2 Riccarton Avenue, Christchurch 8011, New Zealand
[3]School of Biological Sciences, University of Canterbury, Private Bag 4800, Christchurch 8140, New Zealand

Correspondence should be addressed to Kenny Chitcholtan; kenny.chitcholtan@otago.ac.nz

Academic Editor: Curt W. Burger

Resveratrol has aroused significant scientific interest as it has been claimed that it exhibits a spectrum of health benefits. These include effects as an anti-inflammatory and an antitumour compound. The purpose of this study was to investigate and compare any potential antigrowth effects of resveratrol and two of its derivatives, acetyl-resveratrol and polydatin, on 3D cell aggregates of the EGFR/Her-2 positive and negative ovarian cancer cell lines SKOV-3 and OVCAR-8, respectively. Results showed that resveratrol and acetyl-resveratrol reduced cell growth in the SKOV-3 and OVCAR-8 in a dose-dependant manner. The growth reduction was mediated by the induction of apoptosis via the cleavage of poly(ADP-ribose) polymerase (PARP-1). At lower concentrations, 5 and 10 μM, resveratrol, acetyl-resveratrol, and polydatin were less effective than higher concentrations, 50 and 100 μM. In SKOV-3 line, at higher concentrations, resveratrol and polydatin significantly reduced the phosphorylation of Her-2 and EGFR and the expression of Erk. Acetyl-resveratrol, on the other hand, did not change the activation of Her-2 and EGFR. Resveratrol, acetyl-resveratrol, and polydatin suppressed the secretion of VEGF in a dose-dependant fashion. In the OVCAR-8 cell line, resveratrol and acetyl-resveratrol at 5 and 10 μM increased the activation of Erk. Above these concentrations they decreased activation. Polydatin did not produce this effect. This study demonstrates that resveratrol and its derivatives may inhibit growth of 3D cell aggregates of ovarian cancer cell lines via different signalling molecules. Resveratrol and its derivatives, therefore, warrant further *in vivo* evaluation to assess their potential clinical utility.

1. Introduction

Ovarian cancer is a lethal malignancy, and the prognosis is very poor for women who present with an advanced stage of the disease [1]. As chemotherapy is not normally curative in women with advanced ovarian cancers, treatments that can slow the growth of tumours and, hence, prolong the life of those with the disease are of great importance. Advanced ovarian cancer is often associated with ascites, the excess accumulation of the body fluid in the abdominal cavity [2, 3]. The permeability of blood and lymphatic vessels at the peritoneal wall is compromised by high levels of vascular endothelial growth factor (VEGF) and that causes ascites. Ascitic fluid which can move freely around the abdominal cavity contains malignant ovarian cells; these cells can

become deposited on the surface of peritoneal membrane, thereby establishing multiple sites of secondary growth. The floating cancer cells often form small 3D aggregates, which may help them to survive as they circulate in the abdominal cavity [3]. As a result, these 3D cell aggregates may contribute to a likely source of cancer cells that have the ability to form small tumours and later grow in uncontrolled manner. Little is known about how ovarian cancer aggregates survive in ascitic fluid. Also, there have been limited studies that focus on the use of possible therapeutic targets in these ovarian cancer aggregates.

One possible chemotherapeutic target of ovarian cancers would be the inhibition of the tyrosine kinase receptors, ErBb1 (EGFR) and ErBb2 (Her-2). These receptors have been reported to play an important role in a subset of ovarian cancers. The elevated expression of these receptors is typically correlated with a poor prognosis, and thus targeting their activation could potentially affect tumour growth [4]. The activation of EGFR and Her-2 elicits a vast array of signalling proteins responsible for cell proliferation, survival, metastasis, invasion, ECM remodelling, and angiogenesis [5]. The MAPK activation pathway and the production of VEGF are affected by suppressing EGFR/Her-2 activation [5]. However, the role of EGFR and Her-2 in ovarian cancer aggregates is still poorly understood. A compound that has the ability to suppress the activation of these receptors may be of importance in controlling the progression of ovarian cancer aggregates and ascites.

Resveratrol (3,5,4′-trihydroxy-trans-stilbene) (Figure 1(a)) and its derivative compounds, acetyl-resveratrol (3,5,4′-tri-O-acetylresveratrol) (Figure 1(b)) and polydatin (3,5,4′-trihydroxy-stilbene-3-beta-mono-D-glucoside) (Figure 1(c)), are natural occurring polyphenol compounds that have aroused interest due to their potential health benefits. Resveratrol has been shown to affect the activation of EGFR and Her-2 in several types of cancers in preclinical studies [6]. Furthermore, EGFR/Her-2 associated signalling proteins in PI-3K and MAPK pathways have been reported to be affected and responsible for resveratrol's antitumour activities [6]. Despite promising antitumour effects of resveratrol in in vitro studies, its inhibition of tumour progression in animal models is less well defined and is quite variable. Some studies have documented the growth reduction of tumours after a duration of resveratrol ingestion, but others have not noticed any antitumour effects of resveratrol [7, 8]. Furthermore, resveratrol has also been shown to increase tumour growth in certain types of cancers [9]. The discrepancy of antitumour properties of resveratrol between in vitro and in vivo studies may be partly due to the bioavailability of active molecules of resveratrol.

The use of resveratrol as a potential anticancer drug in humans is still controversial [10]. One significant drawback with respect to the clinical use of resveratrol for cancer patients is its typically low bioavailability [11]. Given this, more data with respect to its therapeutic efficacy against specific cancer types are needed to address its potential as a monotherapy or as an adjuvant regimen. Because of the possibility of limited usefulness of resveratrol itself due to the low plasma concentrations, there is a need to investigate compounds that are related to resveratrol and that may have greater bioavailability after ingestion. Two possible candidate compounds are acetyl-resveratrol and polydatin, which are currently under investigation for their cancer preventative properties [12, 13]. Polydatin has shown antitumour activities in in vitro studies [14, 15]. Polydatin has previously been reported to have a greater anti-inflammatory effect than resveratrol in a study of colitis in rats [16]. In animal studies, after ingestion, polydatin is metabolized to resveratrol and glucuronidated resveratrol in the intestines and the liver, respectively [17]. Furthermore, a native polydatin has been shown to be present at significant levels in the plasma of a mouse model [18]. Acetyl-resveratrol is metabolized and converted back to resveratrol that can be detected in plasma of a mouse model [7].

Clearly with respect to ovarian cancer aggregates, there is a need for more studies of the antitumour activities and the possible mechanistic effects of these compounds. Given the above, in this study we investigated whether resveratrol, acetyl-resveratrol, and polydatin elicited antigrowth of 3D cell aggregates of the EGFR/Her-2 positive cell line SKOV-3 and the EGFR/Her-2 negative cell line OVCAR-8. In addition, we presented preliminary studies of the mechanistic looking at the compounds potential modulation via both dependence on and independence of the expression of EGFR/Her-2.

2. Materials and Methods

The human ovarian adenocarcinoma cell line, SKOV-3, used in this project was purchased from ATCC. This cell line has high expression of EGFR and Her-2, PTEN wild type, E-cadherin negative, null *P53*, KRAS wild type, and BRAF wild type [19]. OVCAR-8 was obtained from Dr. Judith McKenzie, Haematology Research Group, University of Otago, Christchurch, New Zealand. This cell line has low expression of EGFR and Her-2, *P53* mutation, and E-cadherin negative [19]. SKOV-3 cells were maintained in Knockout Dulbecco's Modified Eagle Medium (DMEM Catalogue number 10829, GIBCO, ThermoFisher Scientific, New Zealand). This high glucose base medium was supplemented with 10% fetal bovine serum (FBS) (GIBCO, ThermoFisher Scientific, New Zealand), PenStrep (GIBCO, ThermoFisher Scientific, New Zealand) at a working concentration of 100 units/mL penicillin and 100 μg/mL streptomycin, 2 mM GlutaMAX (GIBCO, Invitrogen, New Zealand), and 2 μg/mL fungizone (ThermoFisher Scientific, New Zealand). OVCAR-8 was maintained in similar media, but it contained 5% FBS and 5% serum replacement (ThermoFisher Scientific, New Zealand). The supplemented DMEM media are henceforth referred to as working media. SKOV-3 and OVCAR-8 cells in the respective working media were maintained at 37°C in a humidified 5% CO_2 atmosphere incubator. Both cell lines were continuously maintained in a culture flask.

2.1. Generation of 3D Cell Aggregates. To prevent adhesion of cells to culture plates and to encourage the formation of 3D aggregates, 12-well culture plates were precoated with 24 mg/mL poly-HEMA (Sigma, New Zealand) prior to cell culturing (0.6 mL/well). Prior to coating, poly-HEMA in 95% ethanol at a concentration of 24 mg/mL was heated to approximately 70°C to ensure that the poly-HEMA was fully dissolved. The coated plates were left overnight at 37°C on an orbital shaker. Prior to cell culture, the coated plates were washed once with PBS at pH 7.4. The cell monolayer of the SKOV-3 and OVCAR-8 cell lines was incubated with 1x trypsin-EDTA for 20–30 minutes to detach the cells from the surface of the flask. Cells were counted with a haemocytometer to determine the concentration of cells in the cell suspension. Cells were then plated at a density of 150,000 cells/well and were incubated at 37°C in a humidified 5% CO_2 atmosphere for 6 days during which time the cells became compact aggregates. Over this period the media were removed by aspiration and replaced with 1.5 mL of fresh working media every 2 days for six days.

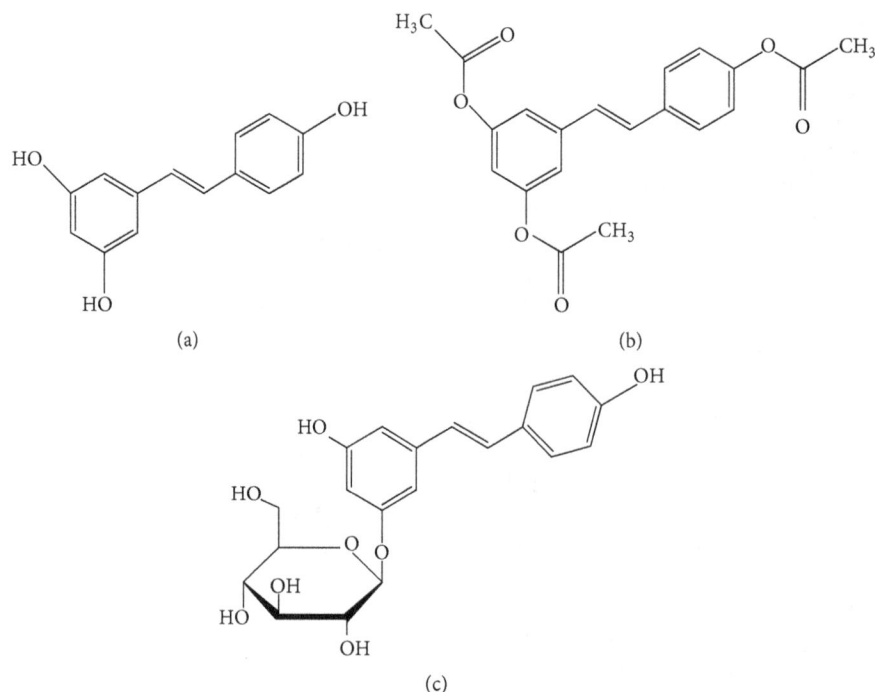

FIGURE 1: The chemical structures of resveratrol (a), acetyl-resveratrol (b), and polydatin (c).

2.2. Treatment with Resveratrol and Derivatives. Resveratrol, acetyl-resveratrol, and polydatin powders were kindly provided by Dr. Saurabh Shah, Biotivia (USA). Acetyl-resveratrol was dissolved in 100% DMSO; polydatin and resveratrol were dissolved in a 50% : 50% combination of PBS and DMSO. For all experiment, the final amount of DMSO in controls and compound treated samples was 0.5% (vol/vol). Fresh working media containing the relevant compounds (at concentrations of 5, 10, 50, and 100 μM) were replaced every 2 days for a total of 6 days. Thus, at the endpoint of cell culturing cells had a total incubation time of 12 days: 6 days for 3D aggregate formation and 6 days for the respective treatments. At least four independent experiments were carried out and each individual experiment was carried out with three replicates.

2.3. Analysis of Cell Cluster Morphology. Following 6 days of incubation to generate the cell aggregates and 6 days of treatment with compounds, images were collected using a camera (Leica DFC310FX, Germany) attached to an inverted light microscope (Leica DMI6000, Germany) with a 10x objective lens in order to assess the SKOV-3 cell aggregate morphology.

2.4. Growth Determination Using the Crystal Violet Assay. Growth of the 3D cell aggregates was quantified indirectly using crystal violet dye staining. In brief, cell aggregates were harvested and incubated with 1x trypsin-EDTA for 20 minutes at 37°C. Cells were washed twice with PBS pH 7.4 and were incubated for a further 30 minutes at 37°C with 2 mg/mL crystal violet in 2% (v/v) ethanol in deionized water. The cells were then washed with deionized water to remove unbound crystal violet dye and were harvested by centrifugation at 1500 rpm for 5 minutes. The supernatant was removed, and

the process was repeated 3–5 times until the supernatant was colourless. Cells were then lysed in 10% (w/v) sodium dodecyl sulphate (SDS) solution. The homogenous cell lysate was diluted 3-fold in deionized water and 200 μL of the samples was loaded onto a 96-well plate. The optical density was determined at 560 nm (OD_{560}) using a microplate reader (SpectraMax M5, Molecular Devices). Measurements for each sample were made in triplicate.

2.5. Cellular Metabolism Determination Using the Alamar Blue Dye Assay. On the 5th day of treatment with compounds, 100 μL of Alamar blue dye (ThermoFisher Scientific, New Zealand) in 1 mL media was added to cell aggregates. Cell aggregates were further incubated with the dye for 20 hours and 200 μL culture media from each well was transferred to a 96-well plate. The absorbance at 570 and 600 nm was measured using a microplate reader (SpectraMax M5, Molecular Devices).

2.6. Detection of Vascular Endothelial Growth Factor (VEGF). After 6 days of respective treatments, the media of the control and treated cells were used to determine secreted VEGF. Analysis of VEGF secretion was carried out using a DuoSet Human VEGF ELISA Kit (R&D Systems, New Zealand). The optical density of each well was measured using a microplate reader (SpectraMax M5, Molecular Devices) at 450 nm. The amount of VEGF in each sample was determined by comparing the absorbance of each of the wells to that of a standard curve. SigmaPlot (Systat Software, San Jose, CA) was used to create a standard curve from which VEGF concentrations of cell media samples were extrapolated.

2.7. Immunoblotting Analysis. Cell clusters were harvested by centrifugation at 1500 rpm for 5 minutes, and the cell pellet was resuspended in cold RIPA buffer containing protease inhibitor cocktail tablets (Complete Mini, Roche, New Zealand). The cell lysates were left on ice for a further 30 minutes to complete total lysis. Sample buffer (0.2% (v/v) bromophenol blue, 25% (v/v) glycerol, 10% SDS in Tris-HCl, and pH 6.8) was added and protein lysates were boiled for 10 minutes. Prior to loading, the cell lysates were mixed and centrifuged at 12,000 rpm for 5 minutes. Protein lysate was loaded and separated by SDS-PAGE using a 5% stacking gel and a 12% separating gel. The SDS-PAGE was run at 120 volts using Tris-glycine running buffer. The SDS-PAGE markers used were MagicMark Western Protein Standard (Invitrogen, New Zealand) and Precision Plus Protein standard (Bio-Rad, Hercules, USA). Separated proteins were electroblotted onto nitrocellulose membranes (0.45 microns, Trans-Blot Nitrocellulose Membrane, Bio-Rad, Hercules, USA). The electroblot was run at 100 Volts for 60 minutes in cold Tris-glycine running buffer containing 10% v/v methanol. The membranes were blocked for 60 minutes with either 5% (w/v) nonfat skim milk (Pams brand, New World, New Zealand) or 1% (w/v) bovine serum albumin (ThermoFisher Scientific, New Zealand) made up in TBS-T buffer or with Pierce Protein-Free Blocking Buffer (Thermo Scientific, New Zealand). Antibodies were diluted from 1 : 500 to 1 : 1000 with the appropriate blocking solution. Membranes were incubated with primary antibodies overnight at 4°C. The membranes were washed with TBS-T buffer on an orbital shaker for 4 × 10 minutes and then incubated with secondary antibody on an orbital shaker for 90 minutes at room temperature. Membranes were subsequently washed a further four times with TBS-T. Antibody localisation was determined using a chemiluminescent detection kit (Amersham ECL Prime Western Blotting Detection Reagent Kit, GE Healthcare). The protein bands were visualized and a densitometry analysis was performed using Alliance 4.7, Unitec (Cambridge, UK). Cell lysates were collected from at least 3 separated cell culture experiments. Antibodies were purchased from Santa Cruz Biotechnology Inc. (Santa Cruz, CA, USA). The primary antibodies used in this study were anti-PARP (sc-25780), anti-GAPDH (sc-25778), anti-pHER2 (sc-12352-R), anti-EGFR (sc-03), anti-pEGFR (sc-101668), anti-ERK (sc-94), and anti-pERK1/2 (sc-7383). Anti-Her-2 was purchased from BD Biosciences (Auckland, New Zealand). The two secondary antibodies used in this study were bovine anti-rabbit IgG-HRP (sc-2385) and bovine anti-mouse IgG-HRP (sc-2380).

2.8. Statistical Analysis. Data were statistically analyzed (SigmaPlot 11) using Student's t-test and ANOVA with $p < 0.05$ was considered to indicate statistical significance. All data are presented as mean ± SEM. Each experiment was repeated at least four times.

3. Results

3.1. Effects of Resveratrol and Its Derivatives on Cell Growth. SKOV-3 cells formed large dense aggregates with circular, oval, and tubular structures in nontreated samples (Figures 2(a), 2(f), and 2(k)). This general morphology and aggregate size were not affected by the lower concentrations (5 μM and 10 μM) of all of the tested compounds. 3D aggregates of control, low concentration treated resveratrol (Figures 2(b) and 2(c)), acetyl-resveratrol (Figures 2(g) and 2(h)), and polydatin (Figures 2(l) and 2(m)) had a smooth rim. However, at the higher concentrations of resveratrol (Figures 2(d) and 2(e)) and acetyl-resveratrol (Figures 2(i) and 2(j)), aggregates had a rough irregular rim. Polydatin treated aggregates also showed an irregular rim, but this was less pronounced than in resveratrol and acetyl-resveratrol treated aggregates.

We further examined the relative growth of cell aggregates using a crystal violet assay. As shown in Figure 2(p), growth was reduced by about 70% with the higher concentrations (50 and 100 μM) of resveratrol and by about 20% with the lower concentration of 10 μM (Figure 2(p)). Similar growth reduction was also obtained with the higher concentrations of acetyl-resveratrol (Figure 2(q)). Polydatin showed less inhibition of growth. At concentrations of 50 and 100 μM, it reduced growth by 20 and 50% (Figure 2(r)), respectively. There was no growth inhibition observed with the lower doses of acetyl-resveratrol and polydatin.

To investigate whether apoptosis facilitating cell death caused the reduction of growth in 3D aggregate cells that were treated with the higher concentrations of the compounds, we examined the expression of the apoptotic marker protein, poly(ADP-ribose) polymerase (PARP). Resveratrol and acetyl-resveratrol increased the fragmentation of PARP giving a band with a molecular weight of 89 kDa; this is consistent with the fact that the reduction of cell number at the higher concentrations of compounds is due to apoptosis (Figures 3(a), 3(b), and 3(c)). The 89 kDa fragmented PARP was also observed in the control in addition to the treated samples, indicative of a baseline level of apoptosis in the cell clusters.

3.2. Effects of Resveratrol, Acetyl-Resveratrol, and Polydatin on Cell Signalling Molecules. Previous work has suggested that the antigrowth effect of resveratrol may be due to its action on a number of intracellular signalling molecules [6]. However, less is known about the effects of acetyl-resveratrol and polydatin on cancer cells, especially in 3D cell aggregates of ovarian cancer cells. We chose the SKOV-3 cell line because it has high expression of the oncogenic EGFR and Her-2 proteins, possible potential targets of the compounds. Resveratrol at 50 and 100 μM was found to reduce the levels of pHer-2 (Figures 4(a) and 4(b)(A)) and pEGFR (Figures 4(a) and 4(b)(C)). There was no marked reduction of pHer-2 and pEGFR at 5 and 10 μM (Figures 4(b)(A) and 4(b)(C)). Higher doses of resveratrol reduced the total expression of Erk1/2 and showed a tendency to suppress pErk1/2 (Figures 4(b)(F) and 4(b)(E)).

In contrast to resveratrol, acetyl-resveratrol did not reduce pHer-2 and pEGFR at the higher concentrations. There was an increase in pHer-2 (Figure 5(b)(A)) at 5 and 10 μM and pEGFR at 10 μM (Figure 5(b)(C)). Acetyl-resveratrol did not modulate the active form of Erk at any

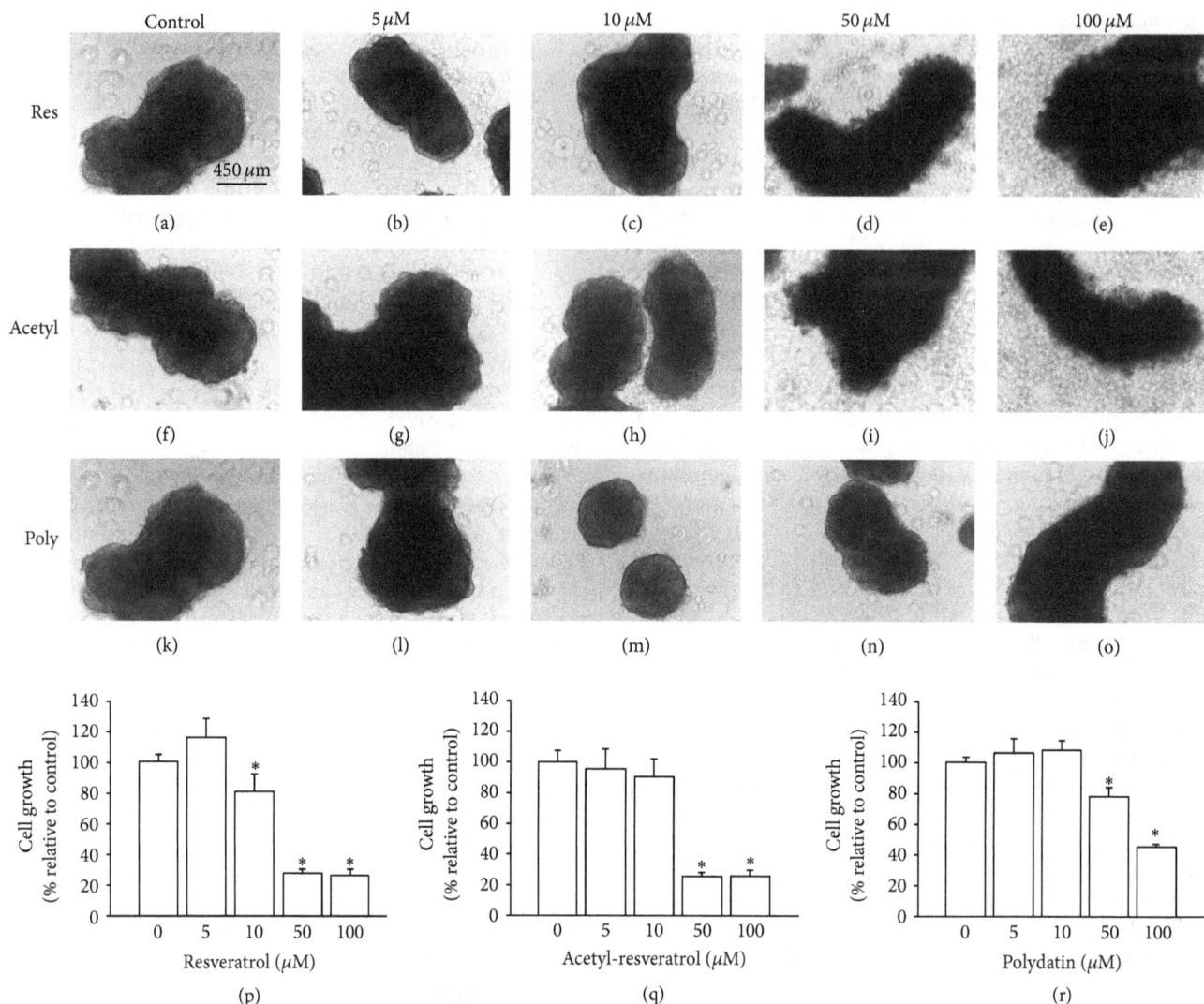

FIGURE 2: Morphological appearance of SKOV-3 cell aggregates with and without treatment. At higher concentrations all three compounds gave aggregates with irregular rims. The effect was more prominent with resveratrol (d, e) and acetyl-resveratrol (i, j) than with polydatin (n, o). The smooth rims of cell aggregates treated with lower concentration were not visibly different from those of control aggregates. Resveratrol significantly reduced cell growth at 10, 50, and 100 μM (p), but acetyl-resveratrol (q) and polydatin (r) only affected growth activity at higher concentrations. $*$ refers to statistically significant as p value less than 0.05 compared to the control.

of the tested concentrations (Figure 5(b)(E)); however the expression of Erk1/2 was reduced at 100 μM (Figure 5(b)(F)). Polydatin at 50 and 100 μM significantly reduced the phosphorylation of Her-2 (Figures 6(a) and 6(b)(A)) and showed a significant reduction of the expression and phosphorylation of EGFR at 100 μM (Figure 6(b)(C)). Polydatin did not alter the expression of Erk1/2.

There have been reports of the association of EGFR and Her-2 with increased expression of angiogenic proteins [5]. Vascular endothelial growth factor (VEGF) is a potent angiogenic peptide, and its elevated levels in women with advanced ovarian cancer are correlated with a poor prognosis [20]. To evaluate the effect of the compounds on secretion of VEGF by SKOV-3 cell aggregates, we performed an ELISA. Resveratrol (Figure 7(a)) and acetyl-resveratrol (Figure 7(b)) at 50 and 100 μM were found to significantly reduce the secretion of

VEGF by SKOV-3 cell aggregates. Again polydatin was less potent, significantly decreasing VEGF secretion only at a concentration of 100 μM (Figure 7(c)).

To investigate the possible mechanistic basis of resveratrol and its derivatives, we also utilized the EGFR and Her-2 negative cell line, OVCAR-8. As shown in Figures 7(d)–7(r), at the higher concentrations of 50 and 100 μM, resveratrol produced an irregular rim of 3D spheroids of OVCAR-8 (Figures 7(g) and 7(h)). Similar effects were observed in spheroids exposed to higher concentrations of acetyl-resveratrol (Figures 7(l) and 7(m)). At the higher concentrations, polydatin did not show any notable effect (Figures 7(q) and 7(r)). At the lower concentrations, all three compounds had no effect on spheroid morphology. Next, we measured cellular metabolism of OVCAR-8 spheroids in the presence of resveratrol and its derivatives. As shown in Figure 8,

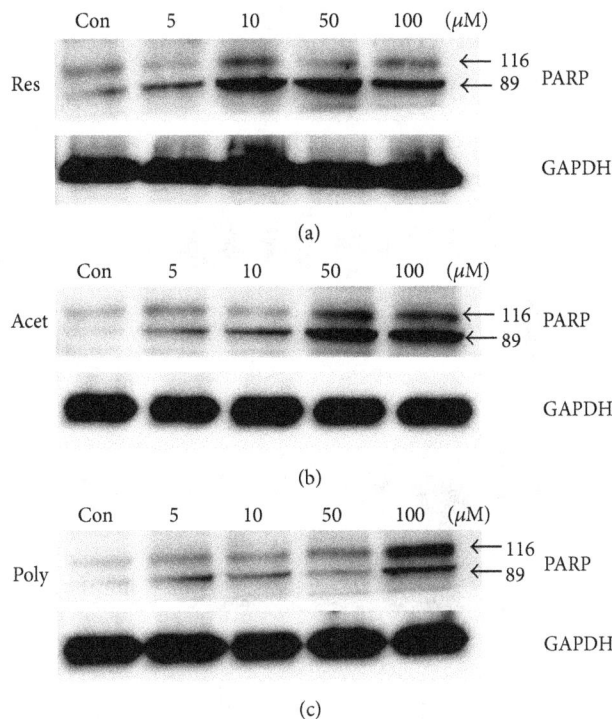

FIGURE 3: The effect of resveratrol (a), acetyl-resveratrol (b), and polydatin (c) on the expression of poly(ADP-ribose) polymerase (PARP) which was used as an indicator of apoptosis in SKOV-3 cell aggregates. At higher concentrations resveratrol, acetyl-resveratrol, and polydatin increased the fragmentation of PARP giving a band of 89 kDa which was indicative of apoptosis. At 10 μM resveratrol induced the fragmentation of PARP. Based line expression of PARP at 116 and 89 kDa was observed in controls and low doses of all compounds.

resveratrol (Figure 8(a)) and acetyl-resveratrol (Figure 8(b)) reduced cellular metabolism in a dose-dependent fashion. Polydatin did not produce this effect. We then examined the growth activity of OVCAR-8 spheroids, and higher concentrations of resveratrol (Figure 8(d)) and acetyl-resveratrol (Figure 8(e)) significantly limited growth activity whereas polydatin had no effect (Figure 8(f)). Next, we investigated the expression of EGFR, Her-2, PARP-1, Erk, and phospho-Erk. OVCAR-8 expressed very low levels of EGFR and Her-2 (data not shown). At higher concentrations, resveratrol (Figure 8(g)) and acetyl-resveratrol (Figure 8(h)) increased the level expression of 89 kDa PARP-1 suggesting that these compounds mediated the apoptotic pathway and facilitate the antigrowth activity. In contrast polydatin did not cause the increased level of PARP-1 (Figure 8(i)). There was lower level of the 89 kDa PARP-1 with the lower concentrations of three compounds. At lower concentrations of 5 and 10 μM resveratrol (Figure 8(g)) and acetyl-resveratrol (Figure 8(h)) increased the activation of Erk, but higher concentrations reduced this effect. Polydatin did not modulate the activation of Erk (Figure 8(i)).

4. Discussion

In this study, we demonstrate antigrowth activity of resveratrol, acetyl-resveratrol, and polydatin against 3D cell aggregates of the SKOV-3 and OVCAR-8 ovarian cancer cell lines. The inhibition of growth appears to be caused by apoptosis and alteration of selective signalling proteins. The effects of these compounds were cell line dependent. In the SKOV-3 cell line, resveratrol and polydatin modulate the activation of EGFR and Her-2, but acetyl-resveratrol does not. Furthermore, secretion of the angiogenic protein, VEGF, in the SKOV-3 cell clusters is reduced in a dose-dependent fashion. In the OVCAR-8 cell line, resveratrol and polydatin modulated the activation of Erk.

Malignant cells in advanced ovarian cancer patients float in ascitic fluid as small cell 3D aggregates [3]. These cancer cell aggregates will regrow at secondary sites such as the peritoneal wall, the omentum, and the surface of internal organs. Therefore, anticancer drugs that prevent growth of aggregates and control ascites could be of great use in the treatment of advanced ovarian cancer. In the present study, we used 3D cell aggregates of the SKOV-3 and OVCAR-8 cell lines, and we have evaluated the antigrowth activity of resveratrol and the derivatives against these cell models. The SKOV-3 cell line has a high expression of the tyrosine kinase receptors, EGFR and Her-2, which have been described to be potential targets of resveratrol. OVCAR-8 cell line has low expression of these receptors, but both cell lines have distinct genetic and molecular profiles [19].

The majority of in vitro studies have evaluated the effects of resveratrol on cell monolayers; a cell culture model is not physiologically relevant and fails to recognize the microenvironment inside tumour tissues. In 3D cell aggregates, there is heterogeneity of cancer cells that may have differing

(a)

(b)

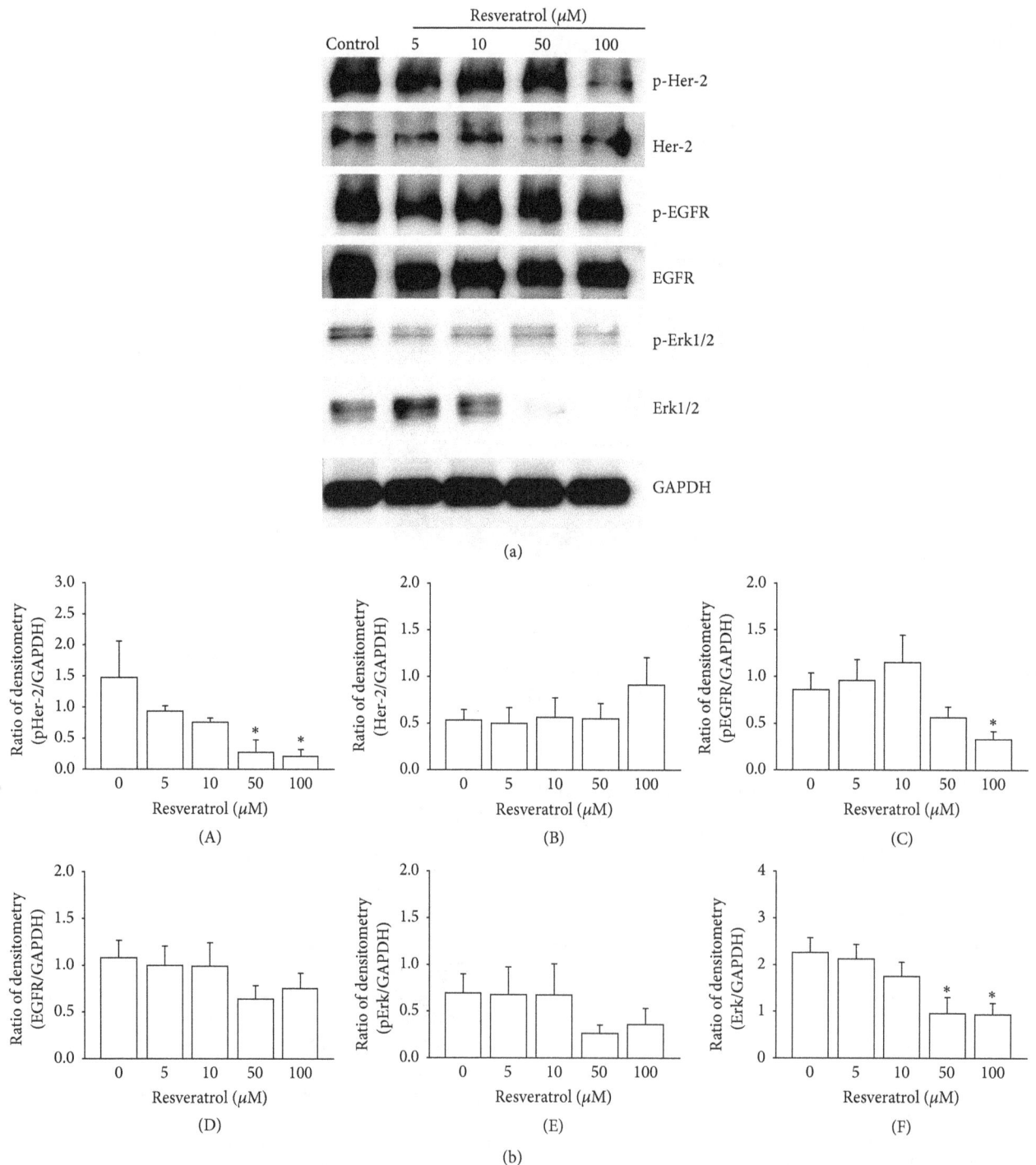

FIGURE 4: The expression and phosphorylation of Her-2, EGFR, Erk1/2, and GAPDH in SKOV-3 cell aggregates after treatment with resveratrol. Higher concentrations of resveratrol reduced the phosphorylation of Her-2 (A) and EGFR (C) and total expression of Erk1/2 (F). * refers to statistically significant as p value less than 0.05 compared to the control.

metabolic activities due to the limitation of nutrient exposure. Furthermore, 3D cell-cell contact may play a crucial role in the autocrine activation. Therefore, this 3D model may be physiologically relevant. Consistent with previous studies, our data show that SKOV-3 and OVCAR-8 cells form large dense cell aggregates when cultured in a nonadherent

condition, which mimics floating cancer cell clusters seen in the ascitic fluid of women with advanced disease [21, 22]. In the present study, we choose a range of concentrations of resveratrol and its derivatives. Concentrations can be considered physiological levels; 5 and 10 μM and can be considered larger than the physiological concentrations, 50

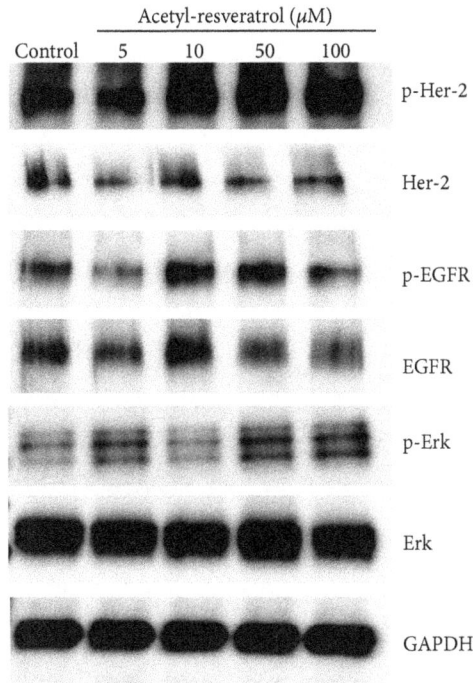

(a)

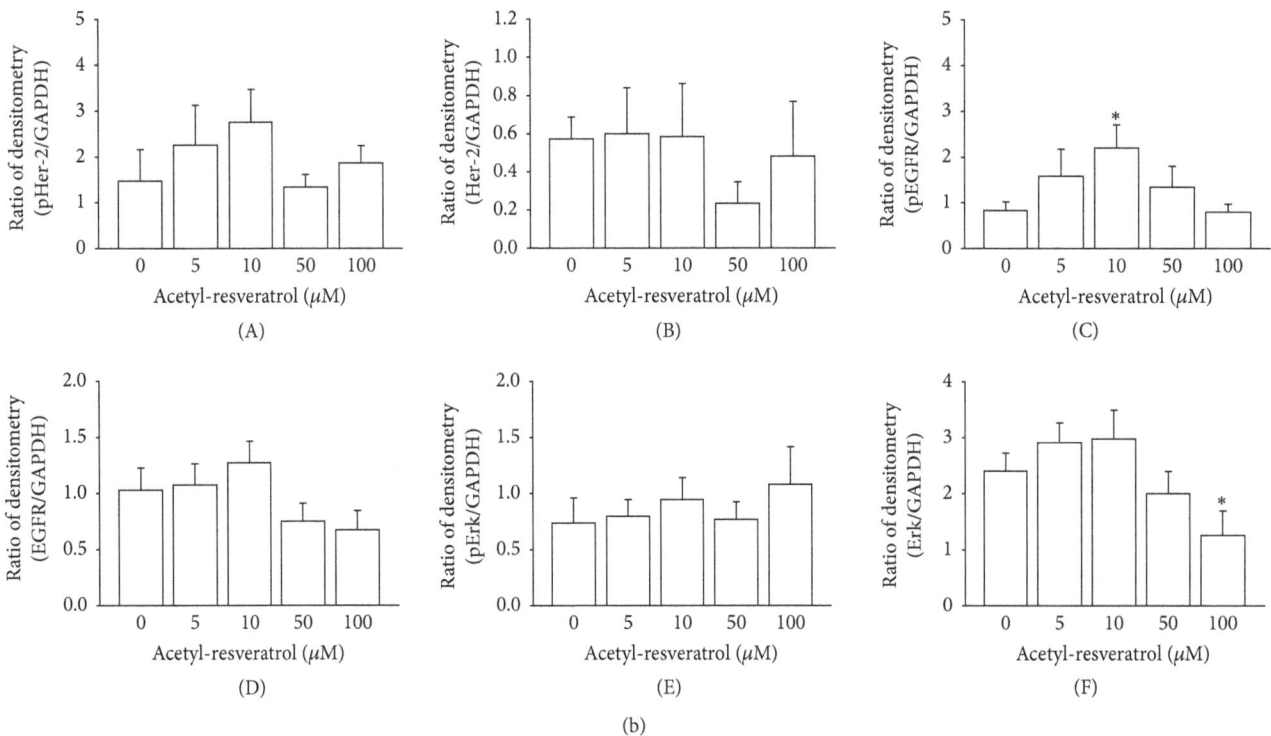

(b)

FIGURE 5: In SKOV-3 cell aggregates, acetyl-resveratrol did not alter the expression of Her-2, but it increased the phosphorylation of EGFR at 10 μM (C). The total expression of Erk was significantly reduced (F). * refers to statistically significant as p value less than 0.05 compared to the control.

and 100 μM. Our results show that the compounds with higher concentrations lead to a decrease in the size of 3D cell aggregates, but at the more physiological concentrations they show no marked measurable effect. At the higher concentrations, the three compounds induce apoptosis in the SKOV-3 cells, but only resveratrol and acetyl-resveratrol exhibit measurable apoptosis in OVCAR-8. Our present study is in line with previous studies that the 3D cell aggregates derived from cancer cells show some inherent apoptosis and that the fraction of apoptotic cells resembles that in a solid

(a)

(b)

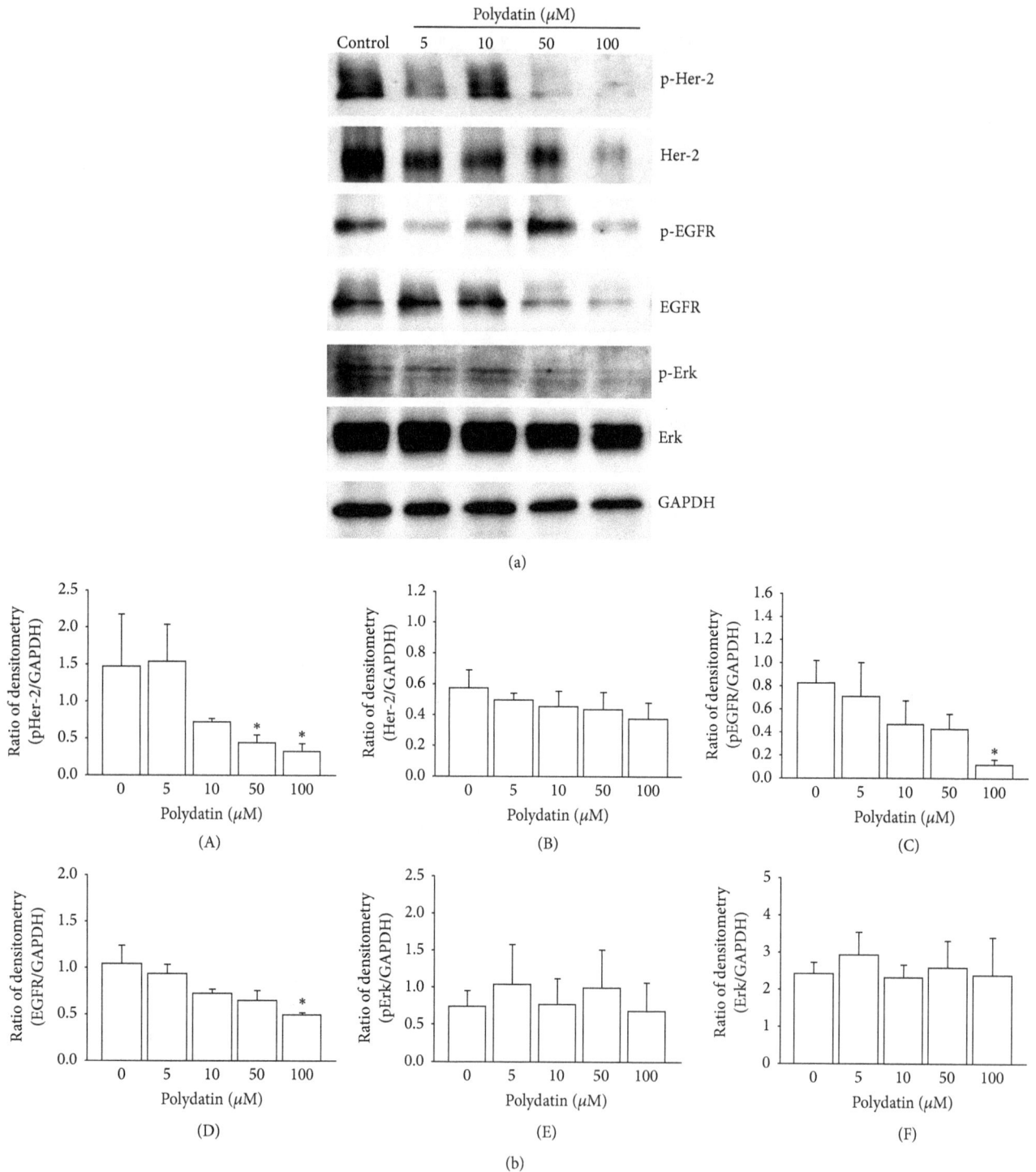

FIGURE 6: In SKOV-3 cell aggregates, the phosphorylation of Her-2 (A) and EGFR (B) was significantly reduced at higher concentrations of polydatin. The total expression of EGFR was significantly reduced with 100 μM polydatin (D). There was no effect on Erk1/2 (E). ∗ refers to statistically significant as p value less than 0.05 compared to the control.

tumour [23, 24]. It has been reported that the status of p53 is a determinant factor of apoptosis. Cancer cells with the p53 wild type are more sensitive to cytotoxic DNA damage and can undergo apoptosis more readily than p53 mutant cells [25]. However, there are also reports that apoptosis is independent of the p53 wild type or mutant [26, 27]. The SKOV-3 cell line has a null $p53$ gene [28] and OVCAR-8 cell line has p53 mutation [19]. Therefore, our data is consistent with those that suggest that resveratrol and its derivatives cause apoptosis by a p53-independent pathway [29, 30].

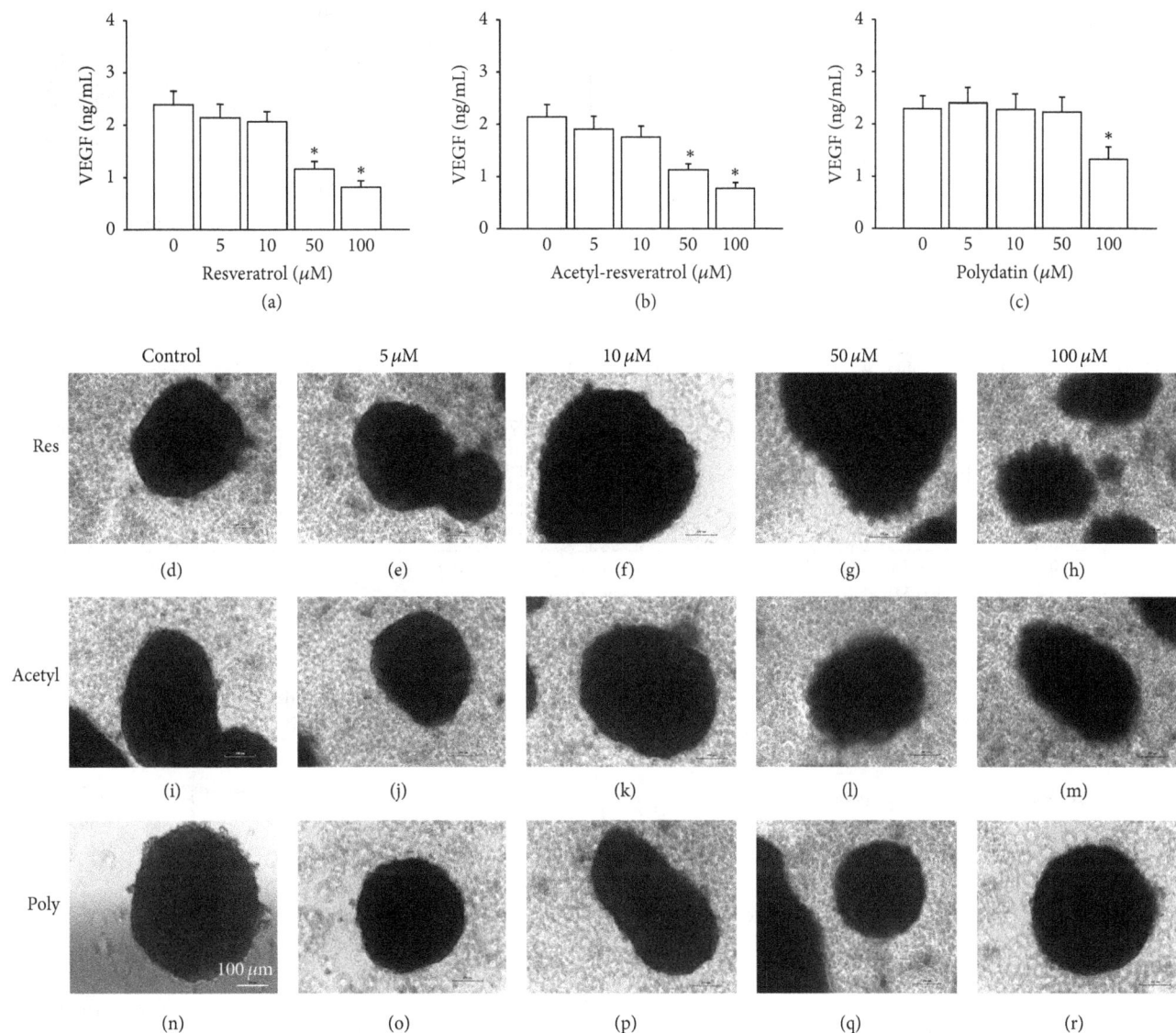

FIGURE 7: The secretion of vascular endothelial growth factor (VEGF) of SKOV-3 cell aggregates (a–c) and the morphology of OVCAR-8 3D spheroids (d–r). Higher doses of resveratrol (a), acetyl-resveratrol (b), and polydatin (c) significantly reduced the secretion of VEGF. High concentrations of resveratrol (g and h) and acetyl-resveratrol (l and m) caused the irregular rims of spheroids. Polydatin (q and r) did not show any effect. ∗ refers to statistically significant as p value less than 0.05 compared to the control.

There are a few reports suggesting effects of resveratrol on 3D cell cultures. Resveratrol has been shown to inhibit growth of 3D cell spheroids of some types of cancers [31–33]. Higher doses of resveratrol compromise the mitochondrial membrane and trigger apoptosis in spheroids of lung cancer [34]. Using the 3D cell aggregates of SKOV-3 and OVCAR-8 cells, our results confirm that at higher concentrations of resveratrol and, for the first time, acetyl-resveratrol and polydatin can alter the profile of some cell signalling molecules. We show that resveratrol and polydatin at higher concentrations can inhibit the activation of Her-2 and EGFR in SKOV-3 line and may affect growth inhibition through the attenuation of MAPK signalling cascade [35, 36]. Acetyl-resveratrol does not have the same effect. In the present study, we also used the EGFR/Her-2 negative cell line, OVCAR-8, to investigate the

effect of resveratrol and its derivatives. Resveratrol and acetyl-resveratrol are able to reduce the activation of Erk following the higher concentrations, but they are likely to increase the activation of Erk at the lower concentrations suggesting that this activity may be EGFR/Her-2 independent. Bifunctional actions of resveratrol have been reported in studies of breast cancer; lower concentrations increase Her-2 expression, but higher doses showed the opposite effect [37]. We observe this effect in resveratrol and acetyl-resveratrol treated OVCAR-8 cells with the modulation of Erk activation. However, our results show that at lower concentrations acetyl-resveratrol increases the active forms of Her-2 and EGFR in SKOV-3 cells.

Differing mechanisms of action of resveratrol have been shown in different cancer cell lines using *in vitro* 2D

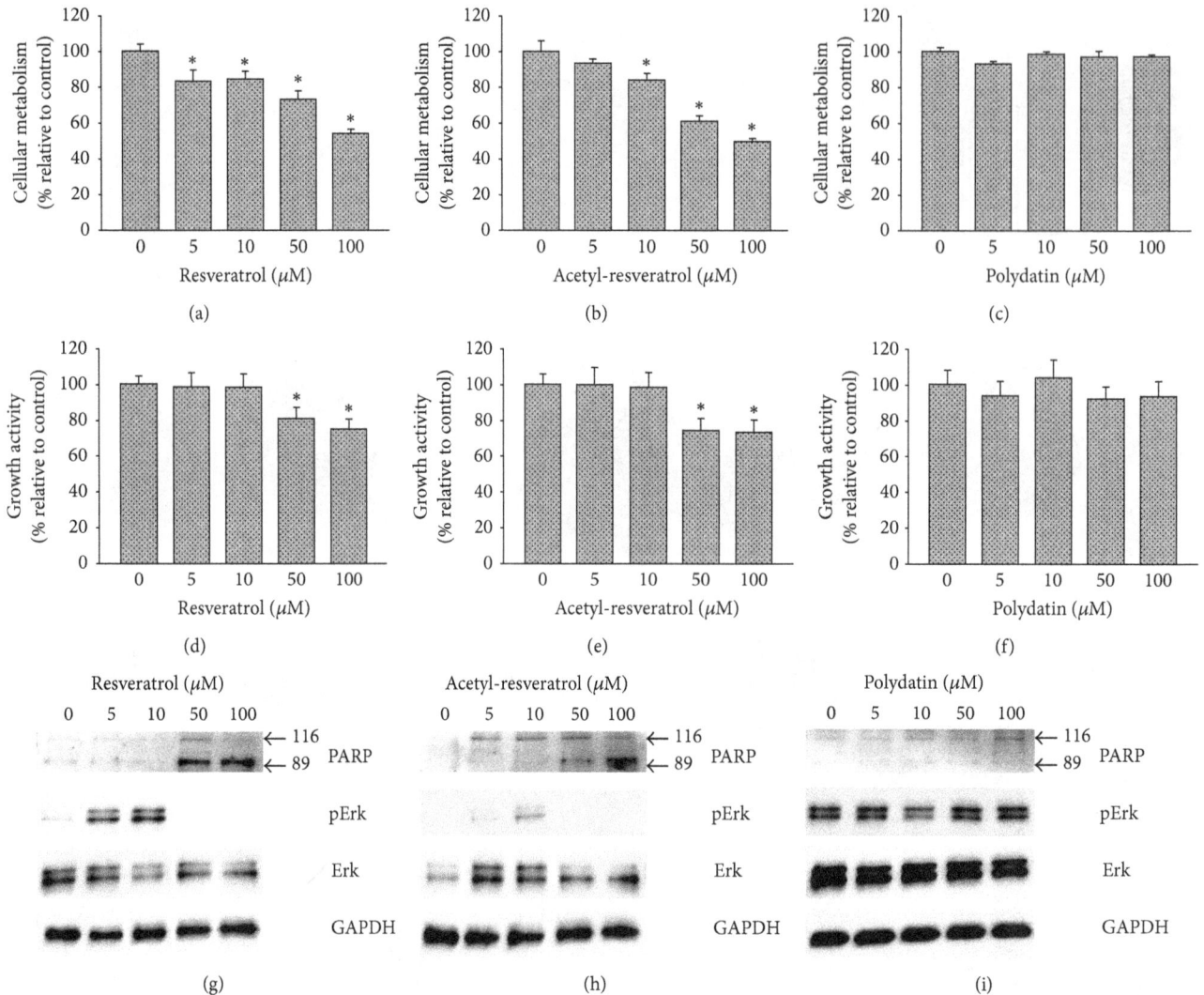

FIGURE 8: The effects of cellular metabolism, growth activity, and modulation of selective proteins following treatment of resveratrol, acetyl-resveratrol, and polydatin in OVCAR-8 spheroids. Resveratrol (a) and acetyl-resveratrol (b) reduced cellular metabolism in a dose-dependent manner. Higher concentrations of both these compounds also reduced growth activity (d and e). Polydatin showed limited effects (c and f). Both resveratrol (g) and acetyl-resveratrol (h) induced the increased expression of 89 kDa PARP-1. The activation of Erk was increased following 5 and 10 μ resveratrol and acetyl-resveratrol exposure. ∗ refers to statistically significant as p value less than 0.05 compared to the control.

cell monolayers. In monolayers, nonphysiological doses of resveratrol show antitumour activity via multiple signalling pathways that regulate cell growth, survival, migration, invasion, and adhesion in various types of cancer cells [6, 8, 35, 38]. There are a few reports showing that physiological concentrations of resveratrol can elicit antitumour activities, but this effect is cancer-cell-type-specific [39]. In cell monolayers of ovarian cancer cell lines, resveratrol at 25 μM did not show any antiproliferative activity [40]. Mitochondrial activity was reduced after 72 hr incubation of OVCAR-3 cell line with 12.5 μM resveratrol, but it did not markedly modulate signalling protein molecules [30]. Raj et al. [41] reported that the continual treatment with 0.5 and 5 μM resveratrol for 6 days significantly reduced the mitochondrial activity in a cell monolayer of SKOV-3 cells but did not

induce apoptosis. Our results show that resveratrol, but not acetyl-resveratrol nor polydatin, elicits antigrowth activity at lower concentrations in SKOV-3 cell aggregates, which is consistent with the previous finding in a colorectal cancer cell model [36]. Furthermore, physiological concentrations of resveratrol and acetyl-resveratrol significantly reduced cellular metabolism in OVCAR-8 spheroids.

In the current study, it is likely that the relative efficacies of resveratrol, acetyl-resveratrol, and polydatin against 3D cell aggregates may be due to their differing functional groups. Resveratrol has three hydroxyl (–OH) functional groups and by replacing these with acetyl groups (–COCH$_3$) to form acetyl-resveratrol this can still elicit growth inhibition in 3D cell aggregates (Figure 1) with a similar degree of potency to resveratrol itself. However, polydatin which contains a large hydrophilic glucose molecule is less potent, and it is possible that the glucose functional group may affect the ability of polydatin to enter the cells. Our results are consistent with another study in which polydatin has been shown to have less potency than resveratrol *in vitro* [38]. Despite this, polydatin has been shown to reduce mitochondrial activity in human nasopharyngeal carcinoma cells at 5 and 10 μM using the MTT assay to demonstrate the effects *in vitro* [14] which may indicate some degree of permeability and it does not inhibit DNA synthesis *in vitro* in Lewis lung carcinoma cell line at concentrations of 10 and 100 μM [15].

There have been limited reports as to the mechanism of action of acetyl-resveratrol both *in vitro* and *in vivo*. Acetyl-resveratrol has been shown to inhibit the cell cycle in established cancer cell lines and have synergistic actions with cytotoxic drugs [42, 43]. At lower concentrations, it can increase the level of mRNA antioxidant proteins, suggesting that acetyl-resveratrol may act as a chemopreventive compound [12]. In a cell-free system, acetyl-resveratrol is converted back to resveratrol by the hydrolysis of the acetyl motif by intracellular esterases. Acetyl-resveratrol is metabolized and converted back to resveratrol that can be detected in plasma of a mouse model [7].

While our results show different antigrowth properties of resveratrol and its derivatives under *in vitro* conditions, their *in vivo* actions are still unknown. Therefore, it is important to confirm the data in an animal model. There are numerous studies showing that metabolized resveratrol can elicit biological activities. In one clinical trial colorectal cancer patients were given 1 gram of resveratrol daily for 8 days prior to surgical removal of the tumour. These showed a reduction of cancer cell proliferation by 5% [44]. However, after ingestion of 5 grams of resveratrol, the bioavailable level in the plasma is between 2.4 and 4.2 μM. This reduces dramatically 60 minutes after ingestion [6, 11]. However, metabolized forms of resveratrol such as resveratrol-sulphate and resveratrol-glucuronide can be found at levels that are significantly higher than the parental compound in the plasma of humans [44]. Resveratrol-sulphate has been shown to inhibit NF-Kb, COX-1 and COX-2 activation in an *in vitro* study [45]. Polydatin has shown promising results in *in vivo* studies. After ingestion of polydatin, resveratrol has been found in the small intestine and faeces, suggesting that the polydatin can be converted to active resveratrol *in vivo* [13]. Polydatin has been shown to reduce the production of inflammatory molecules via the inactivation of NF-kB pathway in mice with ulcerative colitis [16]. The antitumour and antimetastatic activity of polydatin in Lewis lung carcinoma xenografts might be due to the inhibition of angiogenesis of endothelial cells [15].

VEGF is a potent angiogenic peptide secreted from a number of cells in the human body including cancer cells. Women with ovarian cancer produce high levels of VEGF and show signs of tumour progression and typically have a short-term survival [46]. Resveratrol and acetyl-resveratrol show reduction of VEGF secretion at higher concentrations, possibly associated with the reduction of cell numbers. Again, polydatin shows less of an effect. The direct targets of resveratrol with respect to its ability to suppress VEGF in cancer cells are still under investigation. Some studies suggest

that resveratrol may inhibit the NF-kB pathway that may hamper the transcriptional capacity of VEGF gene promoter [6].

5. Conclusion

Taken together, our results suggest that resveratrol and the derivatives, acetyl-resveratrol and polydatin, have antigrowth activities against 3D cell aggregates of ovarian cancer cell lines regardless of the level expression of EGFR and Her-2. The growth inhibition is concentration dependent. The interaction of resveratrol and its derivatives, acetyl-resveratrol and polydatin, with signalling proteins may cause downstream events that lead to apoptosis and growth inhibition. Identification of the exact target molecules is a challenging yet promising area that warrants more research. We conclude that the antigrowth activities of derivatives of resveratrol warrant further studies especially using *in vivo* animal models in order to translate their antitumour effects prior to any clinical trial.

Conflict of Interests

The authors declare that there is no conflict of interests regarding the publication of this paper.

Acknowledgments

This study was supported by the Ovarian Cancer Research Foundation (OCRF), Melbourne, Australia, and internal research grants from the Department of Obstetrics and Gynaecology at the University of Otago, and the University of Canterbury.

References

[1] R. C. Bast Jr., B. Hennessy, and G. B. Mills, "The biology of ovarian cancer: new opportunities for translation," *Nature Reviews Cancer*, vol. 9, no. 6, pp. 415–428, 2009.

[2] E. Lengyel, "Ovarian cancer development and metastasis," *The American Journal of Pathology*, vol. 177, no. 3, pp. 1053–1064, 2010.

[3] S. M. Moghaddam, A. Amini, D. L. Morris, and M. H. Pourgholami, "Significance of vascular endothelial growth factor in growth and peritoneal dissemination of ovarian cancer," *Cancer and Metastasis Reviews*, vol. 31, no. 1-2, pp. 143–162, 2012.

[4] J. S. Nielsen, E. Jakobsen, B. Hølund, K. Bertelsen, and A. Jakobsen, "Prognostic significance of p53, Her-2, and EGFR overexpression in borderline and epithelial ovarian cancer," *International Journal of Gynecological Cancer*, vol. 14, no. 6, pp. 1086–1096, 2004.

[5] P. M. Harari, G. W. Allen, and J. A. Bonner, "Biology of interactions: antiepidermal growth factor receptor agents," *Journal of Clinical Oncology*, vol. 25, no. 26, pp. 4057–4065, 2007.

[6] J. K. Kundu and Y.-J. Surh, "Cancer chemopreventive and therapeutic potential of resveratrol: mechanistic perspectives," *Cancer Letters*, vol. 269, no. 2, pp. 243–261, 2008.

[7] G. W. Osmond, E. M. Masko, D. S. Tyler, S. J. Freedland, and S. Pizzo, "*In vitro* and *in vivo* evaluation of resveratrol and

3,5-dihydroxy-4′-acetoxy-trans-stilbene in the treatment of human prostate carcinoma and melanoma," *Journal of Surgical Research*, vol. 179, no. 1, pp. E141–E148, 2013.

[8] K. S. Stakleff, T. Sloan, D. Blanco, S. Marcanthony, T. Booth, and A. Bishayee, "Resveratrol exerts differential effects *in vitro* and *in vivo* against ovarian cancer cells," *Asian Pacific Journal of Cancer Prevention*, vol. 13, no. 4, pp. 1333–1340, 2012.

[9] J. C. Klink, A. K. Tewari, E. M. Masko et al., "Resveratrol worsens survival in SCID mice with prostate cancer xenografts in a cell-line specific manner, through paradoxical effects on oncogenic pathways," *Prostate*, vol. 73, no. 7, pp. 754–762, 2013.

[10] K. P. L. Bhat and J. M. Pezzuto, "Cancer chemopreventive activity of resveratrol," *Annals of the New York Academy of Sciences*, vol. 957, pp. 210–229, 2002.

[11] D. J. Boocock, G. E. S. Faust, K. R. Patel et al., "Phase I dose escalation pharmacokinetic study in healthy volunteers of resveratrol, a potential cancer chemopreventive agent," *Cancer Epidemiology Biomarkers and Prevention*, vol. 16, no. 6, pp. 1246–1252, 2007.

[12] X.-L. Tan, G. Marquardt, A. B. Massimi, M. Shi, W. Han, and S. D. Spivack, "High-throughput library screening identifies two novel NQO1 inducers in human lung cells," *American Journal of Respiratory Cell and Molecular Biology*, vol. 46, no. 3, pp. 365–371, 2012.

[13] W. Zhang, Q. Li, M. Zhu, Q. Huang, Y. Jia, and K. Bi, "Direct determination of polydatin and its metabolite in rat excrement samples by high-performance liquid chromatography," *Chemical and Pharmaceutical Bulletin*, vol. 56, no. 11, pp. 1592–1595, 2008.

[14] H. Liu, S. Zhao, Y. Zhang et al., "Reactive oxygen species-mediated endoplasmic reticulum stress and mitochondrial dysfunction contribute to polydatin-induced apoptosis in human nasopharyngeal carcinoma CNE cells," *Journal of Cellular Biochemistry*, vol. 112, no. 12, pp. 3695–3703, 2011.

[15] Y. Kimura and H. Okuda, "Effects of naturally occurring stilbene glucosides from medicinal plants and wine, on tumour growth and lung metastasis in lewis lung carcinoma-bearing mice," *Journal of Pharmacy and Pharmacology*, vol. 52, no. 10, pp. 1287–1295, 2000.

[16] J. Yao, J.-Y. Wang, L. Liu et al., "Polydatin ameliorates DSS-induced colitis in mice through inhibition of nuclear factor-kappaB activation," *Planta Medica*, vol. 77, no. 5, pp. 421–427, 2011.

[17] S. Zhou, R. Yang, Z. Teng et al., "Dose-dependent absorption and metabolism of trans-polydatin in rats," *Journal of Agricultural and Food Chemistry*, vol. 57, no. 11, pp. 4572–4579, 2009.

[18] G. Lv, H. Gu, S. Chen, Z. Lou, and L. Shan, "Pharmacokinetic profile of 2,3,5,4′-tetrahydroxystilbene-2-O-β-D-glucoside in mice after oral administration of *Polygonum multiflorum* extract," *Drug Development and Industrial Pharmacy*, vol. 38, no. 2, pp. 248–255, 2012.

[19] S. Domcke, R. Sinha, D. A. Levine, C. Sander, and N. Schultz, "Evaluating cell lines as tumour models by comparison of genomic profiles," *Nature Communications*, vol. 4, article 2126, 2013.

[20] S. Kobold, S. Hegewisch-Becker, K. Oechsle, K. Jordan, C. Bokemeyer, and D. Atanackovic, "Intraperitoneal VEGF inhibition using bevacizumab: a potential approach for the symptomatic treatment of malignant ascites?" *Oncologist*, vol. 14, no. 12, pp. 1242–1251, 2009.

[21] K. L. Sodek, M. J. Ringuette, and T. J. Brown, "Compact spheroid formation by ovarian cancer cells is associated with contractile

behavior and an invasive phenotype," *International Journal of Cancer*, vol. 124, no. 9, pp. 2060–2070, 2009.

[22] J. Myungjin Lee, P. Mhawech-Fauceglia, N. Lee et al., "A three-dimensional microenvironment alters protein expression and chemosensitivity of epithelial ovarian cancer cells *in vitro*," *Laboratory Investigation*, vol. 93, no. 5, pp. 528–542, 2013.

[23] F. Hirschhaeuser, T. Leidig, B. Rodday, C. Lindemann, and W. Mueller-Klieser, "Test system for trifunctional antibodies in 3D MCTS culture," *Journal of Biomolecular Screening*, vol. 14, no. 8, pp. 980–990, 2009.

[24] A. Nyga, U. Cheema, and M. Loizidou, "3D tumour models: novel *in vitro* approaches to cancer studies," *Journal of Cell Communication and Signaling*, vol. 5, no. 3, pp. 239–248, 2011.

[25] A. V. Gudkov and E. A. Komarova, "Pathologies associated with the p53 response," *Cold Spring Harbor Perspectives in Biology*, vol. 2, no. 7, Article ID a001180, 2010.

[26] C. S. Moreno, L. Matyunina, E. B. Dickerson et al., "Evidence that p53-mediated cell-cycle-arrest inhibits chemotherapeutic treatment of ovarian carcinomas," *PLoS ONE*, vol. 2, no. 5, article e441, 2007.

[27] B. Pandit and A. L. Gartel, "Proteasome inhibitors induce p53-independent apoptosis in human cancer cells," *The American Journal of Pathology*, vol. 178, no. 1, pp. 355–360, 2011.

[28] L. Farrand, S. Byun, J. Y. Kim et al., "Piceatannol enhances cisplatin sensitivity in ovarian cancer via modulation of p53, X-linked inhibitor of apoptosis protein (XIAP), and mitochondrial fission," *Journal of Biological Chemistry*, vol. 288, no. 33, pp. 23740–23750, 2013.

[29] A. Kueck, A. W. Opipari Jr., K. A. Griffith et al., "Resveratrol inhibits glucose metabolism in human ovarian cancer cells," *Gynecologic Oncology*, vol. 107, no. 3, pp. 450–457, 2007.

[30] D. Vergara, P. Simeone, D. Toraldo et al., "Resveratrol down-regulates Akt/GSK and ERK signalling pathways in OVCAR-3 ovarian cancer cells," *Molecular BioSystems*, vol. 8, no. 4, pp. 1078–1087, 2012.

[31] L. Roncoroni, L. Elli, E. Dolfini et al., "Resveratrol inhibits cell growth in a human cholangiocarcinoma cell line," *Liver International*, vol. 28, no. 10, pp. 1426–1436, 2008.

[32] S. Günther, C. Ruhe, M. G. Derikito, G. Böse, H. Sauer, and M. Wartenberg, "Polyphenols prevent cell shedding from mouse mammary cancer spheroids and inhibit cancer cell invasion in confrontation cultures derived from embryonic stem cells," *Cancer Letters*, vol. 250, no. 1, pp. 25–35, 2007.

[33] E. Dolfini, L. Roncoroni, E. Dogliotti et al., "Resveratrol impairs the formation of MDA-MB-231 multicellular tumor spheroids concomitant with ceramide accumulation," *Cancer Letters*, vol. 249, no. 2, pp. 143–147, 2007.

[34] X.-X. Wang, Y.-B. Li, H.-J. Yao et al., "The use of mitochondrial targeting resveratrol liposomes modified with a dequalinium polyethylene glycol-distearoylphosphatidyl ethanolamine conjugate to induce apoptosis in resistant lung cancer cells," *Biomaterials*, vol. 32, no. 24, pp. 5673–5687, 2011.

[35] K. J. Jeong, K. H. Cho, N. Panupinthu et al., "EGFR mediates LPA-induced proteolytic enzyme expression and ovarian cancer invasion: inhibition by resveratrol," *Molecular Oncology*, vol. 7, no. 1, pp. 121–129, 2013.

[36] A. P. N. Majumdar, S. Banerjee, J. Nautiyal et al., "Curcumin synergizes with resveratrol to inhibit colon cancer," *Nutrition and Cancer*, vol. 61, no. 4, pp. 544–553, 2009.

[37] H. K. Choi, J. W. Yang, and K. W. Kang, "Bifunctional effect of resveratrol on the expression of ErbB2 in human breast cancer cell," *Cancer Letters*, vol. 242, no. 2, pp. 198–206, 2006.

[38] D. Su, Y. Cheng, M. Liu et al., "Comparision of piceid and resveratrol in antioxidation and antiproliferation activities *in vitro*," *PLoS ONE*, vol. 8, no. 1, Article ID e54505, 2013.

[39] W. Nutakul, H. S. Sobers, P. Qiu et al., "Inhibitory effects of resveratrol and pterostilbene on human colon cancer cells: a side by side comparison," *Journal of Agricultural and Food Chemistry*, vol. 59, no. 20, pp. 10964–10970, 2011.

[40] P. Marimuthu, K. Kaur, U. Kandalam et al., "Treatment of ovarian cancer cells with nutlin-3 and resveratrol combination leads to apoptosis via caspase activation," *Journal of Medicinal Food*, vol. 14, no. 1-2, pp. 46–52, 2011.

[41] M. H. G. Raj, Z. Y. Abd Elmageed, J. Zhou et al., "Synergistic action of dietary phyto-antioxidants on survival and proliferation of ovarian cancer cells," *Gynecologic Oncology*, vol. 110, no. 3, pp. 432–438, 2008.

[42] A.-K. Marel, G. Lizard, J.-C. Izard, N. Latruffe, and D. Delmas, "Inhibitory effects of trans-resveratrol analogs molecules on the proliferation and the cell cycle progression of human colon tumoral cells," *Molecular Nutrition and Food Research*, vol. 52, no. 5, pp. 538–548, 2008.

[43] D. Colin, A. Gimazane, G. Lizard et al., "Effects of resveratrol analogs on cell cycle progression, cell cycle associated proteins and 5fluoro-uracil sensitivity in human derived colon cancer cells," *International Journal of Cancer*, vol. 124, no. 12, pp. 2780–2788, 2009.

[44] K. R. Patel, V. A. Brown, D. J. L. Jones et al., "Clinical pharmacology of resveratrol and its metabolites in colorectal cancer patients," *Cancer Research*, vol. 70, no. 19, pp. 7392–7399, 2010.

[45] B. Calamini, K. Ratia, M. G. Malkowski et al., "Pleiotropic mechanisms facilitated by resveratrol and its metabolites," *Biochemical Journal*, vol. 429, no. 2, pp. 273–282, 2010.

[46] W. A. Spannuth, A. M. Nick, N. B. Jennings et al., "Functional significance of VEGFR-2 on ovarian cancer cells," *International Journal of Cancer*, vol. 124, no. 5, pp. 1045–1053, 2009.

9

Ultrastructure of Placenta of Gravidas with Gestational Diabetes Mellitus

Qian Meng,[1,2] Li Shao,[2] Xiucui Luo,[1] Yingping Mu,[1] Wen Xu,[1] Chao Gao,[2] Li Gao,[2] Jiayin Liu,[2] and Yugui Cui[2]

[1]*Department of Obstetrics, Lianyungang Maternity and Child Health Care Hospital, Lianyungang 222000, China*
[2]*The State Key Laboratory of Reproductive Medicine, Center of Clinical Reproductive Medicine,*
 First Affiliated Hospital of Nanjing Medical University, 300 Guangzhou Road, Nanjing 210029, China

Correspondence should be addressed to Yugui Cui; cuiygnj@njmu.edu.cn

Academic Editor: Gian Carlo Di Renzo

Objectives. Gestational diabetes mellitus (GDM) leads to an abnormal placental environment which may cause some structural alterations of placenta and affect placental development and function. In this study, the ultrastructural appearances of term placentas from women with GDM and normal pregnancy were meticulously compared. *Materials and Methods.* The placenta tissues of term birth from 10 women with GDM and 10 women with normal pregnancy were applied with the signed informed consent. The morphology of fetomaternal interface of placenta was examined using light microscopy (LM) and transmission electron microscopy (TEM). *Results.* On LM, the following morphological changes in villous tissues were found in the GDM placentas when compared with the control placentas: edematous stroma, apparent increase in the number of syncytial knots, and perivillous fibrin deposition. On TEM, the distinct ultrastructural alterations indicating the degeneration of terminal villi were found in the GDM placentas as follows: thickening of the basal membrane (BM) of vasculosyncytial membrane (VSM) and the VSM itself, significantly fewer or even absent syncytiotrophoblastic microvilli, swollen or completely destroyed mitochondria and endoplasmic reticulum, and syncytiotrophoblasts with multiple vacuoles. *Conclusion.* Ultrastructural differences exist between GDM and control placentas. The differences of placenta ultrastructure are likely responsible for the impairment of placental barrier and function in GDM.

1. Introduction

Gestational diabetes mellitus (GDM) is defined as the glucose intolerance with onset or first recognition during pregnancy [1]. GDM affects 4%–7% of pregnant population in the United States [2, 3] and 6.8% in China [4]. GDM is associated with short- and long-term morbidity in both offspring and mother. The short-term adverse outcomes include macrosomia, neonatal hypoglycemia, neonatal jaundice, preeclampsia, preterm delivery, and cesarean delivery, while the long-term complications include obesity, abnormal glucose tolerance and diabetes in adolescence, or early adulthood. Meanwhile, the concept of the fetal origin diseases has been seriously taken including imprinting genes and epigenetics study.

Placenta plays critical roles during pregnancy, including the exchange of nutrients, water, respiratory gases, and waste products and the synthesis of various hormones which regulate the transport of maternal fuels to the fetus and facilitate maternal metabolic adaptation to different pregnancy stages. These functions are determined by the structure, ultrastructure, and function of the placental exchange barrier. The vasculosyncytial membrane (VSM) [5, 6] is an important feature of placental barrier, which is composed of different overlapping structures including a continuous maternal-facing syncytiotrophoblastic layer with multiple apical microvilli, the endothelial lining and underlying basal membrane (BM) of the fetal capillaries, and the villous connective tissue between them. The most significant properties of VSM are to maintain the exchange surface area between the fetomaternal surfaces [7]. The increased thickness of VSM and reduced area of exchange related to fetal hypoxia appear to subject fetus to considerable risks [8].

TABLE 1: Clinical characteristics of women with GDM ($n = 10$) and control group ($n = 10$).

Characteristics	GDM group ($n = 10$)	Control group ($n = 10$)	P value
Maternal age (yr)	30.40 ± 4.90	28.50 ± 3.57	0.34
Weight (kg)	83.55 ± 12.03	73.20 ± 6.52	0.03
Nulliparous (n)	7	8	—
Gestational weeks at delivery	39.00 ± 0.90	39.41 ± 0.96	0.34
Mode of delivery	Caesarean	Caesarean	—
Birth weight (g)	3690 ± 640	3690 ± 390	1.0
Infant sex			
Male	5	4	—
Female	5	6	—

It was found that several ST cells in GDM placentas showed the dilation of rough and smooth endoplasmic reticulum (ER), loss and alteration of microvilli, large vacuoles just beneath the plasma membrane, and mitochondrial irregularities [9]. However, since the placenta is a structurally complex organ composed of many cell types with different origins, it is necessary to obtain the detailed information using systematic ultrastructural examinations. In this study, the morphological and ultrastructural appearances in GDM placentas were investigated using both light microscopy (LM) and transmission electron microscopy (TEM), so as to explore its effect on the placenta functions and fetal development, as well as the fetal origin diseases.

2. Materials and Methods

2.1. Subjects. A 75-goral glucose tolerance test (OGTT) was performed with plasma glucose measurement fasting and at 1 and 2 h for women at 24–28 weeks of gestation who were not previously diagnosed with overt diabetes. The OGTT should be performed in the morning after an overnight fast of at least 8 h. The diagnosis of GDM is made when any of the following plasma glucose values are exceeded based on the American Diabetes Association (2011) [1]: fasting ≥ 5.1 mmol/L (92 mg/dL); 1 hour ≥ 10.0 mmol/L (180 mg/dL); 2 hours ≥ 8.5 mmol/L (153 mg/dL). Women with a history of pregestational diabetes and those with a nonsingleton index pregnancy were excluded. After GDM was diagnosed, those GDM women were asked to control diet in order that their fasting blood glucoses were kept in the satisfying range (3.3 to 5.6 mmol/L). Until delivery, eight GDM women (8/10) kept in the A1 class (fasting glucose less than 5.8 mmol/L, postprandial blood glucose less than 6.7 mmol/L) after good diet control (see Supplemental Table 1 in Supplementary Material available online at http://dx.doi.org/10.1155/2015/283124). Two GDM women (2/10) were classed as A2 (fasting blood glucose higher than or equal to 5.8 mmol/L, postprandial blood glucose higher than or equal to 6.7 mmol/L) because of their poor diet control. The levels of fasting blood glucose and HbA1c in those GDM women with good diet control in the last weeks of gestation were kept in the range of 5.1 to 5.6 mmol/L. However, level of fasting blood glucose (6.1 and 11.3 mmol/L) and level of HbA1c (10.2 and 10.3 mmol/L) in

two GDM women with poor diet control were higher than the satisfactory criteria. The clinical data on maternal age and weight, number of gestational weeks, mode of delivery, birth weight, and weight of placenta were summarized in Table 1. Women with normal pregnancies matched with GDM women for number of gestational weeks, maternal age, and mode of delivery were recruited as control (Supplemental Table 2). In each group, 10 placental samples were collected with the signed infoemed consent. The study procedure was approved by the Ethics Committee of the First Affiliated Hospital of Nanjing Medical University.

2.2. Placental Sample Collection. All selected subjects adopted the cesarean delivery due to other reasons. Placental specimens were weighed and performed on the basis of obstetric indications. The issue specimen was dissected from the placental subchorial zone corresponding to the umbilical cord insertion (~5 cm away from the site of cord insertion), while avoiding area of infarction and hematomas. Placenta with abnormal umbilical cord insertions, such as velamentous cord insertion, was excluded. Fragments from the placenta were cut longitudinally from the maternal side to the fetal side. Placental tissues were divided into three parts, as described by Sood et al. [10]: maternal, middle, and fetal. The middle part, comprising homogeneous villous tissues, was collected and floated in ice-cold phosphate-buffered saline (PBS), cleaned of blood, and immediately cut into double four $1 \times 1 \times 1$ cm fragments, which were fixed either with 4% paraformaldehyde or with 2.5% glutaraldehyde at $4°C$ for further LM and TEM examinations, respectively. To minimize the variation among villous tissue blocks collected from four different placental sites in both groups, four blocks from each placenta were randomly examined.

2.3. LM Examination. Three paraffin-embedded blocks from four paraformaldehyde-fixed tissues and from each placenta were randomly selected. Sections (thickness, 4 μm) were cut from each block and stained with hematoxylin and eosin (HE). The slides were observed under an Axioskop 2 Plus microscope (Carl Zeiss) and photographed. The HE-stained sections were carefully analyzed to provide a general view of the section and to confirm that the sections had appropriate

TABLE 2: Terminal villi were evaluated with respect to cytoplasmic vacuoles, pyknosis, and edema in the stroma, according to the semi-quantitative score based on the degree of ultrastructural change.

Characteristics	0	1	2	3
Cytoplasmic vacuoles	None	Sporadic vacuoles	Moderate degenerative vacuolation	Distinct degenerative vacuolation
Pyknosis	None	Mild pyknosis	Moderate pyknosis	Obvious pyknosis
Stroma edema	None	Mild	Moderate	Massive
Mitochondria	None	Mildly swollen	Obviously swollen	Completely destroyed
Endoplasmic reticulum	None	Mildly swollen	Obviously swollen	Completely destroyed

histological features and were suitable for the subsequent TEM examination.

2.4. TEM Examination. From each placenta, three villous tissue blocks were prepared for ultrastructural examination using TEM. The samples were fixed in 2.5% glutaraldehyde in cacodylate buffer and stored in cacodylate buffer with 0.05 M saccharose (pH, 7.2) at 4°C until processing. The villous tissues were subsequently postfixed in 1% OsO_4 for 2 h at 4°C, routinely processed in a graded series of acetone, infiltrated with acetone-araldite, and embedded in araldite. For orientation, semithin sections (thickness, 1 μm) were stained with thionine. Ultrathin sections (thickness, 80 nm) were treated (double contrast) with uranyl acetate (25 min) and 8% lead nitrate (5 min) and then systematically examined using a JEM-1010 electron microscope (JEOL Ltd.).

Terminal villi were evaluated with respect to the placental blood barrier (thickness of VSM, thickness of syncytiotrophoblast BM, and thickness of endothelial BM), villous stroma (villous edema), and cytotrophoblasts (CTs) and syncytiotrophoblast (ST) along with their substructures (microvillous density per unit surface area, cytoplasmic vacuolization, pyknosis, mitochondria, and ER). Ultrastructural findings were compared with quantitative measured data and assigned a semiquantitative score based on the degree of alteration in the ultrastructure (Table 2). Five fields of vision were randomly selected from each tissue block and systematically investigated at 5,000x, 12,000x, and 25,000x magnification for quantitative analysis. Thus, 15 random fields of vision were recorded and analyzed per placenta to minimize interindividual differences. In each field of vision, the following three measurements were performed: (1) thickness of VSM was measured from the intervillous space to the fetal vessels, perpendicular to the BM, under 5,000x magnification, (2) microvillous density was counted per 10 μm of length under 12,000x magnification, and (3) thickness of the ST BM and endothelial BM was measured under 25,000x magnification. Images were analyzed using the TEM Image Platform (Olympus) to perform random measurements. Two operators severally performed the microscopic analyses and were blinded to the placental groups. The third person collected data from two operators and performed statistical analyses.

2.5. Statistical Analysis. Data were expressed as the mean and standard deviation (SD). Statistical analyses were performed using the SPSS software (Statistical Analysis System, version 17.0 for Windows). Statistical difference between two groups was analyzed using the Student t-test. Statistical significance was set at $P < 0.05$.

3. Results

3.1. Histological Examination. The normal morphophysiological characteristics of term placenta of control group were showed in Figures 1(a) and 1(b). Multigrade branching of villous trees lined with STs was observed. The fetal blood vessels were remarkable with clearly evident erythrocytes inside multiple placental villi. No obvious calcification processes, fibrin deposition, or villous edema was found. Typical morphological figures of term placenta of GDM group were showed in Figures 1(c) and 1(d). In some area of slides of GDM placentas, the following morphological changes in terminal villi were qualitatively showed: edematous stroma, apparent increase in the number of syncytial knots, and perivillous fibrin deposition.

3.2. Ultrastructural Examination. In the control group, the major structure of placental barrier included the STs, endothelium and their underlying BMs were clearly showed in Figures 2(a) to 2(c). The STs were arranged in a monolayer, with multiple nuclei and numerous apical microvilli. The nuclear chromatin distribution was uniform as follows: euchromatin was abundant; heterochromatin was distributed along the nuclear membrane. Mitochondria were usually round or oval, and ERs had developed in the cytoplasm. The BM of STs was continuous, uniform, and thin basal lamina, which was identical to the BM of fetal endothelium. The stroma was the connective tissue core of the chorionic villi between the BMs of STs and fetal endothelium.

In the GDM group, the ultrastructural characteristics of terminal villi that differed from those of the control group were showed in Figures 2(d) to 2(f). The following appearances were found in GDM placentas: the degenerative alterations of terminal villi, the thick BM of VSM and VSM itself, significantly reduced number of or even absent ST microvilli, swollen or even completely destroyed mitochondria, and ERs and STs interspersed with multiple vacuoles. In some areas of GDM placentas, microvilli were completely devoid.

On the TEM, structures of mitochondria, vesica, and endoplasmic reticulum (ER) were further observed. Figures 2(g) to 2(i) showed mitochondria, vesica, and ER in ST cytoplasm of control group. In the GDM group, massive

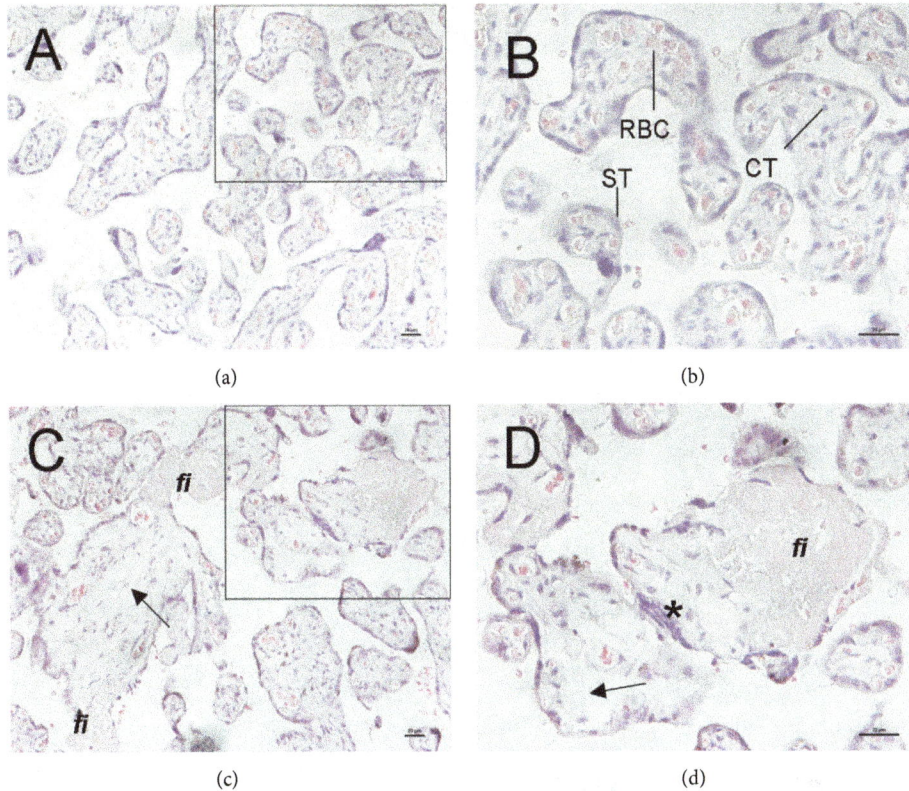

FIGURE 1: Pathological morphology of placentas from control group (a, b) and GDM group (c, d). Placental sections were HE-stained. (a) The normal branching of villous trees. (b) The syncytiotrophoblast (ST) was clearly observed lying outside the villi, with scarce single cells of cytotrophoblast (CT). (c and d) The increased syncytial knotting (∗), villous edema (arrows), and perivillous fibrin (fi) depositions in GDM group. Bar = 20 um.

swelling, even ridge deprivation, and architectural disruption of mitochondria were found (Figure 2(j)), and dilations of cisternae (Figure 2(k)) and ER (Figure 2(l)) were also found.

3.3. Quantitative Assay. Comparisons of semiquantitative parameters (as described in Table 2) of placental ultrastructure between GDM and control group were summarized in Table 3. There were significant differences in those structural characteristics of cytoplasmic vacuoles, stroma edema, mitochondria, and endoplasmic reticulum ($P < 0.01$).

The VSM and BM of ST were significantly thicker in the GDM group ($6,746.15 \pm 1,270.22$ nm and $1,077.49 \pm 194.39$ nm, resp.; Figures 3(a) and 3(d)) than those in the control group ($4,591.34 \pm 1,178.60$ nm and 707.54 ± 256.56, resp.; Figures 3(b) and 3(e)) ($P < 0.05$). The density of ST apical microvilli per unit surface area in the GDM group (44.36 ± 21.95 per 10 μm) was significantly lower than that in the control group (77.13 ± 20.82 per 10 μm) ($P < 0.05$), as showed in Figures 3(g) to 3(i).

4. Discussion

Hyperglycemia and hypoxia are two key factors in the pathophysiological process of GDM complications, and, in GDM, it is hyperglycemia that induces hypoxia and oxidative stress in placenta by several pathways, including leukostasis,

vasoconstriction, and a proinflammatory situation [11–15]. Therefore, hyperglycemia in GDM is a proconstricting [11], procoagulatory [12], proinflammatory [13], proangiogenic [14], and propermeability [15] factor which affects vasculogenesis, angiogenesis and maturation of vascular system, and vascular dysfunction during critical periods of placental development [16]. Some significant changes in the placental barrier in GDM were found, including the thickened placental barrier, decreased density of ST apical microvilli, and increased ST vacuoles, all of which potentially inhibit transplacental transport and exchange. To our knowledge, the present study is the first to investigate systematically the ultrastructural changes in human term placentas derived from women with GDM.

The VSM of terminal villi is the most important structure of placental barrier, which determines the diffusion distance between maternal blood and fetal blood. Mayhew et al. found that those changes in the preeclampsia placenta were related to the fetal intrauterine growth restriction (IUGR), including the exchange surface areas, diffusion distances, and villous membrane diffusive conductance [17]. They found that the IUGR placentas showed the thick BM of ST and VSM itself, which changed the capacity of diffusional transfer across placenta. In addition, the thickening placental barrier is also found in the cases of women who have conceived using assisted reproductive technology [18], who smoke [19],

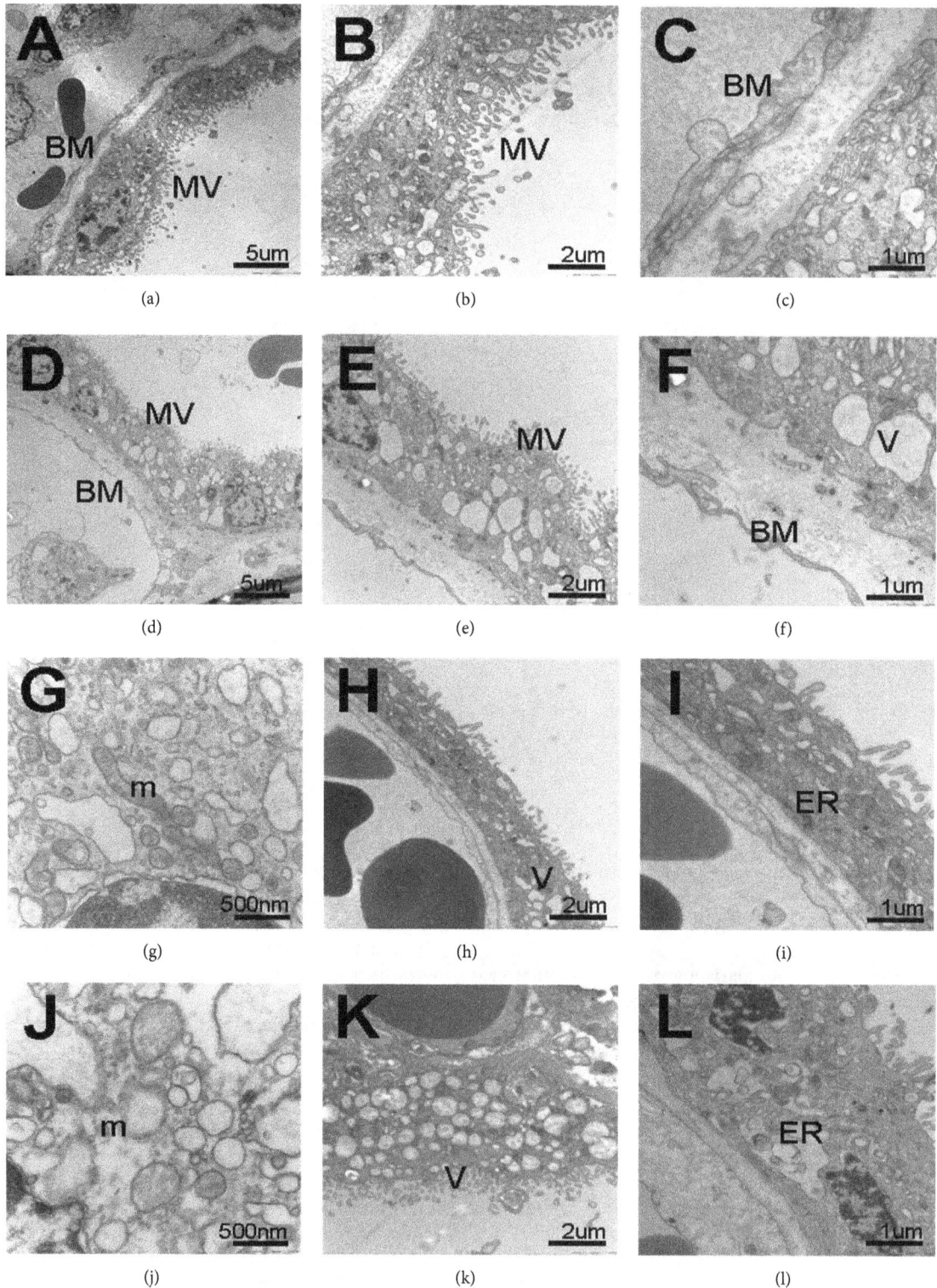

FIGURE 2: Ultrastructure of placentas from control group (a–c, g–i) and GDM group (d–f, j–l) observed using a JEM-1010 electron microscope. TEM images showed at different magnifications (×5000 (a and d), ×12 000 (b and e), and ×25 000 (c and f)). (a–c) Normal placental barriers were displayed in control, VSM, composed of the outer layer ST with a multitude of microvilli (MV) on the surface, fetal capillaries with fetal blood cells inside, and BM and interspaces between them. (d–f) In GDM group, intact placental barriers were apparent along with degenerative alterations of the terminal villi, mainly in VSM and BM, including thicker placental barriers, decreased apical microvilli, and increased multiple vacuoles (V) in ST. Bar = 5 um (a and d), 2 um (b and e), and 1 um (c and f). (g–i) Mitochondria (g), cytoplasmic vacuoles (h), and ER (i) with normal appearance in the cytoplasm of ST in control group. (j) The massive swelling, even ridge deprivation, and architectural disruption of mitochondria (m) in the GDM placenta. (k) The massive cytoplasmic vacuoles accumulation in the ST of GDM placenta. (l) The dilation of endoplasmic reticulum (ER) cisternae in GDM group. Bar = 500 nm (g and j), 2 um (h and k), and 1 um (i and l).

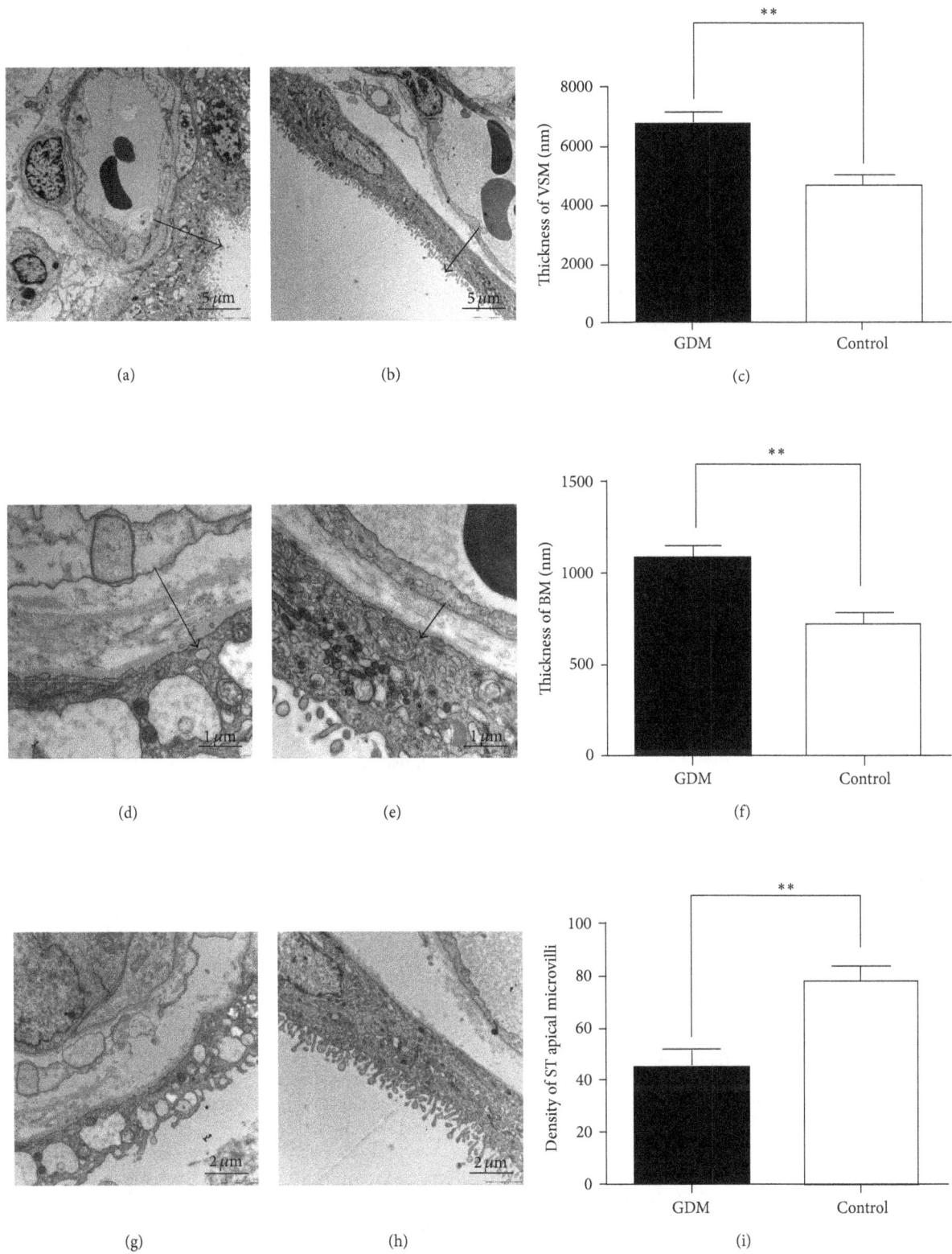

FIGURE 3: Comparison of semiquantitative parameters of placental ultrastructures between GDM and control group. (a–c) The terminal villi of GDM (a) and control (b) placenta. (c) Placental barrier thickness (arrow) of GDM group (6746.15 ± 1270.22 nm, $n = 10$) was significantly thicker than that of control group (4591.34 ± 1178.60 nm, $n = 10$; $P < 0.05$). Bar = 5 um. (d–f) The terminal villi of GDM (d) and control (e) placenta. (f) The BM of ST in GDM group (1077.49 ± 194.39 nm nm, $n = 10$) was thicker than that in control group (707.54 ± 256.56 nm, $n = 10$; $P < 0.05$). Bar = 1 um. (g–i) The density of ST apical microvilli in GDM (g) and control (h) placenta. (i) The density of ST apical microvilli in GDM group (44.36 ± 21.95 per 10 um, $n = 10$) was significantly lower than that in control group (77.13 ± 20.82 per 10 um, $n = 10$; $P < 0.05$) and even microvilli-free in some areas. Bar = 2 um.

TABLE 3: The semiquantitative analysis of placental ultrastructures in the GDM group and control group.

Characteristics	Semiquantitative score	GDM $(n = 150)^{\#}$	Control $(n = 150)^{\#}$	P value
Cytoplasmic vacuoles	0	12 (8%)	75 (50%)	0.000
	1	18 (12%)	30 (20%)	—
	2	42 (28%)	21 (14%)	—
	3	78 (52%)	24 (16%)	—
Pyknosis	0	22 (14.7%)	13 (8.7%)	0.106
	1	35 (23.3%)	73 (48.7%)	—
	2	71 (47.3%)	45 (30%)	—
	3	22 (14.7%)	19 (12.6%)	—
Stroma edema	0	27 (18%)	82 (54.7%)	0.000
	1	28 (18.7%)	35 (23.3%)	—
	2	36 (24%)	21 (14%)	—
	3	59 (39.3%)	12 (8%)	—
Mitochondria	0	11 (7.3%)	79 (52.7%)	0.000
	1	21 (14%)	48 (32%)	—
	2	42 (28%)	16 (10.7%)	—
	3	76 (50.7%)	7 (4.6%)	—
Endoplasmic reticulum	0	24 (16%)	88 (58.7%)	0.000
	1	31 (10.7%)	37 (24.7%)	—
	2	52 (34.7%)	21 (14%)	—
	3	43 (28.6%)	4 (2.6%)	—

$^{\#}$Fifteen fields of vision were randomly recorded and analyzed per placenta in order to minimize the individual differences.

or who have preeclampsia or eclampsia [20]. Vranes et al. observed that the loss of blood vessel elasticity in diabetes was possibly related to the collagen deposition in tunica media [21]. The decreased elasticity of vessel wall leads to vascular hardening and increased susceptibility to atherosclerosis [22], whereas, in the microcirculation, alteration in the BMs of arterioles leads to weakening and dilation of the capillary walls, with a tendency to rupture (microangiopathy) [23, 24]. These changes of the structure and function of villous capillaries in placenta would disrupt the environment of fetus development, such as hypoxia and epigenetic influences [25]. In this study, the thick VSM and BM of VSM were observed in GDM placenta. These changes may adversely affect the transport efficiency of placental vasculature, such as the decreasing transport of oxygen, nutrients, and waste.

The microvilli projecting from the apical portion of ST appear to be highly pleomorphic and show regional variations in distribution. The majority of fetal/maternal exchange occurs at the terminal branches of chorionic villi [26]. The apical microvillous density [27] and the surface area are related to the degree of trophoblastic maturation, and placental maturation is the most discriminative and by far the most important feature that needs to be assessed in diagnosis of the chronic hypoxia in utero [28]. Loss of microvilli and gross thinning of syncytium with distorted microvilli have been reported in the terminal villi of placentas from women with eclampsia [20]. The density of apical microvilli has been observed to be considerably reduced, and the occasional microvilli-free areas have been observed in IUGR and small-for-gestational-age fetuses [29]. These

findings indicated the decreased exchange of gases, nutrients, and waste between maternal and fetal circulatory systems. Previous quantitative studies on the villi of placenta from women with well-controlled diabetes mellitus concluded that normal values were preserved by good glycaemic control regardless of diabetic grouping [30]. Therefore, stereological comparison of 3D spatial relationships involving villi and intervillous pores did not differ significantly in placentas from diabetic subjects with good glycaemic control [31]. Another study presented that uteroplacental blood flows were decreased in women who went on to develop preeclampsia, which indicated that poor glycemic control during pregnancy was associated with the development of preeclampsia [32]. In the present study, our results showed an association between microscopic and ultrastructural changes and the development of diabetes mellitus, which were conflicting with previous reported data. It may be explained by the fact that women in our studies have developed to adverse pregnancy outcome, such as preeclampsia. In the present study, a significantly decreased number of ST microvilli were observed in the GDM placentas. Some STs microvilli appeared to disappear completely. These changes of ultrastructure in GDM placenta would affect transplacental transfer, metabolism, and oxygen-diffusing.

It was also found that there were much more STs vacuolated in GDM placenta when compared with the control group. In the in vitro cultured model of placental villous, ST showed the cytoplasmic vacuolization and subsequent degeneration which was related to preeclampsia [33]. Hyperglycemia and hypoxia in GDM may enhance the lysosome/vacuole functions of ST, which results in the widespread cytoplasmic vacuolization and the altered transplacental metabolic exchange. Mitochondria and ERs are the most vulnerable organelles, which are susceptible to hyperglycemia and hypoxia [34–36]. Mitochondria are double-membrane organelles with multiple essential functions, such as cellular survival, energy metabolism, and intracellular ATP production by oxidative phosphorylation [35, 36]. ER synthesizes many secretary proteins and other factors, lipids, and membrane phospholipids, which participates in steroid synthesis in ST. The dilation and vacuolization of mitochondria and ER were most evident in the in vitro experiments and the in vivo samples of placental tissues from women with preeclampsia combined with IUGR [36]. In our study, we found massive swelling, ridge deprivation, and architectural disruption of the mitochondria and dilation of ER cisternae (Figure 2). The abnormal ultrastructures of mitochondria and ER could have impacts on metabolic functions and synthesis in ST.

In summary, our data showed the distinct alternations in the morphology and ultrastructure of GDM placentas which formed some compensatory mechanism to maintain homeostasis at the maternal-fetal interface in GDM. We assumed that those changes in the placenta and maternal-fetal interface are related to the pregnancy complications, adverse outcomes, and even fetal origin diseases. Moreover, because of the limited sample size, the present study is just the starting point in evaluating pregnancy outcome of GDM. Large-scale analyses and molecular studies are necessary to evaluate the short- and long-term effects of ultrastructural changes of GDM placenta on both offspring and mother.

Conflict of Interests

The authors declare that they have no conflict of interests.

Authors' Contribution

Qian Meng and Li Shao, students of Yugui Cui and Jiayin Liu, carried out the main experiments. Xiucui Luo and Yingping Mu, as clinical doctors, and Chao Gao and Li Gao, as laboratory technicians, took part in some experiments, collection of samples, and discussion. Yugui Cui and Jiayin Liu were the principal investigators. Jiayin Liu worked with group and reviewed the paper. Yugui Cui designed the project and experiments. Qian Meng finished first draft, and Yugui Cui revised the paper. All authors examined the data and read and approved the final paper. Qian Meng and Li Shao contributed equally to this study.

Acknowledgments

The authors sincerely thank Liling Zhou and Qin Lu for their help to prepare TEM samples. They also thank everybody contributing to the study. This work was supported by China 973 Program (2012CB944703, 2012CB944902), a project from State Key Laboratory of Reproductive Medicine, Nanjing Medical University (SKLRM-KF-1110), and Jiangsu Clinical Center Program (BL2012009), China.

References

[1] American Diabetes Association, "Standards of medical care in diabetes—2011," *Diabetes Care*, vol. 34, supplement 1, pp. S11–S61, 2011.

[2] D. Dabelea, J. K. Snell-Bergeon, C. L. Hartsfield, K. J. Bischoff, R. F. Hamman, and R. S. McDuffie, "Increasing prevalence of gestational diabetes mellitus (GDM) over time and by birth cohort: Kaiser Permanente of Colorado GDM screening program," *Diabetes Care*, vol. 28, no. 3, pp. 579–584, 2005.

[3] A. Ferrara, H. S. Kahn, C. P. Quesenberry, C. Riley, and M. M. Hedderson, "An increase in the incidence of gestational diabetes mellitus: Northern California, 1991–2000," *Obstetrics & Gynecology*, vol. 103, pp. 526–533, 2004.

[4] F. Zhang, L. Dong, C. P. Zhang et al., "Increasing prevalence of gestational diabetes mellitus in Chinese women from 1999 to 2008," *Diabetic Medicine*, vol. 28, no. 6, pp. 652–657, 2011.

[5] C. M. Mihu, S. Şuşman, D. R. Ciucă, D. Mihu, and N. Costin, "Aspects of placental morphogenesis and angiogenesis," *Romanian Journal of Morphology and Embryology*, vol. 50, no. 4, pp. 549–557, 2009.

[6] A. L. Kierszenbaum, "An introduction to pathology," in *Histology and Cell Biology*, pp. 635–661, Mosby Elsevier, Philadelphia, Pa, USA, 2nd edition, 2007.

[7] G. J. Burton, D. S. Charnock-Jones, and E. Jauniaux, "Regulation of vascular growth and function in the human placenta," *Reproduction*, vol. 138, no. 6, pp. 895–902, 2009.

[8] H. Fox and N. J. Sebire, *Pathology of the Placenta*, W.B. Saunders, Philadelphia, Pa, USA, 3rd edition, 2007.

[9] M. E. Sak, E. Deveci, M. S. Evsen et al., "Expression of β human chorionic gonadotropin in the placenta of gestational diabetic mothers: an immunohistochemistry and ultrastructural study," *Analytical and Quantitative Cytology and Histology*, vol. 35, no. 1, pp. 52–56, 2013.

[10] R. Sood, J. L. Zehnder, M. L. Druzin, and P. O. Brown, "Gene expression patterns in human placenta," *Proceedings of the National Academy of Sciences of the United States of America*, vol. 103, no. 14, pp. 5478–5483, 2006.

[11] V. P. Singh, B. Le, R. Khode, K. M. Baker, and R. Kumar, "Intracellular angiotensin II production in diabetic rats is correlated with cardiomyocyte apoptosis, oxidative stress, and cardiac fibrosis," *Diabetes*, vol. 57, pp. 3297–3306, 2008.

[12] A. Singh, G. Boden, C. Homko, J. Gunawardana, and A. K. Rao, "Whole-blood tissue factor procoagulant activity is elevated in type 1 diabetes: effects of hyperglycemia and hyperinsulinemia," *Diabetes Care*, vol. 35, no. 6, pp. 1322–1327, 2012.

[13] Z. Yang, V. E. Laubach, B. A. French, and I. L. Kron, "Acute hyperglycemia enhances oxidative stress and exacerbates myocardial infarction by activating nicotinamide adenine dinucleotide phosphate oxidase during reperfusion," *Journal of Thoracic and Cardiovascular Surgery*, vol. 137, no. 3, pp. 723–729, 2009.

[14] C. Ettelaie, S. Su, C. Li, and M. E. W. Collier, "Tissue factor-containing microparticles released from mesangial cells in response to high glucose and AGE induce tube formation in microvascular cells," *Microvascular Research*, vol. 76, no. 3, pp. 152–160, 2008.

[15] S. H. Sung, F. N. Ziyadeh, A. Wang, P. E. Pyagay, Y. S. Kanwar, and S. Chen, "Blockade of vascular endothelial growth factor signaling ameliorates diabetic albuminuria in mice," *Journal of the American Society of Nephrology*, vol. 17, no. 11, pp. 3093–3104, 2006.

[16] L. Myatt, W. Kossenjans, R. Sahay, A. Eis, and D. Brockman, "Oxidative stress causes vascular dysfunction in the placenta," *Journal of Maternal-Fetal Medicine*, vol. 9, no. 1, pp. 79–82, 2000.

[17] T. M. Mayhew, R. Manwani, C. Ohadike, J. Wijesekara, and P. N. Baker, "The placenta in pre-eclampsia and intrauterine growth restriction: studies on exchange surface areas, diffusion distances and villous membrane diffusive conductances," *Placenta*, vol. 28, no. 2-3, pp. 233–238, 2007.

[18] Y. Zhang, W. Zhao, Y. Jiang et al., "Ultrastructural study on human placentae from women subjected to assisted reproductive technology treatments," *Biology of Reproduction*, vol. 85, no. 3, pp. 635–642, 2011.

[19] G. Rath, R. Dhuria, S. Salhan, and A. K. Jain, "Morphology and morphometric analysis of stromal capillaries in full term human placental villi of smoking mothers: an electron microscopic study," *Clinica Terapeutica*, vol. 162, no. 4, pp. 301–305, 2011.

[20] S. S. Salgado and M. K. R. Salgado, "Structural changes in pre-eclamptic and eclamptic placentas—an ultrastructural study," *Journal of the College of Physicians and Surgeons Pakistan*, vol. 21, no. 8, pp. 482–486, 2011.

[21] D. Vranes, M. E. Cooper, and R. J. Dilley, "Cellular mechanisms of diabetic vascular hypertrophy," *Microvascular Research*, vol. 57, no. 1, pp. 8–18, 1999.

[22] S. M. Jin, C. I. Noh, S. W. Yang et al., "Endothelial dysfunction and microvascular complications in type 1 diabetes mellitus," *Journal of Korean Medical Science*, vol. 23, no. 1, pp. 77–82, 2008.

[23] H. Vlassara, M. Brownlee, and A. Cerami, "Accumulation of diabetic rat peripheral nerve myelin by macrophages increases with the presence of advanced glycosylation endproducts," *Journal of Experimental Medicine*, vol. 160, no. 1, pp. 197–207, 1984.

[24] M. Brownlee, "Biochemistry and molecular cell biology of diabetic complications," *Nature*, vol. 414, no. 6865, pp. 813–820, 2001.

[25] C. P. Gheorghe, R. Goyal, A. Mittal, and L. D. Longo, "Gene expression in the placenta: maternal stress and epigenetic responses," *International Journal of Developmental Biology*, vol. 54, no. 2-3, pp. 507–523, 2010.

[26] N. M. Gude, C. T. Roberts, B. Kalionis, and R. G. King, "Growth and function of the normal human placenta," *Thrombosis Research*, vol. 114, no. 5-6, pp. 397–407, 2004.

[27] G. Biagini, V. Vasi, A. Pugnaloni et al., "Morphological development of the human placenta in normal and complicated gestation: a quantitative and ultrastructural study," *Gynecologic and Obstetric Investigation*, vol. 28, no. 2, pp. 62–69, 1989.

[28] T. Y. Khong, A. Staples, R. W. Bendon et al., "Observer reliability in assessing placental maturity by histology," *Journal of Clinical Pathology*, vol. 48, no. 5, pp. 420–423, 1995.

[29] T. I. Ansari, S. Fenlon, S. Pasha et al., "Morphometric assessment of the oxygen diffusion conductance in placentae from pregnancies complicated by intra-uterine growth restriction," *Placenta*, vol. 24, no. 6, pp. 618–626, 2003.

[30] T. M. Mayhew and I. Sisley, "Quantitative studies on the villi, trophoblast and intervillous pores of placentae from women with well-controlled diabetes mellitus," *Placenta*, vol. 19, no. 5-6, pp. 371–377, 1998.

[31] T. M. Mayhew and I. C. Jairam, "Stereological comparison of 3D spatial relationships involving villi and intervillous pores in human placentas from control and diabetic pregnancies," *Journal of Anatomy*, vol. 197, part 2, pp. 263–274, 2000.

[32] V. A. Holmes, I. S. Young, C. C. Patterson et al., "Optimal glycemic control, pre-eclampsia, and gestational hypertension in women with type 1 diabetes in the Diabetes and Pre-Eclampsia Intervention Trial," *Diabetes Care*, vol. 34, no. 8, pp. 1683–1688, 2011.

[33] C. M. Simán, C. P. Sibley, C. J. P. Jones, M. A. Turner, and S. L. Greenwood, "The functional regeneration of syncytiotrophoblast in cultured explants of term placenta," *The American Journal of Physiology—Regulatory Integrative and Comparative Physiology*, vol. 280, no. 4, pp. R1116–R1122, 2001.

[34] D. J. Pagliarini, S. E. Calvo, B. Chang et al., "A mitochondrial protein compendium elucidates complex I disease biology," *Cell*, vol. 134, no. 1, pp. 112–123, 2008.

[35] V. K. Mootha, J. Bunkenborg, J. V. Olsen et al., "Integrated analysis of protein composition, tissue diversity, and gene regulation in mouse mitochondria," *Cell*, vol. 115, no. 5, pp. 629–640, 2003.

[36] C. G. Proud, "Signalling to translation: how signal transduction pathways control the protein synthetic machinery," *Biochemical Journal*, vol. 403, no. 2, pp. 217–234, 2007.

10

Transvaginal Drainage of Pelvic Abscesses and Collections Using Transabdominal Ultrasound Guidance

Kevin C. Ching and Jules H. Sumkin

Department of Radiology, University of Pittsburgh, 200 Lothrop Street, Suite 3950, Presby South Tower, Pittsburgh, PA 15213, USA

Correspondence should be addressed to Kevin C. Ching; kevinchingmd@gmail.com

Academic Editor: Curt W. Burger

Objectives. To evaluate clinical outcomes following transvaginal catheter placement using transabdominal ultrasound guidance for management of pelvic fluid collections. *Methods.* A retrospective review was performed for all patients who underwent transvaginal catheter drainage of pelvic fluid collections utilizing transabdominal ultrasound guidance between July 2008 and July 2013. 24 consecutive patients were identified and 24 catheters were placed. *Results.* The mean age of patients was 48.1 years (range = 27–76 y). 88% of collections were postoperative ($n = 21$), 8% were from pelvic inflammatory disease ($n = 2$), and 4% were idiopathic ($n = 1$). Of the 24 patients, 83% of patients ($n = 20$) had previously undergone a hysterectomy and 1 patient (4%) was pregnant at the time of drainage. The mean volume of initial drainage was 108 mL (range = 5 to 570). Catheters were left in place for an average of 4.3 days (range = 1–17 d). Microbial sampling was performed in all patients with 71% ($n = 17$) returning a positive culture. All collections were successfully managed percutaneously. There were no technical complications. *Conclusions.* Transvaginal catheter drainage of pelvic fluid collections using transabdominal ultrasound guidance is a safe and clinically effective procedure. Appropriate percutaneous management can avoid the need for surgery.

1. Introduction

Percutaneous catheter drainage of abdominal and pelvic fluid collections is a well-established technique used by interventional radiologists for more than 30 years [1–3]. Sampling and drainage of organized fluid collections greatly affect clinical management as these collections may represent seromas, hematomas, or abscesses. Since transabdominal catheter drainage was first described in the 1980s, image-guided catheters are now being placed via transgluteal, transrectal, transperineal, and transvaginal routes using ultrasound and CT guidance [3–5]. While additional techniques for percutaneous catheter placement have become available, draining fluid collections within the pelvis remains a challenging task due to critical intervening structures. The urinary bladder and overlying bowel loops often prevent transabdominal access to fluid collections within the true pelvis. Sciatic neuropathy has been reported in 10% of patients following transgluteal catheter drainage [6]. Transvaginal (TV) catheter drainage of pelvic fluid collections was first described by Nosher et al. utilizing transabdominal (TA) sonography. [7].

A study of 14 patients by VanSonnenberg et al. described both TA and TV ultrasound guidance for transvaginal drainage of pelvic collections. Other than a few case reports, the authors of this paper could not locate a clinical study in the literature assessing patient outcomes following TV catheter placement using TA ultrasound [5, 7]. From our experience, advantages of TV catheter placement using TA ultrasound include excellent visualization of collections within the close confines of the true pelvis, the ability to select the exact location of vaginal puncture, and the ability to perform TV drainage when an endovaginal ultrasound transducer and/or needle guide is not available. This study reports the clinical efficacy and safety of our 5-year experience with transvaginal catheters placed using transabdominal ultrasound guidance for management of pelvic fluid collections.

2. Methods

2.1. Patient Population. The study was approved by the institutional review board and requirement for informed consent was waived. A single-center retrospective review was performed of all consecutive patients who underwent transvaginal drainage using transabdominal ultrasound guidance between July 2008 and July 2013 at a tertiary care women's hospital. Patients who underwent percutaneous drainage using CT guidance or transvaginal ultrasound were excluded. Drainage of nonorganized free pelvic fluid was also excluded. Our preference for the management of pelvic collections is to perform CT or US guided transabdominal drainage when feasible. When contraindicated by intervening structures, a transvaginal route is chosen for catheter drainage. While the decision for TA versus TV US guidance is ultimately attending dependent, almost all TV drainage procedures at our institution are performed using transabdominal US guidance. Antimicrobial therapy is administered prior to drainage in patients with clinical signs and laboratory findings of infection. The microbial culture results obtained from drainage result in discontinuation of antibiotics or tailoring of antibiotics for specific organisms. Patient demographics, procedure reports, clinical notes, and imaging studies were reviewed via the electronic medical record and picture archiving and communication system.

2.2. Study Outcomes. Clinical success was the primary outcome evaluated in this study. This was defined as clinical improvement without the need for surgery or additional percutaneous procedures to manage the pelvic fluid collection. Technical success and complications were studied as secondary outcomes as little data evaluating TA ultrasound for placement of TV catheters exists. Additional data was collected from the medical record including technical details, anesthesia, pelvic anatomy, and microbial specimen analysis.

2.3. Patient Demographics. A total of 24 patients underwent TV catheter placement using TA ultrasound guidance between July 2008 and July 2013. All pelvic fluid collections were diagnosed on computed tomography (CT) studies performed prior to the drainage procedures. The mean age of patients was 48.1 years (range = 27–76 y). In the 24 patients, 24 catheters were placed; however, 4 catheters were immediately removed after postprocedure US showed no residual fluid and the fluid was clear in appearance. All study participants except 1 were inpatients at the time of referral. Pelvic collections were postoperative in 21 patients (88%), were due to pelvic inflammatory disease in 2 patients (8%), and were idiopathic in 1 patient (4%). Of the 21 postoperative collections, 16 (76%) occurred following hysterectomy via transabdominal or transvaginal surgical approaches using traditional, laparoscopic, and robot-assisted techniques. The remaining 5 postoperative collections occurred following surgery for pelvic organ prolapse ($n = 2$), salpingectomy for ectopic pregnancy, laparoscopic appendectomy, and ventral hernia repair each ($n = 1$). Regarding pelvic anatomy, 20 of 24 patients (83%) no longer had a uterus and 1 patient was 11 weeks pregnant at the time of drainage.

2.4. Catheter Placement and Aspiration Procedures. For assessment of technical feasibility, all patients first underwent TA pelvic ultrasound. If the fluid collection was not well

visualized, the urinary bladder was distended with approximately 250 cc of sterile saline to create a sonographic window and improve visualization. The patient was placed in the lithotomy position and a vaginal speculum was inserted. The vagina was then prepped with a povidone-iodine solution. Some patients received moderate conscious sedation when using intravenous midazolam and fentanyl was felt necessary. Using a 3–5 MHz linear ultrasound transducer, longitudinal TA sonography (Figure 1(a)) was performed to visualize the targeted pelvic fluid collection. Locking pigtail universal drainage catheters (Navarre, CR Bard, Inc.) ranging from 6 F to 10 F were placed using Trocar or Seldinger techniques. In our department an ultrasound technologist often scans the patient allowing the radiologist to use both hands for catheter placement; however, the procedure and sonography are easily performed by a single operator. The radiologist can identify the appropriate puncture position by indenting the vaginal mucosa with a blunt instrument such as ring forceps and identifying it with ultrasound. For the Trocar technique instillation of local anesthetic using a 27-gauge needle is made under real-time sonographic guidance, and then a 2 mm nick is made in the posterior fornix or vaginal apex with a standard length 11-blade scalpel. The assembled catheter system is inserted into the collection under real-time TA ultrasound guidance (Figure 1(b)). The inner trocar is removed allowing the pigtail to form and the catheter is then locked (Figure 1(c)). The Seldinger technique is performed similarly; however, initially a 7 inch 18-gauge Quincke spinal needle (BD, Franklin Lake, NJ) is first directed under TA ultrasound guidance into the collection and a 0.035 inch short Rosen J wire is placed through the needle into the collection. A vaginal nick with the scalpel is not necessary when using the Seldinger technique. While 23 of 24 procedures were performed using the Trocar technique, due to equipment availability in our department we use a cystography table so the wire exchange (Seldinger technique) can be performed with fluoroscopic assistance; however, this is not mandatory. The drainage catheter is then inserted over the wire and locked in place. Immediately following catheter placement, as much fluid is aspirated as possible through the catheter and postprocedure transabdominal sonography (Figure 1(d)) is performed to confirm catheter positioning and assess residual fluid. Since a locking catheter is placed, no suture or fixation device was used to secure the catheter. Technique for catheter placement, catheter size, and decision to leave a catheter in place were at the discretion of the treating radiologist. The volume of fluid removed was recorded in procedure notes and fluid specimens were sent for microbial culture. Timing of catheter removal was made by the clinical team and radiology physicians using dwindling catheter output (<10 mL in 24 hours) and clinical improvement as indications for discontinuation. Date of catheter removal was documented in the electronic medical record and the number of catheter days was recorded for the study.

3. Results

Diagnostic workup included CT imaging in all patients (100%) with additional pelvic ultrasound performed in 5

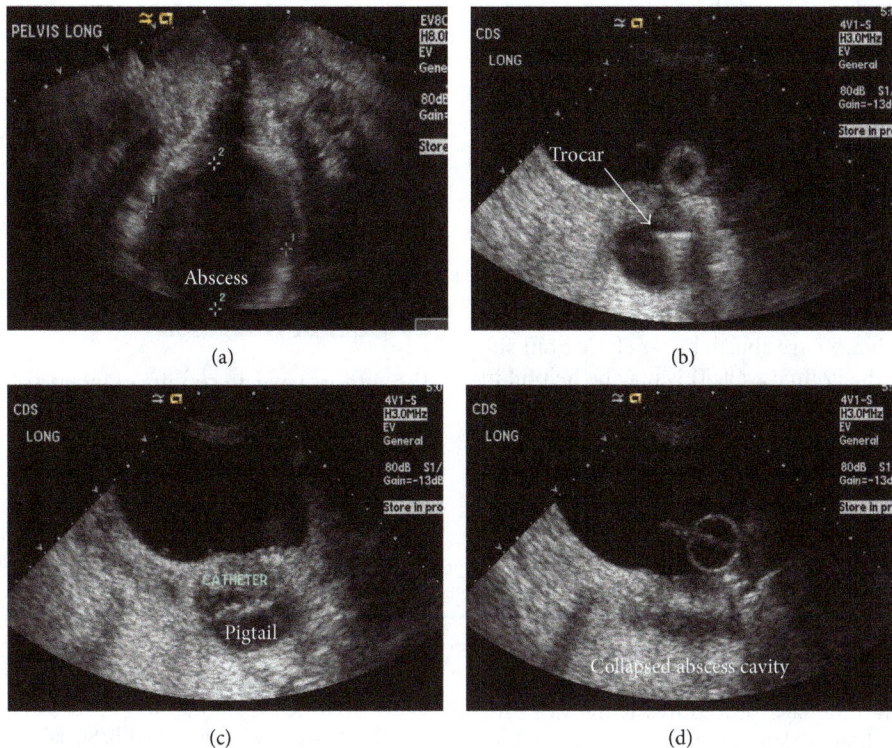

FIGURE 1: (a) Transvaginal ultrasound shows a small collection in the rectouterine space. (b) Sagittal transabdominal ultrasound shows the trocar puncturing inferiorly through the vaginal cuff. (c) 6 F pigtail catheter is advanced into the collection. 45 mL of pus was aspirated with collapse of the abscess cavity (d). The catheter was removed 2 days later and the patient was discharged. Cultures were positive.

patients (21%). In 22 patients (92%), fluid collections were located in the mid deep (true) pelvis within the rectouterine space or rectovesical space. The remaining 2 collections (8%) were left adnexal.

Of the 24 catheters placed, 20 were left to gravity drainage and 4 catheters were immediately removed after sonography revealed sufficient drainage and the fluid was not infected in appearance. The 24 ultrasound guided procedures were performed by 5 attending radiologists. Drainage catheters placed were 6–10 F in size with 8 F being most common (n = 17, 85%). Bladder filling was performed through a Foley catheter in 58% of patients (n = 14) to create a sonographic window. This required Foley catheters to be placed in 11 patients that were immediately removed following the procedure. The remaining 3 patients had an indwelling bladder catheter already in place. 13 of 24 patients (54%) received additional moderate conscious sedation. The Trocar technique was employed for 23 of 24 (96%) catheter placements and the Seldinger technique was used for the remaining patient. Procedure notes documented the volume of fluid initially drained in 22 of 24 patients which averaged 108 mL (range, 5–570 mL). CT or ultrasound was performed in 2 patients (10%) 2 to 14 days following drainage to assess residual fluid prior to catheter removal. Seventeen specimens (71%) returned a positive culture. Catheters were left in place for an average of 4.3 days (range = 1–17 d).

Average length of follow-up was 572 days (range, 1-2,039 d) from the date of percutaneous drainage to the most recent gynecology note in the electronic medical record. All collections were successfully managed with single percutaneous drainage resulting in a clinical success rate of 100%. There were no technical complications. Inadvertent catheter dislodgement occurred in 3 of 20 patients (15%); however, none required catheter replacement or further intervention. No patients required surgery for management of pelvic fluid collections; however, 2 patients were taken to the operating room for repair of fascial dehiscence and debridement of an infected peritoneal chemotherapy catheter.

4. Discussion

Pelvic fluid collections are most commonly postoperative in etiology [1]. As gynecologic surgery is increasingly performed using minimally invasive techniques, open surgical drainage of infected collections would negate the benefits of laparoscopic surgery; therefore nonsurgical percutaneous management is the treatment of choice for draining pelvic collections [8]. Multiple prior studies have reported the efficacy of transvaginal catheter placement for management of pelvic fluid collections [1, 5, 7, 9]. Other than 5 reported cases, these studies utilize TV sonography for imaging guidance [5, 10]. In the study by VanSonnenberg et al. evaluating transvaginal catheter placement in 14 patients, TA ultrasound was used in the first two patients; however the authors noted better visualization with TV sonography which they used for the remaining 12 patients [5]. Distending the urinary bladder improves visualization within the pelvis by creating a sonographic window for TA ultrasound. This was not mentioned in that study. Refinements in ultrasound transducer technology in the 20 years since the reported cases also aid in visualization using the technique we describe.

While this study does not compare the results of TA versus TV ultrasound guidance, the authors believe that there are many benefits to our technique. Using the bladder as a sonographic window, we achieve excellent visualization of deep pelvic fluid collections even when they are small and closely adjacent to bladder and bowel. Also, because only the catheter is placed into the vagina, we are able to better choose our site of puncture through the vaginal wall. This may be helpful in posthysterectomy patients when the vaginal cuff is often friable due to an underlying infection. The pressure exerted by the endovaginal ultrasound probe on the sensitive and healing vaginal cuff when TV sonography was used is also avoided when TA ultrasound is utilized for catheter placement. Having utilized this procedure for many years, the authors believe it is important to be familiar with alternative techniques for transvaginal drainage in the event an endovaginal ultrasound transducer and/or needle guide is not available.

The main disadvantage of using transabdominal sonography for transvaginal drainage procedures is the need for a well-distended bladder. Foley catheters were placed in 46% of patients in our study for bladder filling. While no urinary tract infections (UTI) were documented, bladder catheterization is a risk factor for nosocomial UTI. Bladder distension may also be uncomfortable to patients. In a study comparing TV versus TA ultrasound for embryo transfer, bladder distension was associated with moderate to severe discomfort in 22% of patients [10]. While intraprocedural pain was not reported in our study, moderate IV sedation is well tolerated when additional analgesia is required. Lastly, while the equipment we describe is not available in all departments (cystography table), the majority of procedures in this study were performed using a Trocar technique which do not require fluoroscopy.

Limitations of our study include its retrospective design and lack of a comparison study group using a different method for image guidance. The small sample size also prevented a meaningful statistical analysis from being performed. Our department places transvaginal catheters using transabdominal and transvaginal imaging guidance. When transvaginal catheter placement is indicated the decision for TA versus TV ultrasound guidance is attending dependent. Of note, almost all TV catheters placed in our department are placed using TA ultrasound guidance. In our study the choice of catheter size was also variable ranging from 6 F to 10 F. This may have affected the number of catheter days and rate of clinical improvement as use of larger catheters has been associated with improved clinical outcomes when managing abdominal and pelvic fluid collections [11]. The rate of inadvertent catheter dislodgement was relatively high in our study at 15%; however there was no need for catheter replacement in any of the 3 patients. In addition, dislodgement of transvaginal catheters is an issue independent of whether TV or TA ultrasound guidance was used for the initial placement.

In conclusion, transabdominal sonography for placement of transvaginal catheters is a safe and effective variation of a proven technique for the management of pelvic fluid collections. Our clinical success rate of 100% is comparable to studies using TV ultrasound guidance as well as transgluteal and transabdominal routes for catheter drainage. Physicians may find this technique for TV catheter placement beneficial in postoperative hysterectomy patients or when an endovaginal transducer or needle guide is not available.

Conflict of Interests

The authors have no conflict of interests to declare.

References

[1] A. Saokar Rebello, R. S. Arellano, D. A. Gervais, P. R. Mueller, P. F. Hahn, and S. I. Lee, "Transvaginal drainage of pelvic fluid collections: results, expectations, and experience," *American Journal of Roentgenology*, vol. 191, no. 5, pp. 1352–1358, 2008.

[2] O. Buckley, T. Geoghegan, P. Ridgeway, E. Colhoun, A. Snow, and W. C. Torreggiani, "The usefulness of CT guided drainage of abscesses caused by retained appendicoliths," *European Journal of Radiology*, vol. 60, no. 1, pp. 80–83, 2006.

[3] T. Lorentzen, C. Nolsøe, and B. Skjoldbye, "Ultrasound-guided drainage of deep pelvic abscesses: experience with 33 cases," *Ultrasound in Medicine and Biology*, vol. 37, no. 5, pp. 723–728, 2011.

[4] M. G. Harisinghani, D. A. Gervais, P. F. Hahn et al., "CT-guided transgluteal drainage of deep pelvic abscesses: indications, technique, procedure-related complications, and clinical outcome," *Radiographics*, vol. 22, no. 6, pp. 1353–1367, 2002.

[5] E. VanSonnenberg, H. B. D'Agostino, G. Casola, B. W. Goodacre, R. B. Sanchez, and B. Taylor, "US-guided transvaginal drainage of pelvic abscesses and fluid collections," *Radiology*, vol. 181, no. 1, pp. 53–56, 1991.

[6] B. Robert, C. Chivot, D. Fuks, C. Gondry-Jouet, J. M. Regimbeau, and T. Yzet, "Percutaneous, computed tomography-guided drainage of deep pelvic abscesses via a transgluteal approach: a report on 30 cases and a review of the literature," *Abdominal Imaging*, vol. 38, no. 2, pp. 285–289, 2013.

[7] J. L. Nosher, H. K. Winchman, and G. S. Needell, "Transvaginal pelvic abscess drainage with US guidance," *Radiology*, vol. 165, no. 3, pp. 872–873, 1987.

[8] S. Granberg, K. Gjelland, and E. Ekerhovd, "The management of pelvic abscess," *Best Practice and Research: Clinical Obstetrics and Gynaecology*, vol. 23, no. 5, pp. 667–678, 2009.

[9] T. E. Snyder and S. Faro, "Ultrasound guidance for vaginal drainage of postoperative pelvic hematoma: a case report," *Infectious Diseases in Obstetrics and Gynecology*, vol. 1, no. 6, pp. 293–297, 1994.

[10] D. Bodri, M. Colodrón, D. García, A. Obradors, V. Vernaeve, and O. Coll, "Transvaginal versus transabdominal ultrasound guidance for embryo transfer in donor oocyte recipients: a randomized clinical trial," *Fertility and Sterility*, vol. 95, no. 7, pp. 2263.e1–2268.e1, 2011.

[11] K. C. Ching and H. S. Beasley, "Image-guided drainage of postoperative collections following hyperthermic intraperitoneal chemotherapy: a review of clinical outcomes," *Journal of Vascular and Interventional Radiology*, vol. 25, no. 3, supplement, p. S163, 2014.

11

Effect of Umbilical Cord Entanglement and Position on Pregnancy Outcomes

Natsuko Kobayashi,[1] **Shigeru Aoki,**[1] **Mari S. Oba,**[2]
Tsuneo Takahashi,[1] **and Fumiki Hirahara**[3]

[1]*Perinatal Center for Maternity and Neonates, Yokohama City University Medical Center, 4-57 Urafunecyou, Minami-ku, Yokohama, Kanagawa 232-0024, Japan*
[2]*Department of Biostatistics and Epidemiology, Yokohama City University Graduate School of Medicine and University Medical Center, Yokohama, Japan*
[3]*Department of Obstetrics and Gynecology, Yokohama City University Hospital, Yokohama, Japan*

Correspondence should be addressed to Shigeru Aoki; smyyaoki@yahoo.co.jp

Academic Editor: Everett Magann

Introduction. To investigate the effect of complex umbilical cord entanglement primarily around the trunk on pregnancy outcomes. *Methods.* We studied 6307 pregnant women with singleton pregnancies who underwent vaginal delivery of an infant at ≥37 weeks of gestation. Cases were classified into no cord, nuchal cord, and body cord groups and defined as cases without umbilical cord entanglement, one or more loops of the umbilical cord around the neck only, and umbilical cord around the trunk only, respectively. Pregnancy outcomes were compared among these three groups. *Results.* The no cord, nuchal cord, and body cord group included 4733, 1451, and 123 pregnancies, respectively. Although delivery mode was not significantly different among the three groups, 1-minute Apgar scores <7 and umbilical artery (UA) pH <7.10 were significantly more common in the umbilical cord entanglement groups than in the no cord group. In particular, the frequency of 5-minute Apgar scores <7 was significantly higher ($P = 0.004$), whereas that of UA pH <7.10 tended to be higher ($P = 0.057$) in the body cord group than in the nuchal cord group. *Conclusion.* Compared to nuchal cord, umbilical cord entanglement around the trunk was associated with a higher risk of low Apgar scores and low UA pH.

1. Introduction

Umbilical cord entanglement is the most common pathological condition among umbilical cord abnormalities [1], with an incidence ranging from 14.7% to 33.7% of all deliveries [1–3]. Umbilical cord entanglement reportedly increases the risk of prolonged labor and nonreassuring fetal status due to umbilical cord compression [1, 3–12], while some reports indicate that the risk of cesarean section or forced delivery is not increased [1, 5, 7, 13–16]. Therefore, consensus has not been reached. In addition, to the best of our knowledge, the majority of reports regarding umbilical cord entanglement concern nuchal cord entanglement, with no reported case concerning any other type of umbilical cord entanglement. Therefore, this study aimed to investigate the effect of complex umbilical cord entanglement primarily around the trunk on pregnancy outcome.

2. Materials and Methods

Data were retrospectively analyzed using the medical records of 8636 women with singleton pregnancies who had undergone attempted vaginal delivery at ≥37 gestational weeks between January 2004 and December 2013 at Yokohama City University Medical Center. Women with a serious complication, such as hypertension or diabetes, who delivered a newborn with congenital anomalies or with fetal malpresentation, were excluded. Consequently, 6307 of the 8636 women were included in this study. This study has been approved by the ethics committee of the Yokohama

TABLE 1: Maternal characteristics, compared between the 3 groups.

	No nuchal cord (n = 4733)	Nuchal neck cords (n = 1451)	Nuchal body cords (n = 123)	P value
Maternal age	31.7 ± 5.1	32.0 ± 5.2	32.4 ± 5.3	0.548
Parity				
Primiparous	2356 (49.8%)	773 (53.3%)	64 (52%)	0.272
Multiparous	2377 (50.2%)	678 (46.7%)	59 (48%)	0.882
Gestational age (weeks)	39.6 ± 1.1	39.7 ± 1.1	39.4 ± 1.0	0.064

City University Medical Center. The presence or absence of umbilical cord entanglement was determined at the level of the umbilicus during delivery. The no cord group included cases without umbilical cord entanglement. The nuchal cord group included cases with at least one loop of the umbilical cord around the neck only. The body cord group included cases with the umbilical cord wrapped around the trunk, excluding the neck. Cases with umbilical cord entanglement around multiple parts, such as entanglement around both the neck and trunk or around both the neck and upper/lower limbs, were excluded. Pregnancy outcomes were compared among the 3 groups: no cord, nuchal cord, and body cord groups.

The following maternal characteristics were collected: maternal age at delivery, parity, and gestational age at delivery. The main outcome measures were delivery mode, birth weight, birth height, 1-minute Apgar scores <7, 5-minute Apgar scores <7, umbilical artery (UA) pH <7.1, and an excessively long umbilical cord. An excessively long umbilical cord was defined as an umbilical cord measuring ≥70 cm in length. Data are expressed as mean ± standard deviation or frequency (percentage). The IBM SPSS Statistics version 19 program was used for statistical analyses. Categorical variables were compared using χ^2 tests. Analysis of variance and t-tests were used to compare continuous variables. Statistical tests were considered significant at a P value < 0.05.

3. Results

The no cord group included 4733 pregnancies, the nuchal cord group included 1451 pregnancies, and the body cord group included 123 pregnancies. Table 1 shows the maternal characteristics. No significant difference was observed among the groups in maternal age at delivery, parity, or gestational age.

Table 2 shows the main outcome measures for pregnancy outcomes among the 3 groups. No significant difference in delivery mode was observed among the groups. Moreover, the groups with umbilical cord entanglement, which were the nuchal cord and body cord groups, had significantly longer umbilical cords, compared with the no cord group. In particular, the nuchal cord group had the longest umbilical cord and included significantly more cases of excessively long umbilical cord. Significant differences in the frequencies of 1-minute and 5-minute Apgar scores <7 and <7, respectively, and UA pH <7.1 were observed between the 3 groups, with

higher frequencies observed in the body cord group than in the other 2 groups. Significant differences were observed in neonatal birth weight between the no cord group and umbilical cord entanglement groups (P = 0.004), and birth weight was lower in the nuchal cord and body cord groups than in the no cord group. There were no significant differences in neonatal birth height among the 3 groups.

4. Discussion

Although delivery mode was not significantly different among the 3 groups, the frequencies of 1-minute Apgar scores <7 and UA pH <7.10 were significantly higher in the groups with umbilical cord entanglement than in the no cord group. In particular, the frequency of 5-minute Apgar scores <7 was significantly higher (P = 0.004) and frequency of UA pH <7.10 tended to be higher (P = 0.057) in the body cord group than in the nuchal cord group.

In this study, the presence or absence of umbilical cord entanglement did not affect the delivery mode. This finding is similar to that of the majority of previous studies, in which there were no differences in cesarean section rates based on the presence or absence of umbilical cord entanglement [1, 5, 6, 13–16]. Meanwhile, Larson et al. [4] reported that the instrumental delivery rate was higher in cases with multiple umbilical cord entanglement, but cesarean section rates were not significantly different. Moreover, Bernad et al. [7] reported that umbilical cord entanglement might be a cause of intrauterine fetal death even though there was no difference in forced delivery rates based on cord entanglement. The authors recommended that rigorous management with fetal heart rate monitoring should be conducted during delivery when ultrasonography clearly reveals umbilical cord entanglement and cesarean section should be considered when nonreassuring fetal status is detected.

In the groups with umbilical cord entanglement, the frequencies of 1-minute Apgar scores <7 and UA pH <7.10 were higher than in the no cord group. Assimakopoulos et al. [6] reported that cases with umbilical cord entanglement more frequently had low Apgar scores and low UA pH as have many other studies for either low Apgar scores or low UA pH [1, 4, 6, 8, 10, 12]. The results of the present study also support the findings of these studies and confirm that the presence or absence of umbilical cord entanglement affects neonatal conditions at delivery.

The frequency of 5-minute Apgar scores <7 was significantly higher in the body cord group compared with the

TABLE 2: Comparison of pregnancy outcomes between the 3 groups.

	No nuchal cord ($n = 4733$)	Nuchal neck cords ($n = 1451$)	Nuchal body cords ($n = 123$)	P value
Mode of delivery				
Spontaneous vaginal delivery	4110 (86.8%)	1248 (86.0%)	105 (85.4%)	
Instrumental delivery	298 (6.3%)	89 (6.1%)	7 (5.7%)	0.868
Cesarean delivery	325 (6.9%)	114 (7.9%)	11 (8.9%)	0.605
Excessively long umbilical cord	54 (1.1%)	403 (27.8%)	25 (20.3%)	<0.01
Umbilical cord length (cm)	53.7 ± 8.6	64.1 ± 11.2	61.0 ± 10.8	
Apgar score at 1 min <7	80 (1.7%)	41 (2.8%)	6 (4.9%)	0.002
Apgar score at 5 min <7	9 (0.2%)	6 (0.4%)	3 (2.4%)	<0.01
UApH <7.10	58 (1.2%)	24 (1.6%)	5 (4.1%)	
	7.30 ± 0.070	7.29 ± 0.071	7.28 ± 0.075	0.024
Birth weight (g)	3053 ± 366	3019 ± 369	3008 ± 361	0.004
Birth height (cm)	48.9 ± 1.9	48.8 ± 2.1	48.8 ± 2.0	0.261

UApH: umbilical artery pH.

nuchal cord group in the present study, and the frequency of UA pH <7.10 also tended to be higher. To our knowledge, the majority of studies regarding umbilical cord entanglement concern nuchal cord entanglement, and no previous study has investigated umbilical cord entanglement around the trunk. The lower Apgar scores and UA pH in the body cord group than in the nuchal cord group might be explained by a greater likelihood to suffer umbilical cord compression during uterine contraction in fetuses with umbilical cord entanglement around the trunk compared with nuchal cord entanglement, because a space between the head and trunk is not present in the former but is in the latter.

Neonatal birth weight was 34 g and 45 g lower in the nuchal cord and body cord groups, respectively, than in the no cord group. In a study of neonatal outcomes based on the presence or absence of umbilical cord entanglement in 57853 deliveries, Ogueh et al. [5] reported that the birth weight of fetuses with nuchal cord entanglement was 55 g lower than without nuchal cord entanglement. The authors suggested that chronic intermittent cord compression with hypoxia might lead to fetal growth restriction; alternatively, smaller fetuses have more space to move around in the uterus and are consequently more likely to have umbilical cord entanglement. Meanwhile, Sheiner et al. [1] reported in a similar study which included 166318 deliveries that the birth weight of fetuses with nuchal cord entanglement tended to be higher. Although the results of the present study support those reported by Ogueh et al. [5], further studies are needed to establish firm conclusions regarding the relationship between umbilical cord entanglement and fetal growth.

The present study has several limitations. First, it was conducted with a small sample in a single institution. Second, the effects of nuchal cord entanglement were not evaluated based on the number of loops. Moreover, cases with multiple umbilical cord entanglements involving multiple parts of the body, such as entanglement around both the neck and upper/lower limbs, were excluded.

In conclusion, umbilical cord entanglement is associated with an increased risk of low Apgar scores and low UA pH. The present study suggests that fetuses with complex umbilical cord entanglement primarily around the trunk, but not the neck, are strongly affected by umbilical cord compression during delivery. However, delivery modes were not affected by any type of umbilical cord entanglement, which supports the findings of previous studies. Umbilical cord entanglement is a common pathological condition encountered in daily clinical practice. Although it might affect neonatal conditions during delivery, vaginal delivery can be safely performed in many cases, and undue concern should not be passed on to the mothers, even when ultrasonography reveals the presence of umbilical cord entanglement before delivery.

Conflict of Interests

The authors declare that they have no conflict of interests to declare. The authors confirm that the results of this paper have not been distorted by research funding or conflict of interests.

References

[1] E. Sheiner, J. S. Abramowicz, A. Levy, T. Silberstein, M. Mazor, and R. Hershkovitz, "Nuchal cord is not associated with adverse perinatal outcome," *Archives of Gynecology and Obstetrics*, vol. 274, no. 2, pp. 81–83, 2006.

[2] L. Schäffer, T. Burkhardt, R. Zimmermann, and J. Kurmanavicius, "Nuchal cords in term and postterm deliveries—do we need to know?" *Obstetrics and Gynecology*, vol. 106, no. 1, pp. 23–28, 2005.

[3] C. W. Kong, L. W. Chan, and W. W. K. To, "Neonatal outcome and mode of delivery in the presence of nuchal cord loops: implications on patient counselling and the mode of delivery," *Archives of Gynecology and Obstetrics*, vol. 292, no. 2, pp. 283–289, 2015.

[4] J. D. Larson, W. F. Rayburn, S. Crosby, and G. R. Thurnau, "Multiple nuchal cord entanglements and intrapartum complications," *American Journal of Obstetrics and Gynecology*, vol. 173, no. 4, pp. 1228–1231, 1995.

[5] O. Ogueh, A. Al-Tarkait, D. Vallerand et al., "Obstetrical factors related to nuchal cord," *Acta Obstetricia et Gynecologica Scandinavica*, vol. 85, no. 7, pp. 810–814, 2006.

[6] E. Assimakopoulos, M. Zafrakas, P. Garmiris et al., "Nuchal cord detected by ultrasound at term is associated with mode of delivery and perinatal outcome," *European Journal of Obstetrics Gynecology and Reproductive Biology*, vol. 123, no. 2, pp. 188–192, 2005.

[7] E. S. Bernad, M. Craina, A. Tudor, and S. I. Bernad, "Perinatal outcome associated with nuchal umbilical cord," *Clinical and Experimental Obstetrics and Gynecology*, vol. 39, no. 4, pp. 494–497, 2012.

[8] Y. Narang, N. B. Vaid, S. Jain et al., "Is nuchal cord justified as a cause of obstetrician anxiety?" *Archives of Gynecology and Obstetrics*, vol. 289, no. 4, pp. 795–801, 2014.

[9] S. R. Tamrakar, "Incidence of nuchal cord, mode of delivery and perinatal outcome: a notable experience in Dhulikhel Hospital—Kathmandu University Hospital," *Nepal Medical College Journal*, vol. 15, no. 1, pp. 40–45, 2013.

[10] E. Jauniaux, B. Ramsay, C. Peellaerts, and Y. Scholler, "Perinatal features of pregnancies complicated by nuchal cord," *American Journal of Perinatology*, vol. 12, no. 4, pp. 255–258, 1995.

[11] G. D. V. Hankins, R. R. Snyder, J. C. Hauth, L. C. Gilstrap III, and T. Hammond, "Nuchal cords and neonatal outcome," *Obstetrics and Gynecology*, vol. 70, no. 5, pp. 687–691, 1987.

[12] D. A. Rhoades, U. Latza, and B. A. Mueller, "Risk factors and outcomes associated with nuchal cord: a population-based study," *Journal of Reproductive Medicine for the Obstetrician and Gynecologist*, vol. 44, no. 1, pp. 39–45, 1999.

[13] J. M. Mastrobattista, L. M. Hollier, E. R. Yeomans et al., "Effects of nuchal cord on birthweight and immediate neonatal outcomes," *The American Journal of Perinatology*, vol. 22, no. 2, pp. 83–85, 2005.

[14] G. S. Ghosh and S. Gudmundsson, "Nuchal cord in post-term pregnancy—relationship to suspected intrapartum fetal distress indicating operative intervention," *Journal of Perinatal Medicine*, vol. 36, no. 2, pp. 142–144, 2008.

[15] V. H. González-Quintero, L. Tolaymat, A. C. Muller, L. Izquierdo, M. J. O'Sullivan, and D. Martin, "Outcomes of pregnancies with sonographically detected nuchal cords remote from delivery," *Journal of Ultrasound in Medicine*, vol. 23, no. 1, pp. 43–47, 2004.

[16] W. F. Miser, "Outcome of infants born with nuchal cords," *Journal of Family Practice*, vol. 34, no. 4, pp. 441–445, 1992.

12

In Women with Previous Pregnancy Hypertension, Levels of Cardiovascular Risk Biomarkers May Be Modulated by Haptoglobin Polymorphism

Andreia Matos,[1] **Alda Pereira da Silva,**[1] **Maria Clara Bicho,**[1] **Conceição Afonso,**[1] **Maria José Areias,**[2] **Irene Rebelo,**[3] **and Manuel Bicho**[1,4]

[1] *Genetics Laboratory, Lisbon Medical School, University of Lisbon, 1649-028 Lisbon, Portugal*
[2] *Júlio Diniz Maternity, Maria Pia Hospital, 4050-371 Porto, Portugal*
[3] *Department of Biochemistry, Faculty of Pharmacy and Institute for Molecular and Cell Biology, University of Porto, 4050-313 Porto, Portugal*
[4] *Rocha Cabral Institute, 1250-047 Lisbon, Portugal*

Correspondence should be addressed to Andreia Matos; andreiamatos@fm.ul.pt

Academic Editor: João Bernardes

Preeclampsia (PE) may affect the risk for future cardiovascular disease. Haptoglobin (Hp), an acute phase protein with functional genetic polymorphism, synthesized in the hepatocyte and in many peripheral tissues secondary of oxidative stress of PE, may modulate that risk through the antioxidant, angiogenic, and anti-inflammatory differential effects of their genotypes. We performed a prospective study in 352 women aged 35 ± 5.48 years, which 165 had previous PE, 2 to 16 years ago. We studied demographic, anthropometric, and haemodynamic biomarkers such as C-reactive protein (CRP), myeloperoxidase (MPO), and nitric oxide metabolites (total and nitrites), and others associated with liver function (AST and ALT) and lipid profile (total LDL and cholesterol HDL, non-HDL, and apolipoproteins A and B). Finally, we study the influence of Hp genetic polymorphism on all these biomarkers and as a predisposing factor for PE and its remote cardiovascular disease prognosis. Previously preeclamptic women either hypertensive or normotensive presented significant differences in those risk biomarkers (MPO, nitrites, and ALT), whose variation may be modulated by Hp 1/2 functional genetic polymorphism. The history of PE may be relevant, in association with these biomarkers to the cardiovascular risk in premenopausal women.

1. Introduction

Maternal hypertensive disorders are the most common complications of pregnancy. Pregnancy may be complicated by four distinct forms of hypertension: preeclampsia/eclampsia, chronic hypertension, preeclampsia superimposed on chronic hypertension, and gestational hypertension [1]. Arterial hypertension may be associated with inflammatory and oxidative stress. Preeclampsia as other forms of hypertensive conditions during pregnancy may affect the risk for future cardiovascular disease [2, 3].

Several authors described association between maternal pregnancy complications as preeclampsia—with greater future risk of mother to develop hypertension and atherosclerosis [2, 3]. Indeed, there are biomarkers associated with inflammatory process and blood pressure, which may lead to the future evolution of hypertensive disease of pregnancy and cardiovascular risk in women who previously developed hypertension during pregnancy [4, 5].

Haptoglobin (Hp) is an acute phase $\alpha2$ plasma glycoprotein, synthesized in the hepatocyte and other peripheral tissues, which scavenge free haemoglobin and may modulate differentially cardiovascular risk through its antioxidant and anti-inflammatory different capacities associated with their genotypes [6, 7]. The Hp gene is expressed primarily in hepatocytes but also locally in other tissues or in cells related with inflammatory processes, such as neutrophils [8]. This protein has a pronounced anti-inflammatory action and has high affinity to a specific receptor (CD163) located in circulating monocytes, resident macrophages (M2 type), and liver Kupffer cells [9–11]. The cellular expression of this pathway of Hp, CD163 and hemoxygenase (HO-1), is strongly activated directly or indirectly by cytokines, such as interleukins (IL-6, IL-1), tumor necrosis factor alfa (TNF-α), growth factors (M-CSF) [12], or hormones such as catecholamines and glucocorticoids [13].

Hp may have a role in the pregnant women with hypertension playing a protection role from further cardiovascular risk, once it prevents the formation of free radicals and its accumulation in endothelial cells, catalysed by heme, therefore preventing vessel injury [9, 11, 13].

Hp has a genetic polymorphism (Hp 1.1, 2.1 e 2.2) contributing to the great variability in anti-inflammatory responses; namely, Hp 2.2 phenotype is associated with a lower antioxidant capacity than the other two Hp phenotypes because of its higher molecular mass that restricts its extra vascular diffusion [6, 7, 14]. Also the Hp 2.2/Hb complex scavenges more nitric oxide (NO) than Hp 1.1/Hb due to its longer half-life in circulation [7, 15, 16].

The inhibitory effects on prostaglandin synthesis of Hp 2.2 and Hp 2.1 are less pronounced than those of Hp 1.1 contributing differently for its lower anti-inflammatory action [6, 17, 18]. However, Hp 2.2 is the most angiogenic form in the course of chronic inflammatory processes leading to greater ischemic tissue reparation and promoting of collateral vessel formation than the other two forms [19, 20].

The α-chain of haptoglobin and haptoglobin-related protein (Hpr), belonging to the cluster of Hp in chromosome 16, contains a hydrophobic signal peptide that may explain its association with lipoprotein particles (HDL) or membranes [21].

The objectives of the present work were to evaluate in women with history of hypertension in pregnancy/preeclampsia the susceptibility to develop hypertension in the future and the possible relationship with Hp phenotypes; the second objective was to evaluate the influence of the Hp genetic polymorphism on circulating cardiovascular risk biomarkers and the level of blood pressure in a prospective cohort.

2. Materials and Methods

2.1. Sample Population. We studied 352 women aged 35 ± 5.48 years, and from these, 165 had preeclampsia 2 to 16 (± 6.6) years ago, which was identified from medical records at the Department of Obstetrics and Gynecology from the Júlio Diniz Maternity, Maria Pia Hospital, OPorto. The diagnosis of preeclampsia was based on criteria of the International Society for the Study of Hypertension in Pregnancy (ISSHP) [22]. Women of the control group of the same Hospital were matched for age within group on the study and similarly to the study group. They were firstly interviewed by phone. Then, they were invited to come to the research center during the same phase of their menstrual cycles for sample collection.

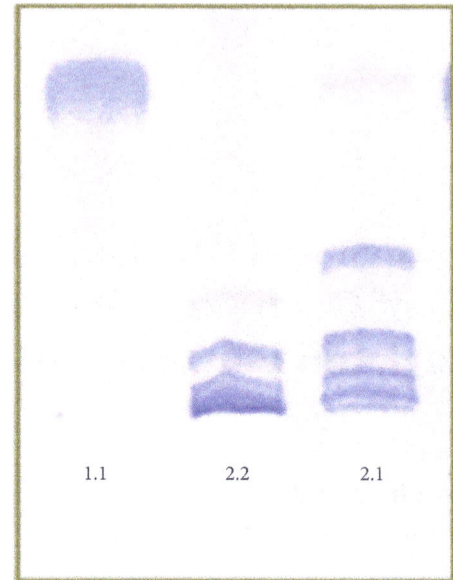

FIGURE 1: Polyacrylamide gel electrophoresis (PAGE) of Hp showing the typical pattern of bands of 1.1, 2.1, and 2.2 phenotypes.

We also evaluated some unhealthy behaviors as smoke and alcoholic habits through a questionnaire that determined women who smoked or drank after pregnancy, respectively.

Women were stratified accordingly to the criteria of the ISSHP [22] in preeclamptic (PE) and normal blood pressure in pregnancy (NBPP); in hypertensive after pregnancy (HTA), and normotensive after pregnancy (NBP), based on the criteria of European Society of Hypertension (ESH) and European Society of Cardiology (ESC) [23].

2.2. Haptoglobin Polymorphism Detection. The three phenotypes of Hp (1.1, 2.1 and 2.2) were separated from plasma using polyacrylamide gel electrophoresis (PAGE) and its presence was detected by the peroxidase activity of the complex haptoglobin—haemoglobin over the colour using substrate of o-dianisidine (Figure 1) [24, 25].

2.3. Circulating Cardiovascular Risk Biomarkers Determination. The different circulating biomarkers were determined by enzyme-linked immunosorbent assay (ELISA—R&D Systems Inc.) such as myeloperoxidase (MPO, ng/mL). Nitric oxide metabolites (NOx, mmol/L) and nitrites (μmol/L), transaminases—AST (Aspartate transaminase, UI/L), and ALT (alanine transaminase, UI/L) were determined by conventional standardized methods. Classical biomarkers as serum lipids and lipoproteins: total cholesterol (t-cholesterol, mg/dl) and HDL and LDL cholesterol, were measured by using automated enzymatic assays (ABX Diagnostic) and apolipoprotein A and B (Apo A and B, mg/dL) by using automated immunoturbidimetric assays (ABX Diagnostic). Serum C-reactive protein (CRP, mg/L) was assessed by an immunoenzymatic method (adaptation of the method of Highton and Hessian, 1984 [26]).

TABLE 1: Distribution of Hp phenotypes in women with normal blood pressure in pregnancy (NBPP) and preeclamptic women (PE).

Phenotype	NBPP $n = 128$ n (%)	PE $n = 137$ n (%)	P value
Hp 1.1	28 (21.9)	22 (16.1)	
Hp 2.1	66 (51.6)	72 (52.5)	0.421
Hp 2.2	34 (26.5)	43 (31.4)	

Chi-square test.

2.4. Blood Pressure and Anthropometric Parameters Evaluation.

Blood pressure in mmHg (BP) was measured by an oscillometric method. Anthropometric parameters such as BMI (body mass index, Kg/m^2) and hip (cm) and waist circumference (WC, cm) were evaluated using classic measurement instruments.

2.5. Statistics Analysis.

In statistical analyses, we included departure from normality according to Kolmogorov Smirnov test and then adequate parametric or nonparametric tests to compare means. We also performed the Chi-square, and for pairwise comparisons between groups we used Student's t test or Mann-Whitney U test, with a probability value of <0.05 considered statistically significant. For this analysis, we used 21 version SPSS programme.

3. Results

The results are shown in two parts. The first one considers the risk of preeclampsia in accordance with Hp phenotype distribution in women during pregnancy (Study 1). The second one observes the susceptibility of cardiovascular risk in women with previous preeclampsia, considering also the influence of circulating cardiovascular risk biomarkers, and Hp phenotype, in a follow-up subsample of 2 to 16 years (Study 2) (Figure 1).

Study 1: Haptoglobin polymorphism and susceptibility for the development of preeclampsia.

Table 1 shows distribution of Hp phenotypes in a population of normotensive (normal blood pressure in pregnancy—NBPP) and hypertensive (Preeclampsia—PE) pregnant women ($N = 265$). The NT women were significantly younger (27.93 ± 4.91, mean ± S.D.) than women with preeclampsia (29.71 ± 5.97, mean ± S.D.) ($P = 0.011$). Most women have over 34 weeks of gestation, independently of hypertension degree, but before or 34 weeks of gestation there were more significantly preeclamptic women (30.3%) ($P < 0.001$) (data not shown).

In our population of 265 Caucasian pregnant women and concerning the Hp phenotype distribution, we found no statistical differences of Hp phenotype distribution (1.1, 2.1, and 2.2) between 128 normotensive women (NT) and 137 PE ($P = 0.421$) (Table 1).

We also evaluated the distribution of Hp phenotype in all preeclamptic women at age of diagnosis between ≤34 weeks

of gestation and >34 weeks of gestation and we observed no significant differences (Table 2).

Study 2: The susceptibility of cardiovascular risk in women with previous preeclampsia and the influence of risk biomarkers and its modulation by the Hp phenotype at long term (2–16 years).

In the follow-up group we evaluated anthropometric and hemodynamic parameters and some biomarkers of cardiovascular risk in a sample of previously preeclamptic women and compared them with normotensive ones adjusted for age at pregnancy. We also study the influence of the Hp phenotype on the levels of biomarkers in circulation.

3.1. Anthropometric and Hemodynamic Parameters.

This sample consisted of 150 women aged 20 to 35 years old (min.: 20–max: 47; 35.24 ± 5.48 (mean ± S.D.) and minimum BMI of 17.1 (underweight) to 42.7 (obesity) (26.39 ± 4.57 Kg/m^2, mean ± S.D.), who were recruited for this prospective study, 2–16 years after delivery. During pregnancy, 60 women were NT and 90 were preeclamptic. In this group, 16.2% have smoke habits and 4.7% consume alcoholic beverages, after pregnancy.

In this sample, when evaluating the values of blood pressure and anthropometric data we observed significantly mean higher values in previously preeclamptic women (PE) for BMI (27.05 ± 4.79, $P = 0.033$), WC (89.54 ± 15.64, $P = 0.004$), systolic blood pressure (134.99 ± 16.50, $P < 0.001$), and diastolic blood pressure (85.93 ± 18.28, $P < 0.001$), when compared with NBPP (Table 3).

3.2. Cardiovascular Risk Circulating Biomarkers.

In order to evaluate biochemical biomarkers potentially implicated in cardiovascular risk, we found statistically significant differences with higher concentrations for previously PE comparing with NBPP, for MPO (85.67 ± 39.39, $P = 0.020$), nitrites (19.12 ± 7.01, $P < 0.001$), ALT (19.00 ± 1.36, $P = 0.003$), and Apo B (0.64 ± 0.14, $P = 0.023$) (Table 4) and slightly higher values for NOx (99.44 ± 39.52, $P = 0.061$).

According to classification during pregnancy [22] and considering the Hp phenotype, we found a variation in anthropometric characteristics and blood pressure and also in the cardiovascular risk biomarkers, classical or not between normotensive and preeclamptic women (Table 5). In women with Hp 1.1 and 2.1 phenotypes, we found significantly higher values in preeclamptic women (PE) in WC (90.78 ± 17.58), systolic and diastolic blood pressures (134.65 ± 18.31 and 86.19 ± 19.42, $P < 0.001$), MPO (94.17 ± 42.14, $P = 0.008$), nitrites (19.98 ± 8.53, $P < 0.001$), ALT (19.98 ± 8.53, $P = 0.005$), and Apo A (0.98 ± 0.16, $P = 0.011$) and also a trend in BMI (26.95 ± 5.46, $P = 0.061$) compared with normotensive ones (Table 5).

On the other hand, for Hp 2.2 phenotype we found also significant differences with higher levels in preeclamptic women, for systolic and diastolic blood pressures (135.61 ± 12.79 and 85.45 ± 16.26, $P < 0.001$) and nitrites (18.01 ± 4.44, $P = 0.007$) compared with normotensive ones (Table 5).

When comparing Hp phenotypes subgroups (1.1 plus 2.1 versus 2.2), within either NBPP or PE groups, we found

TABLE 2: Distribution of Hp phenotypes in the sample of preeclamptic women (PE) stratified by age of gestation at diagnosis.

	Hp 1.1 $n = 19$	Hp 2.1 $n = 66$	Hp 2.2 $n = 42$	P value
≤34 weeks of gestation, n (%)	6 (14.6)	23 (56.1)	12 (29.3)	0.791
>34 weeks of gestation, n (%)	13 (15.1)	43 (50.0)	30 (34.9)	

Chi-square test.
Preeclamptic women (PE) with diagnosis before 34 weeks of gestation (≤34 weeks of gestation) and after 34 weeks of gestation (>34 weeks of gestation).

TABLE 3: Comparison of anthropometric and blood pressure data in women with normal blood pressure in pregnancy (NBPP) and preeclamptic women (PE).

	NBPP n (mean ± SD)	PE n (mean ± SD)	OR	CI (95%)	P value[†]
Age (years)	60 (35.62 ± 5.62)	89 (34.99 ± 5.40)	0.979	(0.922–1.040)	0.492
BMI (Kg/m^2)	59 (25.40 ± 4.05)	88 (27.05 ± 4.79)	1.090	(1.007–1.180)	**0.033**
WC (cm)	56 (82.77 ± 9.85)	88 (89.54 ± 15.64)	1.048	(1.015–1.082)	**0.004**
Systolic BP (mmHg)	58 (118.88 ± 13.38)	88 (134.99 ± 16.50)	1.095	(1.059–1.133)	**<0.001**
Diastolic BP (mmHg)	58 (72.21 ± 10.08)	88 (85.93 ± 18.28)	1.076	(1.043–1.110)	**<0.001**
Pulse pressure	58 (46.67 ± 9.30)	88 (49.06 ± 11.91)	1.021	(0.990–1.053)	0.196

[†]Values adjusted for age (regression binary logistic).
Body mass index (BMI), waist circumference (WC), systolic blood pressure (Systolic BP), diastolic blood (Diastolic BP), and pulse pressure.

TABLE 4: Comparison of cardiovascular risk biomarkers in women with normal blood pressure in pregnancy (NBPP) and women with preeclampsia (PE).

	NBPP n (mean ± SD)	PE n (mean ± SD)	P value
CRP (mg/L)[††]	56 (0.40 ± 0.11)	83 (0.60 ± 0.07)	0.179
MPO (ng/mL)[†]	24 (62.27 ± 30.88)	32 (85.67 ± 39.39)	**0.020**
Nitrites (μmol/L)[†]	25 (10.12 ± 3.80)	32 (19.12 ± 7.01)	**<0.001**
NO$_x$ (μmol/L)[†]	25 (79.18 ± 38.06)	29 (99.44 ± 39.52)	0.061
AST (UI/L)[††]	60 (18.00 ± 0.65)	90 (19.00 ± 0.72)	0.083
ALT (UI/L)[††]	60 (15.50 ± 1.03)	90 (19.00 ± 1.36)	**0.003**
t-Cholesterol (mg/dL)[†]	60 (206.57 ± 34.29)	90 (207.18 ± 39.33)	0.922
Non HDL cholesterol[†]	59 (157.00 ± 35.60)	90 (158.17 ± 37.96)	0.851
LDL (mg/dL)[†]	59 (138.75 ± 32.30)	90 (158.17 ± 37.96)	0.855
HDL (mg/dL)[††]	59 (50.00 ± 1.11)	90 (49.00 ± 0.89)	0.479
Apo A (mg/dL)[†]	58 (0.95 ± 0.20)	87 (0.99 ± 0.17)	0.129
Apo B (mg/dL)[†]	58 (0.59 ± 0.13)	87 (0.64 ± 0.14)	**0.023**

[†]Independent sample t-test; and values are means ± standard deviation (SD).
[††]Mann-Whitney U test; and values are median ± standard error (SE).
C-reactive protein (CRP), Myeloperoxidase (MPO), nitrites, nitric oxide metabolites (NO$_x$), aspartate transaminase (AST), alanine transaminase (ALT), total cholesterol (t-cholesterol), non HDL cholesterol, apolipoprotein A and B (Apo B and Apo A), low density lipoprotein (LDL), and high density lipoprotein (HDL).

significant differences as follows: higher values of Apo A (0.90 ± 0.17 versus 1.07 ± 0.22, $P = 0.002$) and CRP (0.50 ± 0.10 versus 0.70 ± 0.09, $P = 0.026$) associated with Hp 2.2, in NBPP and PE groups, respectively (data not shown).

Women after pregnancy were then stratified accordingly to previously preeclamptic (PE) or normotensive (NBP) women corresponding to reclassifying by the criteria of the ESH/ESC [23]. We found that 47.7% of preeclamptic women developed hypertension (Group 1) and that only 10.3% of normotensive women during pregnancy developed hypertension afterwards, Group 3 as in shown in Figure 2 ($P < 0.001$). Two other groups of women, such as Group 2 of previously preeclamptic women that became normotensive and Group 4 of previously normotensive women that maintain normotensive, were analysed (Figure 2).

When we evaluated circulating cardiovascular risk biomarkers, we found that preeclamptic women that subsequently became normotensive (Group 2, PE > NBP)

TABLE 5: Comparison of blood pressure, anthropometric characteristics, and classic or not biomarkers between women with normal blood pressure in pregnancy (NBPP) and preeclamptic women (PE) according to Haptoglobin phenotype.

	Hp 1.1 plus 2.1			Hp 2.2		
	NBPP	PE	P value	NBPP	PE	P value
	n (mean ± SD)	n (mean ± SD)		n (mean ± SD)	n (mean ± SD)	
BMI (Kg/m²)†	41 (25.18 ± 3.80)	57 (26.95 ± 5.46)	0.061	18 (25.90 ± 4.65)	31 (27.23 ± 3.32)	0.249
WC (cm)†	38 (82.43 ± 10.0)	57 (90.78 ± 17.58)	**0.004**	18 (83.47 ± 9.84)	31 (87.26 ± 11.15)	0.238
Systolic BP (mmHg)†	40 (119.18 ± 13.67)	57 (134.65 ± 18.31)	**<0.001**	18 (118.22 ± 13.01)	31 (135.61 ± 12.79)	**<0.001**
Diastolic BP (mmHg)†	40 (72.80 ± 11.18)	57 (86.19 ± 19.42)	**<0.001**	18 (70.89 ± 7.15)	31 (85.45 ± 16.26)	**<0.001**
Pulse pressure†	40 (46.38 ± 8.12)	57 (48.46 ± 11.89)	0.308	18 (47.33 ± 11.76)	31 (50.16 ± 12.07)	0.429
CRP (mg/L)††	38 (0.40 ± 0.15)	55 (0.50 ± 0.10)	0.697	18 (0.40 ± 0.12)	28 (0.70 ± 0.09)	0.106
MPO (ng/mL)†	17 (57.89 ± 32.47)	18 (94.17 ± 42.14)	**0.008**	7 (72.89 ± 25.64)	14 (74.75 ± 33.89)	0.900
Nitrites (μmol/L)†	18 (9.57 ± 3.19)	18 (19.98 ± 8.53)	**<0.001**	7 (11.54 ± 5.06)	14 (18.01 ± 4.44)	**0.007**
NOx (μmol/L)†	18 (79.04 ± 37.15)	17 (101.32 ± 48.79)	0.141	7 (79.53 ± 43.39)	12 (96.79 ± 22.34)	0.356
AST (UI/L)††	41 (18.00 ± 0.70)	59 (19.00 ± 0.66)	0.084	19 (8.00 ± 1.40)	31 (19.00 ± 1.67)	0.582
ALT (UI/L)††	41 (15.00 ± 1.13)	59 (18.00 ± 1.04)	**0.005**	19 (19.00 ± 2.11)	31 (20.00 ± 3.34)	0.234
t-Cholesterol (mg/dL)†	41 (203.73 ± 33.24)	59 (202.66 ± 38.65)	0.886	19 (212.68 ± 36.63)	31 (215.77 ± 39.81)	0.785
Non HDL cholesterol†	40 (155.58 ± 35.59)	59 (153.97 ± 37.03)	0.830	19 (160.00 ± 36.41)	31 (166.16 ± 39.03)	0.581
LDL (mg/dL)†	40 (137.90 ± 33.04)	59 (133.90 ± 33.04)	0.523	19 (140.53 ± 31.49)	31 (146.29 ± 37.61)	0.579
HDL (mg/dL)†	40 (49.00 ± 1.31)	59 (49.00 ± 1.08)	0.954	19 (56.00 ± 1.95)	31 (49.00 ± 1.59)	0.203
Apo A (mg/dL)†	41 (0.90 ± 0.17)	58 (0.98 ± 0.16)	**0.011**	17 (1.07 ± 0.22)	29 (1.02 ± 0.19)	0.405
Apo B (mg/dL)†	41 (0.58 ± 0.12)	58 (0.62 ± 0.14)	0.122	17 (0.61 ± 0.15)	29 (0.68 ± 0.13)	0.105

†Independent sample t-test; and values are means ± standard deviation (SD).

††Mann-Whitney U test; and values are median ± standard error (SE).

Body mass index (BMI), waist circumference (WC), systolic blood pressure (Systolic BP), diastolic blood (Diastolic BP), pulse pressure, c-reactive protein (CRP), myeloperoxidase (MPO), nitrites, total nitric oxide metabolites (NOx), aspartate transaminase (AST), alanine transaminase (ALT), total cholesterol (t-cholesterol), non HDL cholesterol, low density lipoprotein (LDL), high density lipoprotein (HDL), Apolipoprotein A and B (Apo B and Apo A).

Reclassification of women previously PE and normotensive, 2–16 years after delivery

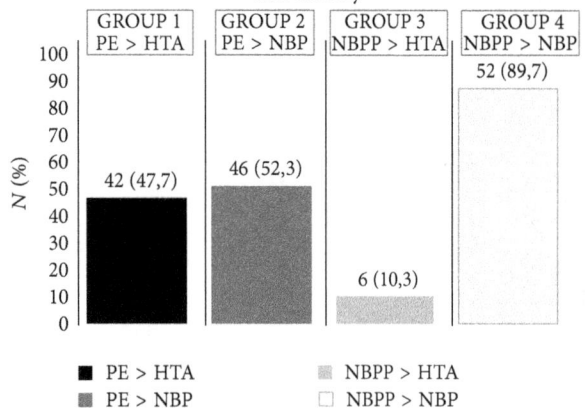

FIGURE 2: Reclassification of women previously PE and normotensive, 2–16 years after delivery. This reclassification took into account the definitions of hypertension according to diastolic and/or systolic pressures during pregnancy and 2–16 years after pregnancy and childbirth. Preeclamptic (PE), normal blood pressure in pregnancy (NBPP), hypertensive after pregnancy (HTA), and normotensive after pregnancy (NBP).

have some clear characteristics of the hypertensive subjects (Group 1, PE > HTA), namely, BMI, WC, pulse pressure, CRP, MPO, nitrites, nitric oxide total metabolites (NOx), transaminases, and lipid profile (Table 6). Moreover the preeclamptic women that developed hypertension were significantly older than the preeclamptic women that did not develop hypertension (Group 1, PE > HTA versus Group 2, PE > NBP) (36.64 ± 5.16 versus 33.50 ± 5.29, $P = 0.008$). The Groups 2 and 3 only differ significantly in systolic and diastolic blood pressures with higher levels for Group 3 (140.00 ± 6.23 and 86.00 ± 5.87, $P < 0.001$ and $P = 0.008$, resp.), and for nitrites with higher levels in Group 2 (18.02 ± 3.89, $P < 0.001$) (Table 6).

The pure normotensive group or Group 4 (NBPP > NBP) differs significantly in BMI (28.71 ± 5.11, $P = 0.033$), systolic (140.00 ± 6.23, $P < 0.001$), diastolic blood pressures (86.00 ± 5.87, $P < 0.001$), and pulse pressure (54.00 ± 9.53, $P = 0.040$) and slightly in CRP (0.70 ± 0.24, $P = 0.055$), when comparing with Group 3, with higher values for the this one (Table 6). When comparing this group (Group 4, NBPP > NBP) with women that became normotensive after a preeclamptic episode (Group 2, PE > NBPP) we found significant differences in BMI (26.85 ± 4.69, $P = 0.033$), WC (88.38 ± 12.01, $P = 0.005$), systolic blood pressure (125.04 ± 8.85, $P < 0.001$), pulse pressure (50.96 ± 8.38, $P = 0.004$), MPO (86.49 ± 44.39, $P = 0.032$), nitrites, (18.02 ± 3.89, $P > 0.001$), ALT (19.00 ± 2.07, $P = 0.021$), and Apo B (0.65 ± 0.13, $P = 0.040$), with higher values for Group 2 (PE > NBP).

Extreme groups (Group 1—PE > HTA and Group 4—NBPP > NBP) differ significantly with higher levels for Group 1 in BMI (27.22 ± 5.00, $P = 0.016$), WC (90.56 ± 18.96, $P = 0.010$), systolic (145.88 ± 16.11, $P < 0.001$), diastolic (98.90 ± 16.26, $P < 0.001$) blood pressures, MPO

(82.74 ± 11.04, $P = 0.010$), nitrites (23.04 ± 13.07, $P = 0.037$), and ALT (19.00 ± 1.85, $P = 0.031$) (Table 6).

We evaluated the distribution of the Hp phenotypes among the four subgroups and we did not find differences between them ($P = 0.273$), even within subgroups of previously preeclamptic or normotensive women considering separately ($P = 0.130$ and 0.185, resp.) (Table 7).

In order to study the influence of the Hp phenotypes (1.1 plus 2.1 versus 2.2) in cardiovascular risk, we analyse in these newly identified four groups the levels of biomarkers and their variation according to Hp phenotype (see Supplementary table in Supplementary Material available online at http://dx.doi.org/10.1155/2014/361727). Relative to individual groups, we found significant differences only in Group 4 (NBPP > NBP, previously normotensive pregnant women that maintain normotensive) with higher levels of Apo A (0.89 ± 0.17 versus 1.07 ± 0.23, $P = 0.003$) and slightly elevated differences for HDL (49.00 ± 1.46 versus 54.20 ± 2.04, $P = 0.068$) associated with Hp 2.2 phenotype.

Considering only the Hp 1.1 plus 2.1 phenotypes, we observed between Groups 1 and 2 (PE > HTA versus PE > NBP) differences for HDL cholesterol with higher values at Group 2 (46.00 ± 1.69 versus 53.00 ± 1.39, $P = 0.053$), and between Groups 2 and 3 (PE > NBP versus NBPP > HTA) we found differences in nitrites (17.90 ± 2.89 versus 9.00 ± 0.00, $P < 0.001$) with higher values for PE > NBP, and between Groups 3 and 4 (NBPP > HTA versus NBPP > NBP) differences were found for BMI (28.71 ± 5.11 versus 24.45 ± 3.22, $P = 0.010$), systolic blood pressure (140.00 ± 6.23 versus 115.50 ± 11.06, $P < 0.001$), diastolic blood pressure (86.00 ± 5.87 versus 70.47 ± 10.26, $P = 0.001$), pulse pressure (54.00 ± 9.53 versus 45.03 ± 7.12, $P = 0.011$), and CRP (0.70 ± 0.24 versus 0.30 ± 0.17, $P = 0.029$), but for WC (89.00 ± 15.11 versus 81.20 ± 8.48, $P = 0.078$) differences were slight. Between Groups 2 and 4 (PE > NBP versus NBPP > NBP) we found significantly mean higher levels for BMI (26.88 ± 5.23 versus 24.45 ± 3.44, $P = 0.026$), WC (88.93 ± 12.51 versus 24.45 ± 3.22, $P = 0.005$), systolic blood pressure (124.56 ± 9.02 versus 115.50 ± 11.06, $P = 0.001$), MPO (96.93 ± 45.84 versus 54.38 ± 30.75, $P = 0.009$), nitrites (17.90 ± 2.89 versus 8.99 ± 2.32, $P < 0.001$), Apo A (0.99 ± 0.15 versus 0.89 ± 0.17, $P = 0.011$), and ALT (18.00 ± 1.65 versus 15.00 ± 1.34, $P = 0.025$). Finally for extreme Groups 1 and 4 (PE > HTA versus NBPP > NBP) there were significant differences in WC (92.74 ± 22.68 versus 81.20 ± 8.47, $P = 0.022$), systolic blood pressure (147.56 ± 19.17 versus 115.50 ± 11.06, $P < 0.001$), diastolic blood pressure (100.92 ± 18.48 versus 70.47 ± 10.26, $P < 0.001$), and MPO (80.33 ± 6.42 versus 54.38 ± 30.75, $P = 0.014$), as well as a trend in BMI (29.97 ± 5.93 versus 24.45 ± 3.22, $P = 0.063$) and ALT (0.45 ± 0.19 versus 0.30 ± 0.17, $P = 0.055$) (supplementary table).

By other hand, when consider only the Hp 2.2 phenotype, we obtained differences between Groups 1 and 2 (PE > HTA versus PE > NBP) with higher values for systolic (143.41 ± 10.12 versus 126.14 ± 8.66, $P < 0.001$) and diastolic (95.94 ± 12.24 versus 72.71 ± 10.37, $P < 0.001$) blood pressures. Between Groups 1 and 4 (PE > HTA versus NBPP > NBP) we found differences in nitrites with higher values in Group 1 (17.53 ± 1.89 versus 11.54 ± 5.06, $P = 0.052$) (data not shown).

TABLE 6: Characterization of four distinguished groups in conformity of hypertension classification and the anthropometric, hemodynamic, cardiovascular risk biomarkers and other biochemical parameters.

	[PE > HTA] (1)	[PE > NBP] (2)	[NBPP > HTA] (3)	[NBPP > NBP] (4)	P value					
					(1)* versus (2)	(1) versus (3)	(2) versus (3)	(2) versus (4)	(3) versus (4)	(1) versus (4)
Age (years)†	42 (36.64 ± 5.16)	46 (33.50 ± 5.29)	6 (36.33 ± 4.97)	52 (35.50 ± 5.78)	**0.008**	0.891	0.220	0.079	0.737	0.320
BMI (Kg/m²)†	42 (27.22 ± 5.00)	45 (26.85 ± 4.69)	6 (28.71 ± 5.11)	51 (24.97 ± 3.83)	0.830	0.500	0.373	**0.033**	**0.033**	**0.016**
WC (cm)†	42 (90.56 ± 18.96)	45 (88.38 ± 12.01)	6 (89.00 ± 15.11)	49 (82.06 ± 9.04)	0.516	0.848	0.908	**0.005**	0.107	**0.010**
Systolic BP (mmHg)†	42 (145.88 ± 16.11)	46 (125.04 ± 8.85)	6 (140.00 ± 6.23)	52 (116.44 ± 11.73)	**<0.001**	0.384	**<0.001**	**<0.001**	**<0.001**	**<0.001**
Diastolic BP (mmHg)†	42 (98.90 ± 16.26)	46 (74.09 ± 10.22)	6 (86.00 ± 5.87)	52 (70.62 ± 9.23)	**<0.001**	0.062	**0.008**	0.080	**<0.001**	**<0.001**
Pulse pressure†	42 (46.98 ± 14.68)	46 (50.96 ± 8.38)	6 (54.00 ± 9.53)	52 (45.83 ± 8.90)	0.144	0.263	0.413	**0.004**	**0.040**	0.658
CRP (mg/L)††	38 (0.60 ± 0.13)	44 (0.60 ± 0.07)	6 (0.70 ± 0.24)	49 (0.40 ± 0.12)	0.388	0.350	0.404	0.079	0.055	0.188
MPO (ng/mL)†	7 (82.74 ± 11.04)	7 (86.49 ± 44.39)	3 (86.83 ± 24.08)	20 (60.86 ± 29.78)	0.781	0.710	0.990	**0.032**	0.167	**0.010**
Nitrites (mol/L)†	7 (23.04 ± 13.07)	25 (18.02 ± 3.89)	3 (9.00 ± 0.00)	21 (9.84 ± 3.56)	0.190	0.110	**<0.001**	**<0.001**	0.693	**0.037**
NO$_x$ (mol/L)†	6 (109.70 ± 40.96)	23 (96.77 ± 39.62)	3 (91.47 ± 63.01)	21 (78.63 ± 35.86)	0.474	0.610	0.839	0.120	0.600	0.134
AST (UI/L)††	42 (19.00 ± 0.84)	46 (20.00 ± 1.19)	6 (17.50 ± 1.25)	52 (18.00 ± 0.66)	0.589	0.190	0.188	0.108	0.564	0.230
ALT (UI/L)††	42 (19.00 ± 1.85)	46 (19.00 ± 2.07)	6 (15.50 ± 1.01)	52 (15.50 ± 1.17)	0.809	0.110	0.121	**0.021**	0.878	**0.031**
t-Cholesterol (mg/dL)†	42 (202.48 ± 42.02)	46 (210.35 ± 37.72)	6 (205.17 ± 14.10)	52 (207.48 ± 36.36)	0.267	0.878	0.739	0.701	0.879	0.538
Non HDL cholesterol†	42 (154.98 ± 38.86)	46 (159.80 ± 37.72)	6 (154.17 ± 15.03)	51 (158.16 ± 37.66)	0.392	0.960	0.721	0.830	0.799	0.690
LDL (mg/dL)†	42 (136.54 ± 37.97)	46 (137.74 ± 40.55)	6 (133.87 ± 10.29)	51 (140.25 ± 34.05)	0.632	0.866	0.818	0.741	0.326	0.690
HDL (mg/dL)††	42 (47.00 ± 1.29)	46 (53.00 ± 1.24)	6 (52.00 ± 3.54)	51 (50.00 ± 1.21)	0.172	0.367	0.878	0.580	0.677	0.130
Apo A (mg/dL)†	40 (0.97 ± 0.18)	45 (1.01 ± 0.16)	6 (0.94 ± 0.17)	50 (0.95 ± 0.21)	0.320	0.698	0.370	0.128	0.952	0.548
Apo B (mg/dL)†	40 (0.63 ± 0.14)	45 (0.65 ± 0.13)	6 (0.60 ± 0.06)	50 (0.59 ± 0.14)	0.704	0.584	0.387	**0.040**	0.866	0.159

†Independent sample t-test; and values are means ± standard deviation (SD); ††Mann-Whitney U test; and values are median ± standard error (SE). Relative to P value of (1) versus (2)*, values were adjusted for age (regression binary logistic).

Preclamptic women (PE); hypertension after pregnancy (HTA), normal blood pressure in pregnancy (NBPP), normotensive after pregnancy (NBP), waist circumference (WC), Body mass index (BMI), systolic blood pressure (systolic BP), diastolic blood pressure (diastolic BP), c-reactive protein (CRP), myeloperoxidase (MPO), nitrites, total nitric oxide (NO$_x$), aspartate transaminase (AST); alanine transaminase (ALT), low density lipoprotein (LDL) and high density lipoprotein (HDL), and apolipoprotein A and B (Apo A and Apo B).

TABLE 7: Comparison of haptoglobin polymorphism between the subgroups.

	Hp 1.1 n (%)	Hp 2.1 n (%)	Hp 2.2 n (%)	P value
[PE > HTA] [1]	9 (21.4)	16 (38.1)	17 (40.5)	0.130
[PE > NBP] [2]	5 (10.9)	27 (58.7)	14 (30.4)	
[NBPP > HTA] [3]	1 (16.7)	5 (83.3)	0 (0.0)	0.185
[NBPP > NBP] [4]	9 (17.3)	25 (48.1)	18 (34.6)	

PE: Preeclamptic women; HTA: hypertension after pregnancy; NBP: normal blood pressure in pregnancy; NBP: normotensive after pregnancy.

4. Discussion

Cardiovascular disease in pre- and postmenopausal women is the most prevalent cause of morbidity including metabolic syndrome with abdominal obesity, dyslipidaemia, insulin resistance, and hypertension.

In the last 10 years, several studies demonstrate that history of preeclampsia increases the risk for development of cardiovascular disease [2, 5]. Hypertensive disease of pregnancy in particular preeclampsia (PE) is characterized by a proinflammatory state of low intensity initiated in the placenta after under-perfusion, hypoxia, and local oxidative stress. This state leads to endothelial dysfunction and secondarily the clinical symptoms of PE [27]. The initial phenomena of ischemia reperfusion of placenta give places probability to the formation and release of advanced glycation end products (AGEs) that secondarily activates the AGE-RAGE (receptor of AGE) axis [28, 29].

AGE-RAGE axis activates an acute phase response locally in placenta or systemically in liver where one of its the components is haptoglobin (Hp) that initiates the axis Hp-CD163-heme oxygenase (HO) that leads to the switch of Th1 to Th2 of acquired immune response [12, 20, 30].

In our present study we did not observe a clear association of the Hp phenotypes with susceptibility to preeclampsia or to its long-term prognosis. But the presence of Hp allele 1 seems to be a protective factor for these outcomes, as it was observed by the other authors [31–33]. For some authors, this can be due to the great immune tolerance potential of the Hp 2.1 phenotype [34, 35]. However, this subject is controversial [36, 37]. The early PE, more characteristics of placenta dysfunction versus late PE, linked to endothelial dysfunction due to constitutional factors such as body mass index (BMI) and metabolic syndrome, cannot be explained by Hp polymorphism (Table 2).

In our cohort, we observed independently of age, significant higher BMI, WC, and systolic and diastolic blood pressure in previously preeclamptic women. The same happens for more elevated MPO, nitrites, ALT, and Apo B concentrations in blood. These results are in accordance with those of other authors [3, 38].

When we analysed those biomarkers (anthropometric, haemodynamic, and circulatory) stratified by Hp phenotypes (Hp 1.1 plus 2.1 versus 2.2), we found significant differences between previously PE versus normotensive (Table 5), respectively, for WC, MPO, ALT, and Apo A (more elevated

in carriers of Hp 1.1 plus 2.1 phenotypes). For lipid profile biomarkers, Hp 2.2 in both NBPP and PE groups has higher values than Hp allele 1 carriers. This can be explained by great expression of Apo A in oxidative condition [21]. Elevated MPO probably is related to NO bioavailability through its oxidation into nitrites, which were also more elevated in previously PE women of both Hp phenotypes [39]. MPO free in plasma or serum represents that one which is mobilized from the vessel wall to the lumen affecting NO bioavailability [40]. After reclassification according to actual blood pressure of previously PE women, in two groups with (Group 1) or without (Group 2) actual hypertension and using the same criteria for previously normotensive women we could have a more real picture of risk of the women having hypertensive disease, years after pregnancy and the natural history of cardiovascular disease in premenopausal women (Figure 2). Between the two subgroups of previously PE women there is a difference in age, with a mean age lower in NBP (Table 6). These women probably became hypertensive later. The same situation relative to age was observed between the two normotensive Groups 3 and 4. Group 3 seems to have characteristics of metabolic syndrome features, like WC, pulse pressure, and CRP. This situation is also observed comparing Group 4 with Group 2 (PE > NBP) and similarly comparing with Group 1 (PE > HTA) as is observed in Table 6.

Finally, haptoglobin polymorphism also did not influence apparently the natural history of previously preeclamptic and normotensive Groups 1 and 2, premenopausal one (Table 7). After our trial to clarify the influence of that polymorphism in some circulating risk biomarkers (supplementary table), in women with Hp 1 allele (Hp 1.1 plus 2.1), we observe a trend for higher values of HDL cholesterol in Group 2 (PE > NBP), compared with women PE > HTA (Group 1), even after adjusting for age.

The difference between groups previously with PE that became hypertensive (Group 1) or yet normotensive (Group 2) and also Group 3 (NBPP > HTA), as compared with Group 4 (NBPP > NBP, previously normotensive pregnant women that maintain normotensive) depends on surrogate biomarkers of metabolic syndrome and NO bioavailability, sustained by Hp 2.2 phenotype.

5. Conclusions

Women with previous preeclampsia and premenopausal, even if became normotensive, presented significant differences compared with previous normotensive women during pregnancy in some classic cardiovascular risk biomarkers as well as in some others, associated with metabolic syndrome, NO bioavaibility and inflammatory process. These biomarkers variation may be modulated by haptoglobin functional genetic polymorphism more relevant in the carriers of haptoglobin 1 allele. The history of hypertensive disease in pregnancy may be relevant, in association with these biomarkers including genetic ones, to the prevention of cardiovascular disease in particular of postmenopausal women.

Conflict of Interests

The authors declare that there is no conflict of interests regarding the publication of this paper.

Authors' Contribution

Andreia Matos and Alda Pereira da Silva contributed equally to the work.

References

[1] M. Noris, N. Perico, and G. Remuzzi, "Mechanisms of disease: pre-eclampsia," *Nature Clinical Practice: Nephrology*, vol. 1, no. 2, pp. 98–120, 2005.

[2] S. Intapad and B. T. Alexander, "Future cardiovascular risk interpreting the importance of increased blood pressure during pregnancy," *Circulation*, vol. 127, no. 6, pp. 668–669, 2013.

[3] S. D. McDonald, J. Ray, K. Teo et al., "Measures of cardiovascular risk and subclinical atherosclerosis in a cohort of women with a remote history of preeclampsia," *Atherosclerosis*, vol. 229, no. 1, pp. 234–239, 2013.

[4] A. C. Staff, "Circulating predictive biomarkers in preeclampsia," *Pregnancy Hypertension*, vol. 1, no. 1, pp. 28–42, 2011.

[5] C. W. Chen, I. Z. Jaffe, and S. A. Karumanchi, "Pre-eclampsia and cardiovascular disease," *Cardiovascular Research*, vol. 101, no. 4, pp. 579–586, 2014.

[6] M. R. Langlois and J. R. Delanghe, "Biological and clinical significance of haptoglobin polymorphism in humans," *Clinical Chemistry*, vol. 42, no. 10, pp. 1589–1600, 1996.

[7] A. P. Levy, R. Asleh, S. Blum et al., "Haptoglobin: basic and clinical aspects," *Antioxidants and Redox Signaling*, vol. 12, no. 2, pp. 293–304, 2010.

[8] K. Theilgaard-Mönch, L. C. Jacobsen, M. J. Nielsen et al., "Haptoglobin is synthesized during granulocyte differentiation, stored in specific granules, and released by neutrophils in response to activation," *Blood*, vol. 108, no. 1, pp. 353–361, 2006.

[9] P. Akila, V. Prashant, M. N. Suma, S. N. Prashant, and T. R. Chaitra, "CD163 and its expanding functional repertoire," *Clinica Chimica Acta*, vol. 413, no. 7-8, pp. 669–674, 2012.

[10] J. H. Graversen, M. Madsen, and S. K. Moestrup, "CD163: a signal receptor scavenging haptoglobin-hemoglobin complexes from plasma," *International Journal of Biochemistry and Cell Biology*, vol. 34, no. 4, pp. 309–314, 2002.

[11] M. J. Nielsen, H. J. Møller, and S. K. Moestrup, "Hemoglobin and heme scavenger receptors," *Antioxidants and Redox Signaling*, vol. 12, no. 2, pp. 261–273, 2010.

[12] E. Gruys, M. J. M. Toussaint, T. A. Niewold, and S. J. Koopmans, "Acute phase reaction and acute phase proteins," *Journal of Zhejiang University: Science*, vol. 6, no. 11, pp. 1045–1056, 2005.

[13] F. Vallelian, C. A. Schaer, T. Kaempfer et al., "Glucocorticoid treatment skews human monocyte differentiation into a hemoglobin-clearance phenotype with enhanced heme-iron recycling and antioxidant capacity," *Blood*, vol. 116, no. 24, pp. 5347–5356, 2010.

[14] H. Van Vlierberghe, M. Langlois, and J. Delanghe, "Haptoglobin polymorphisms and iron homeostasis in health and in disease," *Clinica Chimica Acta*, vol. 345, no. 1-2, pp. 35–42, 2004.

[15] I. Azarov, X. He, A. Jeffers et al., "Rate of nitric oxide scavenging by hemoglobin bound to haptoglobin," *Nitric Oxide—Biology and Chemistry*, vol. 18, no. 4, pp. 296–302, 2008.

[16] A. I. Alayash, "Haptoglobin: old protein with new functions," *Clinica Chimica Acta*, vol. 412, no. 7-8, pp. 493–498, 2011.

[17] P. A. Kendall, S. A. Saeed, and H. O. J. Collier, "Identification of endogenous inhibitor of prostaglandin synthetase with haptoglobin and albumin," *Biochemical Society Transactions*, vol. 7, no. 3, pp. 543–545, 1979.

[18] S. A. Saeed, N. Ahmad, and S. Ahmed, "Dual inhibition of cyclooxygenase and lipoxygenase by human haptoglobin: Its polymorphism and relation to hemoglobin binding," *Biochemical and Biophysical Research Communications*, vol. 353, no. 4, pp. 915–920, 2007.

[19] M. C. Cid, D. S. Grant, G. S. Hoffman, R. Auerbach, A. S. Fauci, and H. K. Kleinman, "Identification of haptoglobin as an angiogenic factor in sera from patients with systemic vasculitis," *Journal of Clinical Investigation*, vol. 91, no. 3, pp. 977–985, 1993.

[20] J. Guetta, M. Strauss, N. S. Levy, L. Fahoum, and A. P. Levy, "Haptoglobin genotype modulates the balance of Th1/Th2 cytokines produced by macrophages exposed to free hemoglobin," *Atherosclerosis*, vol. 191, no. 1, pp. 48–53, 2007.

[21] R. Asleh, R. Miller-Lotan, M. Aviram et al., "Haptoglobin genotype is a regulator of reverse cholesterol transport in diabetes in vitro and in vivo," *Circulation Research*, vol. 99, no. 12, pp. 1419–1425, 2006.

[22] M. A. Brown, M. D. Lindheimer, M. de Swiet, A. van Assche, and J.M. Moutquin, "The classification and diagnosis of the hypertensive disorders of pregnancy: statement from the International Society for the Study of Hypertension in Pregnancy (ISSHP)," *Hypertension in Pregnancy*, vol. 20, no. 1, pp. 9–14, 2001.

[23] "2013 Practice guidelines for the management of arterial hypertension of the European society of hypertension (ESH) and the European society of cardiology (ESC): ESH/ESC task force for the management of arterial hypertension," *Journal of Hypertension*, vol. 31, no. 10, pp. 1925–1938, 2013.

[24] R. P. Linke, "Typing and subtyping of haptoglobin from native serum using disc gel electrophoresis in alkaline buffer: application to routine screening," *Analytical Biochemistry*, vol. 141, no. 1, pp. 55–61, 1984.

[25] A. Guerra, C. Monteiro, L. Breitenfeld et al., "Genetic and environmental factors regulating blood pressure in childhood: prospective study from 0 to 3 years," *Journal of Human Hypertension*, vol. 11, no. 4, pp. 233–238, 1997.

[26] J. Highton and P. Hessian, "A solid-phase enzyme immunoassay for C-reactive protein: clinical value and the effect of rheumatoid factor," *Journal of Immunological Methods*, vol. 68, no. 1-2, pp. 185–192, 1984.

[27] F. J. Valenzuela, A. Pérez-Sepúlveda, M. J. Torres, P. Correa, G. M. Repetto, and S. E. Illanes, "Pathogenesis of preeclampsia: the genetic component," *Journal of Pregnancy*, vol. 2012, Article ID 632732, 8 pages, 2012.

[28] C. M. Cooke, J. C. Brockelsby, P. N. Baker, and S. T. Davidge, "The Receptor for Advanced Glycation End Products (RAGE) is elevated in women with preeclampsia," *Hypertension in Pregnancy*, vol. 22, no. 2, pp. 173–184, 2003.

[29] Q. T. Huang, M. Zhang, M. Zhong et al., "Advanced glycation end products as an upstream molecule triggers ROS-induced sFlt-1 production in extravillous trophoblasts: a novel bridge between oxidative stress and preeclampsia," *Placenta*, vol. 34, no. 12, pp. 1177–1182, 2013.

[30] M. C. Bicho, A. P. da Silva, R. Medeiros, and M. Bicho, "The role of haptoglobin and its genetic polymorphism in cancer: a

review," in *Acute Phase Proteins*, S. Janciauskiene, Ed., InTech, Rijeka, Croatia, 2013.

[31] R. N. Sammour, F. M. Nakhoul, A. P. Levy et al., "Haptoglobin phenotype in women with preeclampsia," *Endocrine*, vol. 38, no. 2, pp. 303–308, 2010.

[32] T. L. Weissgerber, R. E. Gandley, P. L. McGee et al., "Haptoglobin phenotype, preeclampsia risk and the efficacy of vitamin C and E supplementation to prevent preeclampsia in a racially diverse population," *PLoS ONE*, vol. 8, no. 4, Article ID e60479, 2013.

[33] T. L. Weissgerber, J. M. Roberts, A. Jeyabalan et al., "Haptoglobin phenotype, angiogenic factors, and preeclampsia risk," *The American Journal of Obstetrics and Gynecology*, vol. 206, no. 4, pp. 358.e10–358.e18, 2012.

[34] N. Berkova, A. Lemay, D. W. Dresser, J. Fontaine, J. Kerizit, and S. Goupil, "Haptoglobin is present in human endometrium and shows elevated levels in the decidua during pregnancy," *Molecular Human Reproduction*, vol. 7, no. 8, pp. 747–754, 2001.

[35] F. Gloria-Bottini, N. Bottini, M. La Torre, A. Magrini, A. Bergamaschi, and E. Bottini, "The effects of genetic and seasonal factors on reproductive success," *Fertility and Sterility*, vol. 89, no. 5, pp. 1090–1094, 2008.

[36] H. T. Depypere, M. R. Langlois, J. R. Delanghe, M. Temmerman, and M. Dhont, "Haptoglobin polymorphism in patients with preeclampsia," *Clinical Chemistry and Laboratory Medicine*, vol. 44, no. 8, pp. 924–928, 2006.

[37] M. T. Raijmakers, E. M. Roes, R. H. Te Morsche, E. A. Steegers, and W. H. Peters, "Haptoglobin and its association with the HELLP syndrome," *Journal of Medical Genetics*, vol. 40, no. 3, pp. 214–216, 2003.

[38] T. F. McElrath, K. Lim, E. Pare et al., "Longitudinal evaluation of predictive value for preeclampsia of circulating angiogenic factors through pregnancy," *American Journal of Obstetrics and Gynecology*, vol. 207, no. 5, p. 407.e1, 2012.

[39] S. Baldus, T. Heitzer, J. P. Eiserich et al., "Myeloperoxidase enhances nitric oxide catabolism during myocardial ischemia and reperfusion," *Free Radical Biology and Medicine*, vol. 37, no. 6, pp. 902–911, 2004.

[40] S. Baldus, V. Rudolph, M. Roiss et al., "Heparins increase endothelial nitric oxide bioavailability by liberating vessel-immobilized myeloperoxidase," *Circulation*, vol. 113, no. 15, pp. 1871–1878, 2006.

13

Obstetric Characteristics and Management of Patients with Postpartum Psychosis in a Tertiary Hospital Setting

C. E. Shehu[1] and M. A. Yunusa[2]

[1]Department of Obstetrics and Gynaecology, Usmanu Danfodiyo University Teaching Hospital,
 PMB 2370, Sokoto 840001, Sokoto State, Nigeria
[2]Department of Psychiatry, Usmanu Danfodiyo University Teaching Hospital, PMB 2370, Sokoto 840001, Sokoto State, Nigeria

Correspondence should be addressed to C. E. Shehu; doctorkonstance@gmail.com

Academic Editor: Gian Carlo Di Renzo

Background. Postpartum psychosis is the most severe and uncommon form of postnatal affective illness. It constitutes a medical emergency. Acute management emphasizes hospitalization to ensure safety, antipsychotic medication adherence, and treatment of the underlying disorder. *Objective.* The aim of the study was to determine the obstetric characteristics and management of patients with postpartum psychosis in a tertiary centre in North-Western Nigeria. *Methodology.* This was a 10-year retrospective study. Records of the patients diagnosed with postpartum psychosis from January 1st, 2002, to December 31st, 2011, were retrieved and relevant data extracted and analyzed using the SPSS for Windows version 16.0. *Results.* There were 29 cases of postpartum psychosis giving an incidence of 1.1 per 1000 deliveries. The mean age of the patients was 20.6 ± 4 years. Twelve (55%) were primiparae, 16 (72.7%) were unbooked, and 13 (59%) delivered at home. All had vaginal deliveries at term. There were 12 (52.2%) live births, and 11 (47.8%) perinatal deaths and the fetal sex ratio was equal. The most common presentation was talking irrationally. *Conclusion.* There is need for risk factor evaluation for puerperal psychosis during the antenatal period especially in primigravidae and more advocacies to encourage women to book for antenatal care in our environment.

1. Introduction

Postpartum psychosis (or puerperal psychosis) is a severe episode of mental illness which begins suddenly in the days or weeks after delivery. It is a dramatic and severe illness with substantial impact in terms of morbidity, marital relationship, and the infant's psychological development [1]. It is the most severe and uncommon form of postnatal affective illness, with rates of 1-2 episodes per 1000 deliveries [2].

The clinical onset is rapid, with symptoms presenting as early as the first 48 to 72 hours postpartum and the majority of episodes developing within the first 2 weeks after delivery. The presenting symptoms are typically depressed or elated mood, disorganized behaviour, mood lability, delusions, and hallucinations [3]. Puerperal hormone shifts [4], obstetrical complications [5], sleep deprivation [6], and increased environmental stress are possible contributing factors to the onset of the illness. Additional risk factors include primiparous

patient, family history of psychiatric illness, and personal psychiatric history, particularly a history of mania.

Puerperal psychosis is considered an emergency that necessitates an urgent evaluation, psychiatric referral, and possible hospitalization [7]. Differential diagnoses include bipolar disorder, unipolar major depression, obsessive compulsion symptoms, obsessive compulsion disorders, and schizophrenia [8].

Treatment involves the initiation of acute pharmacotherapy, psychoeducation, supportive therapy, and repeatedly assessing of the patient's function and safety status. The medication options include atypical antipsychotic agents and mood stabilizer or antimanic agents, such as lithium or antiepileptic drugs [9]. Electroconvulsive therapy provides a faster and more complete remission of mood and psychotic symptoms with greater reduction in suicidal ideation and is the mainstream treatment for puerperal psychosis especially in women with intolerable drug side effects [10].

Prognosis is good, especially when symptoms emerge less than one month after delivery [11]; however, they are at risk of developing further puerperal and nonpuerperal episodes of bipolar affective disorder [12].

The aim of this study was to review the obstetric characteristics and management of postpartum psychosis in a tertiary hospital in Sokoto, North-Western Nigeria.

2. Methods

This was a 10-year retrospective descriptive study. Case notes of patients diagnosed with postpartum psychosis, using the ICD 10 diagnostic criteria, from January 1st, 2002, to December 31st, 2011, at Usmanu Danfodiyo University Teaching Hospital, Sokoto, were retrieved manually from the health records department. Data relating to age, parity, presentation, risk factors, maternal and foetal morbidity, and mortality were extracted and analyzed using the SPSS for Windows version 16.0. Ethical approval for the study was from the Hospital Ethics Committee.

3. Results

Twenty-five thousand, nine hundred and fifty deliveries occurred in the ten years under review with 29 cases of postpartum psychosis giving an incidence of 1.1 per 1000 deliveries. However, 22 case notes were available for analysis giving a retrieval rate of 75.9%.

The ages of the patients ranged between 16 and 32 years with a mean age of 20.6 ± 4 years (Table 1).

Majority, 20 (91.0%), of the patients were Hausa while other tribes accounted for 2 (9.0%) patients. All the patients were married. Fifteen (68.2%) were in a monogamous setting and 3 (13.6%) were in a polygamous setting while, in 4 (18.2%) patients, the marriage setting was not declared. All the women were housewives and were not gainfully employed and only one woman had formal education up to secondary level (Table 2).

Thirteen (59.1%) were primiparous and 8 (36.4%) were multiparous while 1 (4.5%) was a grand multipara. Sixteen (72.7%) were unbooked and 5 (22.7%) were booked but the booking status of one patient (4.6%) was not stated. Thirteen (59.0%) had unsupervised home delivery and the other 9 (41.0%) delivered in a hospital setting. Majority, 21 (95.4%), had spontaneous vaginal delivery and all the deliveries were at term. There were 12 (52.2%) live births, 8 (34.8%) still births, and 3 (13.0%) early neonatal deaths in the group. One of the women had a set of still born female twins. There were 9 (39.1%) male and 10 (43.5%) female neonates with 4 (17.4%) neonates' sex not stated (Table 3).

The most common clinical presentation was talking irrationally in 86.4% of patients. Other forms of presentation were fever (22.7%), refusal to eat (18.2%), mutism (4.5%), refusal to breastfeed (4.5%), suicidal attempt (4.5%), and infanticidal ideation (4.5%). Eight patients (36.4%) presented to the hospital within 72 hours of onset of symptoms and another 8 presented within the first 2 weeks while the rest presented after 2 weeks of onset of the symptoms.

TABLE 1: Age distribution of the patients.

Age	Number	(%)
15–19	12	54.6
20–24	4	18.2
25–29	5	22.7
30–34	1	4.5
Total	**22**	**100**

TABLE 2: Sociodemographic characteristics of the patients.

Variable	Number	(%)
Ethnic group		
Hausa	20	91.0
Fulani	1	4.5
Igbo	1	4.5
Total	**22**	**100**
Religion		
Islam	21	95.5
Christianity	1	4.5
Total	**22**	**100**
Type of marriage		
Monogamy	15	68.2
Polygamy	3	13.6
Not stated	4	18.2
Total	**251**	**100**
Educational status		
No formal education	21	95.5
Secondary	1	4.5
Total	**22**	**100**

Comorbidities associated with the illness were malaria (22.7%), puerperal sepsis (22.7%), intra-/postpartum eclampsia (22.7%), and severe anaemia (9.2%). Five patients (22.7%) had no comorbidity.

The interval between delivery and onset of postpartum psychosis was 72 hours in 8 (36.3%) patients, within 14 days postpartum in 9 (40.9%) and within the first 4 weeks in the remaining 5 (22.7%) patients (Figure 1).

None of the patients had a prior history of psychiatric illness while 2 (9.1%) had suffered from postpartum psychosis in a previous delivery. Only one woman had a history of chewing *Cola nitida* excessively.

The mainstay of treatment was by the use of pharmacotherapy (imipramine, haloperidol, and benzhexol) in all the patients. However, one patient had electroconvulsive therapy for lack of adequate response to pharmacotherapy. Eleven (50%) patients were discharged home after treatment while the other 11 (50%) were removed from the hospital by their relatives before treatment was completed. There was no maternal mortality recorded among the women.

4. Discussion

This was a retrospective study of case files of women who were diagnosed with postpartum psychosis, using the ICD 10

TABLE 3: Obstetric characteristics of the patients.

Obstetric characteristic	Number	(%)
Parity		
Primipara	13	59.1
Multipara	8	36.4
Grand multipara	1	4.5
Total	**22**	**100**
Booking status		
Booked	5	22.7
Unbooked	16	72.7
Not stated	1	4.6
Total	**22**	**100**
Place of delivery		
Hospital	13	59
Home	9	41
Total	**22**	**100**
Type of delivery		
Spontaneous vaginal delivery	21	95.5
Assisted (vacuum) delivery	1	4.5
Total	**22**	**100**
Neonatal outcome		
Live births	12	52.2
Still births	8	34.8
Early neonatal deaths	3	13.0
Total	**23**	**100**
Neonate's sex		
Female	10	39.1
Male	9	43.5
Not stated	4	17.4
Total	**23**	**100**

Delivery/onset interval

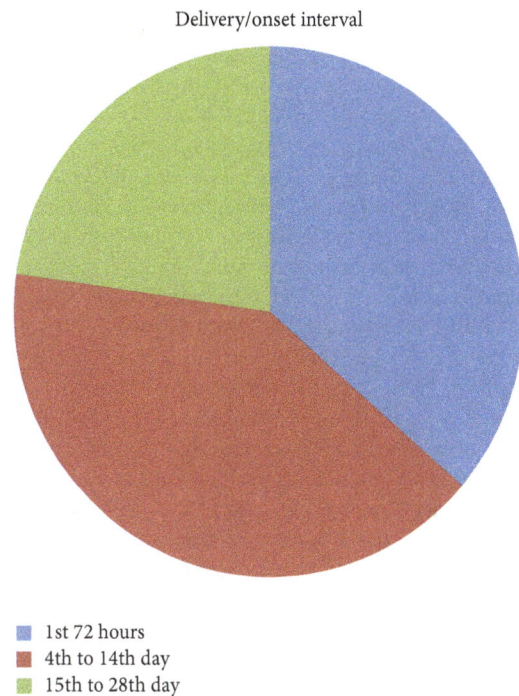

- 1st 72 hours
- 4th to 14th day
- 15th to 28th day

FIGURE 1

diagnostic criteria, Sokoto, North-Western Nigeria. Of the 29 cases recorded, 22 case files were available for analysis. This is one of the limitations of retrospective reviews especially in developing countries where record keeping may be suboptimal.

The incidence of 1.1 per 1000 deliveries found in this study is comparable to that found in other studies [2, 3, 11, 13]; however it was lower than the incidence in Sagamu, South-Western Nigeria [14].

The ages of the patients' ranged between 16 and 32 years with a mean age of 20.63 ± 4 years. This finding differs from that of a study in Sweden which found that older maternal age was associated with increased risk of first hospital admission from postpartum psychosis among first-time mothers [15]. This difference may be because the average age at first birth in Nigeria is less than 19 years [16] and primiparity is reported as a risk factor for postpartum psychosis [1, 5, 6, 14].

All the patients were married with majority in a monogamous setting. All were housewives and were not gainfully employed with only one woman who had formal education up to secondary level. These findings agree with that of studies in Pakistan [17] and Sweden [18] where it was shown that women living in the poorest neighbourhoods exhibited a significantly higher risk of postpartum psychosis than women living in the richest neighbourhoods.

Majority (72.7%) of the women did not have the benefit of antenatal care or delivery by skilled birth attendants either at home or in a hospital setting. This may explain the high perinatal deaths (47.8%) recorded among them as it has been shown that providing skilled care at birth not only reduces maternal mortality but has been found to also reduce perinatal mortality [19]. Furthermore, high perinatal mortality rates are prevalent in our study area even after adjusting for confounders [20]. The infants in this study group were nursed separately at the Special Care Baby Unit of the hospital till their mothers recovered from the acute phase of the illness.

Talking irrationally was the most common form of presentation occurring in 86.4% of patients. This finding was different from what was reported in most literature [2, 3, 11] where the symptoms were depressed or elated mood, disorganized behaviour, delusions, and hallucinations. However, this difference could be because of cultural variations. In Nigeria, child birth is highly celebrated and the new mother is usually expected to be in high spirits especially after a successful delivery. Thus, early symptoms of the illness may go unnoticed and the patient is often brought in with severe psychiatric presentations. Majority of the patients in this study presented after 72 hours of onset of symptoms. This pattern of presentation was a similar finding in an earlier study [5].

The physical comorbidities associated with postpartum psychosis in this study were mostly malaria, puerperal sepsis, and lastly eclampsia. This was in slight contrast to the finding in Tanzania [21] where anaemia topped the list of physical comorbidity followed by infections and preeclampsia. Our findings were not surprising as many of the patients were prone to the morbidities because they had not received antenatal care or delivery by skilled birth attendants.

Postpartum psychosis occurred within the first two weeks of delivery in majority (77.2%) of the patients in this study. However, this finding did not agree with findings from Abeokuta [22] where the illness occurred after this period.

Only two women in this study had a prior history of postpartum psychosis and none had a prior history of psychiatric illness. None also volunteered a family history of psychiatric illness. This is not the usual finding in the literature [5, 14, 16, 20, 23] where the risk of postpartum psychosis has been shown to be increased in families with a history of bipolar disorder. However, a lot of stigmas are attached to psychiatric illnesses in Africa as a whole; thus most people will not willingly volunteer such information. Also, one woman had a history of chewing *Cola nitida* [24] excessively but this has not been listed as a risk factor to the illness in any study yet.

The mainstay of treatment in this study was pharmacotherapy (imipramine, haloperidol, and benzhexol) in all the patients. However, only one patient had electroconvulsive therapy (ECT) for lack of adequate response to pharmacotherapy. ECT becomes the therapeutic option where risk of infanticide, suicide, or refusal to take drugs is high. Some studies advocate the use of ECT as first line treatment in selected cases [25] while others recommend pharmacotherapy [26].

About 50% of the patients were removed from the hospital by their relatives before treatment was completed. This is a common occurrence in the management of psychiatric illnesses in Nigeria where relatives prefer treatment by religious or traditional healers above orthodox medicine [27]. It is noteworthy that there was no maternal mortality recorded among the women who completed treatment and were discharged home.

5. Conclusion

The incidence of postpartum psychosis was 1.1 per 1000 deliveries in our centre. Primiparity appeared to be a risk factor and the illness occurred mainly in unbooked patients who also had unsupervised home deliveries. The most common mode of presentation was irrational talks.

There is need for risk factor evaluation for puerperal psychosis during the antenatal period especially in primigravidae and more advocacies to encourage women to book for antenatal care in our environment.

Conflict of Interests

The authors declare that there is no conflict of interests regarding the publication of this paper.

References

[1] C. W. Allwood, M. Berk, and W. Bodemer, "An investigation into puerperal psychoses in black women admitted to Baragwanath Hospital," *South African Medical Journal*, vol. 90, no. 5, pp. 518–520, 2000.

[2] R. E. Kendell, J. C. Chalmers, and C. Platz, "Epidemiology of puerperal psychoses," *British Journal of Psychiatry*, vol. 150, pp. 662–673, 1987.

[3] I. F. Brockington, K. F. Cernik, E. M. Schofield, A. R. Downing, A. F. Francis, and C. Keelan, "Puerperal psychosis. Phenomena and diagnosis," *Archives of General Psychiatry*, vol. 38, no. 7, pp. 829–833, 1981.

[4] D. A. Sichel and J. W. Driscoll, *Women's Moods*, William Morrow and Company, New York, NY, USA, 1999.

[5] R. O. A. Makanjuola, "Psychotic disorders after childbirth in Nigerian women," *Tropical and Geographical Medicine*, vol. 34, no. 1, pp. 67–72, 1982.

[6] V. Sharma, A. Smith, and M. Khan, "The relationship between duration of labour, time of delivery, and puerperal psychosis," *Journal of Affective Disorders*, vol. 83, no. 2-3, pp. 215–220, 2004.

[7] L. S. Cohen, *Massachusetts General Hospital Handbook of General Hospital Psychiatry*, Mosby Yearbook, St. Louis, Mo, USA, 4th edition, 1997.

[8] C. Jaigobin and F. L. Silver, "Stroke and pregnancy," *Stroke*, vol. 31, no. 12, pp. 2948–2951, 2000.

[9] M. G. Spinelli, "Maternal infanticide associated with mental illness: prevention and the promise of saved lives," *The American Journal of Psychiatry*, vol. 161, no. 9, pp. 1548–1557, 2004.

[10] A. Ciapparelli, L. Dell'Osso, A. Tundo et al., "Electroconvulsive therapy in medication-nonresponsive patients with mixed mania and bipolar depression," *The Journal of Clinical Psychiatry*, vol. 62, no. 7, pp. 552–555, 2001.

[11] M. Britto De Macedo-Soares, R. A. Moreno, S. P. Rigonatti, and B. Lafer, "Efficacy of electroconvulsive therapy in treatment-resistant bipolar disorder: a case series," *Journal of ECT*, vol. 21, no. 1, pp. 31–34, 2005.

[12] J. Schöpf, C. Bryois, M. Jonquière, and P. K. Le, "On the nosology of severe psychiatric post-partum disorders—results of a Catamnestic Investigation," *European Archives of Psychiatry and Neurological Sciences*, vol. 234, no. 1, pp. 54–63, 1984.

[13] B. L. Harlow, A. F. Vitonis, P. Sparen, S. Cnattingius, H. Joffe, and C. M. Hultman, "Incidence of hospitalization for postpartum psychotic and bipolar episodes in women with and without prior prepregnancy or prenatal psychiatric hospitalizations," *Archives of General Psychiatry*, vol. 64, no. 1, pp. 42–48, 2007.

[14] P. O. Adefuye, T. A. Fakoya, O. L. Odusoga, B. O. Adefuye, S. O. Ogunsemi, and R. A. Akindele, "Post-partum mental disorders in sagamu," *East African Medical Journal*, vol. 85, no. 12, pp. 607–611, 2008.

[15] A. Nager, L.-M. Johansson, and K. Sundquist, "Are sociodemographic factors and year of delivery associated with hospital admission for postpartum psychosis? A study of 500,000 first-time mothers," *Acta Psychiatrica Scandinavica*, vol. 112, no. 1, pp. 47–53, 2005.

[16] T. Ayotunde, O. Mary, A. O. Melvin, and F. F. Faniyi, "Maternal age at birth and under-5 mortality in Nigeria," *East African Journal of Public Health*, vol. 6, no. 1, pp. 11–14, 2009.

[17] N. Irfan and A. Badar, "Determinants and pattern of postpartum psychological disorders in Hazara division of Pakistan," *Journal of Ayub Medical College, Abbottabad*, vol. 15, no. 3, pp. 19–23, 2003.

[18] A. Nager, L. M. Johansson, and K. Sundquist, "Neighborhood socioeconomic environment and risk of postpartum psychosis," *Archives of Women's Mental Health*, vol. 9, no. 2, pp. 81–86, 2006.

[19] W. J. Graham Bell, J. S. Bell, and C. H. Bullough, "Can skilled attendance at delivery reduce maternal mortality in developing countries?" in *Safe Motherhood Strategies: A Review of the Evidence*, vol. 17 of *Studies in Health Services Organization and Policy*, pp. 97–130, ITG Press, 2001.

[20] M. B. Suleiman and O. A. Mokuolu, "Perinatal mortality in a Northwestern Nigerian city: a wake up call," *Frontiers in Pediatrics*, vol. 2, article 105, 2014.

[21] N. K. Ndosi and M. L. Mtawali, "The nature of puerperal psychosis at Muhimbili National Hospital: its physical co-morbidity, associated main obstetric and social factors," *African Journal of Reproductive Health*, vol. 6, no. 1, pp. 41–49, 2002.

[22] A. B. Adewunmi and O. Gureje, "Puerperal psychiatric disorders in Nigerian women," *East African Medical Journal*, vol. 68, no. 10, pp. 775–781, 1991.

[23] T. Munk-Olsen, T. M. Laursen, S. Meltzer-Brody, P. B. Mortensen, and I. Jones, "Psychiatric disorders with postpartum onset: possible early manifestations of bipolar affective disorders," *Archives of General Psychiatry*, vol. 69, no. 4, pp. 428–434, 2012.

[24] M. A. Yunusa, A. Obembe, A. Madawaki, and F. Asogwa, "A survey of psychostimulant use among university students in Northwestern Nigeria," *Nigerian Journal of Psychiatry*, vol. 9, no. 3, pp. 40–45, 2011.

[25] G. N. Babu, H. Thippeswamy, and P. S. Chandra, "Use of electroconvulsive therapy (ECT) in postpartum psychosis—a naturalistic prospective study," *Archives of Women's Mental Health*, vol. 16, no. 3, pp. 247–251, 2013.

[26] V. Bergink, K. M. Burgerhout, K. M. Koorengevel et al., "Treatment of psychosis and mania in the postpartum period," *The American Journal of Psychiatry*, vol. 172, no. 2, pp. 115–123, 2015.

[27] F. O. Fatoye and O. B. Fasubaa, "Post-partum mental disorders: pattern and problems of management in Wesley Guild Hospital, Ilesa, Nigeria," *Journal of Obstetrics and Gynaecology*, vol. 22, no. 5, pp. 508–512, 2002.

14

Early Prediction of Preeclampsia

Leona C. Poon and Kypros H. Nicolaides

Harris Birthright Research Centre of Fetal Medicine, King's College Hospital, Denmark Hill, London SE5 9RS, UK

Correspondence should be addressed to Leona C. Poon; chiu_yee_leona.poon@kcl.ac.uk

Academic Editor: Irene Rebelo

Effective screening for the development of early onset preeclampsia (PE) can be provided in the first-trimester of pregnancy. Screening by a combination of maternal risk factors, uterine artery Doppler, mean arterial pressure, maternal serum pregnancy-associated plasma protein-A, and placental growth factor can identify about 95% of cases of early onset PE for a false-positive rate of 10%.

1. Introduction

Preeclampsia (PE) is a major cause of maternal and perinatal morbidity and mortality [1–3] and is thought to be predominantly as the consequence of impaired placentation. Evidence suggests that PE can be subdivided into early onset PE, requiring delivery before 34 weeks' gestation and late onset PE, with delivery at or after 34 weeks, because the former is associated with a higher incidence of adverse outcome [4–7]. A major challenge in modern obstetrics is early identification of pregnancies at high-risk of early onset PE and undertaking the necessary measures to improve placentation and reduce the prevalence of the disease.

The prophylactic use of low-dose aspirin for prevention of PE has an important research question in obstetrics for the last three decades. In 1979, Crandon and Isherwood observed that nulliparous women who had taken aspirin regularly during pregnancy were less likely to have PE than women who did not. Subsequently, more than 50 trials have been carried out throughout the world and a meta-analysis of these studies reported that the administration of low-dose aspirin in high-risk pregnancies is associated with a decrease in the rate of PE by approximately 10% [8]. In most studies that evaluated aspirin for the prevention of PE the onset of treatment was after 16 weeks' gestation. However, recent meta-analyses reported that the prevalence of PE can potentially be halved by the administration of low-dose aspirin started at 16 weeks or earlier [9–11].

Extensive research in the last 20 years, mainly as a consequence of the shift in screening for aneuploidies from the second- to the first-trimester of pregnancy, has identified a series of early biophysical and biochemical markers of impaired placentation [12, 13]. Using a novel Bayes-based method that combines prior information from maternal characteristics and medical history, uterine artery pulsatility index (PI), mean arterial pressure (MAP), and maternal serum pregnancy-associated plasma protein-A (PAPP-A) and placental growth factor (PlGF) at 11–13 weeks' gestation can identify a high proportion of pregnancies at high-risk for early onset PE [12, 13]. The performance of the different methods of screening for PE is summarized in Table 1.

2. Screening by Maternal History

Several professional bodies have issued guidelines on routine antenatal care recommending that, at the booking visit, a woman's level of risk for PE, based on factors in her history, should be determined and women at high-risk are advised to take low-dose aspirin daily from early pregnancy until the birth of the baby (Table 2) [14–17]. However, the performance of screening by the recommended method and the effectiveness of intervention have not been formally evaluated.

The majority of the studies that have reported on the maternal risk factors for the development of PE do not quantify the risk, although some studies do provide relative risks. Most of the available literature is based on retrospective, epidemiological, cohort, or case-control studies though few prospective cohort studies are also reported. Only a few studies have reported on maternal risk factors according to the severity of the disease, that is, early onset PE versus late onset PE.

It has been demonstrated that maternal demographic characteristics, including medical and obstetric history (Table 2), are potentially useful in screening for PE only when the various factors are incorporated into a combined algorithm derived by multivariate analysis [18]. With this approach to screening the effects of variables are expressed as odds ratios for early onset, late onset, or total PE. In general, the maternal risk factor profiles vary between early onset PE and late onset PE. This has led to the view that early and late PE may be different diseases. An alternative view is that PE is a spectrum disorder the degree of which is reflected in gestational age at the time of delivery. Multivariate screening for PE with maternal risk factors has since evolved into a new approach in which the gestation at the time of delivery for PE is treated as a continuous rather than a categorical variable. This approach, which is based on a survival time model, assumes that if the pregnancy was to continue indefinitely, all women would develop PE and whether they do so or not before a specified gestational age depends on a competition between delivery before or after development of PE [12]. In this new approach the effect of various risk factors is to modify the mean of the distribution of gestational age at delivery with PE. In pregnancies at low-risk for PE the gestational age distribution is shifted to the right with the implication that in most pregnancies delivery will actually occur before the development of PE. In high-risk pregnancies the distribution is shifted to the left and the smaller the mean gestational age, the higher the risk for PE (Figure 1).

In this competing risk model the mean gestational age for delivery with PE is 54 weeks with estimated standard deviation of 6.9 weeks. Certain variables, including advancing maternal age over 35 years, increasing weight, Afro-Caribbean and South Asian racial origin, previous pregnancy with PE, conception by in vitro fertilization (IVF) and a medical history of chronic hypertension, preexisting diabetes mellitus, and systemic lupus erythematosus or antiphospholipid syndrome, increase the risk for development of PE. The consequence of this increased risk is a shift to the left of the Gaussian distribution of the gestational age at delivery with PE (Figure 2). Estimated detection rates of PE requiring delivery before 34, 37, and 42 weeks' gestation in screening by maternal factors are about 36%, 33%, and 29%, respectively, at false-positive rate of 5%, and 51%, 43%, and 40%, respectively, at false-positive rate of 10% (Table 1) [12].

3. Screening by Maternal Biophysical Markers

3.1. Uterine Artery Doppler. The most promising screening test for PE is uterine artery Doppler velocimetry. The spiral arteries undergo a series of morphological changes during normal pregnancy [19, 20]. The vessels are firstly invaded

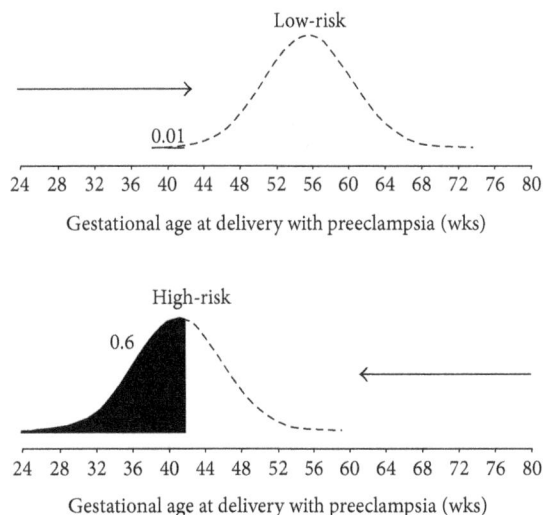

FIGURE 1: Distribution of gestational age at delivery for preeclampsia (PE). In pregnancies at low-risk for PE the gestational age distribution is shifted to the right and in most pregnancies delivery will occur before the development of PE. In pregnancies at high-risk for PE the distribution is shifted to the left. The risk of PE occurring at or before a specified gestational age is given by the area under the distribution curve (black). In the low-risk group the risk of PE at or before 34 weeks' gestation is 0.01 or 1% and in the high-risk group the risk is 0.6 or 60%.

by trophoblast, which then becomes incorporated into the vessel wall and replaces the endothelium and muscular layer. This results in the conversion of the small spiral arteries into vessels of greater diameter with low resistance and high compliance, in absence of maternal vasomotor control. This vascular transformation in the uterus is necessary to ensure a dramatic increase in blood supply to the intervillous space. The underlying mechanism for the development of PE is thought to be impaired trophoblastic invasion of the maternal spiral arteries and their conversion from narrow muscular vessels to wide nonmuscular channels [21–25]. Doppler ultrasound provides a noninvasive method for the assessment of the uteroplacental circulation. The finding that impaired placental perfusion, reflected in increased uterine artery PI, is associated with the development of PE is compatible with the hypothesis that PE is the consequence of impaired placentation and the results of previous first- and second-trimester Doppler studies as well as histological studies of the maternal spiral arteries [26–29]. Pathological studies have demonstrated that the prevalence of placental lesions in women with PE is inversely related to the gestation at delivery [30, 31].

The ability to achieve a reliable measurement of uterine artery PI is dependent on appropriate training of sonographers, adherence to a standard ultrasound technique in order to achieve uniformity of results among different operators. Using transabdominal ultrasonography, a sagittal section of the uterus should be obtained and the cervical canal and internal cervical os are identified. Subsequently, the transducer is gently tilted from side to side and color flow mapping is used to identify each uterine artery along the

TABLE 1: Estimated detection rates of preeclampsia (PE) requiring delivery before 34, 37, and 42 weeks' gestation, at false positive rates (FPR) of 5% and 10%.

Screening test	FPR (%)	Detection rate (%)		
		PE < 34 weeks	PE < 37 weeks	PE < 42 weeks
Maternal characteristics	5.0	36	33	29
	10.0	51	43	40
Uterine artery pulsatility index (Ut-PI)	5.0	59	40	31
	10.0	75	55	42
Mean arterial pressure (MAP)	5.0	58	44	37
	10.0	73	59	54
Pregnancy associated plasma protein-A (PAPP-A)	5.0	44	37	32
	10.0	55	48	42
Placental growth factor (PlGF)	5.0	59	41	29
	10.0	72	54	40
MAP and Ut-PI	5.0	80	55	35
	10.0	90	72	57
PAPP-A and PlGF	5.0	60	43	30
	10.0	74	56	41
Ut-PI, MAP, and PAPP-A	5.0	82	53	36
	10.0	93	75	60
Ut-PI, MAP, and PlGF	5.0	87	61	38
	10.0	96	77	53
Ut-PI, MAP, PAPP-A, and PlGF	5.0	93	61	38
	10.0	96	77	54

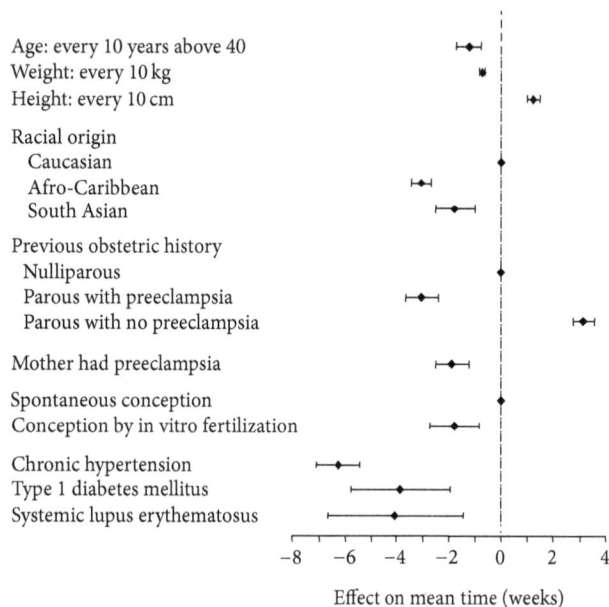

FIGURE 2: Effects of maternal characteristics (with 95% confidence intervals) on the gestational age at delivery for preeclampsia. This effect is expressed as gestational weeks by which the expected gestational age at delivery for preeclampsia is altered.

side of the cervix and uterus at the level of the internal os. Pulsed wave Doppler is then used with the sampling gate set at 2 mm to cover the whole vessel and care should be taken to ensure that the angle of insonation is less than 30°. When three similar consecutive waveforms are obtained the PI is measured and the mean PI of the left and right arteries is calculated. It is important to ensure that the peak systolic velocity is greater than 60 cm/s to ensure that the arcuate artery is not being sampled instead of the uterine artery [29].

First-trimester uterine artery PI has been shown to be affected by gestational age at screening, maternal weight, racial origin, and history of preexisting diabetes mellitus, and consequently it should be expressed as multiple of median (MoM) after adjustment for these factors. The MoM value of uterine artery PI is significantly increased at 11–13 weeks' gestation in women who subsequently develop PE and there is a significant negative linear correlation between the uterine artery PI MoM with gestational age at delivery [12]. Estimated detection rates of PE, at false-positive rate of 5% and 10% in screening by maternal factors with uterine artery PI, are given in Table 1. The addition of uterine artery PI to maternal factors improves the detection rates from 36% to 59% and from 33% to 40%, at false-positive rate of 5%, and from 51% to 75% and from 43% to 55%, at false-positive rate of 10%, for PE requiring delivery before 34 and 37 weeks' gestation, respectively, but not for PE delivering before 42 weeks.

3.2. Blood Pressure. In PE, hypertension develops as a result of vasoconstriction and reduced peripheral vascular compliance [32]. Although hypertension is only a secondary sign of PE, it is an important sign as it is an early indication of the disease. This highlights the importance of accurate

TABLE 2: Recognized maternal risk factors for preeclampsia [14–17].

(i) Previous preeclampsia (PE)

(ii) Previous early onset PE and preterm delivery at <34 weeks' gestation

(iii) PE in more than one prior pregnancy

(iv) Chronic kidney disease

(v) Autoimmune disease such as systemic lupus erythematosis or antiphospholipid syndrome

(vi) Heritable thrombophilias

(vii) Type 1 or type 2 diabetes

(viii) Chronic hypertension

(ix) First pregnancy

(x) Pregnancy interval of more than 10 years

(xi) New partner

(xii) Reproductive technologies

(xiii) Family history of PE (mother or sister)

(xiv) Excessive weight gain in pregnancy

(xv) Infection during pregnancy

(xvi) Gestational trophoblastic disease

(xvii) Multiple pregnancies

(xviii) Age 40 years or older

(xix) Ethnicity: Nordic, Black, South Asian, or Pacific Island

(xx) Body mass index of $35\,kg/m^2$ or more at first visit

(xxi) Booking systolic blood pressure >130 mmHg or diastolic blood pressure >80 mmHg

(xxii) Increased prepregnancy triglycerides

(xxiii) Family history of early onset cardiovascular disease

(xxiv) Lower socioeconomic status

(xxv) Cocaine and methamphetamine use

(xxvi) Nonsmoking

monitoring of blood pressure during antenatal care. Accurate assessment of blood pressure has been hindered by the considerable variability that blood pressure exhibits within each individual. During blood pressure measurement at rest the first recording is often the highest recording, which decreases as the patients become more familiar with the procedure [33]. It is therefore recommended by professional bodies that a series of blood pressure measurements should be made until a prespecified level of stability is achieved [34, 35]. In current clinical practice, the use of mercury sphygmomanometers remains the gold standard for noninvasive blood pressure monitoring, but there are concerns for both the clinical performance and safety of these instruments [36–38]. Observer error is a major limitation of the auscultatory method [39] and terminal digit preference is perhaps the most common manifestation of suboptimal blood pressure determination. Other considerations include the rate of cuff deflation, the use of correct size cuff, the interarm difference in blood pressure, and the arm position and posture that are recognized to have significant effects on blood pressure determination.

The introduction of automated blood pressure monitoring allows simple, standardized, and repeated measurements to be taken. It also addresses many of the errors associated with the conventional sphygmomanometer but their use still requires the selection of the correct cuff size and proper patient positioning if accurate blood pressure is to be obtained. It has therefore been proposed that MAP should be measured by validated automated devices [40], with women in sitting position with back supported and legs uncrossed, that two measurements should be taken from each arm simultaneously with each arm supported at the level of the heart, and that the average of the four measurements should be used [33].

There is substantial evidence demonstrating that an increase in blood pressure in women destined to develop PE can be observed in the first- and second-trimesters of pregnancy [41–75]. Previous studies, including a mixture of prospective and retrospective and cohort and case-control studies and randomized controlled trials, reported widely contradictory results in the performance of screening (detection rate, median 43%, range 5–100%; false-positive rate, median 16%, range 0–66%) as a consequence of major methodological differences. The data from these studies, including more than 60,000 women with 3,300 cases of PE, were compiled into a systematic review, which concluded that the MAP is significantly better than systolic blood pressure or diastolic blood pressure in predicting PE [76].

First-trimester MAP has been shown to be affected by maternal weight, height, age, racial origin, cigarette smoking, family and prior history of PE, and history of chronic hypertension, and consequently it should be expressed as MoM after adjustment for these factors. Similar to the findings with uterine artery PI, the MoM value of MAP is significantly increased at 11–13 weeks' gestation in women who subsequently develop PE and there is a significant negative linear correlation between the MAP MoM with gestational age at delivery [12]. Estimated detection rates of PE, at false-positive rate of 5% and 10% in screening by maternal factors with MAP, are given in Table 1. The addition of MAP to maternal factors improves the detection rates from 36% to 58%, from 33% to 44%, and from 29% to 37%, at false-positive rate of 5%, and from 51% to 73%, from 43% to 59%, and from 40% to 54%, at false-positive rate of 10%, for PE requiring delivery before 34, 37, and 42 weeks' gestation, respectively.

There is a significant association between uterine artery PI and MAP in PE and unaffected pregnancies and therefore when combining the two biophysical markers in calculating the patient specific risk for PE the correlation factors must be taken into consideration to avoid overestimating the contributions from each marker in order to provide accurate risk assessment for PE. Estimated detection rates of PE requiring delivery before 34, 37, and 42 weeks' gestation in screening by maternal factors are 80%, 55%, and 35%, respectively, at false-positive rate of 5% and 90%, 72%, and 57%, respectively, at false-positive rate of 10% (Table 1).

TABLE 3: Proposed maternal biochemical markers for the prediction of preeclampsia.

A disintegrin and metalloprotease 12 (ADAM12)	L-Arginine
Activin-A	L-Homoarginine
Adiponectin	Leptin
Adrenomedullin	Magnesium
Alpha fetoprotein	Matrix metalloproteinase-9
Alpha-1-microglobulin	Microalbuminuria
Ang-2 angiopoietin-2	Microtransferrinuria
Antiphospholipid antibodies	N-Acetyl-β-glucosaminidase
Antithrombin III	Neurokinin B
Atrial natriuretic peptide	Neuropeptide Y
Beta2-microglobulin	Neutrophil gelatinase-associated lipocalin
C-reactive protein	P-Selectin
Calcium	Pentraxin 3
Cellular adhesion molecules	**Placenta growth factor**
Circulating trophoblast	Placental protein 13
Corticotropin release hormone	Plasminogen activator inhibitor-2
Cytokines	Platelet activation
Dimethylarginine (ADMA)	Platelet count
Endothelin	**Pregnancy associated plasma protein-A**
Estriol	Prostacyclin
Ferritin	Relaxin
Fetal DNA	Resistin
Fetal RNA	Serum lipids
Free fetal hemoglobin	Soluble endoglin
Fibronectin	Soluble fms-like tyrosine kinase
Genetic markers	Thromboxane
Haptoglobin	Thyroid function
Hematocrit	Total proteins
Homocysteine	Transferrin
Human chorionic gonadotropin	Tumor necrosis factor receptor-1
Human placental growth hormone	Uric acid
Inhibin A	Urinary calcium to creatinine ratio
Insulin-like growth factor	Urinary kallikrein
Insulin-like growth factor binding protein	Vascular endothelial growth factor
Insulin resistance	Visfatin
Isoprostanes	Vitamin D

4. Screening by Maternal Biochemical Markers

A large number of biochemical markers have been investigated for the prediction of PE (Table 3). Many such markers represent measurable manifestations of impaired placentation due to inadequate trophoblastic invasion of the maternal spiral arteries and reduced placental perfusion leading to placental ischemia related damage with the release of inflammatory factors, platelet activation, endothelial dysfunction, maternal renal dysfunction, or abnormal oxidative stress [19, 21–25]. Maternal serum PAPP-A and PlGF are two biochemical markers that have been investigated extensively and have shown promising results in the early prediction of PE. They have both been shown to be useful in screening for aneuploidies in combination with maternal age, fetal nuchal translucency thickness, and maternal serum free β-human chorionic gonadotropin at 11–13 weeks' gestation [77] and they are now part of the platform of automated machines that provide reproducible results within 30–40 minutes of sampling.

PAPP-A is a syncytiotrophoblast-derived metalloproteinase, which enhances the mitogenic function of the insulin-like growth factors by cleaving the complex formed between such growth factors and their binding proteins [78, 79]. The insulin-like growth factor system is believed to play an important role in placental growth and development; it is therefore not surprising that low serum PAPP-A is associated with a higher incidence of PE. Increased level of maternal serum PAPP-A has been observed in established PE [80–82]. In chromosomally normal pregnancies there is evidence that low maternal serum PAPP-A in the first- and second-trimesters is associated with increased risk for subsequent development of PE. However, measurement of PAPP-A alone is not an effective method of screening for PE because only 8–23% of affected cases have serum levels below the 5th percentile, which is about 0.4 MoM. At the 5th percentile of normal for PAPP-A the reported odds ratios for PE varied between 1.5 and 4.6 [83–89].

PlGF, a glycosylated dimeric glycoprotein, is a member of the vascular endothelial growth factor subfamily. It binds to vascular endothelial growth factor receptor-1 which has been shown to rise in pregnancy. PlGF is synthesized in villous and extravillous cytotrophoblast and has both vasculogenetic and angiogenetic functions. It is believed to contribute a change in angiogenesis from a branching to a nonbranching phenotype controlling the expansion of the capillary network. Its angiogenetic abilities have been speculated to play a role in normal pregnancy and changes in the levels of PlGF or its inhibitory receptor have been implicated in the development of PE [90–93]. PE is associated with reduced placental production of PlGF and several studies reported that during the clinical phase of PE the maternal serum PlGF concentration is reduced. These reduced levels of serum PlGF precede the clinical onset of the disease and are evident from both the first- and second-trimesters of pregnancy [94–102].

In biochemical testing it is necessary to make adjustments in the measured maternal serum metabolite concentration to correct for certain maternal and pregnancy characteristics as well as the machine and reagents used for the assays and is then expressed in MoM of the normal [103]. First-trimester maternal serum concentrations of PAPP-A and PlGF have been shown to be affected by gestational age at screening, maternal weight, racial origin, cigarette smoking, conception by IVF, nulliparity, and preexisting diabetes mellitus [103, 104]. In addition, serum PlGF is also affected by maternal age [104]. Consequently, the measured concentrations of PAPP-A and PlGF must be adjusted for these variables before comparing results with pathological pregnancies. Contrary to the findings with biophysical markers, the MoM values of PAPP-A and PlGF are significantly reduced at 11–13 weeks' gestation in women who subsequently develop PE. There is a significant positive linear correlation between the MoM values of these biochemical markers with gestational age at delivery [13]. This observation further confirms that PE is a single pathophysiological entity with a wide spectrum of severity manifested in gestational age at which delivery becomes necessary for maternal and/or fetal indications.

Estimated detection rates of PE, at false-positive rate of 5% and 10% in screening by maternal factors with biochemical markers, are given in Table 1. The addition of maternal serum PAPP-A and PlGF to maternal factors improves the detection rates from 36% to 60% and from 33% to 43%, at false-positive rate of 5%, and from 51% to 74% and from 43% to 56%, at false-positive rate of 10%, for PE requiring delivery before 34 and 37 weeks' gestation, respectively, but not for PE delivering before 42 weeks.

5. Screening by Maternal Biochemical and Biophysical Markers

Analogous to the effective first-trimester combined screening for aneuploidies, effective screening for PE can also be achieved by a combination of maternal factors and biochemical and biophysical markers. Using the competing risk model, the gestational age at the time of delivery for PE is treated as a continuous variable. Bayes theorem is then used to combine prior information from maternal characteristics and medical history with the MoM values of uterine artery PI, MAP, serum PAPP-A, and PlGF. The major advantage of this model, compared to the other published models [105–107], is that it offers the option to clinicians and researchers to select their own gestational age cut-off to define the high-risk group that could potentially benefit from therapeutic interventions starting from the first-trimester of pregnancy [9–11].

It is important to recognize that there are significant associations between all biophysical and biochemical markers in PE and unaffected pregnancies and therefore when combining the four markers in calculating the patient specific risk for PE the correlation factors are taken into account to provide accurate risk assessment for PE. Estimated detection rates of PE requiring delivery before 34, 37, and 42 weeks' gestation in screening by maternal factors are 93%, 61%, and 38%, respectively, at false-positive rate of 5% and 96%, 77%, and 54%, respectively, at false-positive rate of 10% (Table 1).

6. First-Trimester Screening Followed by Third-Trimester Risk Assessment

Effective screening for early onset PE can be achieved in the first-trimester of pregnancy but late onset PE requiring delivery after 34 weeks' gestation accounting for two-thirds of all PE remains a significant challenge for effective early screening. We have therefore proposed a two-stage strategy for identification of pregnancies at risk of PE. The first stage, at 11–13 weeks, should be primarily aimed at effective prediction of early onset PE, because the prevalence of this condition can be potentially reduced substantially by the prophylactic use of low-dose aspirin started before 16 weeks' gestation [9–11]. The second stage, at 30–33 weeks, should be aimed at effective prediction of PE requiring delivery at or after 34 weeks because close monitoring of such pregnancies for earlier diagnosis of the clinical signs of the disease could potentially improve perinatal outcome through such interventions as the administration of antihypertensive medication and early delivery [108].

A competing risk model, using Bayes theorem, has been developed that combines maternal characteristics and history with biophysical and biochemical markers at 30–33 weeks' gestation to estimate the risk of developing PE requiring delivery within selected intervals from the time of screening. Preliminary results to date confirm that the *a priori* risk for PE depends on maternal characteristics and is increased with increasing maternal age and weight and in women of Afro-Caribbean and South Asian racial origin, in those with personal or family history of PE, and in women with preexisting chronic hypertension, diabetes mellitus, and systemic lupus erythematosus or antiphospholipid syndrome [109]. The third-trimester uterine artery PI and MAP are affected by maternal characteristics and history and the corrected measurements as expressed in MoM values are inversely related to the severity of the disease reflected in the gestational age at delivery. At risk cut-off of 1 : 100, the estimated false-positive and detection rates for PE requiring delivery within the subsequent four weeks were 6% and 91% in screening by a combination of maternal factors, uterine artery PI, and MAP [109].

PE is thought to be the consequence of an imbalance in angiogenic and antiangiogenic proteins [110]. Recent studies have focused on the investigation of pregnancies presenting to specialist clinics with signs of hypertensive disorders with the aim of identifying the subgroup that will develop severe PE requiring delivery within the subsequent 1–4 weeks. In such high-risk pregnancies, measurement of serum PlGF or soluble fms-like tyrosine kinase-1 (sFlt-1) to PlGF ratio is highly accurate in identifying the target group [111–116]. We have demonstrated that serum PlGF decreases with gestational age and maternal weight and is higher in women of Afro-Caribbean and South Asian racial origin than in Caucasians, in parous than nulliparous women, and in smokers than in nonsmokers. Serum sFlt-1 increases with gestational age and maternal age, decreases with maternal weight, is increased in women of Afro-Caribbean racial origin and in pregnancies conceived by IVF, and is lower in parous than nulliparous women [117]. In pregnancies complicated by PE, compared to normal pregnancies, serum PlGF MoM is decreased and sFlt-1 MoM is increased. At risk cut-off of 1 : 100, the estimated false-positive and detection rates for PE requiring delivery within the subsequent four weeks were 4% and 93% in screening by maternal factors, serum PlGF, and sFlt-1 [83] and the false-positive and detection rates improved to 2% and 95% in screening by maternal factors with all biomarkers [118].

7. Conclusion

Effective screening for early onset PE can be achieved in the first-trimester of pregnancy with a detection rate of about 95% and a false-positive rate of 10%. In a proposed new approach to prenatal care the potential value of an integrated clinic at 11–13 weeks' gestation in which maternal characteristics and history are combined with the results of a series of biophysical and biochemical markers to assess the risk for a wide range of pregnancy complications has been extensively documented [119]. In the context of PE the primary aim of such clinic is to identify those cases that would potentially benefit from prophylactic pharmacological interventions to improve placentation; the value of early screening and treatment of the high-risk group with low-dose aspirin is the subject of an ongoing randomized multicentre European study.

It is likely that a similar integrated clinic at 30–33 weeks will emerge for effective prediction of pregnancy complications that develop during the third-trimester. The potential value of such a clinic is to improve perinatal outcome by rationalizing and individualizing the timing and content of subsequent visits for selection of the best time for delivery.

Conflict of Interests

The authors declare that there is no conflict of interests regarding the publication of this paper.

Acknowledgment

This study was supported by a Grant from the Fetal Medicine Foundation (Charity no. 1037116).

References

[1] World Health Organization, *Make Every Mother and Child Count*, World Health Report, 2005, World Health Organization, Geneva, Switzerland, 2005.

[2] Confidential Enquiry into Maternal and Child Health (CEMACH), *Perinatal Mortality 2006. England, Wales and Northern Ireland*, CEMACH, London, UK, 2008.

[3] L. Duley, "The global impact of pre-eclampsia and eclampsia," *Seminars in Perinatology*, vol. 33, no. 3, pp. 130–137, 2009.

[4] C. K. H. Yu, O. Khouri, N. Onwudiwe, Y. Spiliopoulos, and K. H. Nicolaides, "Prediction of pre-eclampsia by uterine artery Doppler imaging: relationship to gestational age at delivery and small-for-gestational age," *Ultrasound in Obstetrics & Gynecology*, vol. 31, no. 3, pp. 310–313, 2008.

[5] A. G. Witlin, G. R. Saade, F. Mattar, and B. M. Sibai, "Predictors of neonatal outcome in women with severe preeclampsia or eclampsia between 24 and 33 weeks' gestation," *The American Journal of Obstetrics and Gynecology*, vol. 182, no. 3, pp. 607–611, 2000.

[6] H. U. Irgens, L. Reisæter, L. M. Irgens, and R. T. Lie, "Long term mortality of mothers and fathers after pre-eclampsia: population based cohort study," *British Medical Journal*, vol. 323, no. 7323, pp. 1213–1216, 2001.

[7] P. von Dadelszen, L. A. Magee, and J. M. Roberts, "Subclassification of Preeclampsia," *Hypertension in Pregnancy*, vol. 22, no. 2, pp. 143–148, 2003.

[8] L. M. Askie, L. Duley, D. J. Henderson-Smart, and L. A. Stewart, "Antiplatelet agents for prevention of pre-eclampsia: a meta-analysis of individual patient data," *The Lancet*, vol. 369, no. 9575, pp. 1791–1798, 2007.

[9] E. Bujold, S. Roberge, Y. Lacasse et al., "Prevention of preeclampsia and intrauterine growth restriction with aspirin started in early pregnancy: a meta-analysis," *Obstetrics and Gynecology*, vol. 116, no. 2, pp. 402–414, 2010.

[10] S. Roberge, P. Villa, K. Nicolaides et al., "Early administration of low-dose aspirin for the prevention of preterm and term preeclampsia: a systematic review and meta-analysis," *Fetal Diagnosis and Therapy*, vol. 31, no. 3, pp. 141–146, 2012.

[11] S. Roberge, Y. Giguère, P. Villa et al., "Early administration of low-dose aspirin for the prevention of severe and mild preeclampsia: a systematic review and meta-analysis," *American Journal of Perinatology*, vol. 29, no. 7, pp. 551–556, 2012.

[12] D. Wright, R. Akolekar, A. Syngelaki, L. C. Poon, and K. H. Nicolaides, "A competing risks model in early screening for preeclampsia," *Fetal Diagnosis and Therapy*, vol. 32, pp. 171–178, 2012.

[13] R. Akolekar, A. Syngelaki, L. Poon, D. Wright, and K. H. Nicolaides, "Competing risks model in early screening for preeclampsia by biophysical and biochemical markers," *Fetal Diagnosis and Therapy*, vol. 33, no. 1, pp. 8–15, 2013.

[14] National Collaborating Centre for Women's and Children's Health (UK), *Hypertension in Pregnancy: The Management of Hypertensive Disorders During Pregnancy*, RCOG Press, London, UK, 2010.

[15] World Health Organization, Department of Reproductive Health and Research, Department of Maternal, Newborn, Child and Adolescent Health, and Department of Nutrition for Health and Development, *WHO Recommendations for Prevention and Treatment of Pre-Eclampsia and Eclampsia*, World Health Organization, 2011.

[16] L. A. Magee, M. Helewa, J. M. Moutquin, and P. von Dadelszen, "Diagnosis, evaluation, and management of the hypertensive disorders of pregnancy," *Journal of Obstetrics & Gynaecology*, vol. 30, no. 3, supplement, pp. S1–S48, 2008.

[17] American College of Obstetricians and Gynecologists, and Task Force on Hypertension in Pregnancy, "Hypertension in pregnancy. Report of the American College of Obstetricians and Gynecologists' Task Force on Hypertension in Pregnancy," *Obstetrics and Gynecology*, vol. 122, no. 5, pp. 1122–1131, 2013.

[18] L. C. Poon, N. A. Kametas, T. Chelemen, A. Leal, and K. H. Nicolaides, "Maternal risk factors for hypertensive disorders in pregnancy: a multivariate approach," *Journal of Human Hypertension*, vol. 24, pp. 104–110, 2010.

[19] R. Pijnenborg, "The placental bed," *Hypertension in Pregnancy*, vol. 15, no. 1, pp. 7–23, 1996.

[20] I. Brosens, W. B. Robertson, and H. G. Dixon, "The physiological response of the vessels of the placental bed to normal pregnancy," *The Journal of Pathology and Bacteriology*, vol. 93, no. 2, pp. 569–579, 1967.

[21] F. de Wolf, W. B. Robertson, and I. Brosens, "The ultrastructure of acute atherosis in hypertensive pregnancy," *The American Journal of Obstetrics and Gynecology*, vol. 123, no. 2, pp. 164–174, 1975.

[22] T. Y. Khong, F. de Wolf, W. B. Robertson, and I. Brosens, "Inadequate maternal vascular response to placentation in pregnancies complicated by pre-eclampsia and by small-for-gestational age infants," *British Journal of Obstetrics & Gynaecology*, vol. 93, no. 10, pp. 1049–1059, 1986.

[23] C. W. G. Redman, "Pre-eclampsia and the placenta," *Placenta*, vol. 12, no. 4, pp. 301–308, 1991.

[24] J. W. Meekins, R. Pijnenborg, M. Hanssens, I. R. McFadyen, and A. van Asshe, "A study of placental bed spiral arteries and trophoblast invasion in normal and severe pre-eclamptic pregnancies," *The British Journal of Obstetrics and Gynaecology*, vol. 101, no. 8, pp. 669–674, 1994.

[25] J. P. Granger, B. T. Alexander, M. T. Llinas, W. A. Bennett, and R. A. Khalil, "Pathophysiology of hypertension during preeclampsia linking placental ischemia with endothelial dysfunction," *Hypertension*, vol. 38, no. 3, pp. 718–722, 2001.

[26] P. Olofsson, R. N. Laurini, and K. Marsal, "A high uterine artery pulsatility index reflects a defective development of placental bed spiral arteries in pregnancies complicated by hypertension and fetal growth retardation," *European Journal of Obstetrics Gynecology and Reproductive Biology*, vol. 49, no. 3, pp. 161–168, 1993.

[27] A. T. Papageorghiou, C. K. H. Yu, S. Cicero, S. Bower, and K. H. Nicolaides, "Second-trimester uterine artery Doppler screening in unselected populations: a review," *Journal of Maternal-Fetal and Neonatal Medicine*, vol. 12, no. 2, pp. 78–88, 2002.

[28] A. M. Martin, R. Bindra, P. Curcio, S. Cicero, and K. H. Nicolaides, "Screening for pre-eclampsia and fetal growth restriction by uterine artery Doppler at 11–14 weeks of gestation," *Ultrasound in Obstetrics and Gynecology*, vol. 18, no. 6, pp. 583–586, 2001.

[29] W. Plasencia, N. Maiz, S. Bonino, C. Kaihura, and K. H. Nicolaides, "Uterine artery Doppler at 11 + 0 to 13 + 6 weeks in the prediction of pre-eclampsia," *Ultrasound in Obstetrics and Gynecology*, vol. 30, no. 5, pp. 742–749, 2007.

[30] J. S. Moldenhauer, J. Stanek, C. Warshak, J. Khoury, and B. Sibai, "The frequency and severity of placental findings in women with preeclampsia are gestational age dependent," *The American Journal of Obstetrics and Gynecology*, vol. 189, no. 4, pp. 1173–1177, 2003.

[31] M. Egbor, T. Ansari, N. Morris, C. J. Green, and P. D. Sibbons, "Morphometric placental villous and vascular abnormalities in early- and late-onset pre-eclampsia with and without fetal growth restriction," *British Journal of Obstetrics and Gynaecology*, vol. 113, no. 5, pp. 580–589, 2006.

[32] S. P. Salas, "What causes pre-eclampsia?" *Bailliere's Best Practice and Research in Clinical Obstetrics and Gynaecology*, vol. 13, no. 1, pp. 41–57, 1999.

[33] L. C. Y. Poon, N. A. Zymeri, A. Zamprakou, A. Syngelaki, and K. H. Nicolaides, "Protocol for measurement of mean arterial pressure at 11-13 weeks' estation," *Fetal Diagnosis and Therapy*, vol. 31, no. 1, pp. 42–48, 2012.

[34] National Heart Foundation of Australia, "Hypertension Management Guide for Doctors," 2004, http://www.heartfoundation.org.au.

[35] T. G. Pickering, J. E. Hall, L. J. Appel et al., "Recommendations for blood pressure measurement in humans and experimental animals: part 1: blood pressure measurement in humans: a statement for professionals from the subcommittee of professional and public education of the American heart association council on high blood pressure research," *Hypertension*, vol. 45, pp. 142–161, 2005.

[36] US Environmental Protection Agency, "Mercury Study Report to Congress. Volume 1: Executive Summary," EPA-452/R-97-003, Environmental Protection Agency, Washington, Wash, USA, 1997.

[37] D. Mion and A. M. G. Pierin, "How accurate are sphygmomanometers?" *Journal of Human Hypertension*, vol. 12, no. 4, pp. 245–248, 1998.

[38] N. D. Markandu, F. Whitcher, A. Arnold, and C. Carney, "The mercury sphygmomanometer should be abandoned before it is proscribed," *Journal of Human Hypertension*, vol. 14, no. 1, pp. 31–36, 2000.

[39] G. Rose, "Standardisation of observers in blood pressure measurement," *The Lancet*, vol. 285, no. 7387, pp. 673–674, 1965.

[40] A. Reinders, A. C. Cuckson, J. T. M. Lee, and A. H. Shennan, "An accurate automated blood pressure device for use in pregnancy and pre-eclampsia: The Microlife 3BTO-A," *BJOG: An International Journal of Obstetrics and Gynaecology*, vol. 112, no. 7, pp. 915–920, 2005.

[41] N. E. Fallis and H. G. Langford, "Relation of second trimester blood pressure to toxemia of pregnancy in the primigravid

patient," *The American journal of obstetrics and gynecology*, vol. 87, pp. 123–125, 1963.

[42] E. W. Page and R. Christianson, "The impact of mean arterial pressure in the middle trimester upon the outcome of pregnancy," *The American Journal of Obstetrics and Gynecology*, vol. 125, no. 6, pp. 740–746, 1976.

[43] E. A. Friedman and R. K. Neff, "Systolic and mean arterial blood pressure," in *Pregnancy Hypertension. A Systematic Evaluation of Clinical Diagnostic Criteria*, E. A. Friedman and R. K. Neff, Eds., pp. 212–219, PSG Publishing, Littleton, Mass, USA, 1977.

[44] D. Robrecht, M. Schriever, and R. Rasenack, "The mean blood pressure in the second trimester (MAP-2) as a valuable aid in the early recognition of the pregnancies with a risk of hypertension," *Geburtshilfe und Frauenheilkunde*, vol. 40, no. 2, pp. 121–124, 1980.

[45] J. M. Moutquin, R. Bilodeau, P. Raynault et al., "A prospective study of blood pressure in pregnancy. Prediction of the complications of hypertension," *Journal de Gynecologie Obstetrique et Biologie de la Reproduction*, vol. 11, no. 7, pp. 833–837, 1982.

[46] T. Oeney, A. Balogh, and H. Kaulhausen, "The predictive value of blood pressure and weight gain during pregnancy for the early diagnosis of gestosis/preeclampsia. Preliminary report," *Fortschritte der Medizin*, vol. 100, no. 7, pp. 277–280, 1982.

[47] I. Mahanna, T. Algeri, C. Cigarini, and G. Zinelli, "Arterial pressure, MAP and dynamic tests in the monitoring of pregnancy," *Annali di Ostetricia, Ginecologia, Medicina Perinatale*, vol. 104, no. 4, pp. 248–255, 1983.

[48] T. Oney and H. Kaulhausen, "The value of the mean arterial blood pressure in the second trimester (MAP-2 value) as a predictor of pregnancy-induced hypertension and preeclampsia. A preliminary report," *Clinical and Experimental Hypertension B*, vol. 2, no. 2, pp. 211–216, 1983.

[49] J. M. Moutquin, C. Rainville, L. Giroux et al., "A prospective study of blood pressure in pregnancy: prediction of preeclampsia," *American Journal of Obstetrics & Gynecology*, vol. 151, no. 2, pp. 191–196, 1985.

[50] R. E. Reiss, R. W. O'Shaughnessy, T. J. Quilligan, and F. P. Zuspan, "Retrospective comparison of blood pressure course during preeclamptic and matched control pregnancies," *The American Journal of Obstetrics and Gynecology*, vol. 156, no. 4, pp. 894–898, 1987.

[51] K. L. Ales, M. E. Norton, and M. L. Druzin, "Early prediction of antepartum hypertension," *Obstetrics and Gynecology*, vol. 73, no. 6, pp. 928–933, 1989.

[52] L. M. A. Villar and B. M. Sibai, "Clinical significance of elevated mean arterial blood pressure in second trimester and threshold increase in systolic or diastolic blood pressure during third trimester," *The American Journal of Obstetrics and Gynecology*, vol. 160, no. 2, pp. 419–423, 1989.

[53] J. M. Moutquin, C. Rainville, L. Giroux et al., "Is a threshold increase in blood pressure predictive of preeclampsia? A prospective cohort study," *Clinical and Experimental Hypertension B*, vol. 9, no. 2, pp. 225–235, 1990.

[54] A. Conde-Agudelo, J. M. Belizan, R. Lede, and E. F. Bergel, "What does and elevated mean arterial pressure in the second half of pregnancy predict—gestational hypertension or preeclampsia?" *The American Journal of Obstetrics and Gynecology*, vol. 169, no. 3, pp. 509–514, 1993.

[55] P. M. Kyle, S. J. Clark, D. Buckley et al., "Second trimester ambulatory blood pressure in nulliparous pregnancy: a useful screening test for pre-eclampsia?" *The British Journal of Obstetrics and Gynaecology*, vol. 100, no. 10, pp. 914–919, 1993.

[56] M. C. Lopez, J. M. Belizan, J. Villar, and E. Bergel, "The measurement of diastolic blood pressure during pregnancy: which Korotkoff phase should be used?" *American Journal of Obstetrics and Gynecology*, vol. 170, no. 2, pp. 574–578, 1994.

[57] M. S. Rogers, T. Chung, and S. Baldwin, "A reappraisal of second trimester mean arterial pressure as a predictor of pregnancy induced hypertension," *Journal of Obstetrics & Gynaecology*, vol. 14, no. 4, pp. 232–236, 1994.

[58] H. Valensise, A. L. Tranquilli, D. Arduini, G. G. Garzetti, and C. Romanini, "Screening pregnant women at 22–24 weeks for gestational hypertension or intrauterine growth retardation by Doppler ultrasound followed by 24-hour blood pressure recording," *Hypertension in Pregnancy*, vol. 14, no. 3, pp. 351–359, 1995.

[59] J. L. Atterbury, L. J. Groome, and S. L. Baker, "Elevated midtrimester mean arterial blood pressure in women with severe preeclampsia," *Applied Nursing Research*, vol. 9, no. 4, pp. 161–166, 1996.

[60] J. R. Higgins, J. J. Walshe, A. Halligan, E. O'Brien, R. Conroy, and M. R. N. Darling, "Can 24-hour ambulatory blood pressure measurement predict the development of hypertension in primigravidae?" *British Journal of Obstetrics and Gynaecology*, vol. 104, no. 3, pp. 356–362, 1997.

[61] A. Konijnenberg, J. A. M. Van der Post, B. W. Mol et al., "Can flow cytometric detection of platelet activation early in pregnancy predict the occurrence of preeclampsia? A prospective study," *The American Journal of Obstetrics and Gynecology*, vol. 177, no. 2, pp. 434–442, 1997.

[62] B. M. Sibai, M. Ewell, R. J. Levine et al., "Risk factors associated with preeclampsia in healthy nulliparous women," *The American Journal of Obstetrics and Gynecology*, vol. 177, no. 5, pp. 1003–1010, 1997.

[63] S. Caritis, B. Sibai, J. Hauth et al., "Predictors of pre-eclampsia in women at high risk," *American Journal of Obstetrics & Gynecology*, vol. 179, no. 4, pp. 946–951, 1998.

[64] M. Knuist, G. J. Bonsel, H. A. Zondervan, and P. E. Treffers, "Risk factors for preeclampsia in nulliparous women in distinct ethnic groups: a prospective cohort study," *Obstetrics and Gynecology*, vol. 92, no. 2, pp. 174–178, 1998.

[65] J. A. Penny, A. W. F. Halligan, A. H. Shennan et al., "Automated, ambulatory, or conventional blood pressure measurement in pregnancy: which is the better predictor of severe hypertension?" *The American Journal of Obstetrics and Gynecology*, vol. 178, no. 3, pp. 521–526, 1998.

[66] J. Bar, R. Maymon, A. Padoa et al., "White coat hypertension and pregnancy outcome," *Journal of Human Hypertension*, vol. 13, no. 8, pp. 541–545, 1999.

[67] R. A. Odegard, L. J. Vatten, S. T. Nilsen, K. A. Salvesen, and R. Austgulen, "Risk factors and clinical manifestations of preeclampsia," *British Journal of Obstetrics and Gynaecology*, vol. 107, no. 11, pp. 1410–1416, 2000.

[68] M. Shaarawy and A.-M. A. Abdel-Magid, "Plasma endothelin-1 and mean arterial pressure in the prediction of pre- eclampsia," *International Journal of Gynecology & Obstetrics*, vol. 68, no. 2, pp. 105–111, 2000.

[69] D. M. Stamilio, H. M. Sehdev, M. A. Morgan, K. Propert, and G. A. Macones, "Can antenatal clinical and biochemical markers predict the development of severe preeclampsia?" *American Journal of Obstetrics and Gynecology*, vol. 182, no. 3, pp. 589–594, 2000.

[70] A. L. Tranquilli, V. Bezzeccheri, S. R. Giannubilo, and E. Garbati, "The "relative weight" of Doppler velocimetry of uterine artery

and ambulatory blood pressure monitoring in prediction of gestational hypertension and prccclanipsia," *Acta Biomedica de l'Ateneo Parmense*, vol. 71, supplement 1, pp. 351–355, 2000.

[71] F. F. Lauszus, O. W. Rasmussen, T. Lousen, T. M. Klebe, and J. G. Klebe, "Ambulatory blood pressure as predictor of preeclampsia in diabetic pregnancies with respect to urinary albumin excretion rate and glycemic regulation," *Acta Obstetricia et Gynecologica Scandinavica*, vol. 80, no. 12, pp. 1096–1103, 2001.

[72] R. Iwasaki, A. Ohkuchi, I. Furuta et al., "Relationship between blood pressure level in early pregnancy and subsequent changes in blood pressure during pregnancy," *Acta Obstetricia et Gynecologica Scandinavica*, vol. 81, no. 10, pp. 918–925, 2002.

[73] A. Ohkuchi, R. Iwasaki, T. Ojima et al., "Increase in systolic blood pressure of ≥ 30 mm Hg and/or diastolic blood pressure of ≥ 15 mm Hg during pregnancy: is it pathologic?" *Hypertension in Pregnancy*, vol. 22, no. 3, pp. 275–285, 2003.

[74] R. Perini, C. Fisogni, R. Bonera et al., "Role of Doppler velocimetry of uterine arteries and ambulatory blood pressure monitoring in detecting pregnancies at risk for preeclampsia," *Minerva Ginecologica*, vol. 56, no. 2, pp. 117–123, 2004.

[75] L. C. Poon, N. A. Kametas, C. Valencia, T. Chelemen, and K. H. Nicolaides, "Systolic diastolic and mean arterial pressure at 11-13 weeks in the prediction of hypertensive disorders in pregnancy: a prospective screening study," *Hypertens Pregnancy*, vol. 30, pp. 93–107, 2011.

[76] J. S. Cnossen, K. C. Vollebregt, N. de Vrieze et al., "Accuracy of mean arterial pressure and blood pressure measurements in predicting pre-eclampsia: systematic review and meta-analysis," *British Medical Journal*, vol. 336, no. 7653, pp. 1117–1120, 2008.

[77] D. Wright, A. Syngelaki, I. Bradbury, R. Akolekar, and K. H. Nicolaides, "First-trimester screening for trisomies 21, 18 and 13 by ultrasound and biochemical testing," *Fetal Diagnosis and Therapy*, vol. 35, no. 2, pp. 118–126, 2014.

[78] M. Bonno, C. Oxvig, G. M. Kephart et al., "Localization of pregnancy-associated plasma protein-a and colocalization of pregnancy-associated plasma protein-a messenger ribonucleic acid and eosinophil granule major basic protein messenger ribonucleic acid in placenta," *Laboratory Investigation*, vol. 71, no. 4, pp. 560–566, 1994.

[79] J. B. Lawrence, C. Oxvig, M. T. Overgaard et al., "The insulin-like growth factor (IGF)-dependent IGF binding protein-4 protease secreted by human fibroblasts is pregnancy-associated plasma protein-A," *Proceedings of the National Academy of Sciences of the United States of America*, vol. 96, no. 6, pp. 3149–3153, 1999.

[80] N. A. Bersinger, A. K. Smárason, S. Muttukrishna, N. P. Groome, and C. W. Redman, "Women with preeclampsia have increased serum levels of pregnancy-associated plasma protein A (PAPP-A), inhibin A, activin A, and soluble E-selectin," *Hypertension in Pregnancy*, vol. 22, no. 1, pp. 45–55, 2003.

[81] N. A. Bersinger and R. A. Ødegård, "Second- and third-trimester serum levels of placental proteins in preeclampsia and small-for-gestational age pregnancies," *Acta Obstetricia et Gynecologica Scandinavica*, vol. 83, no. 1, pp. 37–45, 2004.

[82] K. Deveci, E. Sogut, O. Evliyaoglu, and N. Duras, "Pregnancy-associated plasma protein-A and C-reactive protein levels in pre-eclamptic and normotensive pregnant women at third trimester," *Journal of Obstetrics and Gynaecology Research*, vol. 35, pp. 94–98, 2009.

[83] C. Y. T. Ong, A. W. Liao, K. Spencer, S. Munim, and K. H. Nicolaides, "First trimester maternal serum free *β* human chorionic gonadotrophin and pregnancy associated plasma protein a as predictors of pregnancy complications," *British Journal of Obstetrics and Gynaecology*, vol. 107, no. 10, pp. 1265–1270, 2000.

[84] G. C. S. Smith, E. J. Stenhouse, J. A. Crossley, D. A. Aitken, A. D. Cameron, and J. M. Connor, "Early pregnancy levels of pregnancy-associated plasma protein A and the risk of intrauterine growth restriction, premature birth, preeclampsia, and stillbirth," *The Journal of Clinical Endocrinology & Metabolism*, vol. 87, no. 4, pp. 1762–1767, 2002.

[85] Y. Yaron, S. Heifetz, Y. Ochshorn, O. Lehavi, and A. Orr-Urtreger, "Decreased first trimester PAPP-A is a predictor of adverse pregnancy outcome," *Prenatal Diagnosis*, vol. 22, no. 9, pp. 778–782, 2002.

[86] L. Dugoff, J. C. Hobbins, F. D. Malone et al., "First-trimester maternal serum PAPP-A and free-beta subunit human chorionic gonadotropin concentrations and nuchal translucency are associated with obstetric complications: a population-based screening study (The FASTER Trial)," *American Journal of Obstetrics & Gynecology*, vol. 191, no. 4, pp. 1446–1451, 2004.

[87] K. Spencer, C. K. H. Yu, N. J. Cowans, C. Otigbah, and K. H. Nicolaides, "Prediction of pregnancy complications by first-trimester maternal serum PAPP-A and free *β*-hCG and with second-trimester uterine artery Doppler," *Prenatal Diagnosis*, vol. 25, no. 10, pp. 949–953, 2005.

[88] A. Pilalis, A. P. Souka, P. Antsaklis et al., "Screening for pre-eclampsia and fetal growth restriction by uterine artery Doppler and PAPP-A at 11-14 weeks gestation," *Ultrasound in Obstetrics and Gynecology*, vol. 29, no. 2, pp. 135–140, 2007.

[89] K. Spencer, N. J. Cowans, I. Chefetz, J. Tal, and H. Meiri, "First-trimester maternal serum PP-13, PAPP-A and second-trimester uterine artery Doppler pulsatility index as markers of preeclampsia," *Ultrasound in Obstetrics and Gynecology*, vol. 29, no. 2, pp. 128–134, 2007.

[90] S. E. Maynard, J. Y. Min, J. Merchan et al., "Excess placental soluble fms-like tyrosine kinase 1 (sFlt1) may contribute to endothelial dysfunction hypertension, and proteinuria in preeclampsia," *The Journal of Clinical Investigation*, vol. 111, no. 5, pp. 649–658, 2003.

[91] S. Ahmad and A. Ahmed, "Elevated placental soluble vascular endothelial growth factor receptor-1 inhibits angiogenesis in preeclampsia," *Circulation Research*, vol. 95, no. 9, pp. 884–891, 2004.

[92] R. J. Levine, S. E. Maynard, C. Qian et al., "Circulating angiogenic factors and the risk of preeclampsia," *The New England Journal of Medicine*, vol. 350, no. 7, pp. 672–683, 2004.

[93] H. Stepan, A. Unversucht, N. Wessel, and R. Faber, "Predictive value of maternal angiogenic factors in second trimester pregnancies with abnormal uterine perfusion," *Hypertension*, vol. 49, no. 4, pp. 818–824, 2007.

[94] Y. N. Su, C. N. Lee, W. F. Cheng, W. Y. Shau, S. N. Chow, and F. J. Hsieh, "Decreased maternal serum placenta growth factor in early second trimester and preeclampsia," *Obstetrics and Gynecology*, vol. 97, no. 6, pp. 898–904, 2001.

[95] S. C. Tidwell, H. Ho, W. Chiu, R. J. Torry, and D. S. Torry, "Low maternal serum levels of placenta growth factor as an antecedent of clinical preeclampsia," *American Journal of Obstetrics and Gynecology*, vol. 184, no. 6, pp. 1267–1272, 2001.

[96] M. L. Tjoa, J. M. G. van Vugt, M. A. M. Mulders, R. B. H. Schutgens, C. B. M. Oudejans, and I. J. van Wijk, "Plasma placenta growth factor levels in midtrimester pregnancies," *Obstetrics and Gynecology*, vol. 98, no. 4, pp. 600–607, 2001.

[97] B. M. Polliotti, A. G. Fry, D. N. Saller Jr., R. A. Mooney, C. Cox, and R. K. Miller, "Second-trimester maternal serum placental growth factor and vascular endothelial growth factor for predicting severe, early-onset preeclampsia," *Obstetrics and Gynecology*, vol. 101, no. 6, pp. 1266–1274, 2003.

[98] T. Krauss, H. Pauer, and H. G. Augustin, "Prospective analysis of placenta growth factor (PlGF) concentrations in the plasma of women with normal pregnancy and pregnancies complicated by preeclampsia," *Hypertension in Pregnancy*, vol. 23, no. 1, pp. 101–111, 2004.

[99] R. Thadhani, W. P. Mutter, M. Wolf et al., "First trimester placental growth factor and soluble fms -like tyrosine kinase 1 and risk for preeclampsia," *Journal of Clinical Endocrinology and Metabolism*, vol. 89, no. 2, pp. 770–775, 2004.

[100] R. Akolekar, E. Zaragoza, L. C. Y. Poon, S. Pepes, and K. H. Nicolaides, "Maternal serum placental growth factor at 11 + 0 to 13 + 6 weeks of gestation in the prediction of pre-eclampsia," *Ultrasound in Obstetrics and Gynecology*, vol. 32, no. 6, pp. 732–739, 2008.

[101] F. Crispi, E. Llurba, C. Domínguez, P. Martín-Gallán, L. Cabero, and E. Gratacós, "Predictive value of angiogenic factors and uterine artery Doppler for early- versus late-onset pre-eclampsia and intrauterine growth restriction," *Ultrasound in Obstetrics and Gynecology*, vol. 31, no. 3, pp. 303–309, 2008.

[102] O. Erez, R. Romero, J. Espinoza et al., "The change in concentrations of angiogenic and anti-angiogenic factors in maternal plasma between the first and second trimesters in risk assessment for the subsequent development of preeclampsia and small-for-gestational age," *Journal of Maternal-Fetal and Neonatal Medicine*, vol. 21, no. 5, pp. 279–287, 2008.

[103] K. O. Kagan, D. Wright, K. Spencer, F. S. Molina, and K. H. Nicolaides, "First-trimester screening for trisomy 21 by free beta-human chorionic gonadotropin and pregnancy-associated plasma protein-A: impact of maternal and pregnancy characteristics," *Ultrasound in Obstetrics & Gynecology*, vol. 31, no. 5, pp. 493–502, 2008.

[104] P. Pandya, D. Wright, A. Syngelaki, R. Akolekar, and K. H. Nicolaides, "Maternal serum placental growth factor in prospective screening for aneuploidies at 8–13 weeks' gestation," *Fetal Diagnosis and Therapy*, vol. 31, no. 2, pp. 87–93, 2012.

[105] L. C. Poon, N. A. Kametas, N. Maiz, R. Akolekar, and K. H. Nicolaides, "First-trimester prediction of hypertensive disorders in pregnancy," *Hypertension*, vol. 53, pp. 812–818, 2009.

[106] R. Akolekar, A. Syngelaki, R. Sarquis, M. Zvanca, and K. H. Nicolaides, "Prediction of early, intermediate and late preeclampsia from maternal factors, biophysical and biochemical markers at 11–13 weeks," *Prenatal Diagnosis*, vol. 31, no. 1, pp. 66–74, 2011.

[107] E. Scazzocchio, F. Figueras, F. Crispi et al., "Performance of a first-trimester screening of preeclampsia in a routine care low-risk setting," *The American Journal of Obstetrics and Gynecology*, vol. 208, no. 3, pp. 203.e1–203.e10, 2013.

[108] C. M. Koopmans, D. Bijlenga, H. Groen et al., "Induction of labour versus expectant monitoring for gestational hypertension or mild pre-eclampsia after 36 weeks' gestation (HYPI-TAT): a multicentre, open-label randomised controlled trial," *The Lancet*, vol. 374, no. 9694, pp. 979–988, 2009.

[109] A. Tayyar, S. Garcia-Tizon Larroca, L. C. Poon, D. Wright, and K. H. Nicolaides, " Competing risks model in screening for preeclampsia by mean arterial pressure and uterine artery pulsatility index at 30–33 weeks' gestation," *Fetal Diagnosis and Therapy*, vol. 36, no. 1, pp. 18–27, 2014.

[110] Y. Bdolah, V. P. Sukhatme, and S. A. Karumanchi, "Angiogenic imbalance in the pathophysiology of preeclampsia: newer insights," *Seminars in Nephrology*, vol. 24, no. 6, pp. 548–556, 2004.

[111] S. Verlohren, I. Herraiz, O. Lapaire et al., "The sFlt-1/PlGF ratio in different types of hypertensive pregnancy disorders and its prognostic potential in preeclamptic patients," *The American Journal of Obstetrics and Gynecology*, vol. 206, no. 1, pp. 58.e1–e8.e1, 2012.

[112] S. Rana, C. E. Powe, S. Salahuddin et al., "Angiogenic factors and the risk of adverse outcomes in women with suspected preeclampsia," *Circulation*, vol. 125, no. 7, pp. 911–919, 2012.

[113] T. Chaiworapongsa, R. Romero, Z. A. Savasan et al., "Maternal plasma concentrations of angiogenic/anti-angiogenic factors are of prognostic value in patients presenting to the obstetrical triage area with the suspicion of preeclampsia," *Journal of Maternal-Fetal and Neonatal Medicine*, vol. 24, no. 10, pp. 1187–1207, 2011.

[114] J. Sibiude, J. Guibourdenche, M. Dionne et al., "Placental growth factor for the prediction of adverse outcomes in patients with suspected preeclampsia or intrauterine growth restriction," *PLoS ONE*, vol. 7, no. 11, Article ID e50208, 2012.

[115] L. C. Chappell, S. Duckworth, P. T. Seed et al., "Diagnostic accuracy of placental growth factor in women with suspected preeclampsia: a prospective multicenter study," *Circulation*, vol. 128, no. 19, pp. 2121–2131, 2013.

[116] A. Ohkuchi, C. Hirashima, K. Takahashi, H. Suzuki, S. Matsubara, and M. Suzuki, "Onset threshold of the plasma levels of soluble fms-like tyrosine kinase 1/placental growth factor ratio for predicting the imminent onset of preeclampsia within 4 weeks after blood sampling at 19–31 weeks of gestation," *Hypertension Research*, vol. 36, no. 12, pp. 1073–1038, 2013.

[117] J. Lai, S. Garcia-Tizon Larroca, G. Peeva, L. C. Poon, D. Wright, and K. H. Nicolaides, "Competing risks model in screening for preeclampsia by serum placental growth factor and soluble fms-like tyrosine kinase-1 at 30-33 weeks gestation," *Fetal Diagnosis and Therapy*, vol. 35, no. 4, pp. 240–248, 2014.

[118] S. Garcia-Tizon Larroca, A. Tayyar, L. C. Poon, D. Wright, and K. H. Nicolaides, "Competing risks model in screening for preeclampsia by biophysical and biochemical markers at 30–33 weeks'gestation," *Fetal Diagnosis and Therapy*, vol. 36, no. 1, pp. 9–17, 2014.

[119] K. H. Nicolaides, "Turning the pyramid of prenatal care," *Fetal Diagnosis and Therapy*, vol. 29, no. 3, pp. 183–196, 2011.

15

Management of Fetal Growth Arrest in One of Dichorionic Twins: Three Cases and a Literature Review

Shoji Kaku, Fuminori Kimura, and Takashi Murakami

Department of Obstetrics and Gynecology, Shiga University of Medical Science, Shiga 520-2192, Japan

Correspondence should be addressed to Shoji Kaku; kaku@belle.shiga-med.ac.jp

Academic Editor: Everett Magann

Progressive fetal growth restriction (FGR) is often an indication for delivery. In dichorionic diamniotic (DD) twin pregnancy with growth restriction only affecting one fetus (selective fetal growth restriction: sFGR), the normal twin is also delivered prematurely. There is still not enough evidence about the optimal timing of delivery for DD twins with sFGR in relation to discordance and gestational age. We report three sets of DD twins with sFGR (almost complete growth arrest affecting one fetus for ≥2 weeks) before 30 weeks of gestation. The interval from growth arrest to delivery was 21–24 days and the discordance was 33.7–49.8%. A large-scale study showed no difference of overall mortality or the long-term outcome between immediate and delayed delivery for FGR, while many studies have identified a risk of developmental delay following delivery of the normal growth fetus before 32 weeks. Therefore, delivery of DD twins with sFGR should be delayed if the condition of the sFGR fetus permits in order to increase the gestational age of the normal growth fetus.

1. Introduction

When fetal growth restriction (FGR) is progressive, with no increase of the estimated fetal body weight (EFW) and deterioration of Doppler flow parameters measured at the umbilical artery and ductus venosus, delivery is required. However, there is little consensus about the optimal timing of delivery [1]. Early delivery carries the risks associated with prematurity, but delay may increase hypoxic damage [2]. In monochorionic twins, one fetus may show growth restriction while the growth of the other fetus is normal. This is called selective fetal growth restriction (sFGR) and its frequency is 10–15%. However, there have been no reports about the management of dichorionic diamniotic (DD) twin pregnancy with sFGR. Over the past few decades, the incidence of twin pregnancies has increased by nearly 70% because of the widespread use of assisted reproductive technology [3], which means that DD twin pregnancies have also been increasing. Inde et al. reported that 32.9% of patients who had DD twins received in vitro fertilization [4]. Accordingly, we reviewed our cases and the literature to investigate the management and timing of delivery in DD twins with sFGR and almost complete growth restriction.

2. Case Reports

We searched the clinical records of our hospital from January 2009 to December 2013 for DD twins with sFGR diagnosed before 30 weeks of gestation. Twins were eligible when the EFW of one twin was below the 10th percentile and there was almost complete growth restriction for more than two weeks, while the EFW of the other twin was within the normal range based on a weight nomogram. We excluded cases where the FGR fetus had an abnormal karyotype. Three twin pregnancies were identified that met these criteria. For these fetuses, we examined the period between the diagnosis of growth restriction and delivery in relation to the prognosis of both twins. In all pregnancies, gestational age was confirmed and chorionicity and amnionicity were evaluated prior to 12 weeks. Gestational age was assigned by measurement of crown-rump length. The EFW of the twin with sIUGR was determined by ultrasound once or twice a week with a Voluson E8 (GE Healthcare, Milwaukee, WI).

For management of sFGR in DD twins, the mother was hospitalized. CTG monitoring was performed every day and the EFW was assessed by ultrasound, with both EFW and Doppler examination being done twice a week. If late

(a)

(b)

(c)

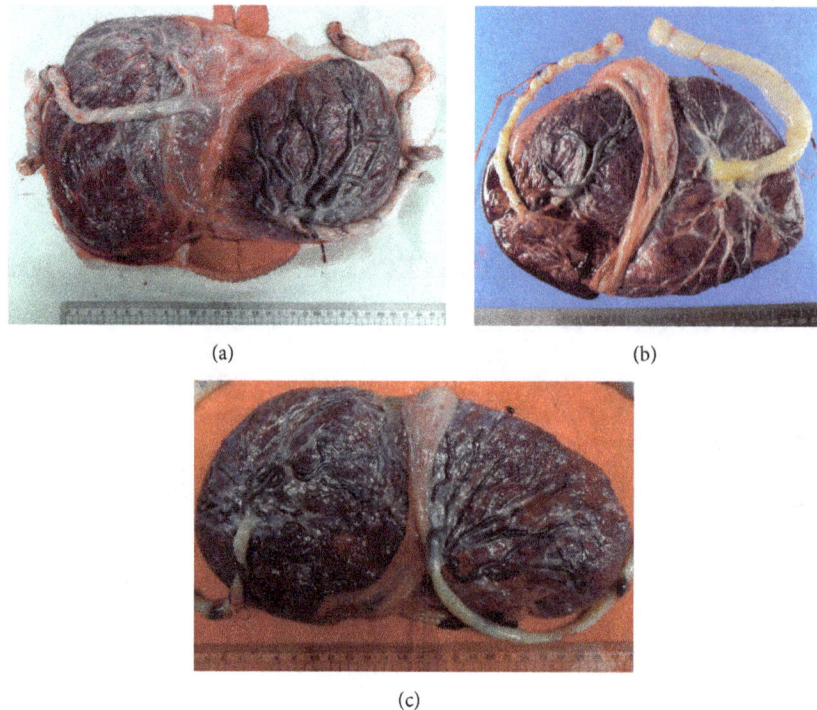

FIGURE 1: Placentas of 3 cases. (a) Placenta of case 1. (b) Placenta of case 2. (c) Placenta of case 3. (a) There is an obvious difference of placental area between the FGR fetus and the normal fetus. (b, c) There is no marked difference of placental area between the FGR fetus and the normal fetus.

deceleration or reduced short-term variation was seen or there was an abnormal UA pulsatility index (more than 2 SD above the normal reference mean) or absence of end-diastolic flow in the UA, we considered delivery if the gestational age was more than 32 weeks. If the gestational age was less than 32 weeks, we increased CTG monitoring to two or three times a day and performed daily ultrasound examination. If late deceleration, absence of short-term variation, or reverse end-diastolic flow (RED) was detected, we considered delivery.

Details of the three cases of sFGR are displayed in Table 1. The gestational age was 27–29 weeks at the detection of almost complete growth restriction persisting for ≥2 weeks, while birth weight discordance was 33.7–49.8% (Table 1). Investigation of the cause of the growth restriction revealed a difference of placental area between the FGR twin and normal twin in case 1 (Figure 1(a)), but there was no significant difference in cases 2 and 3 (Figures 1(b) and 1(c)). In case 2, the FGR fetus showed heterotaxia, but the karyotype was normal. In case 3, the cause of growth restriction was not identified despite prenatal and postnatal investigation. The method of delivery was cesarean section in all three cases. Although we aimed for delivery after 32 weeks of gestation, this was only achieved in case 1. In case 2, RED in the umbilical artery was found at 30 weeks of gestation, and cesarean section was performed three days after the appearance RED. In case 3, labor started at 29 weeks in spite of tocolysis. Accordingly, cesarean section was performed at 29–32 weeks of gestation, and the interval from detection of growth arrest to cesarean section was 21–24 days (median: 22.7 days) (Table 1).

The birth weight of the FGR twin was 778–884 g and that of the normal twin was 1174–1760 g (Table 1). After follow-up of the sFGR infants for one to four years since birth, no major abnormalities have been found other than heterotaxia in case 2. Among the normal growth infants, cerebral hemorrhage was detected in the normal weight twin of case 2 at 4 days after birth and this child requires ongoing treatment.

3. Discussion

When sFGR occurs in DD twins, our objective is to achieve the best outcome for both fetuses. The timing of delivery is generally the major issue in severe FGR and policies about delivery vary widely [5, 6]. A large-scale prospective study showed that the developmental quotient was significantly lower at a corrected age of 2 years after premature delivery of normal growth fetuses between 22 and 32 weeks of gestation [7]. There is no consensus about the management of sFGR in DD twins, including the timing of delivery. Accordingly, we reviewed published reports on the management of sFGR and investigated the timing of delivery in relation to the severity of discordance to determine whether discordance influenced the normal twin because an adverse event occurred in one of our normal growth twins. We also investigated the timing of delivery in relation to the umbilical artery Doppler flow parameters in the sFGR fetus because RED was found in one of our cases.

With regard to the timing of delivery in relation to the severity of discordance, we found that discordance exceeded

TABLE 1

Case number	Age	G	P	Gestational age at detection of growth restriction	Gestational age at delivery	Reason for delivery	Period of growth restriction (days)	Birth weight (g)	Sex	Major sequelae
1	38	0	0	29 w 2 d	32 w 4 d	Planning delivery	24	884	F	—
								1760	M	—
2	30	0	0	27 w 0 d	30 w 1 d	RED of UA	23	838	M	—
								1636	M	Cerebral hemorrhage
3	29	0	0	27 w 0 d	29 w 6 d	Onset of labor	21	778	F	—
								1174	M	—

G: gravidity, P: parity, RED: reverse of end-diastolic flow, UA: umbilical artery, F: female, and M: male.

30% in all 3 of our DD twins. In most studies, the cut-off value is 15%–25%, and it is reported that the risk of morbidity and mortality increases if discordance exceeds that value [8–10]. Unfortunately, there have been no reports focusing on the relation between discordance and prognosis of DD twins, but some studies have investigated the influence of gender. In same sex twins, Demissie et al. reported that greater discordance is associated with an increased risk of intrauterine death for both smaller and larger twin, while intrauterine death and the prognosis of the larger twin are unrelated to discordance when the twins are of different sexes [11]. The same sex twins in these reports included both DD twins and monochorionic twins, while the twins of different sexes would only be DD twins. However, the authors did not distinguish between DD twins of the same and DD twins of different sexes, and the chorionicity and amnionicity are also unclear because the studies were based on twin birth data from the United States [11, 12]. However, we considered that the data for different sex twins corresponded to findings for DD twins.

A few prospective multicenter studies have addressed the timing of delivery based on Doppler flow parameters in the umbilical artery of the FGR fetus. The Growth Restriction Intervention Trial (GRIT) investigated the timing of delivery for FGR [13]. Pregnant women between 24 and 36 weeks of gestation with FGR were randomly assigned to immediate delivery ($n = 296$) or delayed ($n = 291$) delivery if the obstetrician was uncertain about when the FGR fetus should be delivered based on UA Doppler parameters. As a result, there was no difference of overall mortality between the two groups. In addition, 2-year and 6-year follow-up studies showed that there were no significant differences between the two groups with regard to death or disability rates [14, 15]. Although the GRIT study cannot provide us with standard criteria for determining the timing of delivery, the lack of a difference in overall mortality and long-term outcomes of the FGR fetus between immediate and delayed delivery suggests that it may be important for parents or obstetricians to consider prolonging the time in utero for the normal twin of DD twins with sFGR, even for a short period.

When we reassessed our 3 cases based on the literature review, we considered that the timing of delivery should not be decided from the discordance (even though it exceeded 30% in all of our cases), because there is no evidence of a relation between the cut-off value for discordance and the risk of morbidity or mortality in dichorionic twins. Although we aimed for delivery after a gestational age of 32 weeks, delivery was earlier than 32 weeks in 2 cases because of RED and spontaneous onset of labor, respectively, with cerebral hemorrhage occurring in one normal growth twin after premature delivery. In conclusion, there is still not enough evidence about the optimal timing of delivery for DD twins with sFGR in relation to discordance and gestational age, but data from the GRIT study suggest that delivery should be delayed if the condition of the sFGR fetus permits in order to increase the gestational age of the normal growth fetus.

Conflict of Interests

The authors declare that there are no conflict of interests.

References

[1] The GRIT Study Group. Growth Restriction Intervention Trial, "When do obstetricians recommend delivery for a high-risk preterm growth-retarded fetus?" *European Journal of Obstetrics & Gynecology and Reproductive Biology*, vol. 67, pp. 121–126, 1996.

[2] F. L. Gaudier, R. L. Goldenberg, K. G. Nelson et al., "Acid-base status at birth and subsequent neurosensory impairment in surviving 500 to 1000 gm infants," *American Journal of Obstetrics & Gynecology*, vol. 170, no. 1, pp. 48–53, 1994.

[3] Y. M. Lee, J. Cleary-Goldman, and M. E. D'Alton, "The impact of multiple gestations on late preterm (near-term) births," *Clinics in Perinatology*, vol. 33, no. 4, pp. 777–792, 2006.

[4] Y. Inde, M. Satomi, N. Iwasaki et al., "Maternal risk factors for small-for-gestational age newborns in Japanese dichorionic twins," *Journal of Obstetrics and Gynaecology Research*, vol. 37, no. 1, pp. 24–31, 2011.

[5] G. H. A. Visser, R. H. Stigter, and H. W. Bruinse, "Management of the growth-retarded fetus," *European Journal of Obstetrics & Gynecology and Reproductive Biology*, vol. 42, supplement, pp. S73–S78, 1991.

[6] R. Lilford, S. Gudmundsson, D. James et al., "Formal measurement of clinical uncertainty: prelude to a trial in perinatal medicine," *British Medical Journal*, vol. 308, no. 6921, pp. 111–112, 1994.

[7] M. L. Charkaluk, P. Truffert, A. Fily, P. Y. Ancel, and V. Pierrat, "Neurodevelopment of children born very preterm and free of severe disabilities: the Nord-Pas de Calais Epipage Cohort Study," *Acta Paediatrica*, vol. 99, no. 5, pp. 684–689, 2010.

[8] S. Bagchi and H. M. Salihu, "Birth weight discordance in multiple gestations: occurrence and outcomes," *Journal of Obstetrics and Gynaecology*, vol. 26, no. 4, pp. 291–296, 2006.

[9] I. Blickstein, "Growth aberration in multiple pregnancy," *Obstetrics and Gynecology Clinics of North America*, vol. 32, no. 1, pp. 39–54, 2005.

[10] K. E. A. Hack, J. B. Derks, S. G. Elias et al., "Increased perinatal mortality and morbidity in monochorionic versus dichorionic twin pregnancies: clinical implications of a large Dutch Cohort Study," *BJOG*, vol. 115, no. 1, pp. 58–67, 2008.

[11] K. Demissie, C. V. Ananth, J. Martin, M. L. Hanley, M. F. MacDorman, and G. G. Rhoads, "Fetal and neonatal mortality among twin gestations in the United States: the role of intrapair birth weight discordance," *Obstetrics and Gynecology*, vol. 100, no. 3, pp. 474–480, 2002.

[12] C. V. Ananth, K. Demissie, and M. L. Hanley, "Birth weight discordancy and adverse perinatal outcomes among twin gestations in the United States: the effect of placental abruption," *American Journal of Obstetrics & Gynecology*, vol. 188, no. 4, pp. 954–960, 2003.

[13] G. S. Group, "A randomised trial of timed delivery for the compromised preterm fetus: short term outcomes and Bayesian interpretation," *BJOG: An International Journal of Obstetrics & Gynaecology*, vol. 110, no. 1, pp. 27–32, 2003.

[14] J. G. Thornton, J. Hornbuckle, A. Vail et al., "Infant wellbeing at 2 years of age in the Growth Restriction Intervention Trial (GRIT): multicentred randomised controlled trial," *The Lancet*, vol. 364, no. 9433, pp. 513–520, 2004.

[15] D.-M. Walker, N. Marlow, L. Upstone et al., "The growth restriction intervention trial: long-term outcomes in a randomized trial of timing of delivery in fetal growth restriction," *American Journal of Obstetrics & Gynecology*, vol. 204, no. 1, pp. 34.e1–34.e9, 2011.

16

The Importance of the Monitoring of Resuscitation with Blood Transfusion for Uterine Inversion in Obstetrical Hemorrhage

Seishi Furukawa and Hiroshi Sameshima

Department of Obstetrics & Gynecology, Faculty of Medicine, University of Miyazaki, Miyazaki 889-1692, Japan

Correspondence should be addressed to Seishi Furukawa; shiiba46seishi@gmail.com

Academic Editor: Irene Hoesli

Objective. The aim of this study was to describe critical care for obstetrical hemorrhage, especially in cases of uterine inversion. *Study Design.* We extracted data for six patients diagnosed with uterine inversion concerning resuscitation. *Results.* The shock index on admission of the six patients was 1.6 or more on admission. Four of the six experienced delay in diagnosis and received inadequate fluid replacement. Five of the six experienced delay in transfer. Five of the six underwent simultaneous blood transfusion on admission, and the remaining patient experienced a delay of 30 minutes. All six patients successfully underwent uterine replacement soon after admission. One maternal death occurred due to inappropriate practices that included delay in diagnosis, delay in transfer, inadequate fluid replacement, and delayed transfusion. Two patients experiencing inappropriate practices involving delay in diagnosis, delay in transfer, and inadequate fluid replacement survived. *Conclusion.* If a delay in diagnosis occurs simultaneously with a delay in transfer and inadequate fluid replacement, failure in providing a prompt blood transfusion may be critical and result in maternal death. The monitoring of resuscitation with blood transfusion for uterine inversion is essential for the improvement of obstetrical care.

1. Introduction

An autopsy registry survey in Japan indicated that half of the maternal deaths are due to obstetric hemorrhage [1]. In our local survey, uterine inversion accounts for 3.3% of all pregnant women who received any blood transfusion for obstetrical hemorrhage, and the cases of uterine inversion included one maternal death. The incidence of uterine inversion was relatively low, but the prognosis was very poor [2].

Early recognition of uterine inversion is indispensable for early replacement of the inversion to stop the bleeding, and the assessment of vital signs and preparation to prevent hemorrhagic shock are also required. As a consequence, several management protocols for uterine inversion have been proposed [3, 4]. However, despite widespread familiarity with management practices and attention regarding hemorrhage, maternal death still occurs in cases of uterine inversion [2, 5]. The review of individual cases of obstetrical care for uterine inversion is definitely needed to improve maternal outcomes.

Many reports have outlined risk factors concerning the development of uterine inversion [6–8] or useful measures for the replacement of an inverted uterus [5]. However, there is still a lack of clarity regarding the effect of resuscitation failure on mortality and morbidity concerning uterine inversion. In this study, we reviewed the medical records of pregnant patients with uterine inversion. We extracted data concerning resuscitation including condition of the women on admission (shock index: SI), diagnosis, transfer to perinatal center, and clinical practices including uterine replacement, fluid replacement, and blood transfusion therapy. We then compared differences concerning the resuscitation practice within the group of cases involving uterine inversion.

2. Materials and Methods

This study was undertaken retrospectively and obtained approval (#2013-135) from a suitably constituted ethics committee at our institution. We retrospectively reviewed the medical charts of pregnant women with uterine inversion that were admitted to the Perinatal Center of the University of Miyazaki, the Miyazaki Medical Association Hospital, the

TABLE 1: Demographic data of women with uterine inversion. Results are expressed as the number of individuals. GA: gestational age. *Geographical disadvantage for transfer (more than 40 minutes by ambulance car).

Case	Age (ys)	Parity/abortion	Inborn/outborn	GA at delivery (weeks)	Vacuum extraction	Birth weight (g)	Manual removal of placenta
1	33	0/0	Outborn	37	Yes	2836	No
2	28	0/0	Outborn	39	No	3410	No
3*	24	0/1	Outborn	40	Yes	2998	Yes
4	29	0/0	Outborn	37	No	3022	Yes
5	27	0/1	Outborn	41	Yes	3104	No
6	27	0/0	Inborn	39	No	3005	No

Fujimoto General Hospital, or the Nichinan Prefectural Hospital from January 2007 to December 2013. In this study, there were cases of uterine inversion that were also included in our previous study [2]. The Perinatal Center of the University of Miyazaki is a tertiary center, whereas the other hospitals are secondary perinatal centers. These centers mainly deal with high-risk pregnancy. Most parturitions involving low-risk cases are overseen by private clinics. In cases involving an obstetrical emergency, women are referred to a high-order perinatal center dependent on the level of severity [9]. Access to blood products except for platelets is ensured within 60 minutes after a request by any of the centers. A small stock of blood products is available at secondary perinatal centers.

We reviewed the medical records of pregnant patients with uterine inversion and the following maternal characteristics were collected: age, parity (primipara), history of abortion, gestational age at birth, birth weight (g), use of vacuum extraction, and attempted manual removal of the placenta. We checked the following factors related to resuscitation for uterine inversion in each case: inborn or outborn delivery (i.e., private clinic), presence of immediate diagnosis of uterine inversion, SI on admission, presence of prompt transfer to the perinatal center after diagnosis, presence of proper practices including immediate uterine replacement on admission to the perinatal center, adequate fluid replacement before admission to the perinatal center, prompt blood transfusion after admission to the perinatal center, estimated total blood loss within the first 24 hours following delivery, and presence of ICU care. SI was defined as heart rate/systolic blood pressure on admission to the perinatal center [10, 11]. Since a linear relationship between hemorrhage and increasing SI has been recorded [10], in this study we defined inadequate fluid replacement before admission to the perinatal center as less than SI × 1000 mL of crystalloids. As an indicator of prompt transfer to the perinatal center, we investigated the duration from delivery to arrival at the perinatal center. The duration was calculated roughly by increments of 10 minutes from delivery to arrival at each perinatal center. A prompt transfusion therapy was defined as simultaneous blood transfusion on admission to the perinatal center. In cases of a delay in transfusion, the approximate time taken from admission to the start of blood transfusion was extracted from the medical records. The time was also roughly calculated by increments of 10 minutes from admission to the start of the blood transfusion. In

cases involving an inborn delivery, SI on diagnosis was used. A prompt transfusion therapy was defined as rapid blood transfusion soon after diagnosis of uterine inversion (less than 10 minutes). In cases of a delay, the approximate time taken from diagnosis to the start of blood transfusion was extracted from the medical records.

Data are expressed as number (range) or mean ± SD (range).

3. Results

According to the medical records investigated, all six women were primiparous and the average maternal age was 28.0 years (Table 1). The average gestational age at delivery was 38.8 ± 1.6 weeks (37~41 weeks); three of the six cases involved vacuum extraction, and two of the six cases included attempted manual removal of the placenta. Except for cases involved attempting manual removal of placenta, umbilical cord traction was done without an elevation of uterus by the hand. The average birth weight at delivery was 3063 ± 191 g (2998~3410 g). In this study, five of the six cases involved an outborn delivery. Only one clinic was located in a rural area and thereby resulted in a geographical disadvantage for transfer (more than 40 minutes by ambulance). The other clinics were all located near a perinatal center (within 10 minutes by ambulance).

Table 2 shows a comparison of the risk profile among the study group. Two cases involved manual removal of the placenta followed by immediate notice of a mass in the vagina or inverted uterus. At the time of notice, they had severe abdominal pain; however, they did not exhibit shock sign such as loss of conscious or abrupt decline in blood pressure. The other four cases were overlooked at first followed by increasing vaginal bleeding. Five of the six cases showed a delay in transfer (more than 50 minutes after delivery, range: 20–100 minutes) and received inadequate fluid replacement. The SI of all cases was at least 1.6 (range: 1.6–2.7) on admission. Five of the six cases involved simultaneous blood transfusion on admission, and the remaining case showed a delay (30 minutes from admission to start of transfusion). All six cases involved successful uterine replacement soon after admission to the respective perinatal center. Two cases (Cases 1 and 5) received manual replacement without uterine relaxing agent at delivery room; the others received manual replacement in operative room with uterine relaxing agent

TABLE 2: Comparison of the resuscitate profile and outcome among the group with uterine inversion. Results are expressed as the number of individuals. *Geographical disadvantage for transfer (more than 40 minutes by ambulance car). SI: shock index, min.: minutes. Inadequate fluid replacement before admission at the perinatal center was defined as less than SI × 1000 mL of crystalloids.

Case	Delay in diagnosis	Delay in transfer	Inadequate fluid replacement	SI on admission	Delay in blood transfusion	Blood loss (ml)	ICU care	Dead/alive
1	Yes	50 min.	Yes	1.8	30 min.	8367	Yes	Dead
2	Yes	70 min.	Yes	1.6	No	2750	No	Alive
3*	No	70 min.	No	2.1	No	5831	Yes	Alive
4	No	80 min.	No	1.7	No	3800	No	Alive
5	Yes	100 min.	Yes	2.7	No	3121	Yes	Alive
6	Yes	20 min.	Yes	2.1	No	3598	Yes	Alive

either inhaled sevoflurane or low-dose nitroglycerin (0.1 mg increment dose). The average estimated blood loss was 4578± 2143 mL (2750~8367 mL). Four of the six cases included ICU care. Finally, one maternal death occurred due to inappropriate practices that included delay in diagnosis, delay in transfer, inadequate fluid replacement, and delayed transfusion (Case 1). Two patients were subjected to inappropriate practices involving delay in diagnosis, delay in transfer, and inadequate fluid replacement survived (Cases 2 and 5).

4. Discussion

In our region, 80% of deliveries occur at a private clinic [9] and blood products are not located on-site at each clinic. As a consequence, private clinics refer a patient to a high-order perinatal center in the event of postpartum hemorrhage such as uterine inversion. This is the setting of the six cases of uterine inversion investigated in this study. Our six cases included one maternal death that resulted from a delay in diagnosis, delay in transfer, inadequate fluid replacement, and failure of a prompt blood transfusion. On the other hand, two patients were subjected to inappropriate practices involving delay in diagnosis, delay in transfer, and inadequate fluid replacement survived. The difference between survivors and death was the presence of a prompt blood transfusion. In a life-threatening situation involving delay in diagnosis, delay in transfer, and inadequate fluid replacement, the administration of a prompt blood transfusion on-site may be critical. Therefore, problems in our region that affect mortality and morbidity of uterine inversion have emerged from this study.

Despite widespread familiarity with uterine inversion, this condition still occurs at a certain frequency and remains one of the life-threatening causes of obstetrical hemorrhage [5]. Diagnosis of uterine inversion is based on clinical signs such as severe abdominal pain, shock with or without profound bleeding, absence of uterine fundus, or presence of a mass in the vagina by pelvic examination. These clinical signs allow us to identify and undergo early replacement of uterus in most cases, followed by causing in uneventful course [4], but there were still four cases of delayed diagnosis in this study. Delay in diagnosis produced a series of negative responses involving delay in replacement of inverted uterus, transfer, and lack of adequate fluid replacement until admission to the perinatal center. Our study revealed that these factors resulted in a critical condition involving either high SI (2.7) or death. Thus, the primary factor that influences mortality and morbidity is still the early recognition of an inverted uterus [12, 13]. However, it is well known that neurogenic shock as one of the early signs of uterine inversion contributes increasing the number of mortality and morbidity [14]. In our study, there were no cases of neurogenic shock at the time of notice. Accordingly, we could not define the importance of neurogenic shock for major factors to define the prognosis in this study.

In general, practitioners had little experience with this condition due to its rarity and therefore did not recognize signs of uterine inversion [15]. Furthermore, most private clinics in Japan have inadequate obstetric services in terms of medical staff [16]. The presence of fewer obstetricians in clinics might therefore reduce the possibility of early recognition. In particular, because of those, it is crucial to recognize the importance of appropriate management of third stage of labor such as avoiding umbilical cord traction, prompt diagnosis, and prompt replacement of inverted uterus. Those practices will yield an uneventful course. It is therefore necessary to create disease-specific guidelines for rare events in obstetrical hemorrhage such as uterine inversion or amniotic fluid embolism.

In cases of a life-threatening situation involving a delay in diagnosis, delay in transfer, and inadequate fluid replacement, the administration of a prompt blood transfusion on-site may be critical. It has also been proposed that a delay in blood transfusion results in coagulopathy and organ failure [17]. Bonnet and colleagues reported that a delay in blood transfusion was associated with a series of maternal deaths from postpartum hemorrhage [18]. They indicated that there is a room for improvement concerning blood transfusion in terms of timing and reported that 79% of the maternal deaths occurred in clinics with an on-site blood bank. In our study, every perinatal center had access to blood products. One facility started blood transfusion with blood-type compatible products following a delay in transfusion (30 minutes from admission to the start of transfusion). The others started blood transfusion with O-group blood that may be transfused into people of all (blood) groups. According to the guidelines of the Royal College of Obstetricians and Gynecologists, O Rh D negative red cells can be given to patients in extreme situations [19]. Therefore, it is assumed that the decision regarding timing and transfusion using O-group blood is the important factor that determines the outcomes. However, our study involved a small number of cases. There is therefore a need to expand the survey of mothers suffering from uterine inversion.

In conclusion, we demonstrated the importance of the monitoring of critical care for uterine inversion in obstetrical hemorrhage. In case of a delayed diagnosis, the findings of our study will result in better obstetrical practices. A delay in diagnosis of inverted uterus results in a life-threatening situation involving a delay in early replacement, transfer, and inadequate fluid replacement. In the case of a life-threatening situation, a prompt blood transfusion using O-group blood on-site is a critical factor that determines the outcome of uterine inversion.

Conflict of Interests

The authors declare that the contents of their paper are not fully presented elsewhere and that there is no financial or other relationship that might lead to a conflict of interests.

References

[1] N. Kanayama, J. Inori, H. Ishibashi-Ueda et al., "Maternal death analysis from the Japanese autopsy registry for recent 16 years: significance of amniotic fluid embolism," *Journal of Obstetrics and Gynaecology Research*, vol. 37, no. 1, pp. 58–63, 2011.

[2] K. Furuta, S. Furukawa, U. Hirotoshi, K. Michikata, K. Kai, and H. Sameshima, "Differences in maternal morbidity concerning risk factors for obstetric hemorrhage," *Austin Journal of Obstetrics and Gynecology*, vol. 1, no. 5, p. 5, 2014.

[3] D. L. Ripley, "Uterine emergencies: atony, inversion, and rupture," *Obstetrics and Gynecology Clinics of North America*, vol. 26, no. 3, pp. 419–434, 1999.

[4] P. J. Wendel and S. M. Cox, "Emergent obstetric management of uterine inversion," *Obstetrics and Gynecology Clinics of North America*, vol. 22, no. 2, pp. 261–274, 1995.

[5] D. R. Hostetler and M. F. Bosworth, "Uterine inversion: a life-threatening obstetric emergency," *Journal of the American Board of Family Practice*, vol. 13, no. 2, pp. 120–123, 2000.

[6] T. Witteveen, G. van Stralen, J. Zwart, and J. van Roosmalen, "Puerperal uterine inversion in the Netherlands: a nationwide cohort study," *Acta Obstetricia et Gynecologica Scandinavica*, vol. 92, no. 3, pp. 334–337, 2013.

[7] S. P. Rachagan, V. Sivanesaratnam, K. P. Kok, and S. Raman, "Acute puerperal inversion of the uterus—an obstetric emergency," *Australian and New Zealand Journal of Obstetrics and Gynaecology*, vol. 28, no. 1, pp. 29–32, 1988.

[8] W. K. Lee, M. S. Baggish, and M. Lashgari, "Acute inversion of the uterus," *Obstetrics & Gynecology*, vol. 51, no. 2, pp. 144–147, 1978.

[9] S. Tokunaga, H. Sameshima, and T. Ikenoue, "Applying the ecology model to perinatal medicine: from a regional population-based study," *Journal of Pregnancy*, vol. 2011, Article ID 587390, 4 pages, 2011.

[10] M. Allgöwer and C. Burri, ""Shock index"," *Deutsche Medizinische Wochenschrift*, vol. 92, no. 43, pp. 1947–1950, 1967.

[11] R. W. King, M. C. Plewa, N. M. F. Buderer, and F. B. Knotts, "Shock index as a marker for significant injury in trauma patients," *Academic Emergency Medicine*, vol. 3, no. 11, pp. 1041–1045, 1996.

[12] P. Watson, N. Besch, and W. A. Bowes Jr., "Management of acute and subacute puerperal inversion of the uterus," *Obstetrics and Gynecology*, vol. 55, no. 1, pp. 12–16, 1980.

[13] R. Keriakos and S. R. Chaudhuri, "Managing major postpartum haemorrhage following acute uterine inversion with rusch balloon catheter," *Case Reports in Critical Care*, vol. 2011, Article ID 541479, 3 pages, 2011.

[14] A. J. Thomson and I. A. Greer, "Non-haemorrhagic obstetric shock," *Best Practice & Research Clinical Obstetrics & Gynaecology*, vol. 14, no. 1, pp. 19–41, 2000.

[15] R. F. Leal, R. Luz, J. de Almeida, V. Duarte, and I. Matos, "Total and acute uterine inversion after delivery: a case report," *Journal of Medical Case Reports*, vol. 8, article 347, 2014.

[16] K. Nagaya, M. D. Fetters, M. Ishikawa et al., "Causes of maternal mortality in Japan," *The Journal of the American Medical Association*, vol. 283, no. 20, pp. 2661–2667, 2000.

[17] T. C. Nunez and B. A. Cotton, "Transfusion therapy in hemorrhagic shock," *Current Opinion in Critical Care*, vol. 15, no. 6, pp. 536–541, 2009.

[18] M.-P. Bonnet, C. Deneux-Tharaux, and M.-H. Bouvier-Colle, "Critical care and transfusion management in maternal deaths from postpartum haemorrhage," *European Journal of Obstetrics Gynecology and Reproductive Biology*, vol. 158, no. 2, pp. 183–188, 2011.

[19] https://www.rcog.org.uk/globalassets/documents/guidelines/gtg-47.pdf.

17

Prognostic Value of Residual Disease after Interval Debulking Surgery for FIGO Stage IIIC and IV Epithelial Ovarian Cancer

Marianne J. Rutten,[1] **Gabe S. Sonke,**[2] **Anneke M. Westermann,**[3] **Willemien J. van Driel,**[4] **Johannes W. Trum,**[4,5] **Gemma G. Kenter,**[1] **and Marrije R. Buist**[1]

[1]*Centre for Gynaecologic Oncology Amsterdam, Academic Medical Centre, Amsterdam, Netherlands*
[2]*Department of Medical Oncology, Netherlands Cancer Institute, P.O. Box 22700, 1100 DE Amsterdam, Netherlands*
[3]*Department of Medical Oncology, Academic Medical Centre, Amsterdam, Netherlands*
[4]*Centre for Gynaecologic Oncology Amsterdam, Netherlands Cancer Institute, Netherlands*
[5]*Centre for Gynaecologic Oncology Amsterdam, Free University Medical Centre, Amsterdam, Netherlands*

Correspondence should be addressed to Marianne J. Rutten; m.j.rutten@amc.uva.nl

Academic Editor: Enrique Hernandez

Although complete debulking surgery for epithelial ovarian cancer (EOC) is more often achieved with interval debulking surgery (IDS) following neoadjuvant chemotherapy (NACT), randomized evidence shows no long-term survival benefit compared to complete primary debulking surgery (PDS). We performed an observational cohort study of patients treated with debulking surgery for advanced EOC to evaluate the prognostic value of residual disease after debulking surgery. All patients treated between 1998 and 2010 in three Dutch referral gynaecological oncology centres were included. The prognostic value of residual disease after surgery for disease specific survival was assessed using Cox-regression analyses. In total, 462 patients underwent NACT-IDS and 227 PDS. Macroscopic residual disease after debulking surgery was an independent prognostic factor for survival in both treatment modalities. Yet, residual tumour less than one centimetre at IDS was associated with a survival benefit of five months compared to leaving residual tumour more than one centimetre, whereas this benefit was not seen after PDS. Leaving residual tumour at IDS is a poor prognostic sign as it is after PDS. The specific prognostic value of residual tumour seems to depend on the clinical setting, as minimal instead of gross residual tumour is associated with improved survival after IDS, but not after PDS.

1. Introduction

Advanced epithelial ovarian cancer (EOC) is the leading cause of gynaecologic cancer death. It is treated with a combination of cytoreductive surgery and chemotherapy. Despite advances in chemotherapeutic agents and more radical surgery, there has been little improvement in overall survival in the past decades [1]. A randomised trial showed similar survival rates between patients with advanced stage EOC treated with neoadjuvant chemotherapy and interval debulking surgery (NACT-IDS) or primary debulking surgery (PDS) and adjuvant chemotherapy [2]. However, complete resection of all macroscopic tumour at debulking surgery showed to be the single most important independent

prognostic factor in advanced ovarian carcinoma [2–6]. The primary objective of debulking surgery in ovarian cancer is complete removal of all visible disease [3, 7]. As the result of surgery is a very important and modifiable prognostic factor, no macroscopic residual disease should be pursued to obtain the best prognosis [3, 7–10]. Although this is more often achieved at IDS, it does not result in appreciably better overall survival. Thus, the prognostic value of tumour residual at debulking surgery appears different in patients who received NACT compared to PDS [3, 11, 12].

In this study we evaluated the prognostic significance of residual disease after primary debulking surgery and after interval debulking surgery.

2. Methods

2.1. Patients. Consecutive patients who underwent cytoreductive surgery at one of three oncologic centres in the north western part of Netherlands (Academic Medical Centre, Free University Medical Centre, and Netherlands Cancer Institute) for primary epithelial ovarian, fallopian tube, or peritoneal cancer (EOC) FIGO stage IIIC/IV between January 1998 and August 2010 were identified from a prospective clinical cancer registry.

All patients underwent surgery by gynaecologic oncologists. Patients referred from a nononcologic centre after prior suboptimal surgery by a general gynaecologist were excluded. Staging of disease was done according to FIGO (2006) criteria for ovarian carcinoma. Every operative cytoreductive procedure was performed with the aim of leaving NRD. PDS was performed if in the opinion of the multidisciplinary team, consisting of gynaecologic oncologists, medical oncologists, and a dedicated radiologist, debulking surgery of all visible tumour to less than one centimetre in diameter was possible. Patients with more extensive disease and those unable to undergo surgery started neoadjuvant chemotherapy. Patients who underwent exploratory laparotomy for diagnostic biopsy or oophorectomy without debulking were analysed in the IDS group.

Results of surgery were qualified as no residual disease (NRD), minimal residual disease (MRD; deposits of residual tumour <1 cm), or gross residual disease (GRD; deposits of residual tumour >1 cm).

Standard procedures at PDS as well as at IDS included midline laparotomy, hysterectomy, bilateral salpingooophorectomy, infragastric omentectomy, and removal of all macroscopic tumour if possible. Surgery was classified as extensive if additional interventions such as diaphragmatic and peritoneal stripping, (partial) liver resection, splenectomy, bowel resection, or pelvic- and para-aortic lymphadenectomy were performed to achieve at least MRD. This was performed when it was thought to aid in cytoreductive outcome to at least MRD. Patient data were abstracted from the clinical cancer registry. Information included demographic data, laboratory results, surgical findings, interventions at surgery and results, pathology, treatment, and follow-up data.

2.2. Analysis. Treatment characteristics were compared using chi-square and Student's *t*-test or Mann-Whitney *U* test when appropriate. Progression-free survival and disease specific survival were calculated from the date of first surgery, or start of chemotherapy in case of NACT, to the documented date of progression, respectively, death or last follow-up, whichever occurred first. Impact of surgery result on survival was assessed by constructing Kaplan-Meier curves with a log-rank test. Cox-regression analyses were performed to assess the influence of residual disease in combination with other prognostic factors on survival. All reported significance was 2-tailed at a level of 0.05. Statistical analysis was performed using SPSS statistical software, version 20.

3. Results

In the study period 689 patients were surgically treated for primary EOC FIGO stage IIIC or stage IV. The characteristics of the patients are shown in Table 1. Mean age of all patients was 62 years. The majority of patients had FIGO stage IIIC disease, serous histology, and grade 3 tumour. Median follow-up was 62 months (range 0.9–165 months).

In total, 462 patients were treated with NACT and IDS. The remaining 227 patients were treated with primary debulking surgery. Within the group of patients treated with NACT-IDS, 134 underwent an explorative laparotomy or laparoscopy before start of chemotherapy to assess the operability and to obtain histology for diagnosis, but without debulking surgery.

There were 41 patients in the PDS group who underwent IDS after 2-3 courses of chemotherapy because of GRD after PDS. No difference in survival was observed between patients with GRD after PDS who subsequently had IDS compared to those who did not. Therefore patients who underwent PDS as well as IDS were analysed in the PDS group. Median disease specific survival of the total population was 35 months.

Of all patients, 254 had extensive surgery. This percentage did not differ between patients treated with PDS or IDS. NRD was achieved at debulking surgery in 36% and 46% of patients in the PDS and IDS group, respectively (Table 2). At IDS this was more often achieved without extensive surgery.

Chemotherapy mostly was administered as a carboplatin/paclitaxel combination, although single agent carboplatin and other combinations were sometimes administered (Table 1). In both treatment groups patients received a median of six cycles of chemotherapy (range 0–13). Before IDS patients received 3 (range 1–10) cycles of chemotherapy.

3.1. Prognostic Factors for Survival after PDS. Median follow-up for patients treated with PDS was 74 months (range 1–152). Mortality within 30 days after surgery was less than one percent. Progression within six months after the last cycle of chemotherapy was seen in 32% of patients treated with PDS (Table 3). Median progression-free survival (PFS) was 17 months and median disease specific survival (DSS) 40 months (Figure 1).

Completeness of surgery was an important prognostic factor. DSS with NRD was 57 months compared with 36 months after both MRD and GRD (HR MRD versus NRD 1.5 (95% CI 1.0–2.2), HR GRD versus NRD 1.6 (95% CI 1.1–2.4)). MRD did not result in prolonged survival compared to GRD. The adjusted HR for MRD versus GRD was HR 0.9 (95% CI 0.6–1.3). In multivariable analysis residual disease was an independent prognostic factor. The corresponding HRs were 2.0 (95% CI 1.1–3.8) and 1.8 (95% CI 1.1–3.2). Other independent predictors for DSS were performance status (HR 2.0 (95% CI 1.3–3.1)) and mucinous or clear cell histology versus others (HR 2.9 95% CI 1.4–6.2 and 2.7; 95% CI 1.3–5.6 resp.). Extensive surgery did not result in prolonged survival (HR 0.8 (95% CI 0.6–1.3)). The results of the univariable and multivariable analysis are presented in Table 4(a).

TABLE 1: Baseline characteristics.

	All patients (*n* = 689)	PDS (*n* = 227)	IDS (*n* = 462)
Age; mean (SD)	61.5 (10.7)	59.4 (31–86)	62.5 (29–83)
WHO performance status, number (%)			
0	310 (45.0)	122 (53.7)	188 (40.7)
1	218 (31.6)	63 (27.7)	155 (33.5)
2	53 (7.7)	13 (5.6)	40 (8.7)
3	9 (1.3)	2 (0.1)	7 (1.5)
Missing	99 (14.4)	27 (11.9)	72 (15.6)
ASA-score, number (%)			
1	198 (28.7)	62 (27.4)	136 (29.4)
2	370 (53.7)	119 (52.4)	251 (54.2)
3	88 (12.8)	35 (15.4)	53 (11.5)
Missing	34 (4.9)	11 (4.8)	23 (4.9)
FIGO stage, number (%)			
IIIC	543 (78.8)	209 (92.1)	334 (72.3)
IV	146 (21.2)	18 (7.9)	128 (27.7)
Histologic type, number (%)			
Serous	502 (72.9)	156 (68.7)	346 (74.8)
Mucinous	24 (3.5)	12 (5.3)	12 (2.6)
Endometrioid	47 (6.8)	29 (12.8)	18 (3.9)
Clear cell	20 (2.9)	11 (4.8)	9 (2.0)
Undifferentiated	86 (12.5)	12 (5.3)	74 (16.1)
Mixed/other	10 (1.5)	7 (3.0)	3 (0.6)
Histologic grade, number (%)			
Well differentiated	32 (4.6)	15 (6.6)	17 (3.7)
Moderately differentiated	103 (14.9)	47 (20.7)	56 (12.1)
Poorly differentiated	373 (54.1)	141 (62.1)	232 (50.2)
Missing	181 (26.3)	24 (10.6)	157 (34.0)
CA 125 before treatment; median (range)	908.0 (12–67448)	807.5 (12–67448)	1041 (15–42077)
Ascites at surgery (ml); median (range)	500 (0–70000)	200 (0–12000)	500 (0–70000)
Cycles of chemotherapy	6 (0–13)	6 (0–9)	6 (0–13)
Type of chemotherapy			
Carboplatin/paclitaxel	641 (93)	197 (87)	444 (96)
Multidrug without platinum	10 (1.5)	3 (1)	7 (2)
Single drug platinum	27 (3.9)	17 (8)	10 (2)
No chemotherapy received	8 (1.2)	8 (4)	0 (0.0)
Missing	3 (0.4)	2 (1)	1 (0)

TABLE 2: Treatment results according to treatment group. Values given are numbers (%).

	PDS patients (*n* = 227)	IDS patients (*n* = 462)
Residual disease		
No macroscopic tumour	81 (36)	213 (46)
Minimal residual (<1 cm)	67 (30)	187 (41)
Gross residual (>1 cm)	79 (35)	60 (13)
Missing	0 (0)	2 (0)
Extensive surgery	85 (39)	169 (38)
Missing	9 (4)	19 (4)

3.2. Prognostic Factors for Survival after IDS. Median follow-up for patients with IDS was 55 months (range 3–165). Mortality within 30 days after surgery was less than one percent. Progression within six months after the last cycle of chemotherapy was seen in 40% of patients after IDS (Table 2). Median progression-free survival (PFS) was 14 months and median disease specific survival (DSS) 33 months (Figure 1).

Completeness of surgery was the most important prognostic factor. DSS with NRD was 44 months compared with 27 months with MRD and 22 months with GRD (HR MRD versus NRD 1.9 (95% CI 1.5–2.4), HR GRD versus NRD 3.4 (95% CI 2.5–4.7)). The results of the univariable and

TABLE 3: Survival outcome according to timing of surgical treatment. Values given are numbers (%) or months (SE) for DSS and PFS.

Survival	PDS patients ($n = 227$)	IDS patients ($n = 462$)
Mortality < 30 days after surgery (%)	2 (1)	2 (0)
DSS in months		
NRD	59.2 (7)	43.6 (3)
MRD	36.7 (3)	26.7 (3)
GRD	35.6 (4)	21.5 (2)
PFS in months		
NRD	23.7 (4)	17.4 (1)
MRD	16.7 (2)	11.9 (1)
GRD	12.5 (1)	9.0 (1)
Progression within 6 months after last cycle of chemotherapy	68 (32)	182 (40)

DSS: disease specific survival; PFS: progression-free survival; NRD: no residual disease; MRD: minimal residual disease (deposits of residual tumour <1 cm); GRD: gross residual disease (deposits of residual tumour >1 cm).

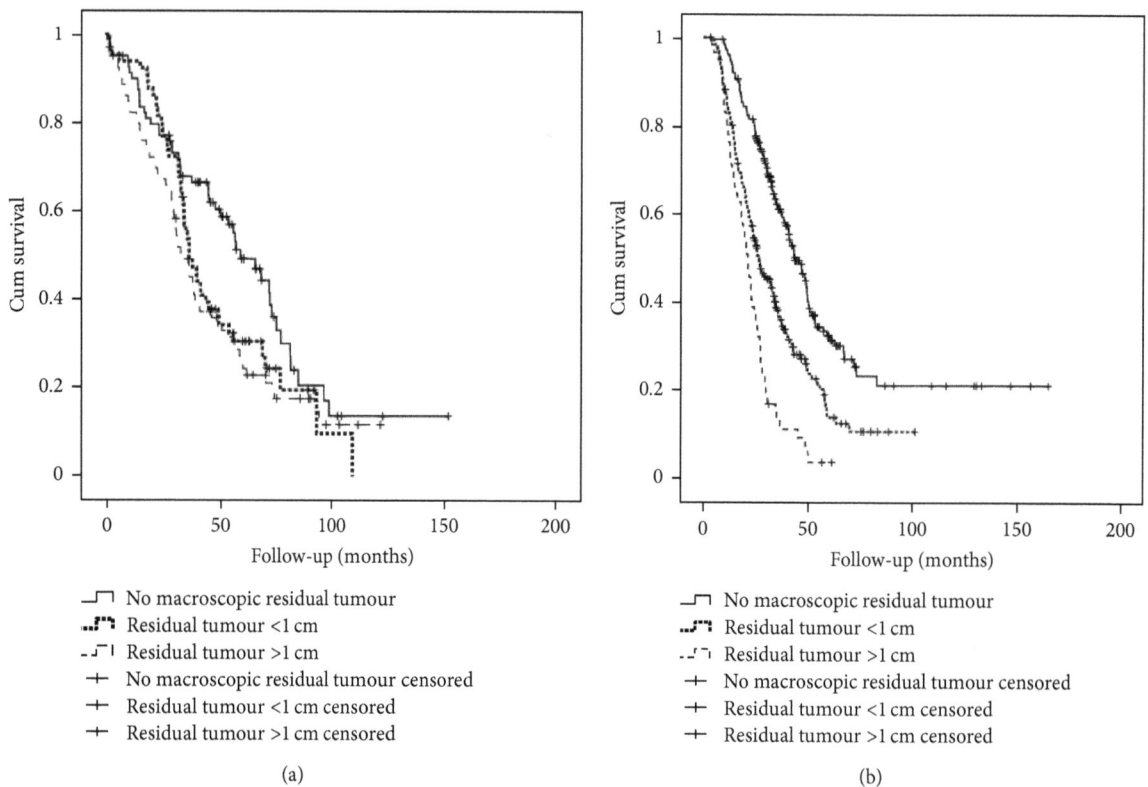

FIGURE 1: Disease specific survival according to surgery result for (a) primary debulking surgery (PDS) and (b) interval debulking surgery (IDS).

multivariable analysis are presented in Table 4(b). In multi-variable analyses residual disease was the only independent prognostic factor. The corresponding HRs were 1.8 (95% CI 1.3–2.5) and 3.1 (95% CI 2.0–4.8). The adjusted HR for MRD versus GRD was 0.6 (95% CI 0.4–0.8). Although at univariable analysis large volume ascites predicted worse prognosis, it was not an independent predictor. Extensive surgery at interval debulking surgery did not result in better survival (HR 1.1 (95% CI 0.9–1.4)).

4. Discussion

To our knowledge this is the largest cohort analysing prognostic factors in patients treated with NACT-IDS for EOC outside the realm of a clinical trial. Absence of residual disease after debulking surgery was confirmed to be a strong prognostic marker for disease specific survival after IDS as it is after PDS. Yet, the prognostic value of residual disease depends on the clinical setting. Patients selected for PDS

TABLE 4: Prognostic factors for disease specific survival after primary debulking surgery (a) and after interval debulking surgery (b).

(a)

	Univariable analysis			Multivariable analysis		
	HR	95% CI	p value	HR	95% CI	p value
Age (years)	1.00	0.99–1.02	0.55	1.01	0.99–1.03	0.47
FIGO stage IV	1.46	0.82–2.58	0.20	1.06	0.45–2.47	0.90
WHO performance ≥ 1	2.02	1.44–2.85	<0.001	**2.01**	**1.32–3.07**	**<0.001**
ASA ≥ 2	1.10	0.78–1.56	0.59	0.80	0.38–0.80	0.38
Histology						
HGS and undifferentiated	1			1		
Low grade serous	0.39	0.10–1.58	0.19	0.19	0.03–1.45	0.11
Mucinous	1.93	1.04–3.60	0.04	**2.93**	**1.38–6.20**	**0.01**
Endometrioid	0.83	0.50–1.36	0.46	0.81	0.41–1.62	0.56
Clear cell	1.81	0.95–3.48	0.07	**2.69**	**1.29–5.62**	**0.01**
CA 125 before treatment	1.07	0.98–1.18	0.15	0.97	0.84–1.11	0.63
Intraoperative ascites > 500 ml	1.35	0.97–1.06	0.08	0.89	0.56–1.41	0.61
Extensive surgery	0.85	0.61–1.18	0.34	0.84	0.55–1.27	0.41
Residual disease						
NRD	1			1		
MRD	1.48	0.99–2.21	0.05	**2.04**	**1.11–3.76**	**0.02**
GRD	1.64	1.13–2.39	0.01	**1.84**	**1.05–3.21**	**0.03**

(b)

	Univariable analysis			Multivariable analysis		
	HR	95% CI	p value	HR	95% CI	p value
Age (years)	**1.01**	**1.00–1.02**	**0.03**	1.02	0.99–1.03	0.06
FIGO stage IV	1.09	0.85–1.38	0.51	1.17	0.80–1.71	0.41
WHO performance ≥ 1	**1.32**	**1.03–1.68**	**0.03**	0.96	0.70–1.32	0.80
ASA ≥ 2	1.19	0.93–1.53	0.16	1.06	0.75–1.49	0.75
Histology						
HGS and undifferentiated	1			1		
Low grade serous	0.66	0.29–1.49	0.32	0.34	0.11–1.08	0.08
Mucinous	1.49	0.74–3.03	0.27	2.05	0.74–5.73	0.17
Endometrioid	0.77	0.41–1.46	0.43	1.24	0.64–2.40	0.53
Clear cell	1.08	0.51–2.31	0.83	1.48	0.60–3.71	0.40
CA 125 before treatment				0.94	0.84–1.05	0.25
Intraoperative ascites > 500 ml	**1.68**	**1.26–2.24**	**<0.001**	1.41	0.93–2.15	0.10
Extensive surgery	0.92	0.73–1.16	0.49	1.09	0.86–1.37	0.08
Residual disease						<0.001
NRD	1			1		
MRD	**1.87**	**1.47–2.39**	**<0.001**	**1.79**	**1.26–2.53**	**<0.001**
GRD	**3.42**	**2.48–4.72**	**<0.001**	**3.11**	**2.01–4.81**	**<0.001**

HR: hazard ratio, CI: confidence interval, HGS: high grade serous, NRD: no residual disease, MRD: minimal residual disease (deposits of residual tumour <1 cm), and GRD: gross residual disease (deposits of residual tumour >1 cm).

left without residual disease after debulking surgery have the longest survival. Even so, NRD at IDS results in longer survival than leaving any residual disease. Furthermore, achievement of minimal rather than gross residual disease at IDS results in significantly prolonged survival, whereas this effect was not confirmed for PDS.

In accordance with other studies, NRD was achieved more often in the IDS group than in the PDS group, although this did not confer a survival benefit [12, 13]. A likely explanation for this discrepancy in our cohort study is the selection of patients for NACT-IDS based on tumour load and comorbidity. Another possible explanation is the induction of fibrosis with NACT, which might masquerade tumour deposits and thus lead to an overestimation of the completeness of surgery [14–16]. This hypothesis is supported by the findings of Hynninen et al. [11], who recently reported a lower sensitivity for identifying malignant sites after NACT than at primary debulking surgery [9]. Finally, the development of platinum resistance during NACT has been suggested by exposing larger tumour volumes to chemotherapy [17, 18].

Chang et al. [19] previously stated that radical surgery leads to better overall survival when patients are treated with PDS. We could not confirm this in our PDS group, which could be due to the size of our population. Yet, patients with extensive disease diagnosed on computed tomography imaging or at diagnostic surgery were not randomly selected for NACT and no effort to perform extensive primary surgery was made in this group, resulting in selection bias.

The long and near-complete follow-up with known cause of death for all deceased patients is a strength of this study. However, patients were not followed from first date of visiting the Outpatient Department, but from start of treatment, respectively, first surgery, either diagnostic or therapeutic, or start of NACT. We have chosen this moment of start of follow-up because a number of patients were referred to our centres for treatment and their first date of contact in hospitals elsewhere was not known. Yet, since moment of start of the treatment strategies was calculated in the same way, it is unlikely that bias is introduced within the treatment groups regarding survival.

As in any observational study, formal comparison of outcome between treatment groups is hampered by confounding by indication and therefore invalid. PDS was performed if, in the opinion of the multidisciplinary team, debulking surgery of all visible tumour to less than one centimetre in diameter was possible. Patients with more extensive disease and patients unfit to undergo surgery started neoadjuvant chemotherapy. Therefore, in our series, patients receiving NACT had more extensive disease and generally worse performance status. The value of prognostic markers such as the degree of residual disease after surgery, however, can be compared. We showed that patients who have no residual disease after NACT-IDS or PDS and adjuvant chemotherapy have the best prognosis. This is consistent with published studies. Moreover, if at PDS it is not feasible to achieve NRD there is a higher chance to obtain this at IDS, and this will improve prognosis [2, 12, 20].

If at IDS NRD cannot be achieved, all possible effort, including extensive surgery, should be performed to achieve at least residual disease of less than one centimeter. Current diagnostic work-up is not adequate and new diagnostic tools are needed to optimize selection of patients for primary surgery or NACT [21]. Laparoscopy is currently studied in a randomised trial of patient selection [6].

In conclusion, NRD should be the goal of all cytoreductive surgery in ovarian cancer. Therefore selection of patients for treatment is of utmost importance.

Conflict of Interests

The authors declare that there is no conflict of interests regarding the publication of this paper.

References

[1] M. P. Coleman, D. Forman, H. Bryant et al., "Cancer survival in Australia, Canada, Denmark, Norway, Sweden, and the UK, 1995–2007 (the international cancer benchmarking partnership): an analysis of population-based cancer registry data," *The Lancet*, vol. 377, no. 9760, pp. 127–138, 2011.

[2] I. Vergote, C. G. Tropé, F. Amant et al., "Neoadjuvant chemotherapy or primary surgery in stage IIIC or IV ovarian cancer," *The New England Journal of Medicine*, vol. 363, no. 10, pp. 943–953, 2010.

[3] I. Vergote, A. Du Bois, F. Amant, F. Heitz, K. Leunen, and P. Harter, "Neoadjuvant chemotherapy in advanced ovarian cancer: on what do we agree and disagree?" *Gynecologic Oncology*, vol. 128, no. 1, pp. 6–11, 2013.

[4] S. M. Eisenkop, R. L. Friedman, and H.-J. Wang, "Complete cytoreductive surgery is feasible and maximizes survival in patients with advanced epithelial ovarian cancer: a prospective study," *Gynecologic Oncology*, vol. 69, no. 2, pp. 103–108, 1998.

[5] A. du Bois, A. Reuss, E. Pujade-Lauraine, P. Harter, I. Ray-Coquard, and J. Pfisterer, "Role of surgical outcome as prognostic factor in advanced epithelial ovarian cancer: a combined exploratory analysis of 3 prospectively randomized phase 3 multicenter trials: by the Arbeitsgemeinschaft Gynaekologische Onkologie Studiengruppe Ovarialkarzinom (AGO-OVAR) and the Groupe d'Investigateurs Nationaux Pour les Etudes des Cancers de l'Ovaire (GINECO)," *Cancer*, vol. 115, no. 6, pp. 1234–1244, 2009.

[6] M. J. Rutten, K. N. Gaarenstroom, T. Van Gorp et al., "Laparoscopy to predict the result of primary cytoreductive surgery in advanced ovarian cancer patients (LapOvCa-trial): a multicentre randomized controlled study," *BMC Cancer*, vol. 12, article 31, 2012.

[7] A. Elattar, A. Bryant, B. A. Winter-Roach, M. Hatem, and R. Naik, "Optimal primary surgical treatment for advanced epithelial ovarian cancer," *Cochrane Database of Systematic Reviews*, no. 8, Article ID CD007565, 2011.

[8] D. S. Chi, F. Musa, F. Dao et al., "An analysis of patients with bulky advanced stage ovarian, tubal, and peritoneal carcinoma treated with primary debulking surgery (PDS) during an identical time period as the randomized EORTC-NCIC trial of PDS vs neoadjuvant chemotherapy (NACT)," *Gynecologic Oncology*, vol. 124, no. 1, pp. 10–14, 2012.

[9] I. Zapardiel, M. Peiretti, V. Zanagnolo et al., "Diaphragmatic surgery during primary cytoreduction for advanced ovarian cancer: peritoneal stripping versus diaphragmatic resection," *International Journal of Gynecological Cancer*, vol. 21, no. 9, pp. 1698–1703, 2011.

[10] S. Polterauer, I. Vergote, N. Concin et al., "Prognostic value of residual tumor size in patients with epithelial ovarian cancer FIGO stages IIA-IV: analysis of the OVCAD data," *International Journal of Gynecological Cancer*, vol. 22, no. 3, pp. 380–385, 2012.

[11] J. Hynninen, M. Lavonius, S. Oksa, S. Grénman, O. Carpén, and A. Auranen, "Is perioperative visual estimation of intra-abdominal tumor spread reliable in ovarian cancer surgery after neoadjuvant chemotherapy?" *Gynecologic Oncology*, vol. 128, no. 2, pp. 229–232, 2013.

[12] M. Luyckx, E. Leblanc, T. Filleron et al., "Maximal cytoreduction in patients with figo stage iiic to stage IV ovarian, fallopian, and peritoneal cancer in day-to-day practice: a retrospective french multicentric study," *International Journal of Gynecological Cancer*, vol. 22, no. 8, pp. 1337–1343, 2012.

[13] C. L. Fago-Olsen, B. Ottesen, H. Kehlet et al., "Neoadjuvant chemotherapy as ovarian cancer treatment: ever more used with major regional differences," *Danish Medical Bulletin*, vol. 59, no. 8, p. A4477, 2012.

[14] W. G. McCluggage, R. W. Lyness, R. J. Atkinson et al., "Morphological effects of chemotherapy on ovarian carcinoma," *Journal of Clinical Pathology*, vol. 55, no. 1, pp. 27–31, 2002.

[15] K. Miller, J. H. Price, S. P. Dobbs, R. H. McClelland, K. Kennedy, and W. G. McCluggage, "An immunohistochemical and morphological analysis of post-chemotherapy ovarian carcinoma," *Journal of Clinical Pathology*, vol. 61, no. 5, pp. 652–657, 2008.

[16] D. Samrao, D. Wang, F. Ough et al., "Histologic parameters predictive of disease outcome in women with advanced stage ovarian carcinoma treated with neoadjuvant chemotherapy," *Translational Oncology*, vol. 5, no. 6, pp. 469–474, 2012.

[17] J. A. Rauh-Hain, C. C. Nitschmann, M. J. Worley Jr. et al., "Platinum resistance after neoadjuvant chemotherapy compared to primary surgery in patients with advanced epithelial ovarian carcinoma," *Gynecologic Oncology*, vol. 129, no. 1, pp. 63–68, 2013.

[18] C. G. Tropé, M. B. Elstrand, B. Sandstad, B. Davidson, and H. Oksefjell, "Neoadjuvant chemotherapy, interval debulking surgery or primary surgery in ovarian carcinoma FIGO stage IV?" *European Journal of Cancer*, vol. 48, no. 14, pp. 2146–2154, 2012.

[19] S. J. Chang, R. E. Bristow, and H. S. Ryu, "Impact of complete cytoreduction leaving no gross residual disease associated with radical cytoreductive surgical procedures on survival in advanced ovarian cancer," *Annals of Surgical Oncology*, vol. 19, no. 13, pp. 4059–4067, 2012.

[20] J. Sehouli, K. Savvatis, E.-I. Braicu, S.-C. Schmidt, W. Lichtenegger, and C. Fotopoulou, "Primary versus interval debulking surgery in advanced ovarian cancer: results from a systematic single-center analysis," *International Journal of Gynecological Cancer*, vol. 20, no. 8, pp. 1331–1340, 2010.

[21] M. J. Rutten, M. M. Leeflang, G. G. Kenter, B. W. Mol, and M. Buist, "Laparoscopy for diagnosing resectability of disease in patients with advanced ovarian cancer," *Cochrane Database of Systematic Reviews*, vol. 2, Article ID CD009786, 2014.

18

Prevention of Ovarian Hyperstimulation Syndrome: A Review

Vinayak Smith,[1] Tiki Osianlis,[2] and Beverley Vollenhoven[2,3,4]

[1]Alice Springs Hospital, Department of Obstetrics and Gynaecology, Alice Springs, NT 0870, Australia
[2]Monash IVF, 252 Clayton Road, Clayton, VIC 3168, Australia
[3]Monash Health, Women's and Children's Program, Monash Medical Centre, Clayton Road, Clayton, VIC 3168, Australia
[4]Department of Obstetrics and Gynaecology, Monash University, Clayton, VIC 3168, Australia

Correspondence should be addressed to Vinayak Smith; smith.vinayak@gmail.com

Academic Editor: Curt W. Burger

The following review aims to examine the available evidence to guide best practice in preventing ovarian hyperstimulation syndrome (OHSS). As it stands, there is no single method to completely prevent OHSS. There seems to be a benefit, however, in categorizing women based on their risk of OHSS and individualizing treatments to curtail their chances of developing the syndrome. At present, both Anti-Müllerian Hormone and the antral follicle count seem to be promising in this regard. Both available and upcoming therapies are also reviewed to give a broad perspective to clinicians with regard to management options. At present, we recommend the use of a "step-up" regimen for ovulation induction, adjunct metformin utilization, utilizing a GnRH agonist as an ovulation trigger, and cabergoline usage. A summary of recommendations is also made available for ease of clinical application. In addition, areas for potential research are also identified where relevant.

1. Introduction

Ovarian hyperstimulation syndrome (OHSS) is encountered in practice as an iatrogenic complication of controlled ovarian stimulation (COS). COS is aimed at producing multiple ovarian follicles during assisted conception cycles in hope of increasing the number of oocytes available for collection. OHSS, however, is characterised by an exaggerated response to this process [1, 2].

The incidence of moderate to severe OHSS is between 3.1 and 8% of in vitro fertilization (IVF) cycles but can be as high as 20% in high risk women [3, 4]. Typically, OHSS is a phenomenon which is associated with gonadotrophin use during COS. There are instances, however, where OHSS has been documented to arise spontaneously either in conjunction with clomiphene or with gonadotrophin releasing hormone use [2, 5]. This review aims to examine the pathophysiology of OHSS and the evidence behind the various methods employed by clinicians to prevent its occurrence.

2. Methods

A literature search was carried out on the following electronic databases (until December 2014): MEDLINE, EMBASE, and The Cochrane Central Register of Controlled Trials. Only articles in English were taken into consideration and abstracts were excluded. A combination of text words or Medical Subject Headings (MeSH) terms were subsequently utilized to generate a list of citations: ("OHSS" OR "ovarian hyperstimulation syndrome") AND ("prevention"). Articles and their references were then examined in order to identify other potential studies which could provide perspective for the following review.

Systematic reviews, meta-analyses, and randomized controlled trials (RCTs) were then preferentially selected over other forms of data where feasible in order to formulate the following review and recommendations.

3. Results and Discussion

3.1. Pathophysiology. OHSS is theorized to manifest systemically as a result of vasoactive mediators being released from hyperstimulated ovaries. As a result, capillary permeability is increased which causes the extravasation of fluid from the intravascular compartment into the third space. The haemoconcentration which ensues results in complications such as hypercoagulability and reduced end organ perfusion [6, 7].

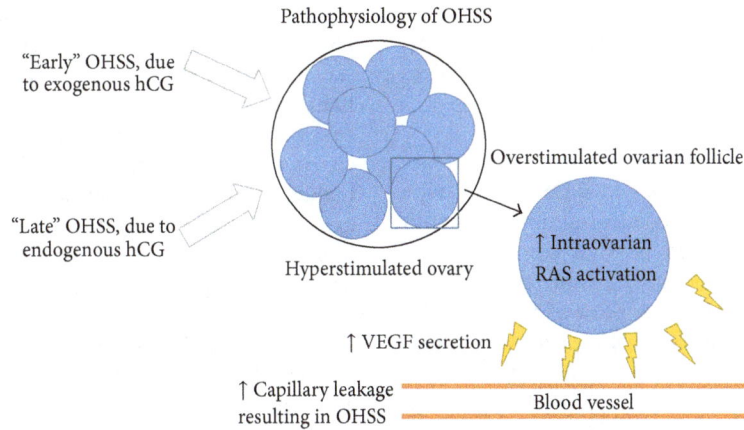

FIGURE 1: Graphical representation of the pathophysiology of ovarian hyperstimulation syndrome (OHSS).

There is currently no consensus on the exact cause of OHSS. Human Chorionic Gonadotrophin (hCG) exposure, however, is thought to be a critical mediator of the syndrome. This is based on the findings that OHSS does not develop when hCG is withheld as an ovulatory trigger during COS and also that increased hCG exposure is associated with an increased risk of OHSS [8, 9].

The role of hCG can be further elucidated via the two distinct clinical presentations observed in OHSS: the "early" and "late" forms. "Early" OHSS occurs within 9 days of hCG being administered as an ovulatory trigger and reflects the effect of exogenous hCG on ovaries that have already been hyperstimulated by gonadotrophins. "Late" OHSS, on the other hand, occurs more than 10 days after the use of hCG as an ovulatory trigger (in the absence of luteal hCG support) and demonstrates the ovarian response to endogenous hCG produced by the trophoblast [9].

hCG is thought to play a key role in the pathophysiological mechanism of OHSS by mediating the release of vascular endothelial growth factor-A (VEGF-A). VEGF-A, through its interactions with the VEGF receptor-2 (VEGFR-2), promotes angiogenesis and vascular hyperpermeability. Its overexpression, therefore, characterises the increased vascular permeability observed in OHSS [10, 11]. VEGF-A concentrations have been demonstrated to be elevated after hCG administration and in women with or at risk of OHSS [12, 13].

Another pathophysiological mechanism implicated in OHSS is the intraovarian renin angiotensin system (RAS). The ovarian RAS is involved in regulating vascular permeability, angiogenesis, endothelial proliferation, and prostaglandin release. hCG causes a strong activation of the RAS, evidenced by high renin activity in the follicular fluid of women with OHSS [11, 14]. Overstimulation of this cascade, together with increasing VEGF levels, is postulated to synergistically potentiate OHSS (Figure 1) [15, 16].

3.2. Prevention of OHSS. As the old adage goes, prevention is better than cure. As it stands, there is no perfect strategy which completely eliminates OHSS. There are factors however which we can take into consideration in order to reduce its incidence.

3.2.1. Identifying the "At Risk" Woman. Being aware of the risk factors for OHSS will allow clinicians to preempt its occurrence and thereby reduce its incidence during ovulation induction with gonadotrophins.

(A) Primary Risk Factors. Preexisting risk factors for OHSS include young age, low body weight, polycystic ovarian syndrome (PCOS), and a previous history of OHSS [3, 17, 18].

Hormonal markers are also increasingly being utilized in predicting ovarian response to stimulation. Anti-Müllerian Hormone (AMH) in particular is a marker which shows much promise. Gnoth et al., in their prospective study of 316 women, have demonstrated that AMH [AMH ≤ 0.18 pmol/L (1.26 ng/mL)] can identify normal responders (≥ 4 oocytes retrieved) to COS with a success rate of 98% [19]. This predictive capacity extends to identifying women at risk of developing OHSS as well. Using receiver operating characteristics (ROC) curves, Lee et al. have identified a high pretreatment basal AMH concentration [AMH > 0.47 pmol/L (3.36 ng/mL)] as a useful predictor of developing OHSS (sensitivity 90.5%, specificity 81.3%). Moreover, AMH performed better than weight, age, or ovarian response markers in identifying these women [20]. Given its low inter- and intracycle variability, AMH has the potential to become an excellent predictive tool should issues surrounding its validity be completely resolved [21].

Absolute serum oestradiol (E_2) concentrations, however, have performed poorly in identifying women at risk of developing OHSS. This can mostly be attested to the marked heterogeneity in studies with regard to the threshold E_2 levels used to define high risk women [8, 22].

Ultrasonographic markers, such as the antral follicle count (AFC), are also another facet worthy of mention in the prediction of OHSS. Available evidence suggests that the AFC is equally predictive of excessive response to COS and OHSS as the basal serum AMH [23–25]. Jayaprakasan et al., in their prospective study of 1012 subjects, noted an AFC ≥ 24 to be correlated with an increased risk of moderate to severe OHSS in comparison to an AFC < 24 (8.6% versus 2.2%) [26]. These findings are mirrored by Delvigne and Rozenberg and Papanikolaou et al. who cite an increased risk of OHSS with an AFC (2–8 mm) $\geq$ 12. There are, however, variances amongst the studies regarding the definition of what constitutes antral follicles on ultrasound which limits their applicability [3, 27].

(B) Secondary Risk Factors. Secondary risk factors examine ovarian response parameters related to COS in the hope of predicting OHSS. During COS, ultrasound and serum E_2 monitoring are considered to be vital components of surveillance for OHSS. Based on this, parameters such as a rapidly rising E_2 level, a large number of developing follicles on the day of hCG administration (>14 follicles with a diameter of 11 mm), and a large number of oocytes retrieved have been proposed as risk factors for developing OHSS [17, 28]. None of the above predictors, however, have been shown to be independently predictive of OHSS and can be considered to be moderate at best given the wide variation in cut-off levels being utilized [1, 3, 29].

In combination, however, Papanikolaou et al. in their prospective cohort of 2524 GnRH antagonist cycles have identified the combination of $\geq$18 follicles on ultrasound (diameter $\geq$ 11 mm) and $E_2 \geq 5000$ ng/L on the day of hCG trigger to be more useful (sensitivity 83%, specificity 84%) than E_2 concentrations alone in the prediction of severe OHSS [28].

It also should be noted, however, that women without any risk factors can develop OHSS as there is some degree of hyperstimulation in all stimulation protocols. The possibility of OHSS therefore should always remain at the back of the clinicians mind in any woman undergoing COS [29].

3.2.2. Risk Stratification. Prevention strategies for OHSS are broadly classified as both primary and secondary in nature. Primary prevention classifies a person based on their risk factors into high, normal, or low risk for OHSS, then individualizing treatment regimens to them on that basis. Secondary prevention, on the other hand, focuses on methods used in patients who have displayed an excessive response to ovarian stimulation during a cycle and aims to prevent progression to OHSS [1].

3.2.3. Primary Prevention. In women who are identified as being at a high risk of OHSS, treatment regimens need to be modified in view of curtailing an overexcessive ovarian response.

(A) Targeting Unifollicular Ovulation. As previously highlighted, women with PCOS are at an increased risk for OHSS. Since 4–8% of women worldwide have the syndrome, this is a major subpopulation towards whom primary prevention should be directed. The goal of therapy therefore in this subgroup of women is to induce unifollicular ovulation through ovulation induction (OI) and thereby prevent progression to OHSS [30]. With this in mind, aspects which deserve consideration are as follows.

(i) Reducing the Gonadotrophin Dose. The best evidence suggests that the minimum gonadotrophin dose should be used for OI given its lower risk of OHSS. This favours a "step-up" regimen over a "step-down" regimen. In the "step-up"

regimen, ovarian stimulation is initiated with a low dose of FSH (i.e., 75 IU), which is subsequently increased every 7 days (i.e., 37.5 IU) until an ovarian response is noted (follicle > 10 mm). This dose is then continued until the criteria for an ovulatory trigger are met [2, 18]. This regimen is associated with a lower risk of OHSS, cycle cancellation, and a higher rate of unifollicular development in contrast to other low dose/step-down protocols. In a "step-down" regimen, a higher starting FSH dose is used which is downtitrated based on ovarian response [31, 32].

(ii) Avoiding Adjunct GnRH Agonist (GnRHa) Utilization. During OI in women with PCOS, GnRHa is concomitantly administered with gonadotrophins to downregulate the endogenous pituitary secretion of LH in hope of preventing premature luteinisation. This process, however, seems to increase the dose of exogenous gonadotrophins required [1]. In their Cochrane Review, Nugent et al. highlighted the sequelae of this through the higher overstimulation rate (OR 3.15; 95% CI 1.48–6.70). This coupled with the increased cost and additional inconvenience without an increase in pregnancy rates prompted them to make a recommendation against its use [33].

(iii) Reducing the Gonadotrophin Duration. There is consensus on the fact that reducing the duration of gonadotrophin exposure reduces the risk of OHSS. One way this is achieved is through "mild" stimulation protocols which delay the administration of FSH till the mid or late follicular phase [1, 34]. Previously, a major issue associated with this was early cycle cancellation due to premature luteinisation and lower pregnancy rates. However, the addition of GnRH antagonists for late cycle suppression of gonadotrophin release has resulted in improved clinical outcomes, a lower risk of OHSS, and multiple pregnancies and made it cost effective as well. On a side note, the pooled data of 3 RCTs have shown mild stimulation to be less effective than conventional "long" regimens in terms of the pregnancy rates per cycle (15% versus 29%) [35–38].

(iv) Utilising Adjuvant Metformin Therapy. Metformin is theorized to exert its influence in preventing OHSS by inhibiting the secretion of vasoactive molecules, such as VEGF, during OI and thereby modulates vascular permeability [39]. In the recent Cochrane Review by Tso et al., based upon 8 RCTs with 798 women, it was noted that there was a lower risk of OHSS with metformin use (OR 0.29; 95% CI 0.18–0.49). It was also of note that metformin reduced the risk of OHSS by 63% and increased the clinical pregnancy rate (OR 1.52; 95% CI 1.07–2.15) [40] without an effect on live birth rates. These findings were consistent with an earlier systemic review by Palombo et al., which described a significantly lower OHSS rate with metformin administration too (0.27; 95% CI 0.16–0.46).

Based on the studies, a daily dose between 1000 and 2000 mg at least 2 months prior to COS is recommended for the purpose of preventing OHSS [41–43].

(v) Utilising Aromatase Inhibitors (AIs) for Ovulation Induction. AIs, such as letrozole, function by downregulating oestrogen production through inhibition of cytochrome P450

enzymes. This causes an increase in pituitary secretion of FSH which promotes folliculogenesis. In addition, the central negative feedback mechanisms still remain intact, which leads to the theory that it may reduce the incidence of OHSS during OI [44]. A recent Cochrane Review by Franik et al., however, failed to show any difference in OHSS rates through utilization of AIs in contrast to other methods of OI [45].

As such, AIs are not routinely recommended.

(B) Individualizing IVF Treatment Regimens. There is increasing evidence to suggest that individualised COS (iCOS) can reduce OHSS and associated cycle cancellations [46, 47]. iCOS entails identifying women at risk of an overexcessive response through various biomarkers, of which the combination of both AFC and AMH seems to be the most promising [24, 48]. The means of COS (e.g., starting FSH dose or tailored GnRH antagonist protocol) can then be decided based on an algorithm of these biomarkers. One example of this can be seen through the study by La Marca et al., where an algorithm was formulated based on age, AFC, and FSH to calculate the FSH starting dose. This algorithm was able to accurately predict ovarian sensitivity and account for 30% of the variability of ovaries to FSH. In addition, it was also a model that had easy applicability in clinical practice [49]. The CONSORT study also serves as another good illustration of this concept, with adequate oocyte yield and good pregnancy rates (34.2%) [50]. Findings from the ongoing multicentre OPTIMIST study will also be welcome in order to shed light on the cost effectiveness associated with iCOS as well [51].

As it stands, however, iCOS shows a lot of promise in curtailing OHSS through tailored COS regimens and seems to be the initial steps towards an ART of the near future.

(C) Avoiding hCG for Luteal Phase Support (LPS). During COS, endogenous LH concentrations are markedly lower due to the negative feedback caused by the supraphysiological progesterone (P_4) concentrations maintained by the multiple corpora lutea. This results in a shortened luteal phase and poor endometrial receptivity resulting in reduced implantation and pregnancy rates. As such luteal phase support is imperative to improve these parameters [52–54]. hCG, which is similar to LH in its physiological actions, has been used effectively in this scenario. A Cochrane Review, however, noted that it potentiated the risk of OHSS (OR 3.62; 95% CI 1.85–7.06) and also showed no effect on live birth rate (LBR) and clinical pregnancy rate (CPR). In contrast, the use of progesterone (P) halves the OHSS risk while significantly improving the LBR (OR 2.95; 95% CI 1.02–8.56) and CPR (OR 1.83; 95% CI 1.29–2.61) [55].

On the basis of these findings, the routine use of progesterone over hCG is recommended for LPS.

(D) Considering Alternatives for Triggering Ovulation. The agent of choice for triggering ovulation should be picked based on the risk of the woman for developing OHSS. No agent, however, completely eliminates the risk of OHSS.

(i) *Exogenous hCG* has long been used to mimic the ovulatory LH surge. Its long half-life (2.32 days) however causes prolonged luteotrophic effects, multiple corpora lutea development, and higher luteal phase P_4 and E_2 concentrations. Hence, given its higher risk of potentiating OHSS it should be either used at the lowest possible dose (i.e., 5000 IU) or altogether avoided in high risk women [29, 56]. It is of note that the use of lower hCG doses as an ovulation trigger, in contrast to the conventional dose of 10,000 IU, has not impacted clinical outcomes but questions do remain over its capacity to reduce the risk of OHSS [57, 58].

(ii) *GnRH agonists (GnRHa)* produce a more tempered and shorter midcycle gonadotrophin surge (24–36 hours) in contrast to hCG by stimulating pituitary LH secretion. Theoretically, this LH surge should just be sufficient to induce ovulation without being prolonged enough to induce hyperstimulation. The available data supports this notion by demonstrating that OHSS is virtually eliminated with GnRHa utilization (in a "freeze all" approach) which mandates its consideration in the high risk woman [59–61]. This however should be taken in the context of the IVF regimen utilized as well. For instance, with the recent increase in proponents of dual trigger regimens (addition of 1–2000 IU of hCG to a GnRHa trigger) for its improved pregnancy and implantation and live birth rates, the propensity for OHSS remains very possible. It should also be noted that OHSS can occur de novo as part of GnRHa triggered cycles but the incidence of this is limited to a handful of case studies [62–64].

(iii) *Recombinant LH (rhLH)* use is also another possible prevention strategy in the high risk woman by attempting to mimic the endogenous LH surge. With a half-life of 10 hours, and a shorter and/or lower LH peak, it is expected that there should be minimal risk of causing OHSS. A Cochrane Review by Youssef et al. however did not show any difference in the risk for severe OHSS between rhLH and urinary hCG. Furthermore, it has also been associated with a lower pregnancy rate and a poor cost benefit ratio. Its routine use therefore cannot be recommended [65, 66].

3.2.4. Secondary Prevention. Secondary prevention is extended to women who have undergone COS and subsequently mounted an exaggerated response. The aim of interventions in these circumstances is to prevent progression to OHSS.

(A) Coasting. Coasting is a preventative strategy by which gonadotrophins are withdrawn when a certain E_2 concentration and/or a critical number of follicles are reached. hCG trigger is subsequently delayed until E_2 levels significantly decrease or plateau. Once the E_2 reaches a "safe" level, hCG is administered followed by oocyte retrieval and embryo transfer or freezing depending on the E_2 concentration. It is generally employed for a period less than 3 days [29, 67].

Coasting is a commonly used first line secondary prevention strategy by clinicians [68]. Question marks remain however about the evidence behind the procedure. D'Angelo et al., in their Cochrane Review, identified 4 RCTs which highlighted that there was no difference in the incidence of moderate and severe OHSS (OR 0.53, 95% CI 0.44–1.08) with coasting. In addition, a lower number of oocytes were retrieved from the coasting group which prompted them to recommend that there was no benefit of coasting in comparison to other interventions [69]. An earlier meta-analysis also came to the conclusion that coasting may decrease the risk of OHSS in high risk women but does not completely prevent it. Coasting, however, seems to have no effect on live birth rates and clinical pregnancy rates [67, 70].

As it stands, there is not much strong evidence to back its routine use and no specific criteria about commencing and discontinuing coasting given the wide heterogeneity in study protocols, control groups, and definition of OHSS classes as well [1, 67].

(B) Cryopreservation of Embryos. During cryopreservation, COS and subsequent oocyte retrieval is performed followed by the cryopreservation of embryos. These are then transferred in a subsequent unstimulated IVF cycle where the woman's ovarian response to hCG has normalized [71]. A Cochrane Review only identified 2 RCTs for analysis and came to the conclusion that there was insufficient evidence to support routine cryopreservation [72]. Recent evidence however strongly supports the use of a GnRHa trigger followed by cryopreservation as being the most effective method in preventing OHSS, best illustrated by Devroey and colleagues through their OHSS-Free Clinic [73].

Another dogma which previously surrounded cryopreserved embryos was the lower pregnancy rates in contrast to fresh embryo transfers related to older slow freezing methods [74]. With the advent of modern techniques such as vitrification, however, there is convincing evidence to suggest that cryopreservation has better pregnancy rates (32% increase) than fresh embryo transfer as well [75–77].

Based on these findings, we recommend the use of a GnRHa trigger followed by cryopreservation for averting OHSS.

(C) Cycle Cancellation. Cycle cancellation and withholding of hCG are the only definite methods of preventing OHSS [78, 79]. However, it must be taken in context with the high financial impact and psychological distress that it causes to women. It is therefore, in many cases, a last resort for clinicians [1, 29].

3.2.5. Alternative Methods of Prevention

(A) Colloid Infusion. Colloid infusions are administered around the time of oocyte retrieval as they are theorized to prevent OHSS by binding to and deactivating the vasoactive mediators of OHSS.

(i) Albumin. A Cochrane Review by Youssef et al. noted that there was borderline statistically lower incidence of severe OHSS with albumin utilization but there was marked heterogeneity in the studies (8 RCTs; OR 0.67; 95% CI 0.04–0.40; $I^2 = 62\%$). A subsequent sensitivity analysis performed after excluding 2 unpublished studies, however, showed no significant alteration in the results (OR 0.75; 95% CI 0.47–1.21)

[80]. Another systematic review by Jee et al. also found that intravenous (IV) albumin did not reduce the rate of severe OHSS (RR 0.80; 95% CI 0.57–1.12) and also raised concerns regarding significantly reduced pregnancy rates (RR 0.85, 95% CI 0.74–0.98) [81]. The lack of prevention against severe OHSS was further reiterated in the systemic review by Venetis et al. (OR 0.80; 95% CI 0.52–1.22) as well. In addition, factors such as the possibility of transmission of viral infections (i.e., hepatitis B/C/HIV) and prion disease through albumin as well as its propensity to cause anaphylactic reactions are risks that should not be overlooked [82].

On the basis of these factors, the routine use of IV albumin to prevent OHSS cannot be recommended.

(ii) Hydroxyethyl Starch (HES). HES is a plasma expander that has been mooted as an alternative to albumin as it is non-biological and therefore negates the above-mentioned risks associated with albumin use. The evidence behind its benefit is certainly more robust as well. The Cochrane Review by Youssef et al. noted that there was a statistically significant decrease in severe OHSS (OR 0.12; 95% CI 0.04–0.40) with HES use without any effect on pregnancy rates (OR 1.20; 95% CI 0.49–2.95) [80].

It must be borne in mind that these findings were based on only 3 RCTs and more compelling evidence should be sought prior to recommending its routine use.

(iii) Cabergoline. Cabergoline is a dopamine antagonist which prevents the excessive increase in VEGF mediated vascular permeability encountered with OHSS through its antiangiogenic properties [83]. Tang et al. in their Cochrane Review of 230 women in 2 RCTs found cabergoline to be effective in significantly reducing the incidence of moderate OHSS (OR 0.38; 95% CI 0.19–0.78) with no significant effect on clinical pregnancy rate and miscarriage rates. This protective effect, however, did not extend to severe OHSS, possibly due to the number of studies available for comparison [84]. A recent systemic review by Leitao at el. on the issue, which took 7 RCTs into consideration, has further established its efficacy in preventing the occurrence of moderate and severe OHSS (RR 0.38; 95% CI 0.29–0.51) as well as without a negative impact on clinical pregnancy or oocytes retrieved [85].

Therefore, the use of cabergoline is recommended and it is suggested that treatment be commenced on the day of hCG trigger at a dose of 0.5 mg for 8 days [86].

(C) Vasopressin Induced VEGF Secretion Blockade. Amongst the novel therapies being investigated for the prevention of OHSS, the vasopressin V1a receptor antagonist, relcovaptan, has been studied for its ability to inhibit VEGF by modulating vasoconstriction and vascular smooth muscle proliferation. Relcovaptan, in the hyperstimulated rat model, has shown lower concentrations of VEGF-A in the peritoneal fluid and lesser ovarian weight gain significant decreases in the number of corpora lutea in contrast to control groups. Further research in this area remains rather promising and may broaden the management protocols which clinicians have for OHSS in the near future [87].

TABLE 1: Summary of recommendations for strategies to prevent OHSS.

Intervention	Recommendation	Effect of intervention	Level of evidence
Reducing gonadotrophin dose	Recommended	"Step-up regimen" has a lower risk of OHSS, cycle cancellation from hyperstimulation, and higher rate of monofollicular ovulation in contrast to other protocols	1b, 4
Reducing gonadotrophin duration	Utilized as clinically appropriate	"Mild" stimulation protocol with GnRH antagonist for late suppression has a lower risk of OHSS and multiple pregnancies and is cost effective	1b
		It also is less effective in terms of pregnancy rates than "long" protocols	1a
Individualized COS (iCOS)	Further research required	iCOS can reduce OHSS rates and associated cycle cancellations. It also produces a significant oocyte yield and good pregnancy rates	1b, 2a
GnRHa as an ovulation trigger	Recommended	GnRHa use virtually eliminates OHSS rates	1b
hCG as an ovulation trigger	Further research required	Lowest dose of hCG does not seem to reduce OHSS rates	2a, 2b, 4
Adjuvant metformin therapy	Recommended	Metformin is associated with a lower risk of OHSS and increased clinical pregnancy rate	1a, 4
Cabergoline	Recommended	Cabergoline reduces the incidence of OHSS without an effect on pregnancy rates	1a
Hydroxyethyl starch	Utilized as clinically appropriate	HES causes a decrease in OHSS without an effect on pregnancy rates	1a
Coasting	Further research required	Coasting does not completely prevent OHSS, is associated with a lower oocyte yield, and has no benefit in contrast to other interventions. The protocols are also very diverse	1a, 4
Cryopreservation	Utilized as clinically appropriate	Cryopreservation alone does not reduce rates of OHSS	1a
		GnRHa followed by cryopreservation virtually eliminates OHSS	1b
Cycle cancellation	Utilized as clinically appropriate	Cancellation completely eliminates risk of OHSS but has a high financial and emotional burden	4
Adjunct GnRHa use	Not recommended	GnRHa use increases the associated costs and rate of OHSS while lowering the pregnancy rates	1a
Aromatase inhibitors for OI	Not recommended	AIs have shown no reduction in rates of OHSS in contrast to other methods of OI	1a
rhLH	Not recommended	rhLH use does not reduce the risk of OHSS and has higher costs and lower pregnancy rates	1a, 1b
hCG for luteal phase support	Not recommended	Progesterone significantly reduces the risk of OHSS with improved clinical pregnancy rates and live birth rates in comparison to hCG for LPS	1a
Albumin infusion	Not recommended	Albumin does not reduce OHSS rates and may cause lower pregnancy rates. There are also associated risks with anaphylaxis and disease transmission	1a
Vasopressin V1a receptor antagonist	Further research required	It appears to reduce the ovarian weight gain and multiple corpus luteum development in OHSS	2b

Glossary for levels of evidence, 1a: systematic review and/or meta-analysis; 1b: ≥one RCT; 2a: ≥1 well-designed controlled study without randomization; 2b: ≥1 well-designed quasi experimental study; 3: ≥1 well-designed descriptive study; 4: committee or expert opinions.

4. Conclusion

OHSS is a complication associated with COS which clinicians have no complete way of preventing at present. Through the various prevention strategies reviewed in this paper (summarized in Table 1), there are avenues by which its incidence can be greatly reduced. This begins with the identification of the "high risk" woman through to the woman who is "at risk" and subsequently initiating the appropriate therapies. It is also an avenue towards which further research initiatives should be directed in a bid to strengthen the preexisting evidence base for available therapies and to develop novel techniques to aid in the prevention of OHSS.

Conflict of Interests

The authors declare that there is no conflict of interests, be it financial or in any other form.

Authors' Contribution

All authors substantially contributed to the conception and design of the following review and were involved in the collection of data to that effect. The data was then collectively examined and critically appraised in order to formulate the above-mentioned review and subsequent recommendations. All authors were in agreement with the final version of this review submitted for publication.

References

[1] P. Humaidan, J. Quartarolo, and E. G. Papanikolaou, "Preventing ovarian hyperstimulation syndrome: guidance for the clinician," *Fertility and Sterility*, vol. 94, no. 2, pp. 389–400, 2010.

[2] B. K. Tan and R. Mathur, "Management of ovarian hyperstimulation syndrome. Produced on behalf of the BFS policy and practice committee," *Human Fertility*, vol. 16, no. 3, pp. 151–159, 2013.

[3] A. Delvinge and S. Rozenberg, "Epidemiology and prevention of ovarian hyperstimulation syndrome (OHSS): a review," *Human Reproduction Update*, vol. 8, no. 6, pp. 559–577, 2002.

[4] C. O. Nastri, D. M. Teixeira, R. M. Moroni, V. M. Leitao, and W. P. Martins, "Ovarian hyperstimulation syndrome: pathophysiology, staging, prediction and prevention," *Ultrasound in Obstetrics & Gynecology*, vol. 45, no. 4, pp. 377–393, 2015.

[5] C. Di Carlo, F. Savoia, C. Ferrara, G. A. Tommaselli, G. Bifulco, and C. Nappi, "Case report: a most peculiar family with spontaneous, recurrent ovarian hyperstimulation syndrome," *Gynecological Endocrinology*, vol. 28, no. 8, pp. 649–651, 2012.

[6] M. P. Goldsman, A. Pedram, C. E. Dominguez, I. Ciuffardi, E. Levin, and R. H. Asch, "Increased capillary permeability induced by human follicular fluid: a hypothesis for an ovarian origin of the hyperstimulation syndrome," *Fertility and Sterility*, vol. 63, no. 2, pp. 268–272, 1995.

[7] A. Tollan, N. Holst, F. Forsdahl, H. O. Fadnes, P. Oian, and J. M. Maltau, "Transcapillary fluid dynamics during ovarian stimulation for in vitro fertilization," *The American Journal of Obstetrics and Gynecology*, vol. 162, no. 2, pp. 554–558, 1990.

[8] M. A. Aboulghar and R. T. Mansour, "Ovarian hyperstimulation syndrome: classifications and critical analysis of preventive measures," *Human Reproduction Update*, vol. 9, no. 3, pp. 275–289, 2003.

[9] R. S. Mathur, A. V. Akande, S. D. Keay, L. P. Hunt, and J. M. Jenkins, "Distinction between early and late ovarian hyperstimulation syndrome," *Fertility and Sterility*, vol. 73, no. 5, pp. 901–907, 2000.

[10] D. O. Bates and S. J. Harper, "Regulation of vascular permeability by vascular endothelial growth factors," *Vascular Pharmacology*, vol. 39, no. 4-5, pp. 225–237, 2002.

[11] N. Naredi, P. Talwar, and K. Sandeep, "VEGF antagonist for the prevention of ovarian hyperstimulation syndrome: current status," *Medical Journal Armed Forces India*, vol. 70, no. 1, pp. 58–63, 2014.

[12] S. R. Soares, R. Gómez, C. Simón, J. A. García-Velasco, and A. Pellicer, "Targeting the vascular endothelial growth factor system to prevent ovarian hyperstimulation syndrome," *Human Reproduction Update*, vol. 14, no. 4, pp. 321–333, 2008.

[13] T.-H. Wang, S.-G. Horng, C.-L. Chang et al., "Human chorionic gonadotropin-induced ovarian hyperstimulation syndrome is associated with up-regulation of vascular endothelial growth factor," *Journal of Clinical Endocrinology and Metabolism*, vol. 87, no. 7, pp. 3300–3308, 2002.

[14] M. Kasum, "New insights in mechanisms for development of ovarian hyperstimulation syndrome," *Collegium Antropologicum*, vol. 34, no. 3, pp. 1139–1143, 2010.

[15] D. Herr, I. Bekes, and C. Wulff, "Local Renin-Angiotensin system in the reproductive system," *Frontiers in Endocrinology*, vol. 4, article 150, 2013.

[16] L. Schwentner, A. Wöckel, D. Herr, and C. Wulff, "Is there a role of the local tissue RAS in the regulation of physiologic and pathophysiologic conditions in the reproductive tract?" *Journal of the Renin-Angiotensin-Aldosterone System*, vol. 12, no. 4, pp. 385–393, 2011.

[17] ASRM, "Ovarian hyperstimulation syndrome," *Fertility and Sterility*, vol. 90, no. 5, supplement, pp. S188–S193, 2008.

[18] Joint SOGC-CFAS Clinical Practice Guideline, "The diagnosis and management of ovarian hyperstimulation syndrome," *Journal of Obstetrics and Gynaecology Canada*, vol. 2068, pp. 1156–1162, 2011.

[19] C. Gnoth, A. N. Schuring, K. Friol, J. Tigges, P. Mallmann, and E. Godehardt, "Relevance of anti-Mullerian hormone measurement in a routine IVF program," *Human Reproduction*, vol. 23, no. 6, pp. 1359–1365, 2008.

[20] T.-H. Lee, C.-H. Liu, C.-C. Huang et al., "Serum anti-Müllerian hormone and estradiol levels as predictors of ovarian hyperstimulation syndrome in assisted reproduction technology cycles," *Human Reproduction*, vol. 23, no. 1, pp. 160–167, 2008.

[21] D. Dewailly, C. Y. Andersen, A. Balen et al., "The physiology and clinical utility of anti-Müllerian hormone in women," *Human Reproduction Update*, vol. 20, no. 3, pp. 370–385, 2014.

[22] R. Orvieto, "Ovarian hyperstimulation syndrome- an optimal solution for an unresolved enigma," *Journal of Ovarian Research*, vol. 6, no. 1, article 77, 2013.

[23] A. Aflatoonian, H. Oskouian, S. Ahmadi, and L. Oskouian, "Prediction of high ovarian response to controlled ovarian hyperstimulation: anti-Müllerian hormone versus small antral follicle count (2–6 mm)," *Journal of Assisted Reproduction and Genetics*, vol. 26, no. 6, pp. 319–325, 2009.

[24] S. L. Broer, M. Dólleman, B. C. Opmeer, B. C. Fauser, B. W. Mol, and F. J. M. Broekmans, "AMH and AFC as predictors of excessive response in controlled ovarian hyperstimulation: a meta-analysis," *Human Reproduction Update*, vol. 17, no. 1, pp. 46–54, 2011.

[25] P. Ocal, S. Sahmay, M. Cetin, T. Irez, O. Guralp, and I. Cepni, "Serum anti-Müllerian hormone and antral follicle count as predictive markers of OHSS in ART cycles," *Journal of Assisted Reproduction and Genetics*, vol. 28, no. 12, pp. 1197–1203, 2011.

[26] K. Jayaprakasan, Y. Chan, R. Islam et al., "Prediction of in vitro fertilization outcome at different antral follicle count thresholds in a prospective cohort of 1,012 women," *Fertility and Sterility*, vol. 98, no. 3, pp. 657–663, 2012.

[27] E. G. Papanikolaou, P. Humaidan, N. P. Polyzos, and B. Tarlatzis, "Identification of the high-risk patient for ovarian hyperstimulation syndrome," *Seminars in Reproductive Medicine*, vol. 28, no. 6, pp. 458–462, 2010.

[28] E. G. Papanikolaou, C. Pozzobon, E. M. Kolibianakis et al., "Incidence and prediction of ovarian hyperstimulation syndrome in women undergoing gonadotropin-releasing hormone antagonist in vitro fertilization cycles," *Fertility and Sterility*, vol. 85, no. 1, pp. 112–120, 2006.

[29] R. S. Mathur and B. K. Tan, "British fertility society policy and practice committee: prevention of ovarian hyperstimulation syndrome," *Human Fertility*, vol. 17, no. 4, pp. 257–268, 2014.

[30] I. Tummon, L. Gavrilova-Jordan, M. C. Allemand, and D. Session, "Polycystic ovaries and ovarian hyperstimulation syndrome: a systematic review," *Acta Obstetricia et Gynecologica Scandinavica*, vol. 84, no. 7, pp. 611–616, 2005.

[31] S. Christin-Maitre, J. N. Hugues, and Recombinant FSH Study Group, "A comparative randomized multicentric study comparing the step-up versus step-down protocol in polycystic ovary syndrome," *Human Reproduction*, vol. 18, no. 8, pp. 1626–1631, 2003.

[32] R. Homburg, T. Levy, and Z. Ben-Rafael, "A comparative prospective study of conventional regimen with chronic low-dose administration of follicle-stimulating hormone for anovulation associated with polycystic ovary syndrome," *Fertility and Sterility*, vol. 63, no. 4, pp. 729–733, 1995.

[33] D. Nugent, P. Vandekerckhove, E. Hughes, M. Arnot, and R. Lilford, "Gonadotrophin therapy for ovulation induction in subfertility associated with polycystic ovary syndrome.," *Cochrane Database of Systematic Reviews*, no. 4, Article ID CD000410, 2000.

[34] N. Mahajan, "Should mild stimulation be the order of the day?" *Journal of Human Reproductive Sciences*, vol. 6, no. 4, pp. 220–226, 2013.

[35] F. P. Hohmann, N. S. Macklon, and B. C. J. M. Fauser, "A randomized comparison of two ovarian stimulation protocols with gonadotropin-releasing hormone (GnRH) antagonist cotreatment for in vitro fertilization commencing recombinant follicle-stimulating hormone on cycle day 2 or 5 with the standard long GnRH agonist protocol," *Journal of Clinical Endocrinology and Metabolism*, vol. 88, no. 1, pp. 166–173, 2003.

[36] M. J. Pelinck, N. E. A. Vogel, A. Hoek, E. G. J. M. Arts, A. H. M. Simons, and M. J. Heineman, "Minimal stimulation IVF with late follicular phase administration of the GnRH antagonist cetrorelix and concomitant substitution with recombinant FSH: a pilot study," *Human Reproduction*, vol. 20, no. 3, pp. 642–648, 2005.

[37] A. Revelli, S. Casano, F. Salvagno, and L. Delle Piane, "Milder is better? advantages and disadvantages of 'mild' ovarian stimulation for human in vitro fertilization," *Reproductive Biology and Endocrinology*, vol. 9, article 25, 2011.

[38] M. A. Karimzadeh, S. Ahmadi, H. Oskouian, and E. Rahmani, "Comparison of mild stimulation and conventional stimulation in ART outcome," *Archives of Gynecology and Obstetrics*, vol. 281, no. 4, pp. 741–746, 2010.

[39] E. M. Elia, R. Quintana, C. Carrere et al., "Metformin decreases the incidence of ovarian hyperstimulation syndrome: an experimental study," *Journal of Ovarian Research*, vol. 6, no. 1, article 62, 2013.

[40] L. O. Tso, M. F. Costello, L. E. Albuquerque, R. B. Andriolo, and C. R. Macedo, "Metformin treatment before and during IVF or ICSI in women with polycystic ovary syndrome," *Cochrane Database of Systematic Reviews*, vol. 11, Article ID Cd006105, 2014.

[41] S. Palomba, A. Falbo, and G. B. la Sala, "Effects of metformin in women with polycystic ovary syndrome treated with gonadotrophins for in vitro fertilisation and intracytoplasmic sperm injection cycles: a systematic review and meta-analysis of randomised controlled trials," *BJOG: An International Journal of Obstetrics & Gynaecology*, vol. 120, no. 3, pp. 267–276, 2013.

[42] Y. El-Faissal, "Approaches to complete prevention of OHSS," *Middle East Fertility Society Journal*, vol. 19, no. 1, pp. 13–15, 2014.

[43] M. F. Costello, M. Chapman, and U. Conway, "A systematic review and meta-analysis of randomized controlled trials on metformin co-administration during gonadotrophin ovulation induction or IVF in women with polycystic ovary syndrome," *Human Reproduction*, vol. 21, no. 6, pp. 1387–1399, 2006.

[44] V. C. Y. Lee and W. Ledger, "Aromatase inhibitors for ovulation induction and ovarian stimulation," *Clinical Endocrinology*, vol. 74, no. 5, pp. 537–546, 2011.

[45] S. Franik, J. A. Kremer, W. L. Nelen, and C. Farquhar, "Aromatase inhibitors for subfertile women with polycystic ovary syndrome," *Cochrane Database of Systematic Rev*, vol. 2, Article ID CD010287, 2014.

[46] A. La Marca and S. K. Sunkara, "Individualization of controlled ovarian stimulation in IVF using ovarian reserve markers: from theory to practice," *Human Reproduction Update*, vol. 20, no. 1, Article ID dmt037, pp. 124–140, 2014.

[47] K. Fiedler and D. Ezcurra, "Predicting and preventing ovarian hyperstimulation syndrome (OHSS): the need for individualized not standardized treatment," *Reproductive Biology and Endocrinology*, vol. 10, article 32, 2012.

[48] E. Bosch and D. Ezcurra, "Individualised controlled ovarian stimulation (iCOS): maximising success rates for assisted reproductive technology patients," *Reproductive Biology and Endocrinology*, vol. 9, article 82, 2011.

[49] A. La Marca, V. Grisendi, S. Giulini et al., "Individualization of the FSH starting dose in IVF/ICSI cycles using the antral follicle count," *Journal of Ovarian Research*, vol. 6, no. 1, article 11, 2013.

[50] F. Olivennes, C. M. Howles, A. Borini et al., "Individualizing FSH dose for assisted reproduction using a novel algorithm: the CONSORT study," *Reproductive BioMedicine Online*, vol. 18, no. 2, pp. 195–204, 2009.

[51] T. C. van Tilborg, M. J. C. Eijkemans, J. S. E. Laven et al., "The OPTIMIST study: optimisation of cost effectiveness through individualised FSH stimulation dosages for IVF treatment. A randomised controlled trial," *BMC Women's Health*, vol. 12, article 29, 2012.

[52] E. A. Pritts and A. K. Atwood, "Luteal phase support in infertility treatment: a meta-analysis of the randomized trials," *Human Reproduction*, vol. 17, no. 9, pp. 2287–2299, 2002.

[53] H. M. Fatemi, E. M. Kolibianakis, M. Camus et al., "Addition of estradiol to progesterone for luteal supplementation in patients stimulated with GnRH antagonist/rFSH for IVF: a randomized controlled trial," *Human Reproduction*, vol. 21, no. 10, pp. 2628–2632, 2006.

[54] S. L. Young, "Oestrogen and progesterone action on endometrium: a translational approach to understanding endometrial receptivity," *Reproductive BioMedicine Online*, vol. 27, no. 5, pp. 497–505, 2013.

[55] M. van der Linden, K. Buckingham, C. Farquhar, J. A. Kremer, and M. Metwally, "Luteal phase support for assisted reproduction cycles," *Cochrane Database of Systematic Reviews*, no. 10, Article ID CD009154, 2011.

[56] M. D. Damewood, W. Shen, H. A. Zacur, W. D. Schlaff, J. A. Rock, and E. E. Wallach, "Disappearance of exogenously administered human chorionic gonadotropin," *Fertility and Sterility*, vol. 52, no. 3, pp. 398–400, 1989.

[57] E. M. Kolibianakis, E. G. Papanikolaou, H. Tournaye, M. Camus, A. C. van Steirteghem, and P. Devroey, "Triggering final oocyte maturation using different doses of human chorionic gonadotropin: a randomized pilot study in patients with polycystic ovary syndrome treated with gonadotropin-releasing hormone antagonists and recombinant follicle-stimulating hormone," *Fertility and Sterility*, vol. 88, no. 5, pp. 1382–1388, 2007.

[58] S. Kashyap, K. Parker, M. I. Cedars, and Z. Rosenwaks, "Ovarian hyperstimulation syndrome prevention strategies: reducing the human chorionic gonadotropin trigger dose," *Seminars in Reproductive Medicine*, vol. 28, no. 6, pp. 475–485, 2010.

[59] J.-C. Emperaire and A. Ruffie, "Triggering ovulation with endogenous luteinizing hormone may prevent the ovarian hyperstimulation syndrome," *Human Reproduction*, vol. 6, no. 4, pp. 506–510, 1991.

[60] J. Itskovitz, R. Boldes, J. Levron, Y. Erlik, L. Kahana, and J. M. Brandes, "Induction of preovulatory luteinizing hormone surge and prevention of ovarian hyperstimulation syndrome by gonadotropin-releasing hormone agonist," *Fertility and Sterility*, vol. 56, no. 2, pp. 213–220, 1991.

[61] S. Kol and P. Humaidan, "GnRH agonist triggering: recent developments," *Reproductive BioMedicine Online*, vol. 26, no. 3, pp. 226–230, 2013.

[62] H. M. Fatemi, B. Popovic-Todorovic, P. Humaidan et al., "Severe ovarian hyperstimulation syndrome after gonadotropin-releasing hormone (GnRH) agonist trigger and 'freeze-all' approach in GnRH antagonist protocol," *Fertility and Sterility*, vol. 101, no. 4, pp. 1008–1011, 2014.

[63] D. Griffin, C. Benadiva, N. Kummer, T. Budinetz, J. Nulsen, and L. Engmann, "Dual trigger of oocyte maturation with gonadotropin-releasing hormone agonist and low-dose human chorionic gonadotropin to optimize live birth rates in high responders," *Fertility and Sterility*, vol. 97, no. 6, pp. 1316–1320, 2012.

[64] S. van der Meer, J. Gerris, M. Joostens, and B. Tas, "Triggering of ovulation using a gonadotrophin-releasing hormone agonist does not prevent ovarian hyperstimulation syndrome," *Human Reproduction*, vol. 8, no. 10, pp. 1628–1631, 1993.

[65] European Recombinant LH Study Group, "Human recombinant luteinizing hormone is as effective as, but safer than, urinary human chorionic gonadotropin in inducing final follicular maturation and ovulation in *in vitro* fertilization procedures: results of a multicenter double-blind study," *The Journal of Clinical Endocrinology & Metabolism*, vol. 86, no. 6, pp. 2607–2618, 2001.

[66] M. A. Youssef, H. G. Al-Inany, M. Aboulghar, R. Mansour, and A. M. Abou-Setta, "Recombinant versus urinary human chorionic gonadotrophin for final oocyte maturation triggering in IVF and ICSI cycles," *Cochrane Database of Systematic Reviews*, no. 4, Article ID CD003719, 2011.

[67] A. Delvigne and S. Rozenberg, "A qualitative systematic review of coasting, a procedure to avoid ovarian hyperstimulation syndrome in IVF patients," *Human Reproduction Update*, vol. 8, no. 3, pp. 291–296, 2002.

[68] A. Delvigne' and S. Rozenberg, "Preventive attitude of physicians to avoid OHSS in IVF patients," *Human Reproduction*, vol. 16, no. 12, pp. 2491–2495, 2001.

[69] A. D'Angelo, J. Brown, and N. N. Amso, "Coasting (withholding gonadotrophins) for preventing ovarian hyperstimulation syndrome," *Cochrane Database of Systematic Reviews*, vol. 2, no. 6, Article ID Cd002811, 2011.

[70] R. Mansour, M. Aboulghar, G. Serour, Y. Amin, and A. M. Abou-Setta, "Criteria of a successful coasting protocol for the prevention of severe ovarian hyperstimulation syndrome," *Human Reproduction*, vol. 20, no. 11, pp. 3167–3172, 2005.

[71] A. D'Angelo, "Ovarian hyperstimulation syndrome prevention strategies: cryopreservation of all embryos," *Seminars in Reproductive Medicine*, vol. 28, no. 6, pp. 513–518, 2010.

[72] A. D'Angelo and N. Amso, "Embryo freezing for preventing ovarian hyperstimulation syndrome," *Cochrane Database of Systematic Reviews*, no. 3, Article ID Cd002806, 2007.

[73] P. Devroey and P. Adriaensen, "OHSS free clinic," *Facts, Views & Vision in ObGyn*, vol. 3, no. 1, pp. 43–45, 2011.

[74] L. Herrero, M. Martínez, and J. A. Garcia-Velasco, "Current status of human oocyte and embryo cryopreservation," *Current Opinion in Obstetrics and Gynecology*, vol. 23, no. 4, pp. 245–250, 2011.

[75] M. Dolmans, M. Marotta, C. Pirard, J. Donnez, and O. Donnez, "Ovarian tissue cryopreservation followed by controlled ovarian stimulation and pick-up of mature oocytes does not impair the number or quality of retrieved oocytes," *Journal of Ovarian Research*, vol. 7, no. 80, 2014.

[76] M. Roque, "Freeze-all policy: is it time for that?" *Journal of Assisted Reproduction and Genetics*, vol. 32, no. 2, pp. 171–176, 2015.

[77] M. Roque, K. Lattes, S. Serra et al., "Fresh embryo transfer versus frozen embryo transfer in in vitro fertilization cycles: a systematic review and meta-analysis," *Fertility and Sterility*, vol. 99, no. 1, pp. 156–162, 2013.

[78] R. Mathur and W. Sumaya, "Prevention and management of ovarian hyperstimulation syndrome," *Obstetrics, Gynaecology and Reproductive Medicine*, vol. 18, no. 1, pp. 18–22, 2008.

[79] J. G. Schenker and D. Weinstein, "Ovarian hyperstimulation syndrome: a current survey," *Fertility and Sterility*, vol. 30, no. 3, pp. 255–268, 1978.

[80] M. A. Youssef, H. G. Al-Inany, J. L. Evers, and M. Aboulghar, "Intra-venous fluids for the prevention of severe ovarian hyperstimulation syndrome," *Cochrane Database of Systematic Reviews*, no. 2, Article ID CD001302, 2011.

[81] B. C. Jee, C. S. Suh, Y. B. Kim et al., "Administration of intravenous albumin around the time of oocyte retrieval reduces pregnancy rate without preventing ovarian hyperstimulation syndrome: a systematic review and meta-analysis," *Gynecologic and Obstetric Investigation*, vol. 70, no. 1, pp. 47–54, 2010.

[82] C. A. Venetis, E. M. Kolibianakis, K. A. Toulis, D. G. Goulis, I. Papadimas, and B. C. Tarlatzis, "Intravenous albumin administration for the prevention of severe ovarian hyperstimulation syndrome: a systematic review and metaanalysis," *Fertility and Sterility*, vol. 95, no. 1, pp. 188.e3–196.e3, 2011.

[83] J. A. Garcia-Velasco, "How to avoid ovarian hyperstimulation syndrome: a new indication for dopamine agonists," *Reproductive BioMedicine Online*, vol. 18, no. 2, pp. S71–S75, 2009.

[84] H. Tang, T. Hunter, Y. Hu, S. D. Zhai, X. Sheng, and R. J. Hart, "Cabergoline for preventing ovarian hyperstimulation syndrome," *Cochrane Database of Systematic Reviews*, no. 2, Article ID CD008605, 2012.

[85] V. M. S. Leitao, R. M. Moroni, L. M. D. Seko, C. O. Nastri, and W. P. Martins, "Cabergoline for the prevention of ovarian hyperstimulation syndrome: systematic review and meta-analysis of randomized controlled trials," *Fertility and Sterility*, vol. 101, no. 3, pp. 664–675.e7, 2014.

[86] M. Kasum, H. Vrčić, P. Stanić et al., "Dopamine agonists in prevention of ovarian hyperstimulation syndrome," *Gynecological Endocrinology*, vol. 30, no. 12, pp. 845–849, 2014.

[87] C. Cenksoy, P. O. Cenksoy, O. Erdem, B. Sancak, and R. Gursoy, "A potential novel strategy, inhibition of vasopressin-induced VEGF secretion by relcovaptan, for decreasing the incidence of ovarian hyperstimulation syndrome in the hyperstimulated rat model," *European Journal of Obstetrics Gynecology and Reproductive Biology*, vol. 174, no. 1, pp. 86–90, 2014.

19

Maternal and Pediatric Health Outcomes in relation to Gestational Vitamin D Sufficiency

Stephen J. Genuis

Faculty of Medicine, University of Calgary and University of Alberta, 2935-66 Street, Edmonton, AB, Canada T6K 4C1

Correspondence should be addressed to Stephen J. Genuis; sgenuis@ualberta.ca

Academic Editor: W. T. Creasman

Juxtaposed with monumental improvement in maternal-fetal outcomes over the last century, there has been the recent emergence of rising rates of gestational complications including preterm birth, operative delivery, and gestational diabetes. At the same time, there has been a burgeoning problem with widespread vitamin D deficiency among populations of many developed nations. This paper provides a brief review of potential health outcomes recently linked to gestational vitamin D deficiency, including preterm birth, cesarean delivery, and gestational diabetes. Although immediate costs for obstetric complications related to gestational vitamin D insufficiency may be modest, the short- and long-term costs for pediatric healthcare resulting from such gestational complications may be enormous and present an enduring burden on healthcare systems. With increasing evidence pointing to fetal origins of some later life disease, securing vitamin D sufficiency in pregnancy appears to be a simple, safe, and cost-effective measure that can be incorporated into routine preconception and prenatal care in the offices of primary care clinicians. Education on gestational nutritional requirements should be a fundamental part of medical education and residency training, instruction that has been sorely lacking to date.

1. Introduction and Background

In the early and mid-1800s, the maternal mortality rate in some European obstetrical clinics approached 1 in 5 women as a result of puerperal fever [1]. With the epic discovery of the origins of this "childbed fever" by Ignaz Philipp Semmelweis in the mid-19th century and the eventual knowledge translation of his simple hand washing technique into the clinical domain, rates of postpartum mortality eventually decreased [1]. Over the subsequent century, there continued to be monumental advances in many areas of Maternal-Fetal Medicine. Along with a profound decline in maternal mortality from 7.2 deaths per 1000 births in the early 1900s to 0.08 by the end of 2000 [2, 3], there was a concomitant decline in infant mortality from 96 to less than 7 deaths per 1000 live births [2, 3]. With ongoing research and study over the last decades, remarkable advances have continued to be made in the assessment and management of a variety of gestational and perinatal challenges. Despite much success, however, there are new and emerging concerns in the early 21st century within the field of Maternal-Fetal Medicine.

Along with an astonishing rise in the rate of cesarean delivery with attendant complications to the human microbiome [4, 5], we have witnessed a concerning escalation in preterm birth [6], a complication associated with higher rates of long-term physical and mental health problems in the offspring [6–8]. The Institute of Medicine (IOM) estimated the annual costs for the burden of morbidity, disability, and mortality associated with preterm birth in the United States to be at least $26.2 billion [9]. Furthermore, the costs associated with neonatal intensive care, healthcare now required by an increasing percentage of the newborn population [10], are staggering [11]. It is also evident that maternal complications do not necessarily stop with giving birth. Rates of serious obstetrical complications such as postpartum depression, for example, extract enormous personal cost and remain a serious and widespread problem [12].

In addition, there is increasing discussion in the literature about fetal origins of pediatric and adult disease [13, 14], resulting from potentially modifiable gestational determinants such as disordered maternal nutrition [15] and toxic exposures [16–18]. As this is a new area of study, however, the extent of sequelae associated with modifiable gestational determinants is yet unrecognized; it is thus not possible to assign precise costs associated with long-term outcomes. It is important, however, to explore and implement clinical approaches during the preconception and gestational period which address determinants of suboptimal outcomes in order to maximize the enduring health of mothers and their offspring.

2. Modifiable Gestational Determinants and Illness

With recent attention to epigenetic research, it is becoming apparent that virtually all disease, including affliction in the gestational period, is the result of the interaction between our genes and the environment [19]. In fact, rather than genetic predestination [20], recent evidence confirms that modifiable environmental factors appear to be responsible for 70–90 percent of clinical illness [21]. Yet within the environmental domain, there appear to be only two determinants which make up the environment sphere. (i) Are we getting what we need? (ii) Are we being exposed to things that are toxic? [19]. Accordingly, it appears that the bulk of human disease, including problems in pregnancy, is related to deficiency and toxicity [19].

Evidence in the obstetric literature appears to support this contention and provides opportunity to make advances with regard to maternal and fetal well-being. In fact, medical intervention and maternal education delivered prior to conception (preconception care) to secure nutritional adequacy and preclude toxic exposures are being extolled as the next frontier of maternal and child healthcare [31]. The March of Dimes, a nonprofit organization dedicated to the health of mothers and babies, suggests that "the [physician] must take advantage of every health encounter to provide preconception care and risk reduction before and between conceptions—the time when it really can make a difference" [32]. With the evident link between fetal determinants and later onset disease, measures to secure an optimal gestational environment can have a profound impact on maternal and pediatric health with enormous personal, social, and financial savings.

There is considerable attention in the literature to the direct link between assorted toxicants in pregnancy and adverse maternal and fetal outcomes [16]. Most recently, FIGO (The International Federation of Obstetrics and Gynecology) released a special communication highlighting the urgent need to address the issue of widespread toxicant exposure and bioaccumulation in reproductive aged women [18]. In addition, it is becoming increasingly apparent that various nutritional deficiencies are widespread and may have an enormous impact on subsequent maternal and fetal health. Increasing evidence appears to confirm that at no point throughout the life cycle is it more important to secure adequate nutrient intake than in pregnancy [26]. This fact, for example, accounts for the emphasis on folate sufficiency in early gestation [33] as well as the increased study into the outcomes related to gestational deficiency of required omega-3 fatty acids [34] and magnesium [35].

With the emerging evidence that vitamin D acts epigenetically in the regulation of over 2700 different genes [36], there has been much recent research exploring the widespread prevalence of vitamin D deficiency through the continuum of life, including the gestational and neonatal period. This paper is designed to review the literature findings about the enduring impact of gestational vitamin D sufficiency on maternal and pediatric health and well-being.

3. Methods

This brief review was prepared by assessing available medical and scientific literature from Medline as well as by reviewing several books, nutritional journals, conference proceedings, government publications, and nutrition related periodicals. Terms searched included gestational vitamin D, pregnancy and vitamin D, fetus and vitamin D, nutrition in pregnancy, as well as pediatric health and vitamin D. Relevant references found in these publications were also searched in order to glean pertinent information. A primary observation, however, was that limited scientific literature is available on the issue of gestational vitamin D insufficiency as it relates to long-term health outcomes.

The format of a traditional integrated narrative review was chosen as such reviews play a pivotal role in scientific research and professional practice in medical issues spanning different medical disciplines, in this case obstetrics, pediatrics, and general medicine. Furthermore, this type of publication approach seemed apposite when endeavoring to answer specific clinical questions in a field with limited primary study [37]. Finally, it was deemed that a traditional integrated review paper might be optimal when exploring a myriad range of health outcomes, both short and long term.

4. Clinical Relevance of Vitamin D Sufficiency in Reproductive Healthcare

The widespread clinical importance of determining the correlation between vitamin D levels and reproductive outcomes is evident. The medical literature has achieved general consensus that vitamin D levels throughout much of the globe, as reflected by population measurements of $25(OH)D_3$ levels, are generally inadequate [38]. About 2/3 of the population in northern climates are considered deficient with average $25(OH)D_3$ levels in one study of 67 nmol/L [39], well below the 120–150 nmol/L level that has recently been associated with preferred health [24] (Table 1). With such widespread deficiency, it is vital to determine whether or not low gestational levels of vitamin D are a significant determinant of reproductive and pediatric health outcomes.

The need for clarity on this issue has also been recognized because of disparity about recommended dosing among esteemed medical groups. While the Institute of Medicine (IOM) agrees that 4,000 IU of vitamin daily is allowable and nontoxic, their actual recommended daily intake has been limited to 600 IU daily in general and 400 IU/day during gestation [40, 41]. These IOM recommendations for required vitamin D intake have been put into serious question [42], however, as a significant statistical error has been identified

TABLE 1: Optimal adult levels of vitamin D (as reflected by 25(OH)D levels) from different sources.

Source	Vitamin D level (nmol/L)	Vitamin D level (ng/mL)
Holick (2010) [22]	100–150	40–60
Endocrine Society (2011) [23]	At least >75, aim for 100	At least >30, aim for 40
Amrein et al. (2014) [24]	120–150	48–60
Schwalfenberg and Genuis (2015) [25]	120–150	48–60

No consensus on a specific optimal 25(OH)D level in pregnancy has been achieved.

Emerging agreement that supplemental vitamin D_3 at a dosage of 4000 IU/day throughout pregnancy may be safe and effective [26–30].

in the way their recommendations were arrived at [43]. Accordingly, exploration of consensus findings on the clinical benefits of vitamin D supplementation is in order in all medical disciplines including reproductive healthcare.

5. Limitations of Vitamin D Research as Related to Gestational Outcomes

Although maternal-fetal outcomes in the presence of adequate gestational vitamin D are generally favorable as reported in the medical literature, some reports have been inconsistent and cast doubt on the link between gestational vitamin D sufficiency and health. Specifically, supplementation of vitamin D in pregnancy in some studies appears to suggest marked benefit while research in other publications does not appear to confer significant improvement in maternal-fetal outcomes [44]. For example, a systematic review and meta-analysis by Pérez-López et al. found that gestational vitamin D supplementation was associated with increased birth weight and birth length but, unlike some other research, was not associated with other beneficial maternal and neonatal outcomes such as reductions in preeclampsia, gestational diabetes, small for gestational age infants, preterm birth, or rates of cesarean delivery [44]. The apparent disparity between findings in various studies has caused some to reflexively conclude that vitamin D status in pregnancy is irrelevant to maternal-fetal outcomes.

Studies on reproductive outcomes related to vitamin D supplementation, however, are inherently plagued by a number of common confounders which cloud the picture. It is important to realize that vitamin D status is very different from whether or not someone is consuming vitamin D supplementation. Many factors may affect the resultant status of vitamin D in the body (as reflected by measurement of 25(OH)D levels) after ingested supplementation. Dosing of supplements, body weight, levels of various toxicants, and individual metabolism can all be factors in consequent vitamin D indices after supplementation. Many of the recent publications challenging the efficacy of gestational vitamin D sufficiency have been meta-analyses which attempt to synthesize diverse data from numerous observational and

supplementation studies which do not necessarily incorporate individual differences in these central determinants.

Specific concerns about several vitamin D meta-analyses can account for the varying outcomes reported from this type of research. (i) There is wide heterogeneity of studied populations with variations in vitamin D supplement dosing, geophysical location, social and dietary conditions, and other factors in studied groups [45]. Supplementation at varying doses (e.g., 400 IU/day versus 4000 IU/day), for example, may achieve remarkably different levels of serum 25(OH)D and thus different outcomes. (ii) Commencement of supplementation at differing times during the gestation may miss critical periods when vitamin D may play a pivotal role. (iii) Different types of vitamin D (vitamin D_2 versus vitamin D_3) have different physiological impact. And (iv) various methodological concerns are evident [46], such as the lack of standardized assays.

In addition, it is well recognized in healthcare that regardless of how compelling the evidence on a specific scientific or medical issue, introduction of doubt can be a potent impediment to the implementation of effective public health and clinical measures [47, 48]. Accordingly, a critical appraisal of such meta-analyses is in order to achieve an accurate perspective on the efficacy of gestational vitamin D supplementation.

6. Gestational Vitamin D Status and Obstetrical Outcomes

The list of adverse gestational outcomes in pregnancy associated with vitamin D insufficiency continues to mount. Early in pregnancy, for example, an increased risk of first trimester miscarriage has been linked to inadequate maternal vitamin D levels [49]. Interestingly, one study demonstrated that nearly half the women assessed with habitual miscarriage were found to have 25(OH)D levels below 75 nmol/L [50]. This research found that lower vitamin D levels were associated with immune dysregulation in a number of ways, including differences in indices involving natural killer cells, various cytokines, and certain regulatory proteins, when compared to those with sufficient vitamin D levels [50]. The authors of this study also noted that women with lower vitamin D levels had higher degrees of various autoantibodies including antiphospholipid antibody [50], a clinical state that has been associated with fetal death, recurrent early miscarriage, preeclampsia, and placental insufficiency [51].

A number of papers have confirmed an increased risk of developing gestational diabetes in those with inadequate vitamin D levels [52, 53]. Vitamin D sufficiency in pregnancy appears to be related to improved insulin levels, as well as better glucose regulation as reflected by HbA1c levels [54]. As pregnancies complicated by gestational diabetes present risks for assorted adverse sequelae, efforts to avoid dysregulated sugar control in pregnancy are worthwhile. Obesity presents a confounding influence in this discussion, however, as a greater BMI is associated with lower vitamin D levels as well as greater insulin resistance and risk for gestational diabetes. Numerous studies have also correlated low levels of vitamin D with the development of preeclampsia [52, 53, 55, 56], perhaps through immune mechanisms involving antiphospholipid antibody [51], and/or inflammatory mechanisms involving cytokines [56].

Of particular significance is the reality that preterm birth before 37 weeks of gestation remains the leading cause of neonatal morbidity and mortality [57]. Escalating evidence in the literature confirms a protective association between maternal vitamin D sufficiency and the incidence of preterm birth [58–60]. A recent study found that the rate of occurrence of preterm birth appeared to be inversely parallel to the maternal serum 25-hydroxyvitamin D levels [58]. The authors report that the incidence of preterm birth at less than 37 weeks of gestation was (i) 11.3%, (ii) 8.6%, and (iii) 7.3% among mothers with respective serum 25-hydroxyvitamin D levels of (i) less than 50, (ii) between 50 and 74.9, and (iii) 75 nmol/L or greater. Another study found that infants born before 32 weeks of gestation were 2.4 times more likely to have vitamin D levels below 50 nmol/L when compared with those born after 32 weeks of gestation [61].

Other gestational issues also appear to be influenced by maternal vitamin D levels. Vitamin D insufficiency, for example, has also been correlated with maternal periodontal disease [62], a higher likelihood of small for gestational age infants [63, 64], and an increased risk of bacterial vaginosis [65].

As well as individual studies, systematic reviews exploring association between vitamin D sufficiency and health outcomes have also been illuminating. A systematic review and meta-analysis of 24 studies suggested that low maternal vitamin D levels in pregnancy may be associated with an increased risk of small for gestational age infants, as well as being linked to preeclampsia, gestational diabetes, and preterm birth [66]. Another systematic review and meta-analysis published in the *British Medical Journal* also linked vitamin D insufficiency with an increased risk of gestational diabetes, preeclampsia, and small for gestational age infants [65].

Vitamin D status also appears to influence modes of delivery. Vitamin D deficiency has been linked to increased odds of primary cesarean delivery [67] as well as a higher likelihood of emergency cesarean section [68]. In one study, women with vitamin D levels below 37.5 nmol/L were almost four times as likely to require a primary cesarean delivery as women with higher levels [67]. Through the evolving work on the Human Microbiome Project, it has recently been found that the infant's journey through the birth canal is instrumental in shaping a healthy microbiome, a feature which appears to be a determinant of subsequent health and which may be compromised by cesarean delivery [69]. Accordingly, efforts to diminish the high rates of Cesarean delivery are warranted.

Gestational vitamin D status also appears to influence outcomes beyond the pregnancy and delivery. A very challenging problem for many new mothers is postpartum depression. There is escalating evidence in general that low vitamin D levels are correlated with higher risk for a variety of mental health problems including depressive illness [70], as vitamin D is known to play an important role in activating genes that release neurotransmitters such as dopamine

and serotonin [70, 71]. Intervention to normalize levels of vitamin D appears to be successful in restoring mental health [72]. In particular, in relation to maternal health, a recent study published in the *British Journal of Obstetrics and Gynecology* reported that serum 25[OH]D levels in women with no postpartum depression were significantly higher than those in women suffering with postpartum depression [73].

7. Gestational Vitamin D Status and Later Life Outcomes

Although research into fetal origins of disease in later life remains in its infancy, there is increasing suspicion that gestational nutritional sufficiency may be a determinant of health in later life. For example, preliminary evidence suggests that insufficient levels of prenatal vitamin D may be a factor in the development of autism [74] and lower respiratory infections [75]. A Spanish study to this end found that mothers who had gestational vitamin D levels above 75 nmol/L had offspring with a one-third lower rate of acute respiratory tract infections during the first year of life [76].

A recent body of work has begun to suggest that lower gestational vitamin D levels may also be associated with higher rates of pediatric atopic disease [77], food sensitivities [78], atopic dermatitis [79], eczema [80], asthma [81], impaired lung function [82], allergic disease [83], and other conditions frequently characterized by a hypersensitive immune state. It appears that fetal vitamin D levels may play a modulating role in immune functions involved in atopic disorders. As hypersensitivity outcomes may also be seen in those children born to mothers contaminated with assorted xenobiotics in pregnancy [84–89], however, it is not known whether the immune dysregulation and hypersensitivity may be the consequence of a primary gestational insufficiency of vitamin D, or whether various chemical toxicants might play a role by impairing vitamin D uptake, renal synthesis, and assimilation [25, 90] while at the same time inducing immune compromise and hypersensitivity through other mechanisms [91].

Maternal vitamin D status during gestation also appears to have influence on many other health indices in the future of the offspring. For example, gestational vitamin D status directly correlates with subsequent whole-body and lumbar spine bone mineral content in progeny at 9 years of age [92]. Furthermore, an interesting cohort study correlating maternal vitamin D deficiency at 18 weeks of pregnancy and health outcomes of progeny found that gestational vitamin D deficiency was associated with impaired lung development in 6-year-old offspring, neurocognitive difficulties at age 10, increased risk of eating disorders in adolescence, and lower peak bone mass at 20 years [93]. The authors state that "vitamin D may have an important, multifaceted role in the development of fetal lungs, brain, and bone" [93]. Finally, gestational vitamin D levels may impact adult health as there is early evidence that vitamin D sufficiency in pregnancy may have a protective role in the development of adult onset multiple sclerosis [94].

8. Economic Burden of Gestational Vitamin D Deficiency

The economic impact of vitamin D deficiency as it relates to maternal-fetal health is difficult to objectively quantify as insufficient evidence has accumulated thus far on the totality of short- and long-term sequelae of vitamin D insufficiency. Furthermore, current appraisals tend to underestimate the extent of the required resource utilization for specific conditions associated with vitamin D insufficiency. For example, cost estimates for the immediate care involved with the increase in cesarean delivery rates can be calculated, but these do not at all take into account unexpected surgical complications [95] that may arise in the future or the enormous potential cost impact from enduring microbiome changes resulting from operative delivery [69, 96]. The reality is that adverse gestational complications do not end with the pregnancy and can result in morbidity and resource utilization extending throughout the life of the offspring.

This is also demonstrated by the challenge of preterm birth, as premature birth results in significant morbidity, mortality, healthcare utilization, and associated costs starting in infancy and extending for years to come [97]. This can be quite a burden on national healthcare systems. In Canada, for example, the estimated additional 10-year cost to care for the children born prematurely each year is hundreds of millions of dollars [98]. Furthermore, many health problems sustained by children born prematurely continue far beyond their tenth birthday with a consequent and sometimes ongoing economic burden placed on health, education, and social service resources. With regard to economic challenges associated with vitamin D insufficiency, suffice it to say that there are considerable costs potentially associated with gestational vitamin D insufficiency [99] as well as corresponding benefits and cost savings resulting from inexpensive supplementation with this essential nutrient [99].

9. Conclusion

There is escalating attention in the scientific literature to the association between myriad nutrients and health outcomes [100, 101]. Training in clinical nutritional biochemistry, nonetheless, still remains woefully inadequate or nonexistent in most medical education programs [102, 103]. As a result, there are ongoing calls of late for curriculum revision to incorporate practical training in clinical nutrition [103, 104]. It is apparent that training is required to establish clinical competency in (i) understanding of the role of various nutrients in human health, (ii) how to assess nutritional biochemistry in patients, and (iii) and how to intervene to secure nutrient sufficiency for individuals and population groups

With the mounting evidence of several health sequelae associated with gestational vitamin D deficiency, the value of preconception education and care by health providers and public health bodies to secure vitamin D sufficiency throughout gestation is evident. As pregnant women [105], particularly those with dark skin [106], are at considerable risk for experiencing vitamin D insufficiency [39], it is important to have a high index of suspicion and to effectively preclude, assess for, and manage vitamin D inadequacy, as would be done with other biochemical irregularities.

Although (to the author's knowledge) there are no specific target levels for 25(OH)D during the various stages of pregnancy that correlate with optimal results in relation to maternal and pediatric health outcomes, some authors have made recommendations for supplemental levels that appear to be safe and effective. These recommendations range from 600 IU/day from the Institute of Medicine [41] to 2000 IU/day from the Canadian Pediatric Society [107], to 4000 IU/daily from various researchers who have concluded that the latter dose is both efficacious and safe [26–30]. One researcher has suggested that the dietary requirement during pregnancy and lactation may actually be as high as 6000 IU/day [108], but most researchers have concluded, with our current knowledge, that a supplemental vitamin D intake of 4000 IU/day is optimal [30]. As discussed, individual vitamin D indices can be influenced by various determinants despite specific levels of supplementation; it is thus the author's recommendation that a personalized medical approach be taken via individual screening for 25(OH)D as a routine part of preconception and prenatal care.

With evidence that a major proportion of the adult population [38], particularly in northern climates [39], is potentially deficient in vitamin D, it appears that, at minimum, one out of every few expectant mothers will have inadequate levels of this essential nutrient. With the recognition that vitamin D plays an essential role in myriad genes that encode for health and well-being in the offspring, it behooves the medical and public health community to endeavor to secure vitamin D adequacy in the gestational period. The ongoing personal health burden associated with gestational vitamin D insufficiency throughout many parts of the world has the potential to be ameliorated considerably by straightforward educational and healthcare measures in the preconception and prenatal period to secure vitamin D sufficiency throughout pregnancy. It is time for maternity health providers to be apprised of the potential for improved and enduring health and well-being associated with inexpensive measures to secure vitamin D nutritional adequacy during gestation, the most vulnerable time in the life cycle of the developing child.

Conflict of Interests

There is no conflict of interests.

References

[1] H. F. Spirer and L. Spirer, "Death and numbers: Semmelweis the statistician," *Physicians for Social Responsibility Quarterly*, vol. 1, pp. 43–52, 1991.

[2] United States Department of Health Education and Welfare, *Infant, Fetal, and Maternal Mortality: United States—1963*, United States Department of Health, Washington, DC, USA, 1966, http://www.cdc.gov/nchs/data/series/sr_20/sr20_003acc.pdf.

[3] United States Department of Health and Human Services, Health—United States 2004, Hyattsville, Md, USA, http://www.cdc.gov/nchs/data/hus/hus04.pdf.

[4] G. Biasucci, M. Rubini, S. Riboni, L. Morelli, E. Bessi, and C. Retetangos, "Mode of delivery affects the bacterial community in the newborn gut," *Early Human Development*, vol. 86, supplement 1, pp. S13–S15, 2010.

[5] S. Dogra, O. Sakwinska, S. Soh et al., "Dynamics of infant gut microbiota are influenced by delivery mode and gestational duration and are associated with subsequent adiposity," *mBio*, vol. 6, no. 1, Article ID e02419-14, 2015.

[6] E. R. B. McCabe, G. E. Carrino, R. B. Russell, and J. L. Howse, "Fighting for the next generation: US prematurity in 2030," *Pediatrics*, vol. 134, no. 6, pp. 1193–1199, 2014.

[7] R. W. Loftin, M. Habli, C. C. Snyder, C. M. Cormier, D. F. Lewis, and E. A. Defranco, "Late preterm birth," *Reviews in Obstetrics & Gynecology*, vol. 3, no. 1, pp. 10–19, 2010.

[8] M. C. McCormick, "The contribution of low birth weight to infant mortality and childhood morbidity," *The New England Journal of Medicine*, vol. 312, no. 2, pp. 82–90, 1985.

[9] R. E. Behrman, A. S. Butler, and Institute of Medicine (US) Committee on Understanding Premature Birth and Assuring Healthy Outcomes, *Preterm Birth: Causes, Consequences, and Prevention*, National Academies Press, Washington, DC, USA, 2007.

[10] W. Harrison and D. Goodman, "Epidemiologic trends in neonatal intensive care, 2007–2012," *JAMA Pediatrics*, vol. 169, no. 9, pp. 855–862, 2015.

[11] A. Ramachandrappa and L. Jain, "Health issues of the late preterm infant," *Pediatric Clinics of North America*, vol. 56, no. 3, pp. 565–577, 2009.

[12] T. Cristescu, S. Behrman, S. V. Jones, L. Chouliaras, and K. P. Ebmeier, "Be vigilant for perinatal mental health problems," *Practitioner*, vol. 259, no. 1780, pp. 19–23, 2015.

[13] S. Visentin, F. Grumolato, G. B. Nardelli, B. Di Camillo, E. Grisan, and E. Cosmi, "Early origins of adult disease: low birth weight and vascular remodeling," *Atherosclerosis*, vol. 237, no. 2, pp. 391–399, 2014.

[14] R. H. Lane, "Fetal programming, epigenetics, and adult onset disease," *Clinics in Perinatology*, vol. 41, no. 4, pp. 815–831, 2014.

[15] M. Weber, J. M. Ayoubi, and O. Picone, "Nutrition of pregnant women: consequences for fetal growth and adult diseases," *Archives de Pédiatrie*, vol. 22, no. 1, pp. 116–118, 2015.

[16] S. J. Genuis, "The chemical erosion of human health: adverse environmental exposure and in-utero pollution—determinants of congenital disorders and chronic disease," *Journal of Perinatal Medicine*, vol. 34, no. 3, pp. 185–195, 2006.

[17] D. A. Rossignol, S. J. Genuis, and R. E. Frye, "Environmental toxicants and autism spectrum disorders: a systematic review," *Translational Psychiatry*, vol. 4, no. 2, article e360, 2014.

[18] G. C. Di Renzo, J. A. Conry, J. Blake et al., "International federation of gynecology and obstetrics opinion on reproductive health impacts of exposure to toxic environmental chemicals," *International Journal of Gynecology & Obstetrics*, vol. 131, no. 3, pp. 219–225, 2015.

[19] S. J. Genuis, "What's out there making us sick?" *Journal of Environmental and Public Health*, vol. 2012, Article ID 605137, 10 pages, 2012.

[20] S. J. Genuis, "Our genes are not our destiny: incorporating molecular medicine into clinical practice," *Journal of Evaluation in Clinical Practice*, vol. 14, no. 1, pp. 94–102, 2008.

[21] S. M. Rappaport and M. T. Smith, "Epidemiology. Environment and disease risks," *Science*, vol. 330, no. 6003, pp. 460–461, 2010.

[22] M. F. Holick, "Vitamin D and health: evaluation, biologic functions, and recommended dietary intake for vitamin D," in *Vitamin D: Physiology, Molecular Biology, and Clinical Applications*, pp. 3–35, Springer, New York, NY, USA, 2010.

[23] M. F. Holick, N. C. Binkley, H. A. Bischoff-Ferrari et al., "Evaluation, treatment, and prevention of vitamin D deficiency: an Endocrine Society clinical practice guideline," *The Journal of Clinical Endocrinology & Metabolism*, vol. 96, no. 7, pp. 1911–1930, 1911.

[24] K. Amrein, S. A. Quraishi, A. A. Litonjua et al., "Evidence for a U-shaped relationship between prehospital vitamin D status and mortality: a cohort study," *The Journal of Clinical Endocrinology & Metabolism*, vol. 99, no. 4, pp. 1461–1469, 2014.

[25] G. K. Schwalfenberg and S. J. Genuis, "Vitamin D, essential minerals, and toxic elements: exploring interactions between nutrients and toxicants in clinical medicine," *The Scientific World Journal*, vol. 2015, Article ID 318595, 8 pages, 2015.

[26] B. W. Hollis, D. Johnson, T. C. Hulsey, M. Ebeling, and C. L. Wagner, "Vitamin D supplementation during pregnancy: double-blind, randomized clinical trial of safety and effectiveness," *Journal of Bone and Mineral Research*, vol. 26, no. 10, pp. 2341–2357, 2011.

[27] A. Dawodu, H. F. Saadi, G. Bekdache, Y. Javed, M. Altaye, and B. W. Hollis, "Randomized controlled trial (RCT) of vitamin D supplementation in pregnancy in a population with endemic vitamin D deficiency," *Journal of Clinical Endocrinology and Metabolism*, vol. 98, no. 6, pp. 2337–2346, 2013.

[28] C. L. Wagner, R. B. McNeil, D. D. Johnson et al., "Health characteristics and outcomes of two randomized vitamin D supplementation trials during pregnancy: a combined analysis," *The Journal of Steroid Biochemistry and Molecular Biology*, vol. 136, pp. 313–320, 2013.

[29] C. L. Wagner, R. McNeil, S. A. Hamilton et al., "A randomized trial of vitamin D supplementation in 2 community health center networks in South Carolina," *American Journal of Obstetrics and Gynecology*, vol. 208, no. 2, pp. 137.e1–137.e13, 2013.

[30] A. Mithal and S. Kalra, "Vitamin D supplementation in pregnancy," *Indian Journal of Endocrinology and Metabolism*, vol. 18, no. 5, pp. 593–596, 2014.

[31] H. K. Atrash, K. Johnson, M. Adams, J. F. Cordero, and J. Howse, "Preconception care for improving perinatal outcomes: the time to act," *Maternal and Child Health Journal*, vol. 10, supplement 1, pp. S3–S11, 2006.

[32] March of Dimes Birth Defects Foundation, "March of dimes updates: is early prenatal care too late?" *Contemporary OB/GYN*, vol. 12, pp. 54–72, 2002.

[33] G. Barkai, S. Arbuzova, M. Berkenstadt, S. Heifetz, and H. Cuckle, "Frequency of Down's syndrome and neural-tube defects in the same family," *The Lancet*, vol. 361, no. 9366, pp. 1331–1335, 2003.

[34] K. A. Mulder, D. J. King, S. M. Innis, and H. R. Baradaran, "Omega-3 fatty acid deficiency in infants before birth identified using a randomized trial of maternal DHA supplementation in pregnancy," *PLoS ONE*, vol. 9, no. 1, Article ID e83764, 2014.

[35] J. Takaya and K. Kaneko, "Small for gestational age and magnesium in cord blood platelets: intrauterine magnesium deficiency may induce metabolic syndrome in later life," *Journal of Pregnancy*, vol. 2011, Article ID 270474, 5 pages, 2011.

[36] S. V. Ramagopalan, A. Heger, A. J. Berlanga et al., "A ChIP-seq defined genome-wide map of vitamin D receptor binding: associations with disease and evolution," *Genome Research*, vol. 20, no. 10, pp. 1352–1360, 2010.

[37] M. P. Dijkers, "The value of traditional reviews in the era of systematic reviewing," *American Journal of Physical Medicine & Rehabilitation*, vol. 88, no. 5, pp. 423–430, 1963.

[38] M. F. Holick and T. C. Chen, "Vitamin D deficiency: a worldwide problem with health consequences," *The American Journal of Clinical Nutrition*, vol. 87, no. 4, pp. 1080S–1086S, 2008.

[39] S. J. Genuis, G. K. Schwalfenberg, M. N. Hiltz, and S. A. Vaselenak, "Vitamin D status of clinical practice populations at higher latitudes: analysis and applications," *International Journal of Environmental Research and Public Health*, vol. 6, no. 1, pp. 151–173, 2009.

[40] A. C. Ross, J. E. Manson, S. A. Abrams et al., "The 2011 report on dietary reference intakes for calcium and vitamin D from the Institute of Medicine: what clinicians need to know," *The Journal of Clinical Endocrinology & Metabolism*, vol. 96, no. 1, pp. 53–58, 2011.

[41] Institute of Medicine, *Dietary Reference Intakes for Calcium and Vitamin D*, National Academies Press, Washington, DC, USA, 2010.

[42] G. K. Schwalfenberg and S. J. Whiting, "A Canadian response to the 2010 Institute of Medicine vitamin D and calcium guidelines," *Public Health Nutrition*, vol. 14, no. 4, pp. 746–748, 2011.

[43] P. J. Veugelers and J. P. Ekwaru, "A statistical error in the estimation of the recommended dietary allowance for vitamin D," *Nutrients*, vol. 6, no. 10, pp. 4472–4475, 2014.

[44] F. R. Pérez-López, V. Pasupuleti, E. Mezones-Holguin et al., "Effect of vitamin D supplementation during pregnancy on maternal and neonatal outcomes: a systematic review and meta-analysis of randomized controlled trials," *Fertility and Sterility*, vol. 103, no. 5, pp. 1278.e4–1288.e4, 2015.

[45] S. N. Karras, P. Anagnostis, S. A. Paschou, E. Kandaraki, and D. G. Goulis, "Vitamin D status during pregnancy: time for a more unified approach beyond borders?" *European Journal of Clinical Nutrition*, vol. 69, no. 8, pp. 874–877, 2015.

[46] S. N. Karras, P. Anagnostis, A. Petroczi, C. Annweiler, D. P. Naughton, and D. P. Goulis, "Maternal vitamin D status in pregnancy: a critical appraisal of current analytical data on maternal and neonatal outcomes," *Hormones*, vol. 14, no. 2, pp. 224–231, 2015.

[47] D. Michaels, *Doubt Is Their Product: How Industry's Assault on Science Threatens Your Health*, Oxford University Press, New York, NY, USA, 2008.

[48] S. J. Genuis and C. T. Lipp, "Electromagnetic hypersensitivity: fact or fiction?" *The Science of the Total Environment*, vol. 414, pp. 103–112, 2012.

[49] L. B. Andersen, J. S. Jørgensen, T. K. Jensen et al., "Vitamin D insufficiency is associated with increased risk of first-trimester miscarriage in the Odense Child Cohort," *The American Journal of Clinical Nutrition*, vol. 102, no. 3, pp. 633–638, 2015.

[50] K. Ota, S. Dambaeva, A.-R. Han, K. Beaman, A. Gilman-Sachs, and J. Kwak-Kim, "Vitamin D deficiency may be a risk factor for recurrent pregnancy losses by increasing cellular immunity and autoimmunity," *Human Reproduction*, vol. 29, no. 2, pp. 208–219, 2014.

[51] R. A. Levy, F. C. Dos Santos, G. R. de Jesus, and N. R. de Jesus, "Antiphospholipid antibodies and antiphospholipid syndrome during pregnancy: diagnostic concepts," *Frontiers in Immunology*, vol. 6, article 205, 2015.

[52] D. K. Dror, "Vitamin D status during pregnancy: maternal, fetal, and postnatal outcomes," *Current Opinion in Obstetrics & Gynecology*, vol. 23, no. 6, pp. 422–426, 2011.

[53] P. M. Brannon, "Vitamin D and adverse pregnancy outcomes: beyond bone health and growth," *Proceedings of the Nutrition Society*, vol. 71, no. 2, pp. 205–212, 2012.

[54] A. El Lithy, R. M. Abdella, Y. M. El-Faissal, A. M. Sayed, and R. M. Samie, "The relationship between low maternal serum vitamin D levels and glycemic control in gestational diabetes assessed by HbA1c levels: an observational cross-sectional study," *BMC Pregnancy and Childbirth*, vol. 14, article 362, 2014.

[55] L. M. Bodnar, J. M. Catov, H. N. Simhan, M. F. Holick, R. W. Powers, and J. M. Roberts, "Maternal vitamin D deficiency increases the risk of preeclampsia," *Journal of Clinical Endocrinology and Metabolism*, vol. 92, no. 9, pp. 3517–3522, 2007.

[56] D. Barrera, L. Díaz, N. Noyola-Martínez, and A. Halhali, "Vitamin D and inflammatory cytokines in healthy and preeclamptic pregnancies," *Nutrients*, vol. 7, no. 8, pp. 6465–6490, 2015.

[57] Y. J. Heng, S. Liong, M. Permezel, G. E. Rice, M. K. Di Quinzio, and H. M. Georgiou, "Human cervicovaginal fluid biomarkers to predict term and preterm labor," *Frontiers in Physiology*, vol. 6, article 151, 2015.

[58] L. M. Bodnar, R. W. Platt, and H. N. Simhan, "Early-pregnancy vitamin D deficiency and risk of preterm birth subtypes," *Obstetrics & Gynecology*, vol. 125, no. 2, pp. 439–447, 2015.

[59] T. Zhu, T. J. Liu, X. Ge, J. Kong, L. J. Zhang, and Q. Zhao, "High prevalence of maternal vitamin D deficiency in preterm births in northeast China, Shenyang," *International Journal of Clinical and Experimental Pathology*, vol. 8, no. 2, Article ID 25973031, pp. 1459–1465, 2015.

[60] C. L. Wagner, C. Baggerly, S. McDonnell et al., "Post-hoc analysis of vitamin D status and reduced risk of preterm birth in two vitamin D pregnancy cohorts compared with South Carolina March of Dimes 2009–2011 rates," *The Journal of Steroid Biochemistry and Molecular Biology*, 2015.

[61] H. H. Burris, L. J. Van Marter, T. F. McElrath et al., "Vitamin D status among preterm and full-term infants at birth," *Pediatric Research*, vol. 75, no. 1, pp. 75–80, 2014.

[62] K. A. Boggess, J. A. Espinola, K. Moss, J. Beck, S. Offenbacher, and C. A. Camargo Jr., "Vitamin D status and periodontal disease among pregnant women," *Journal of Periodontology*, vol. 82, no. 2, pp. 195–200, 2011.

[63] Y. H. Chen, L. Fu, J. H. Hao et al., "Maternal vitamin D deficiency during pregnancy elevates the risks of small for gestational age and low birth weight infants in Chinese population," *The Journal of Clinical Endocrinology & Metabolism*, vol. 100, no. 5, pp. 1912–1919, 2015.

[64] P. Zhu, S.-L. Tong, W.-B. Hu et al., "Cord blood 25-hydroxyvitamin D and fetal growth in the China-Anhui birth cohort study," *Scientific Reports*, vol. 5, Article ID 14930, 2015.

[65] F. Aghajafari, T. Nagulesapillai, P. E. Ronksley, S. C. Tough, M. O'Beirne, and D. M. Rabi, "Association between maternal serum 25-hydroxyvitamin D level and pregnancy and neonatal outcomes: systematic review and meta-analysis of observational studies," *The BMJ*, vol. 346, article f1169, 2013.

[66] S. Q. Wei, H. P. Qi, Z. C. Luo, and W. D. Fraser, "Maternal vitamin D status and adverse pregnancy outcomes: a systematic review and meta-analysis," *The Journal of Maternal-Fetal & Neonatal Medicine*, vol. 26, no. 9, pp. 889–899, 2013.

[67] A. Merewood, S. D. Mehta, T. C. Chen, H. Bauchner, and M. F. Holick, "Association between vitamin D deficiency and primary cesarean section," *The Journal of Clinical Endocrinology & Metabolism*, vol. 94, no. 3, pp. 940–945, 2009.

[68] S. L. Loy, N. Lek, F. Yap et al., "Association of maternal vitamin D status with glucose tolerance and caesarean section in a

multi-ethnic Asian cohort: the growing up in Singapore towards healthy outcomes study," *PLoS ONE*, vol. 10, no. 11, Article ID e0142239, 2015.

[69] I. Solt, "The human microbiome and the great obstetrical syndromes: a new frontier in maternal-fetal medicine," *Best Practice & Research Clinical Obstetrics & Gynaecology*, vol. 29, no. 2, pp. 165–175, 2015.

[70] W. J. G. Hoogendijk, P. Lips, M. G. Dik, D. J. H. Deeg, A. T. F. Beekman, and B. W. J. H. Penninx, "Depression is associated with decreased 25-hydroxyvitamin D and increased parathyroid hormone levels in older adults," *Archives of General Psychiatry*, vol. 65, no. 5, pp. 508–512, 2008.

[71] D. Eyles, J. Brown, A. Mackay-Sim, J. McGrath, and F. Feron, "Vitamin D3 and brain development," *Neuroscience*, vol. 118, no. 3, pp. 641–653, 2003.

[72] R. Vieth, S. Kimball, A. Hu, and P. G. Walfish, "Randomized comparison of the effects of the vitamin D3 adequate intake versus 100 mcg (4000 IU) per day on biochemical responses and the wellbeing of patients," *Nutrition Journal*, vol. 3, article 8, 2004.

[73] C. W. Fu, J. T. Liu, W. J. Tu, J. Q. Yang, and Y. Cao, "Association between serum 25-hydroxyvitamin D levels measured 24 hours after delivery and postpartum depression," *BJOG*, vol. 122, no. 12, pp. 1688–1694, 2015.

[74] E. Fernell, S. Bejerot, J. Westerlund et al., "Autism spectrum disorder and low vitamin D at birth: a sibling control study," *Molecular Autism*, vol. 6, article 3, 2015.

[75] M. C. Magnus, L. C. Stene, S. E. Haberg et al., "Prospective study of maternal mid-pregnancy 25-hydroxyvitamin D level and early childhood respiratory disorders," *Paediatric and Perinatal Epidemiology*, vol. 27, no. 6, pp. 532–541, 2013.

[76] E. Morales, I. Romieu, S. Guerra et al., "Maternal vitamin D status in pregnancy and risk of lower respiratory tract infections, wheezing, and asthma in offspring," *Epidemiology*, vol. 23, no. 1, pp. 64–71, 2012.

[77] C.-Y. Chiu, S.-Y. Huang, Y.-C. Peng et al., "Maternal vitamin D levels are inversely related to allergic sensitization and atopic diseases in early childhood," *Pediatric Allergy and Immunology*, vol. 26, no. 4, pp. 337–343, 2015.

[78] C.-Y. Chiu, T.-S. Yao, S.-H. Chen et al., "Low cord blood vitamin D levels are associated with increased milk sensitization in early childhood," *Pediatric Allergy and Immunology*, vol. 25, no. 8, pp. 767–772, 2014.

[79] N. Baïz, P. Dargent-Molina, J. D. Wark, J.-C. Souberbielle, and I. Annesi-Maesano, "Cord serum 25-hydroxyvitamin D and risk of early childhood transient wheezing and atopic dermatitis," *Journal of Allergy and Clinical Immunology*, vol. 133, no. 1, pp. 147–153, 2014.

[80] D. J. Palmer, T. R. Sullivan, C. M. Skeaff, L. G. Smithers, and M. Makrides, "Higher cord blood 25-hydroxyvitamin D concentrations reduce the risk of early childhood eczema: in children with a family history of allergic disease," *World Allergy Organization Journal*, vol. 8, no. 1, article 28, 2015.

[81] T. Gazibara, H. T. den Dekker, J. C. de Jongste et al., "Associations of maternal and fetal 25-hydroxyvitamin D levels with childhood lung function and asthma. The Generation R Study," *Clinical & Experimental Allergy*, 2015.

[82] G. R. Zosky, P. H. Hart, A. J. O. Whitehouse et al., "Vitamin D deficiency at 16 to 20 weeks' gestation is associated with impaired lung function and asthma at 6 years of age," *Annals of the American Thoracic Society*, vol. 11, no. 4, pp. 571–577, 2014.

[83] C. Benetti, P. Comberiati, C. Capristo, A. L. Boner, and D. G. Peroni, "Therapeutic effects of vitamin D in asthma and allergy," *Mini-Reviews in Medicinal Chemistry*, vol. 15, no. 11, pp. 935–943, 2015.

[84] W. Jedrychowski, A. Galas, A. Pac et al., "Prenatal ambient air exposure to polycyclic aromatic hydrocarbons and the occurrence of respiratory symptoms over the first year of life," *European Journal of Epidemiology*, vol. 20, no. 9, pp. 775–782, 2005.

[85] W. Jedrychowski, F. Perera, U. Maugeri et al., "Intrauterine exposure to lead may enhance sensitization to common inhalant allergens in early childhood: a prospective prebirth cohort study," *Environmental Research*, vol. 111, no. 1, pp. 119–124, 2011.

[86] P. Grandjean, L. K. Poulsen, C. Heilmann, U. Steuerwald, and P. Weihe, "Allergy and sensitization during childhood associated with prenatal and lactational exposure to marine pollutants," *Environmental Health Perspectives*, vol. 118, no. 10, pp. 1429–1433, 2010.

[87] E. Okada, S. Sasaki, Y. Saijo et al., "Prenatal exposure to perfluorinated chemicals and relationship with allergies and infectious diseases in infants," *Environmental Research*, vol. 112, pp. 118–125, 2012.

[88] C. Miyashita, S. Sasaki, Y. Saijo et al., "Effects of prenatal exposure to dioxin-like compounds on allergies and infections during infancy," *Environmental Research*, vol. 111, no. 4, pp. 551–558, 2011.

[89] S. B. Stolevik, U. C. Nygaard, E. Namork et al., "Prenatal exposure to polychlorinated biphenyls and dioxins is associated with increased risk of wheeze and infections in infants," *Food and Chemical Toxicology*, vol. 49, no. 8, pp. 1843–1848, 2011.

[90] J. Moon, "The role of vitamin D in toxic metal absorption: a review," *Journal of the American College of Nutrition*, vol. 13, no. 6, pp. 559–564, 1994.

[91] S. J. Genuis, "Sensitivity-related illness: the escalating pandemic of allergy, food intolerance and chemical sensitivity," *The Science of the Total Environment*, vol. 408, no. 24, pp. 6047–6061, 2010.

[92] M. K. Javaid, S. R. Crozier, N. C. Harvey et al., "Maternal vitamin D status during pregnancy and childhood bone mass at age 9 years: a longitudinal study," *The Lancet*, vol. 367, no. 9504, pp. 36–43, 2006.

[93] P. H. Hart, R. M. Lucas, J. P. Walsh et al., "Vitamin D in fetal development: findings from a birth cohort study," *Pediatrics*, vol. 135, no. 1, pp. e167–e173, 2015.

[94] F. Mirzaei, K. B. Michels, K. Munger et al., "Gestational vitamin D and the risk of multiple sclerosis in offspring," *Annals of Neurology*, vol. 70, no. 1, pp. 30–40, 2011.

[95] N. Al-Asmari and T. Tulandi, "The relevance of post-cesarean adhesions," *Surgical Technology International*, vol. 22, pp. 177–181, 2012.

[96] J. Sonnenburg and E. Sonnenburg, *The Good Gut: Taking Control of Your Weight, Your Mood, and Your Long-Term Health*, Bantam Press, London, UK, 2015.

[97] S. Beck, D. Wojdyla, L. Say et al., "The worldwide incidence of preterm birth: a systematic review of maternal mortality and morbidity," *Bulletin of the World Health Organization*, vol. 88, no. 1, pp. 31–38, 2010.

[98] K. M. Johnston, K. Gooch, E. Korol et al., "The economic burden of prematurity in Canada," *BMC Pediatrics*, vol. 14, article 93, 2014.

[99] W. B. Grant, G. K. Schwalfenberg, S. J. Genuis, and S. J. Whiting, "An estimate of the economic burden and premature deaths due to vitamin D deficiency in Canada," *Molecular Nutrition & Food Research*, vol. 54, no. 8, pp. 1172–1181, 2010.

[100] S. M. Solon-Biet, S. J. Mitchell, R. de Cabo, D. Raubenheimer, D. G. Le Couteur, and S. J. Simpson, "Macronutrients and caloric intake in health and longevity," *Journal of Endocrinology*, vol. 226, no. 1, pp. R17–R28, 2015.

[101] S. J. Genuis, "Nutritional transition: a determinant of global health," *Journal of Epidemiology and Community Health*, vol. 59, no. 8, pp. 615–617, 2005.

[102] J. Crowley, L. Ball, C. Wall, and M. Leveritt, "Nutrition beyond drugs and devices: a review of the approaches to enhance the capacity of nutrition care provision by general practitioners," *Australian Journal of Primary Health*, vol. 18, no. 2, pp. 90–95, 2012.

[103] M. Castillo, R. Feinstein, J. Tsang, and M. Fisher, "Basic nutrition knowledge of recent medical graduates entering a pediatric residency program," *International Journal of Adolescent Medicine and Health*, 2015.

[104] C. Lo, "Integrating nutrition as a theme throughout the medical school curriculum," *The American Journal of Clinical Nutrition*, vol. 72, no. 3, supplement, pp. 882S–889S, 2000.

[105] D. C. Lehotay, P. Smith, J. Krahn, M. Etter, and J. Eichhorst, "Vitamin D levels and relative insufficiency in Saskatchewan," *Clinical Biochemistry*, vol. 46, no. 15, pp. 1489–1492, 2013.

[106] M. Aucoin, R. Weaver, R. Thomas, and L. Jones, "Vitamin D status of refugees arriving in Canada: findings from the calgary refugee health program," *Canadian Family Physician*, vol. 59, no. 4, pp. e188–e194, 2013.

[107] Canadian Pediatric Society, "Vitamin D supplementation: recommendations for Canadian mothers and infants," *Paediatrics & Child Health*, vol. 12, no. 7, pp. 583–598, 2007.

[108] B. W. Hollis, "Vitamin D requirement during pregnancy and lactation," *Journal of Bone and Mineral Research*, vol. 22, supplement 2, pp. V39–V44, 2007.

20

Serum hCG Levels following the Ovulatory Injection: Associations with Patient Weight and Implantation Time

Dorette J. Noorhasan,[1,2,3] **Peter G. McGovern,**[1,2,4] **Michael Cho,**[1,2] **Aimee Seungdamrong,**[1,2] **Khaliq Ahmad,**[2,5] **and David H. McCulloh**[1,2,6]

[1]*Division of Reproductive Endocrinology and Infertility, Department of Obstetrics, Gynecology and Women's Health, New Jersey Medical School, UMDNJ, Newark, NJ 07103, USA*

[2]*University Reproductive Associates, Hasbrouck Heights, NJ 07604, USA*

[3]*Fertility Specialists of Texas, 5757 Warren Parkway, Suite No. 300, Frisco, TX 75034, USA*

[4]*Department of Obstetrics and Gynecology, Saint Luke's Roosevelt Hospital, New York, NY 10019, USA*

[5]*Department of Obstetrics and Gynecology, Texas Tech University Health Sciences Center School of Medicine, Lubbock, TX 79430, USA*

[6]*NYU Fertility Center, New York University Langone Medical Center, New York, NY 10016, USA*

Correspondence should be addressed to Peter G. McGovern; pmcgovern@uranj.com

Academic Editor: Curt W. Burger

Objective. To test if serum hCG levels the morning after the ovulatory hCG injection correlate with (1) retrieval efficiency, (2) oocyte maturity, (3) embryo quality, (4) pregnancy, and/or (5) time to implantation in patients undergoing in vitro fertilization (IVF) with intracytoplasmic sperm injection (ICSI). *Design*. Retrospective cohort analysis. *Setting*. University-based IVF clinic. *Patient(s)*. All IVF/ICSI cycles from April 2005 to February 2008 whose hCG administration was confirmed (*n* = 472 patients). *Intervention(s)*. Serum hCG was measured the morning following the ovulatory injection, on the 16th day following retrieval, and repeated on day 18 for those with positive results. *Main Outcome Measure(s)*. Number of follicles on the day of hCG injection, number of oocytes retrieved, maturity of oocytes, embryo quality, pregnancy outcome, and time to implantation. *Result(s)*. hCG levels did not correlate with retrieval efficiency, oocyte maturity, embryo quality, or pregnancy. Postinjection hCG levels were inversely associated with patient weight and time to implantation. *Conclusion(s)*. No correlation was found between hCG level and any parameter of embryo quality. Patient weight affected hCG levels following hCG injection and during the early period of pregnancy following implantation. No association between postinjection hCG level and time of implantation (adjusted for patient weight) was apparent.

1. Introduction

Traditionally 10,000 IU of hCG is administered to cause final oocyte maturation and ovulation in patients undergoing in vitro fertilization (IVF). It is well established that hCG can mimic the midcycle LH surge [1]. It is clear that the ovulatory injection of hCG is required to assure that oocytes will be retrieved at time of retrieval [2–5], thus avoiding "empty follicle syndrome." In our practice, we have patients returning the morning after administering 10,000 IU of hCG so that we may assess their serum hCG level and to help determine if the patients correctly administered the injection. Although

it is clear that some level of serum hCG after the ovulatory injection is necessary for oocyte retrieval, it is not clear whether a specific threshold level of serum hCG is required to permit successful IVF outcome. In addition, we chose to examine if the patient's weight (a correlate of the patient's volume of distribution) for this fixed dose of administration and for any endogenous hCG production affects circulating hCG levels and outcomes.

The objectives of this study were to evaluate if the serum hCG levels in blood drawn the morning following ovulatory injection of hCG correlate with (1) retrieval efficiency, (2) maturity of the retrieved oocytes, (3) embryo developmental extent and quality, (4) incidence of pregnancy, and/or (5) time to implantation in patients undergoing in vitro fertilization (IVF) with intracytoplasmic sperm injection (ICSI).

2. Materials and Methods

2.1. Study Population. The Rutgers-New Jersey Medical School (formerly UMDNJ) Institutional Review Board approved this study (IRB # 0120070090). A retrospective chart review of all patients undergoing IVF with ICSI between April 2005 and February 2008 at a university-affiliated reproductive endocrinology clinic was conducted. Follicular growth was monitored by ultrasound and serum estradiol measurements. Follicular growth was considered sufficient when ultrasound monitoring revealed at least 2 follicles with a mean diameter of 16 mm or larger. Each patient was instructed to administer an intramuscular injection of 10,000 IU of hCG later that night for final oocyte maturation and ovulatory stimulation. Oocyte retrieval was scheduled for 34 hours after the injection. All patients were instructed to return for a blood draw between 7:00 and 8:00 am on the morning following the injection, to confirm that the hCG medication had been properly administered (6 ± 2 hours later). Serum hCG was assessed by chemiluminescent assay (Immulite 1000, Siemens, Deerfield, IL). A total of 472 IVF cycles in 367 patients were found to have confirmatory values of serum hCG determined the morning after the hCG injection. Of these 367 patients, 280 underwent only one retrieval, 72 patients underwent 2 cycles, 12 patients underwent 3 retrievals, and 3 patients underwent 4 retrievals. Records were reviewed to determine the number of follicles (~10 mm and larger) seen on ultrasound monitoring the morning prior to hCG injection, the oocytes that did not contain a germinal vesicle (GV) (i.e., mature oocytes), the developmental extent and quality of embryos that were transferred, and the incidence of pregnancy.

2.2. Retrieval Efficiency. The number of oocytes retrieved was divided by the number of follicles observed in the ovaries on the final day of ultrasound monitoring (the morning prior to injection of hCG). This ratio served to estimate the efficiency of retrieving oocytes from the follicles (the proportion of follicles yielding oocytes).

2.3. Oocyte Maturity. The number of oocytes with a germinal vesicle at the time of oocyte clean-up prior to intracytoplasmic sperm injection (ICSI) was determined. The percentage of oocytes that did *not* contain a germinal vesicle was used as an estimate of the number of mature oocytes (that had begun the maturation), since this was the only criterion that we used to determine the oocytes on which we performed ICSI.

2.4. Embryo Developmental Extent and Quality. The developmental extent as well as embryo quality was assessed for all embryos transferred back to the patient's uterus. For embryos transferred on day 3, the number of cells was counted and served as an indicator of the extent of embryo development. Grades for embryos transferred on day 3 (A, B, and C) were based on a combination of cell sizes (appropriate equality of divisions) and on fragmentation (less fragmentation leading to higher scores). For embryos transferred on day 5, the extent of blastocyst development was determined: morulae (M) with no sign of blastocele formation, blastocysts (B) with a blastocele that had not begun to expand, blastocysts that had expanded (XB), and blastocysts undergoing hatching (H). In addition, scores indicative of blastocyst quality were evaluated using a two-letter grade indicative of the number of cells in the inner cell mass (A > 7, B 4–7, and C < 4) and the number of cells seen in one focal plane at the equator of the blastocyst (A > 8, B 4–8, and C < 4). The first letter presented in Figure 1(c) denotes the number of cells in the inner cell mass.

2.5. Incidence of Clinical Pregnancy. Serum hCG levels were determined on the 16th day following oocyte retrieval to determine if pregnancy had occurred. If the value on day 16 following oocyte retrieval was greater than 5.3 mIU/mL (the threshold of the assay for detecting pregnancy), serum hCG level was repeated on the 18th day following oocyte retrieval to look for a rise in serum hCG values 2 days after the initial measurement. An ultrasound examination was performed 4 weeks following the oocyte retrieval if hCG levels continued to rise after days 16 and 18. Clinical pregnancy was defined as the presence of at least one fetal sac in the uterus detected using ultrasound.

2.6. Time to Implantation. Only those patients with hCG levels that increased between day 16 and day 18 were evaluated for time of implantation (n = 113). The time of implantation was determined by extrapolation of the linear regression line relating the two ln [hCG]'s (for day 16 and 18 serum hCG values) versus time to the value at which [hCG] equaled 10 mIU/mL for each fetal sac seen, similar to a method reported previously [6]. A serum hCG value of 10 mIU/mL was arbitrarily chosen for each fetal sac because, in previous examinations, this choice of threshold yielded a relative minimum in the standard deviation of estimated implantation times (it is also about twice the manufacturer's lower limit of detecting a pregnancy (5.2 IU/L)).

2.7. Statistical Analysis. Linear regression analyses were performed to evaluate the correlation between serum hCG and the number of oocytes retrieved per follicle scanned, maturity of the oocytes, clinical pregnancy rate, and time to implantation. Contingency Chi Squared tests were performed to evaluate the association between serum hCG and embryo quality. A p value of <0.05 was considered to be statistically significant.

3. Results

Serum hCG levels determined the morning following the hCG injection averaged 202 ± 122 IU/L. Values of serum hCG varied widely ranging from 35 to 623 IU/L.

3.1. Efficiency of Oocyte Retrieval. The percentage of oocytes retrieved per follicle scanned was 89 ± 29% (Figure 1). Values

(a)

(b)

(c)

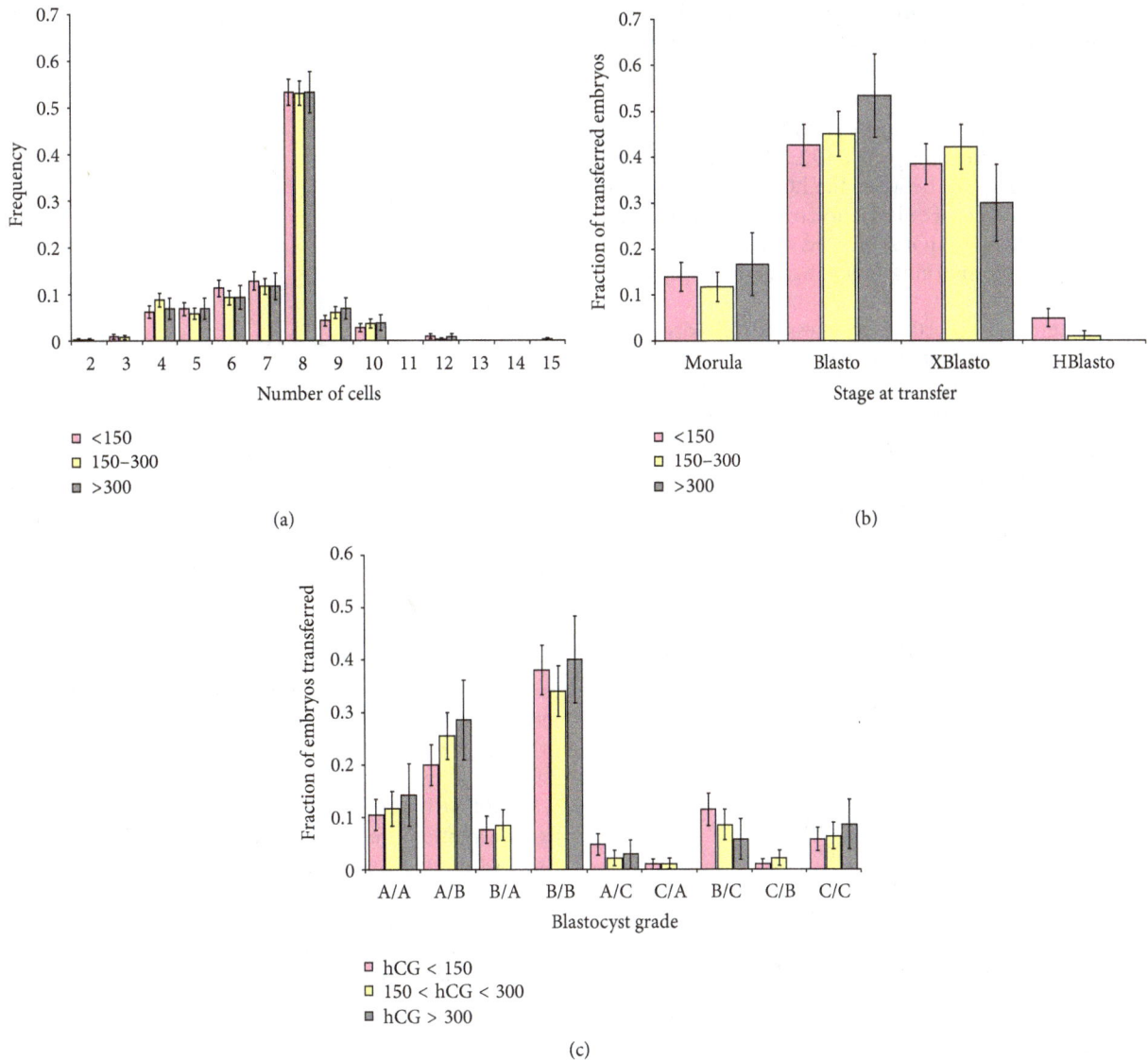

FIGURE 1: Postovulatory serum hCG levels and embryo quality. Bars indicate the incidence (frequency) of embryos with specified numbers of cells transferred on day 3 (a), embryo stage transferred on day 5 (b), and embryo grade transferred on day 5 (c). Error bars represent standard error. Postovulatory serum hCG levels were not associated with the number of cells in day 3 embryos (Contingency Chi Squared, $p = 0.972$) (a), the embryo stage in day 5 transfers (Contingency Chi Squared, $p = 0.399$) (b), nor the blastocyst grade in day 5 transfers (Contingency Chi Squared, $p = 0.933$).

for efficiency of oocyte retrieval varied widely from 27% to 260%. (Values exceeding 100% probably occurred due to difficulty with ultrasound visualization of the ovaries.) Values for efficiency of oocyte retrieval were not significantly associated with the serum hCG level determined the morning following the hCG injection ($R = 0.073$; $p = 0.37$).

3.2. Oocyte Maturity. The percentage of mature oocytes was $88 \pm 13.5\%$. The percentage of oocytes that were mature varied widely and ranged from 43% to 100%. Values for the percentage of oocytes that were mature were not significantly associated with the serum hCG levels determined the morning following the hCG injection ($R = 0.11$; $p = 0.18$).

3.3. Embryo Developmental Extent and Quality. Of the 472 patients, 343 patients underwent embryo transfer (total of 822 embryos) on day 3 and 129 underwent embryo transfer (total of 234 embryos) on day 5. Based upon the distribution of hCG values, we divided the patients undergoing day 3 transfer into three categories representing three groups defined as low, moderate, and high levels of hCG (<150 mIU/mL with 134 patients and 318 embryos, 150–300 mIU/mL with 156 patients and 376 embryos, and >300 mIU/mL with 53 patients and 128 embryos). The number of cells in each embryo was assessed for embryos transferred on day 3. The distribution of cell numbers, indicative of developmental extent, is shown in Figure 1(a). Embryos with 8 cells were most common in all 3 categories with other cell numbers less represented in all categories (Figure 1(a)). The similarity of the three hCG categories suggests that there was no significant difference in the developmental extent in the three groups. The distributions were not significantly different when compared using Contingency Chi Squared: $\chi^2 = 4.5$ with 12 degrees of freedom; $p = 0.972$. This indicates that there was no association between the hCG groups and the distribution of numbers of cells. Hence, in day 3 embryos, the developmental extent was not associated with the serum hCG level determined the morning following the hCG injection (Figure 1(a)).

Embryo grades, reflecting evenness of cell divisions, and lack of fragmentation were compared for the same three groups of patients examined for cell numbers. The distributions of grades were not significant (Contingency Chi Squared: $\chi^2 = 4.5$ with 3 degrees of freedom; $p = 0.2$).

Similarly, the extent of blastocyst development was assessed for embryos transferred on day 5. Blastocysts that had no expanded blastocele (Blasto) and blastocysts that had expanded blastocele (XBlasto) were predominant in all three categories. Comparison of the distributions of blastocyst development yielded no significant differences (Contingency Chi Squared: $\chi^2 = 6.22$ with 6 degrees of freedom; $p = 0.399$). Therefore, the stages of the blastocysts transferred on day 5 were not associated with the hCG groups. Hence, blastocyst stages were not associated with serum hCG levels determined the morning following the hCG injection (Figure 1(b)).

The quality of blastocysts was assessed for embryos transferred on day 5. Based upon the distribution of hCG values, we divided the 129 patients undergoing day 5 transfer into three categories representing three groups defined as low, moderate, and high levels of hCG (<150 mIU/mL with 59 patients with 105 embryos, 150–300 mIU/mL with 52 patients with 94 embryos, and >300 mIU/mL with 18 patients with 35 embryos). Blastocysts graded A/B and B/B were predominant in all three hCG categories. Comparison of the distributions of blastocyst grades yielded no significant differences (Contingency Chi Squared: $\chi^2 = 8.48$ with 16 degrees of freedom; $p = 0.933$). Therefore, the grades of the blastocysts transferred on day 5 were not associated with the hCG groups. Hence, blastocyst grades were not associated with serum hCG levels determined the morning following the hCG injection (Figure 1(c)).

3.4. Clinical Pregnancy.

Two hundred five of the retrievals resulted in clinical pregnancy (205/472 = 43.4%). Clinical pregnancy was not significantly correlated with hCG levels determined the morning following the hCG injection ($R = 0.088$, $p = 0.28$) (Figure 2). In addition, there is no apparent threshold for postovulatory serum hCG levels that will predict pregnancy. The four lowest serum hCG values (35.6, 37.5, 43.7, and 46.6 mIU/mL) were all associated with a clinical pregnancy (4 adjacent points, upper left in Figure 2).

3.5. Time of Implantation.

The mean time to implantation was 8.6 ± 2.3 days. Implantation times ranged from 3.2 to 14.9 days after oocyte retrieval. Roughly 72% of the implantations

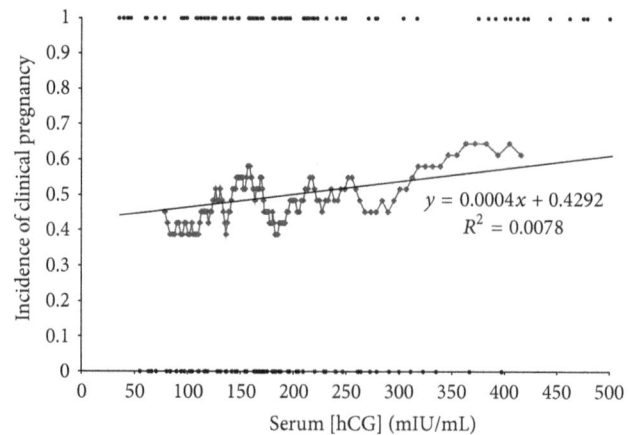

FIGURE 2: Postovulatory serum hCG level and pregnancy rate. The incidence of pregnancy was 50%. Serum hCG levels the morning after ovulatory injection did not correlate with incidence of clinical pregnancy ($R = 0.088$). Patients who were pregnant were considered a value of 1 and patients who were not pregnant were considered a value of 0. Straight line is the regression line for all patients. The blue tracing displays a rolling average of the patients.

occurred on day 6, 7, 8, 9, or 10. The mean time to implantation was later (9.5–10 days) when the postinjection serum hCG level was low (~100 mIU/mL) when compared to 8 days when the postinjection serum hCG level was higher (250–400 mIU/mL). Despite the wide degree of variability of implantation times, the trend toward earlier implantation time with higher serum levels of hCG seems apparent even in the raw data points. A semilogarithmic best-fit line fits the raw data well and mirrors the trend present in the rolling average. This inverse relationship between logarithm of time to implantation and serum hCG level yielded a significant correlation coefficient ($R = -0.335$; $p < 0.001$) (Figure 3).

3.6. Association between Time of Implantation and Postinjection Serum hCG Levels and Patient Weight.

HCG levels varied from patient to patient. One possible contributor to the variation in hCG levels was the final volume of dilution within the patient, a value proportional to 1/patient weight. Serum hCG levels were significantly correlated with 1/patient weight ($r = 0.62$, $p < 0.001$). In addition, the time of implantation was significantly correlated with 1/patient weight ($r = 0.36$, $p < 0.001$). Therefore, 1/patient weight, postinjection hCG levels, and the time of implantation were all significantly associated.

In order to attempt to discern if dilution factor could explain both the postinjection hCG levels and the estimate of implantation time (based on serum levels of hCG), we corrected the implantation time estimates by using individualized thresholds of serum hCG for each patient. These individualized thresholds were determined by multiplying the original threshold (10 mIU/mL per fetal sac) by the dilution factor, 156.27 lb/patient weight (a dimensionless factor obtained by dividing the average weight of all patients (156.27 lb) by the specific patient's weight). When this correction was applied, the association between postinjection hCG

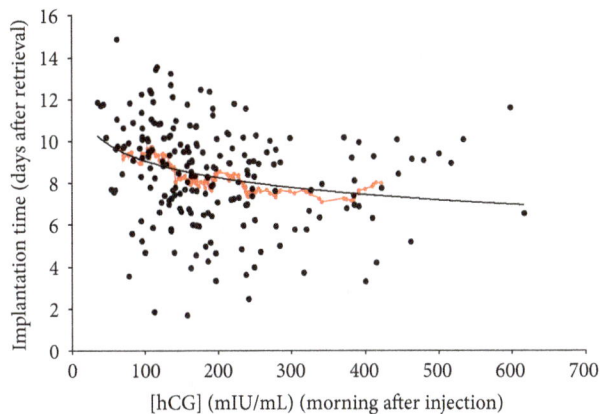

FIGURE 3: Time to implantation (days) as a function of serum hCG level the morning after 10 000 units ovulatory injection. The mean time to implantation was 8.6 ± 2.3 days ($n = 113$). There was an inverse correlation between implantation time and serum hCG ($R = -0.335$). A rolling average of the implantation time (red circles) was longer (9–10.5 days) when the postinjection serum hCG levels were lower (~100 mIU/mL) when compared to an implantation time of ~8 days when the postinjection serum hCG levels were higher (250–400 mIU/mL). There was a significant inverse association (regression equation, smooth line) between implantation time and serum hCG level ($p = 9 \times 10^{-7}$).

level and corrected implantation time was not significant ($r = -0.07$, $p = 0.31$)

4. Discussion

To our knowledge, this is the second published report examining postinjection serum β-hCG levels and IVF outcome. It has been previously reported that improper administration of the ovulatory hCG results in a serum hCG level of zero and the empty follicle syndrome where no oocytes are obtained at retrieval [2–5]. One might expect that different serum levels of hCG could lead to different rates of ovulation, different attainment of maturation by oocytes, and possibly different rates of embryonic development.

The time of implantation was significantly associated with serum hCG level the morning following hCG injection. This novel observation is particularly revealing in consideration of the observation that there were no significant differences in embryonic development. The actual time to implantation cannot be determined accurately without the use of histological examination, impossible to perform during a cycle of conception. Hence, hCG level evaluation (serum and/or urine) has traditionally been used as secondary variable to evaluate time of implantation [6–10].

Our observations reveal an expected relationship between weight and dilution of administered drug. Causal roles of weight versus hCG level on implantation time are difficult to establish when multiple variables are associated with the outcome as well as with each other. One prior study (Shah et al., [11]) found no significant association between obesity status and hCG levels following intramuscular injection examining smaller numbers of subjects. While

it is plausible that weight was a major determinant of serum hCG level, and that postinjection hCG levels were determinants of the time of implantation, it is not possible to establish from these data whether implantation time was affected by the hCG level attained following hCG injection, or by patient weight or some other unidentified factor that may be associated with one, two, or all three of these parameters. This work suggests that patient weight may be a confounding factor in the use of this technique to estimate the time of implantation. The observation that correction of the implantation time by adjusting the hCG threshold for the dilution factor suggests that the same dilution effect that occurs for exogenous injection of hCG may occur with the endogenous release of hCG. When adjustment for this was applied, the association of implantation time with postinjection hCG level was not significant, suggesting that the serum hCG levels shortly following implantation are diluted to the same extent as injected hCG. Further, this suggests that the hCG levels expected during pregnancy should be adjusted by patient weight. Dismissal of a pregnancy as unsuccessful based on a single low serum hCG level in a heavy patient may lead to poor patient management.

Despite the initial β-hCG and appropriate doubling in forty-eight hours, the exact time of implantation is still quite unpredictable. Previously, several studies have been conducted to shed light on this phenomenon. Wilcox et al. collected daily urinary hCG samples for six months in 221 women attempting natural conception [7]. In 199 natural conceptions, they found that implantation day (the first day that hCG appeared in the woman's urine) ranged from day 6 to day 18 after ovulation and that 84% of the women had implantation on day 8, 9, or 10 following ovulation [7]. The risk of early pregnancy loss increased with later implantations [7]. The range of implantation times that we report after oocyte retrieval (3.2 to 14.9 days after oocyte retrieval) is quite similar to the range of implantation days after ovulation reported by Wilcox et al. [7]. Our observation that 72% of the implantations occurred on day 6, 7, 8, 9, or 10 also suggests that implantation following IVF occurs with a similar interval after hCG injection as implantation occurs following the LH surge in the natural cycles observed by Wilcox et al. [7].

In laboratory animals it has been demonstrated that the endometrium goes through several phases: (1) neutral toward implantation, (2) receptive window of implantation, and (3) refractory phase to implantation [12, 13]. It is still unclear exactly what histological and morphological endometrial change as well as what hormonal milieu is optimal for implantation. Generally, based on donor and frozen embryo transfer cycles, it is clear that some level of endometrial receptivity (endometrial histologic readiness in the right hormonal milieu) is necessary for implantation to occur. Based on our findings here, embryo developmental extent and quality were not associated with serum hCG levels the morning following the hCG injection. However, time to implantation was inversely related to these serum hCG values. This may suggest that that the hCG levels attained following the ovulatory injection of hCG affect the endometrial window of receptivity (and hence time to implantation).

We did not evaluate if postinjection serum hCG values or if time to implantation was affected by the type of stimulation protocol. However, it has been previously reported that time to implantation is not affected by the type of IVF stimulation protocol used. It was previously demonstrated that implantation time did not differ among women using protocols of (a) IVF stimulation without a GnRH agonist, (b) long GnRH agonist protocol and embryo transfer on day 2, (c) long GnRH agonist protocol and embryo transfer on day 3, and (d) GnRH flare protocol [6].

In summary, we found that postinjection serum hCG levels did *not* correlate with number of oocytes retrieved per follicle scanned, maturity of the retrieved oocytes, embryo development or quality, or incidence of pregnancy confirming the results of Levy et al. [14].

Postinjection serum hCG levels determined were inversely correlated with both the time of implantation and patient weight. Higher serum hCG levels were associated with earlier implantation times. However, the lack of significant correlation when implantation time was corrected using individualized hCG thresholds adjusted for patient weight suggests that the association between implantation time and postinjection serum hCG levels may be due to similar dilution of exogenous and endogenous hCG levels. Since the extent of embryonic development was not different at different serum hCG levels, we propose that embryonic developmental rate or quality observed at the time of embryo transfer was not responsible for these differences in the time of implantation. We propose a larger series to confirm these observations, along with further investigations to better determine the exact mechanism(s) of this phenomenon, before this information might be used in attempts to improve clinical outcomes.

Capsule

Postinjection serum hCG level predicts neither embryo quality nor IVF outcome. However, it is closely associated with implantation time, and with patient weight. After correction for patient weight in calculations for implantation time, the association of implantation time with the postinjection hCG level is no longer significant, suggesting that serum hCG levels are dependent upon patient weight both following hCG injection and during endogenous rises of hCG during early pregnancy.

Disclosure

The data is the result of original research. The data on serum hCG and IVF outcome were presented at the American Society for Reproductive Medicine 64th annual meeting, San Francisco, CA (P # 37). The data on serum hCG and implantation time were presented at the Society for Gynecologic Investigation 56th annual meeting, Glasgow, Scotland (P # 708).

Conflict of Interests

Peter G. McGovern, M.D., has past research funding support from NIH, Merck, EMDSerono and Ferring Pharmaceuticals.

David H. McCulloh, Ph.D., has received an honorarium from Columbia Laboratories. There was no third party financial support for conducting this study.

References

[1] I. Boime, V. Garcia-Campayo, and A. J. W. Hsueh, *Yen and Jaffe's Reproductive Endocrinology*, Elsevier Saunders, Philadelphia, Pa, USA, 5th edition, 2004.

[2] C. J. Quintans, M. J. Donaldson, L. A. Blanco, and R. S. Pasqualini, "Empty follicle syndrome due to human errors: its occurrence in an in-vitro fertilization programme," *Human Reproduction*, vol. 13, no. 10, pp. 2703–2705, 1998.

[3] T. G. Zreik, J. A. Garcia-Velasco, T. M. Vergara, A. Arici, D. Olive, and E. E. Jones, "Empty follicle syndrome: evidence for recurrence," *Human Reproduction*, vol. 15, no. 5, pp. 999–1002, 2000.

[4] A. Kourtis, D. Rousso, and D. Panidis, "The empty follicle syndrome," *Journal of Endocrinological Investigation*, vol. 27, no. 2, pp. 187–191, 2004.

[5] T. L. Stevenson and H. Lashen, "Empty follicle syndrome: the reality of a controversial syndrome, a systematic review," *Fertility and Sterility*, vol. 90, no. 3, pp. 691–698, 2008.

[6] M.-I. Hsu, P. Kolm, J. Leete, K. W. Dong, S. Muasher, and S. Oehninger, "Analysis of implantation in assisted reproduction through the use of serial human chorionic gonadotropin measurements," *Journal of Assisted Reproduction and Genetics*, vol. 15, no. 8, pp. 496–503, 1998.

[7] A. J. Wilcox, D. D. Baird, and C. R. Weinberg, "Time of implantation of the conceptus and loss of pregnancy," *The New England Journal of Medicine*, vol. 340, no. 23, pp. 1796–1799, 1999.

[8] H.-C. Liu, J. Cohen, M. Alikani, N. Noyes, and Z. Rosenwaks, "Assisted hatching facilitates earlier implantation," *Fertility and Sterility*, vol. 60, no. 5, pp. 871–875, 1993.

[9] P. A. Nepomnaschy, C. R. Weinberg, A. J. Wilcox, and D. D. Baird, "Urinary hCG patterns during the week following implantation," *Human Reproduction*, vol. 23, no. 2, pp. 271–277, 2008.

[10] P. A. Bergh and D. Navot, "The impact of embryonic development and endometrial maturity on the timing of implantation," *Fertility and Sterility*, vol. 58, no. 3, pp. 537–542, 1992.

[11] D. K. Shah, S. A. Missmer, K. F. B. Correia, and E. S. Ginsburg, "Pharmacokinetics of human chorionic gonadotropin injection in obese and normal-weight women," *Journal of Clinical Endocrinology and Metabolism*, vol. 99, no. 4, pp. 1314–1321, 2014.

[12] K. Yoshinaga, "Uterine receptivity for blastocyst implantation," *Annals of the New York Academy of Sciences*, vol. 541, pp. 424–431, 1988.

[13] A. Psychoyos, "Hormonal control of uterine receptivity for nidation," *Journal of Reproduction and Fertility. Supplement*, vol. 25, pp. 17–28, 1976.

[14] G. Levy, M. J. Hill, C. Ramirez et al., "Serum human chorionic gonadotropin levels on the day before oocyte retrieval do not correlate with oocyte maturity," *Fertility and Sterility*, vol. 99, no. 6, pp. 1610–1614, 2013.

21

Practical Advice for Emergency IUD Contraception in Young Women

Norman D. Goldstuck[1] and Dirk Wildemeersch[2]

[1]Department of Obstetrics and Gynaecology, Faculty of Medicine and Health Sciences, Stellenbosch University and Tygerberg Hospital, Western Cape, South Africa
[2]Gynecological Outpatient Clinic and IUD Training Center, Rooseveltlaan 43/44, 9000 Ghent, Belgium

Correspondence should be addressed to Norman D. Goldstuck; nahumzh@yahoo.com

Academic Editor: John R. Van Nagell

Too few women are aware of the very high efficacy of intrauterine copper devices (IUDs) to prevent pregnancy after unprotected intercourse. Women who frequently engage in unprotected intercourse or seek emergency contraception (EC) are at high risk of unplanned pregnancy and possible abortion. It is therefore important that these women receive precise and accurate information about intrauterine devices as they may benefit from using an IUD for EC as continuing contraception. Copper IUDs should be used as first choice options given their rapid onset of action and their long-term contraceptive action which require minimal thought or intervention on the part of the user. In the United States, there is only one copper IUD presently available which limits treatment options. There are numerous copper IUDs available for use in EC, however, their designs and size are not always optimal for use in nulliparous women or women with smaller or narrower uteruses. Utilization of frameless IUDs which do not require a larger transverse arm for uterine retention may have distinct advantages, particularly in young women, as they will be suitable for use in all women irrespective of uterine size. This paper provides practical information on EC use with emphasis on the use of the frameless IUD.

1. Emergency Contraceptive Methods

Most women are aware of the existence of emergency contraceptive pills; however, many do not know their mechanism of action, when or how to take them, and their overall effectiveness and may inadvertently rely on them as their principal means of contraception. Given the lack of information available on both the use of copper IUDs as EC and its long-term contraceptive benefits, it is safe to assume that the knowledge of both patients and physicians on the benefits of copper releasing IUDs is even lower.

2. Oral Emergency Contraceptives

There are two available oral methods for EC, 1.5 mg levonorgestrel (LNG) (e.g., Plan B, Norlevo and Levonelle) and 30 mg ulipristal acetate (UPA) (e.g., Ella and EllaOne). They work through delaying ovulation and are effective up to 5 days after unprotected intercourse although the efficacy of LNG decreases close to the time of ovulation. Once ovulation has occurred, EC pills are likely to be ineffective to prevent pregnancy. The overall efficacy for women taking oral EC during their fertile window (from 5 days before ovulation to 1 day after ovulation) was 60–68% in two studies evaluating these methods [1, 2]. Taking oral EC after unprotected intercourse prior to the fertile period appears to be optimal. The pregnancy rates were 4 times higher in women taking oral LNG or UPA EC who had unprotected intercourse the day prior to ovulation compared to those who had sex outside the fertile period [3].

Oral EC has the advantage of being easily obtainable although the cost may be expensive. There are also disadvantageous which should be realized as the oral EC methods have a higher pregnancy rate in women who have unprotected sex in the fertile window. EC pills also appear to be less effective in overweight women, especially LNG, with a pregnancy risk

Highest risk (day 12–16)
Levonorgestrel (up to day 10)
Ulipristal acetate (up to day 12)
Intrauterine device (up to day 18–20)

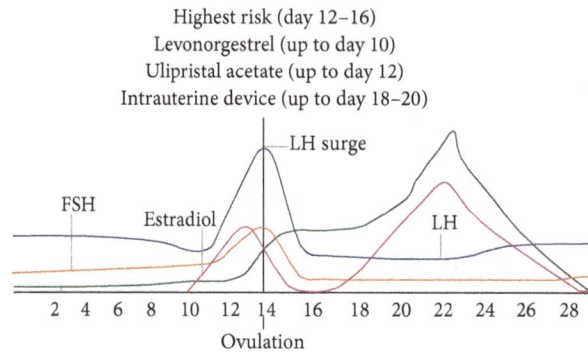

FIGURE 1: Fertility risk and window of action of different methods of emergency contraception.

in the higher weight categories (women weighing between 70 and 80 kg or more and body mass index (BMI) over 35) similar to expected rates in the absence of contraception [4]. Ulipristal acetate may be considered in these women as the impact of BMI appears less pronounced than with LNG [2]. Repeated acts of unprotected intercourse also appear to be a risk factor [2]. Furthermore, some drugs (e.g., anticonvulsants, antituberculosis drugs) may reduce the concentration of levonorgestrel and ulipristal. Ulipristal should not be used in women taking drugs that can reduce its absorption (e.g., antacids, H2 receptor antagonists, and proton pump inhibitors) or reduce its systemic concentration by inducing liver enzymes [5].

3. Intrauterine Devices

3.1. Effectiveness of Copper IUDs for Emergency Contraception. Oral EC methods are useful to prevent pregnancy after unprotected intercourse but they do not contribute to lowering the number of future unintended pregnancies and induced abortions [7]. Copper-releasing IUDs, on the other hand, are not only more effective than oral EC methods, but they also contribute significantly to reducing future unintended pregnancies and abortions. Copper ions are toxic to sperm and to the ovum. They alter motility and function of sperm and ova and cause alterations in the uterus and oviducts. As such, they prevent fertilization. When inserted after ovulation, they usually prevent implantation [8].

Copper IUDs have three main advantages over oral EC. (1) The efficacy of copper IUDs has been clearly established. A recent systematic review of 42 studies reported a pregnancy rate of 0.09% which is 10 times better than oral ECs [9]. (2) Currently, it is recommended that a copper IUD can be inserted up to 5–7 days after unprotected intercourse or up to 5 days after the earliest estimated day of ovulation. In this situation, the copper IUD may act by preventing implantation; when used in the usual manner, it usually prevents fertilization [10]. For the sake of clarity, in the event when sex occurred more than 5 days prior to the subject presenting, but the expected ovulation date was 5 days or less than 5 days ago, a copper IUD can still be inserted because of its preimplantation effect as implantation may occur only 6 days after ovulation [11]. In line with this, official guidelines

by WHO and other organizations (American College of Obstetricians and Gynecologists (ACOG) and the Royal College of Obstetricians and Gynaecologists of the United Kingdom) advise that copper IUDs be used within 5 days of unprotected intercourse in order to avoid IUD insertion after implantation which is viewed as the start of pregnancy. However, this viewpoint has no scientific basis. It is based on the assumption that insertion of an IUD at the time or a day or more after possible implantation is forbidden. There are two reasons for this. The first is that disrupting a newly implanted conceptus is viewed as not being morally correct. However, this is a philosophical problem not a scientific one [12]. The second is that, in the same way as an IUD may predispose to infection during an established intrauterine pregnancy where it remains *in situ*, the same may analogously be true for a pregnancy of only a few cells in size and which is only a few days old. There is no evidence at all for this prejudicial approach. In fact, there is evidence that IUDs as EC are effective and safe after this time [13] and that they may be inserted at any time of the cycle if a high sensitivity pregnancy test is negative [14]. This approach is evidence based and reduces possible errors in that the subject does not have to accurately remember the day of last menstrual period or the day(s) of unprotected coitus and makes the decision to insert an emergency IUD more objective. (3) Once inserted, an IUD can provide ongoing contraception for 5 years or more. A recent study suggested that women appear to have interest in "same-day" IUD insertion following unprotected intercourse, particularly better educated young women and those who had a prior unwanted pregnancy [15].

Furthermore, IUDs are unaffected by BMI, timing of unprotected intercourse, or additional sex after IUD placement. Figure 1 shows the window of action of different emergency contraceptive methods in relation to ovulation.

3.2. Insertion-Related Aspect. The IUD is an extremely safe method but requires placement by an appropriately trained health care provider. Placement may often be difficult and present a challenge especially in adolescent and nulliparous women or it is required by physicians with limited experience. In a study of women who were scheduled for IUD insertion for EC, 19% had a failed insertion, meaning that the provider was unable to insert the IUD and these women received oral

EC instead [16]. There are however a number of practical points which could help in facilitating insertion. Information should be provided about the insertion procedure and measures taken to reduce discomfort associated with IUD insertion. Also information about the benefits and risks of IUD use should be given. Attention to comfort is very important as many women may refuse an IUD purely because of fear for pain. Insertion pain cannot be predicted. Ultrasonography does not give additional information to predict pain. According to Kaislasuo et al., dysmenorrhea is the only predictor of severe or intolerable insertion pain due to increased uterine/cervical contractility [17]. Utilizing means of sufficient analgesia, especially in nulliparous women, is important. Equally important is an appropriate patient-friendly setting accommodated with soft ambient light. Not to be forgotten is the use of a narrow and short speculum in young women to facilitate access to the cervix. A 1.0–1.5 cm wide speculum is sometimes necessary in young women. A too large speculum often causes more pain than the IUD insertion procedure. Listening to music during the procedure decreases procedural pain [18].

The injection of a small amount of lidocaine or mepivacaine in the anterior lip of the cervix before placement of (preferably) atraumatic forceps is a good habit, especially if the patient is anxious, or if slow closing of the Allis forceps causes pain, or prior to placement of a toothed forceps (e.g., Pozzi forceps). The use of a dental syringe with extrafine needle is highly practical and can also be used for local or locoregional anesthesia.

After disinfection and gentle straightening of the uterus, a "cotton swab test" (soaked in antiseptic solution) can be performed to test the tightness of the internal cervical os and to obtain information on pain sensation. If the test provokes severe pain, additional local anesthesia can be provided prior to sounding the uterus.

Many believe that the use of misoprostol greatly facilitates IUD insertion as it dilates the cervix [19]. We recommend the use of 200–400 μg of misoprostol, orally or vaginally, 3 hours before IUD insertion. Others prefer to place the tablets vaginally in the posterior fornix the night before the procedure (9–12 hours before) but one hour sublingually before placement of the IUD may also be a good alternative (unpublished observations). Despite conflicting published data about the benefits of misoprostol, significant differences were found in nulliparous women between groups using misoprostol, 400 μg vaginally, 4 hours before insertion, compared to placebo with less difficulty and less moderate-to-severe pain at IUD insertion [20]. It may be that the vaginal route could be preferable as plasma concentrations of misoprostol remain substantially higher than that when administered by the oral or sublingual routes. However, most women prefer the oral route to vaginal application [21]. It is recommended that a nonsteroidal analgesic should be added to reduce its prostaglandin-mediated side effects and uterine cramping. Some physicians claim that applying heat to the lower abdomen (using electric heating pad or a microwave-heated cherry seed pillow) may significantly reduce painful sensations [22]. If the patient is having severe discomfort with the insertion of the sound or requires cervical dilation,

then the administration of a paracervical block or even conscious sedation (such as propofol or midazolam) can be used. However, this is rarely necessary and perhaps only in extremely anxious women.

3.3. Safety of Intrauterine Devices. The risk of pelvic infection, which may lead to infertility, ectopic pregnancy, and chronic pelvic pain, remains one of the major concerns of IUD providers as well as of women. There is good scientific evidence that the risk of pelvic inflammatory disease (PID) is not increased after the first month following insertion of the IUD. Investigations by WHO showed that the risk of PID is limited to the first 20 days after insertion [23]. Cervicitis at the time of insertion is not absolute contraindication and patients can be treated and the IUD is placed as the risk of developing pelvic inflammatory disease remains very low.

Many practitioners however remain concerned about PID, especially in higher risk populations. WHO suggests that the benefits of IUDs generally outweigh the risks in women of any age, whether parous or not, and that IUDs can be inserted in women younger than 20, provided that these women are at low risk of sexually transmitted infections. Rates of PID may vary between 0.6 and 1.6 per 1000 woman-years [23]. However, WHO also advises against the use of IUDs in women who have had PID in the previous 3 months [24]. ACOG recommends screening all adolescents at the time of or before IUD insertion. A practical solution is to test all high risk patients and to place the IUD on the same day. If the test results are positive, then treatment should be administered immediately (a single oral dose of 1 g of azithromycin or 2 × 100 mg of oral doxycycline for 7 days). Women who develop symptoms of PID after IUD insertion can be safely treated with antibiotics without removing the IUD.

3.4. Dimensional Aspects Related to IUD Use. Despite the fact that many women would select an IUD for EC if an IUD was proposed to them, the continuation rates in those who selected the IUD are rather poor. In a study conducted in the US using TCu380A (ParaGard), approximately 40% of IUDs were removed during the first year due to side effects indicating the need for newer IUD designs and better tolerated IUDs [25].

Researchers have stressed the importance of an optimal interrelationship between the IUD and the uterine cavity for many decades in an attempt to have fewer side effects and greater acceptability [26]. They found that pain and abnormal bleeding during use of the IUD is related to the disparity between the size of the uterine cavity and that of the IUD. The width of the uterine cavity appeared to be most important in relation to IUD side effects. In a study in Finland conducted on 165 young nulliparous women, the uterine cavity width was measured with 3D ultrasound and found a *median* transverse fundal diameter of the uterine cavity of 24.4 mm. One hundred and one (62.7%) women had a transverse diameter at the fundus of less than 24.4 mm (Table 3). Thus, a very large segment of the female population have substantially smaller uterine widths. The smallest diameter observed in the study was 13.8 mm [27]. Figure 2 illustrates

TABLE 1: Fundal transverse diameter (mm) in 165 Finnish nulliparous women [6].

	Range	50th percentile measure	No (%) under 50th percentile
Fundal width (mm)	13.8–35.0	24.4	101 (62.7)

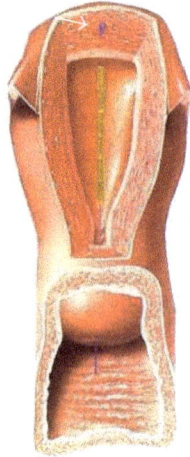

FIGURE 2: Illustration of the frameless GyneFix IUD anchored in the fundus of the uterus (see arrow). The anchoring knot is inserted in the fundus with a specially designed inserter.

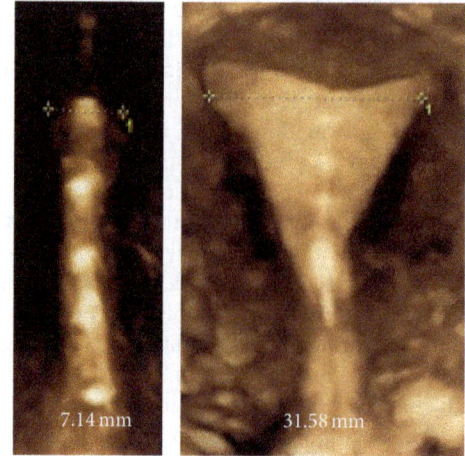

FIGURE 3: 3D illuatration in two women fitted with a frameless IUD showing the disparity in width of the IUD which varies in these women between 7.14 and 31.58 mm.

the frameless IUD inserted in the uterus and Figure 3 shows the disparity in cavity width in two nulliparous women.

The great disparity in size and shape of the uterine cavity in nulliparous women is shown in Table 1.

The mean transverse uterine cavity dimension in nulliparous women is far less than the length of the transverse arm of most conventional IUDs (e.g., ParaGard), which is 32 mm, resulting often in distortion, displacement, embedment, and expulsion of the IUD. In order to circumvent this spatial incompatibility, researchers adapted T-shaped IUDs. It was found that the fundal transverse dimension is of paramount importance with respect to IUD acceptance, as women tolerated the IUD much better [28]. An optimal IUD-cavity relationship also promotes IUD retention and stability while minimizing endometrial/myometrial trauma.

Frameless copper IUDs could be the optimal design from a dimensional point of view. The copper 330 frameless IUD has been used with good results in EC studies [6]. Due to its absence of a horizontal transverse arm and its flexibility, the device adapts to uterine cavities of every size and shape. These characteristics eliminate the ability of the uterus to exert expulsive forces on frameless IUDs, in contrast to that seen with the framed T-shape designed IUDs, and result in high efficacy, low expulsion rate, reduced bleeding, reduced or no pain complaints, long duration of action, and most importantly long-term comfort. The design characteristics of the frameless IUD would be attractive as a first choice method for many women and for young

women requesting EC, especially for those with a small (e.g., nulliparous women) or distorted uterine cavity, and for women who have experienced problems with framed IUDs. The one-dimensional design of the frameless LNG-IUS explains its high acceptability and high continuation of use (over 90% at 5 years) [29, 30]. Figure 3 illustrates the dimensional compatibility even in women with very narrow uterine cavities.

The small size of the frameless IUD also results in a reduced effect on the amount of menstrual blood lost. It does not significantly increase menstrual blood loss, as may occur with framed IUDs due to its overall small size. This is important as heavy menstrual bleeding is the most common reason for IUD discontinuation. Table 2 is a short list of questions which are relevant to patients requesting EC.

4. Conclusion

Adolescents and young nulliparous women are the groups that are most likely to be EC users. Yet, they are the least well-informed groups about EC in general and the use of an IUD for EC in particular. This paper offers practical information which may be helpful to choose the best option for women. Figure 1 could be used as a poster for health care providers as well as women as it clearly visualizes the fertility risk and window of action of different methods of emergency contraception.

Key Message Points

(i) In real life, IUDs are much more effective than the pill, contraceptive patch, and vaginal ring, especially in young women.

(ii) The copper IUD is the most effective method for EC, significantly more effective than oral EC.

(iii) A copper IUD can be inserted up to 5 days after unprotected intercourse or 5 days after the calculated

TABLE 2: Short questionnaire to help select the EC method for the individual patient.

Question	Comment
(1) Which contraceptive method did you use up to now?	The pill, contraceptive patch, and the vaginal ring have a typical failure rate of 9% during the first year of use.
(2) When did your last menstrual period start?	Calculating the expected date of ovulation is important to select the EC method.
(3) When did you have unprotected sex?	All oral EC methods can be used up to day 10–12 of the menstrual cycle with preference for UPA close to ovulation. Oral ECs may not be safe 1 or 2 days before ovulation and are not effective after ovulation.
(4) Do you want to use a long-acting method of contraception?	An IUD should be the method of choice because of its high EC efficacy and ongoing protection.
(5) Do you have a stable relationship?	Women in a stable relationship have a low risk whilst women having sexual relations with different partners over the last month are at higher risk.
(6) Have you been treated for a sexually transmitted disease over the past 3 months?	IUD insertion may be performed immediately following screening tests and antibiotics should be prescribed if tests are positive.

TABLE 3: Uterine width measured by ultrasound in 165 nulliparous women. Note wide in uterine width as the high number of women with a uterine cavity less than 24 mm [28].

	Range	50th percentile measure	N (%) under 50th percentile
Fundal width (mm)	13.8–35.0 mm	24.4 mm	101 (62.7)

ovulation day or anytime in the cycle if a high sensitivity pregnancy test is negative.

(iv) Copper IUDs are effective regardless of overweight or obesity and frequency of intercourse in the cycle.

(v) IUDs provide long-term contraception but not all IUDs fit in young nulliparous and adolescent women.

(vi) Women are interested in safe, effective, well-tolerated, and long-acting contraception; the frameless IUD would appeal to them as its acceptability is high.

(vii) Clinicians who lack training for IUD insertion should refer women requesting an IUD in a timely manner.

Disclosure

Dr. Dirk Wildemeersch has been involved in the optimization of new, innovative, drug delivery systems for use in the uterus. He is currently advisor in devising new concepts in controlled release for contraception, gynecological treatment, and prevention of infectious diseases.

Conflict of Interests

Dr. Norman D. Goldstuck has no conflict of interests regarding the publication of this paper.

References

[1] C. B. Polis, K. Schaffer, K. Blanchard, A. Glasier, C. C. Harper, and D. A. Grimes, "Advance provision of emergency contraception for pregnancy prevention (full review)," *The Cochrane Database of Systematic Reviews*, no. 2, Article ID CD005497, 2007.

[2] A. Glasier, S. T. Cameron, D. Blithe et al., "Can we identify women at risk of pregnancy despite using emergency contraception? Data from randomized trials of ulipristal acetate and levonorgestrel," *Contraception*, vol. 84, no. 4, pp. 363–367, 2011.

[3] G. Noé, H. B. Croxatto, A. M. Salvatierra et al., "Contraceptive efficacy of emergency contraception with levonorgestrel given before or after ovulation," *Contraception*, vol. 84, no. 5, pp. 486–492, 2011.

[4] N. Kapp, J. L. Abitbol, H. Mathé et al., "Effect of body weight and BMI on the efficacy of levonorgestrel emergency contraception," *Contraception*, vol. 91, no. 2, pp. 97–104, 2015.

[5] HRA Pharma UK, EllaOne: summary of product characteristics, 2011, http://www.medicines.org.uk/EMC/medicine/22280/SPC/ellaOne+30+mg/.

[6] R. E. D'Souza, T. Masters, W. Bounds, and J. Guillebaud, "Randomised controlled trial assessing the acceptability of GyneFix versus Gyne-T380S for emergency contraception," *Journal of Family Planning and Reproductive Health Care*, vol. 29, no. 2, pp. 23–29, 2003.

[7] A. I. Dermish and D. K. Turok, "The copper intrauterine device for emergency contraception: an opportunity to provide the optimal emergency contraception method and transition to highly effective contraception," *Expert Review of Medical Devices*, vol. 10, no. 4, pp. 477–488, 2013.

[8] M. E. Ortiz and H. B. Croxatto, "Copper-T intrauterine device and levonorgestrel intrauterine system: biological bases of their mechanism of action," *Contraception*, vol. 75, no. 6, supplement, pp. S16–S30, 2007.

[9] K. Cleland, H. Zhu, N. Goldstuck, L. Cheng, and J. Trussell, "The efficacy of intrauterine devices for emergency contraception: a systematic review of 35 years of experience," *Human Reproduction*, vol. 27, no. 7, pp. 1994–2000, 2012.

[10] D. R. Mishell Jr., "Intrauterine devices: mechanisms of action, safety, and efficacy," *Contraception*, vol. 58, no. 3, pp. 45S–53S, 1998.

[11] A. J. Wilcox, D. D. Baird, and C. R. Weinberg, "Time of implantation of the conceptus and loss of pregnancy," *The New England Journal of Medicine*, vol. 340, no. 23, pp. 1796–1799, 1999.

[12] N. D. Goldstuck, "Emergency contraception: history, methods, mechanisms, misconceptions and a philosophical evaluation," *Gynecology & Obstetrics*, vol. 4, no. 5, 2014.

[13] N. D. Goldstuck, "Delayed postcoital IUD insertion," *Contraceptive Delivery Systems*, vol. 4, no. 4, pp. 293–296, 1983.

[14] D. K. Turok, E. M. Godfrey, D. Wojdyla, A. Dermish, L. Torres, and S. C. Wu, "Copper T380 intrauterine device for emergency contraception: highly effective at any time in the menstrual cycle," *Human Reproduction*, vol. 28, no. 10, pp. 2672–2676, 2013.

[15] E. B. Schwarz, M. Kavanaugh, E. Douglas, T. Dubowitz, and M. D. Creinin, "Interest in intrauterine contraception among seekers of emergency contraception and pregnancy testing," *Obstetrics and Gynecology*, vol. 113, no. 4, pp. 833–839, 2009.

[16] A. I. Dermish, D. K. Turok, J. C. Jacobson, M. E. S. Flores, M. McFadden, and K. Burke, "Failed IUD insertions in community practice: an under-recognized problem?" *Contraception*, vol. 87, no. 2, pp. 182–186, 2013.

[17] J. Kaislasuo, O. Heikinheimo, P. Lähteenmäki, and S. Suhonen, "Predicting painful or difficult intrauterine device insertion in nulligravid women," *Obstetrics & Gynecology*, vol. 124, no. 2, pp. 345–353, 2014.

[18] R. Angioli, C. De Cicco Nardone, F. Plotti et al., "Use of music to reduce anxiety during office hysteroscopy: prospective randomized trial," *Journal of Minimally Invasive Gynecology*, vol. 21, no. 3, pp. 454–459, 2014.

[19] K. Ward, J. C. Jacobson, D. K. Turok, and P. A. Murphy, "A survey of provider experience with misoprostol to facilitate intrauterine device insertion in nulliparous women," *Contraception*, vol. 84, no. 6, pp. 594–599, 2011.

[20] A. Scavuzzi, A. S. R. Souza, A. A. R. Costa, and M. M. R. Amorim, "Misoprostol prior to inserting an intrauterine device in nulligravidas: a randomized clinical trial," *Human Reproduction*, vol. 28, no. 8, pp. 2118–2125, 2013.

[21] C. Arvidsson, M. Hellborg, and K. Gemzell-Danielsson, "Preference and acceptability of oral versus vaginal administration of misoprostol in medical abortion with mifepristone," *European Journal of Obstetrics & Gynecology and Reproductive Biology*, vol. 123, no. 1, pp. 87–91, 2005.

[22] M. D. Akin, K. W. Weingand, D. A. Hengehold, M. B. Goodale, R. T. Hinkle, and R. P. Smith, "Continuous low-level topical heat in the treatment of dysmenorrhea," *Obstetrics & Gynecology*, vol. 97, no. 3, pp. 343–349, 2001.

[23] T. M. M. Farley, M. J. Rosenberg, P. J. Rowe, J.-H. Chen, and O. Meirik, "Intrauterine devices and pelvic inflammatory disease: an international perspective," *The Lancet*, vol. 339, no. 8796, pp. 785–788, 1992.

[24] World Health Organization, *Medical Eligibility Criteria for Contraceptive Use*, World Health Organization, 4th edition, 2010, http://whqlibdoc.who.int/publications/2010/9789241563888_eng.pdf.

[25] D. K. Turok, S. E. Gurtcheff, E. Handley, S. E. Simonsen, C. Sok, and P. Murphy, "A pilot study of the Copper T380A IUD and oral levonorgestrel for emergency contraception," *Contraception*, vol. 82, no. 6, pp. 520–525, 2010.

[26] S. Tejuja and P. K. Malkani, "Clinical significance of correlation between size of uterine cavity and IUCD: a study by planimeter-hysterogram technique," *The American Journal of Obstetrics and Gynecology*, vol. 105, no. 4, pp. 620–627, 1969.

[27] J. Kaislasuo, O. Heikinheimo, P. Lähteenmäki, and S. Suhonen, "Predicting painful or difficult intrauterine device insertion in nulligravid women," *Obstetrics and Gynecology*, vol. 124, no. 2, pp. 345–353, 2014.

[28] K. H. Kurz, "Cavimeter uterine measurements and IUD clinical correlation," in *Intrauterine Contraception: Advances and Future Prospects*, G. I. Zatuchni, A. Goldsmith, and J. J. Sciarra, Eds., pp. 142–162, Harper & Row, Philadelphia, Pa, USA, 1984.

[29] D. Wildemeersch, A. Pett, S. Jandi, T. Hasskamp, P. Rowe, and M. Vrijens, "Precision intrauterine contraception may significantly increase continuation of use: a review of long-term clinical experience with frameless copper-releasing intrauterine contraception devices," *International Journal of Women's Health*, vol. 5, no. 1, pp. 215–225, 2013.

[30] D. Wildemeersch, S. Jandi, A. Pett, K. Nolte, T. Hasskamp, and M. Vrijens, "Use of frameless intrauterine devices and systems in young nulliparous and adolescent women: results of a multicenter study," *International Journal of Women's Health*, vol. 6, pp. 727–734, 2014.

22

Cattle Uterus: A Novel Animal Laboratory Model for Advanced Hysteroscopic Surgery Training

Ayman A. A. Ewies and Zahid R. Khan

Department of Obstetrics and Gynaecology, Birmingham City Hospital, Birmingham, West Midlands B18 7QH, UK

Correspondence should be addressed to Ayman A. A. Ewies; aymanewies@hotmail.com

Academic Editor: Thomas Herzog

In recent years, due to reduced training opportunities, the major shift in surgical training is towards the use of simulation and animal laboratories. Despite the merits of Virtual Reality Simulators, they are far from representing the real challenges encountered in theatres. We introduce the "Cattle Uterus Model" in the hope that it will be adopted in training courses as a low cost and easy-to-set-up tool. It adds new dimensions to the advanced hysteroscopic surgery training experience by providing tactile sensation and simulating intraoperative difficulties. It complements conventional surgical training, aiming to maximise clinical exposure and minimise patients' harm.

1. Introduction

Advanced hysteroscopic surgical procedures such as transcervical resection of endometrium (TCRE), transcervical resection of polyp (TCRP), transcervical resection of fibroid (TCRF), and septum resection are minimally invasive procedures which have a slow learning curve and a narrow margin for error. Good training is conducive to sound practice, and the gynaecological surgeon will ultimately grasp the skills, hand-eye coordination, and manual dexterity to enable competent performance of these procedures in a shorter operating time [1].

Traditionally, surgical training in hysteroscopy takes place in the operating room where trainees first observe the procedure performed and then take on increasing roles in surgical cases under direct supervision [2]. However, the time required to perfect the required skills is no longer available to current generations of trainees given their overall shorter training period. With the implementation of the European Working Time Directive (EWTD), trainees in obstetrics and gynaecology now work a maximum of 48 hours per week, approximately half that of their predecessors, thus limiting their exposure to surgical procedures. Therefore, to minimise patient's harm and maximise surgical exposure, trainers are obliged to use other methods that replace real experience with ones that evoke or replicate substantial aspects of the real world in a fully interactive manner such as simulation or animal laboratories [3]. As early as 1927, Mayo, one of the founders of the renowned Mayo Clinic, argued that "there is no excuse for the surgeon to learn on the patients" [4]. The logical sequence of events is that one has to crawl before he or she can walk; therefore, skills need to be performed well and practiced thoroughly before one contemplates doing them on patients [1].

Apart from the "Pig Bladder Model" for training of basic hysteroscopic surgical skills and VersaPoint polypectomy [2], there is a paucity of soft tissue models that could be used for training of procedures such as TCRE, TCRP, TCRF, and septum resection. In this paper, we introduce the "Cattle Uterus Model" for advanced hysteroscopic surgery training in the hope that it will be adopted in various training courses in the UK and worldwide.

2. Materials and Methods

2.1. The Cattle Uterus

2.1.1. Anatomy. The cattle uterus consists of a septate uterine body which is 4 to 5 cm long and two uterine horns 15 to

25 cm in length each (Figure 1). The uterus is suspended by the broad ligament in a coiled or curled manner. Each horn has its own oviduct. There is only one cervix which has 3–5 muscular cartilaginous transverse annular folds [5].

2.1.2. Why Did We Choose the Cattle Uterus? On exploring available options, various animals' uteri were considered inappropriate either because of the small size or having an anatomy which does not fit the purpose. The pig uterus, for example, consists mainly of two long horns 60–90 cm in length each with a small uterine body at the junction of both horns [6]. The advantages of using the cattle uterus as an animal laboratory model for the purpose of advanced hysteroscopic surgery training are the similarity in size of the uterine body with the human uterus, the realistic tissue resistance and tactile sensation that created a genuine training model which cannot be provided by the "Pig Bladder" model or simulation, and the presence of a uterine septum that allows training in septum resection, a surgical skill that is difficult to obtain given its rarity of occurrence in human.

2.1.3. Supply. The cattle uteri are supplied by Wetlab-Medmeat (Kenilworth, Warwickshire, UK) which provides various types of tissue to aid surgical simulation. The products are derived from healthy animals which are intended for human consumption and humanely slaughtered in abattoirs in accordance with European Economic Community (EEC) regulations. These regulations under The Animal Health Veterinary Laboratories Agency (AHVLA) and EEC regulation 142/2011 allow for providing animal tissue material for educational purposes [7].

2.2. Developing the "Cattle Uterus Model". The skills to perform advanced hysteroscopic surgery are often acquired by attending workshops that comprise didactic lectures and hands-on components with the aim of improving theoretical knowledge, enhancing clinical judgment, and initiating and upscaling manual dexterity [1]. We organised a three-day international hands-on advanced hysteroscopic surgery workshop at the Sandwell and West Birmingham Hospitals NHS Trust, UK. 14 consultants and senior trainees in gynaecology from the United Kingdom and overseas attended the workshop.

The "Cattle Uterus Model" was used for the first time where every candidate was trained on one uterus. The two uterine horns were clamped as close as possible to the uterine body using adjustable cable ties. The cervical canal of all uteri was wider than 10 mm; therefore, similar cable tie was used to squeeze the cervix to be fluid tight. Each uterus was fixed to a purpose built plastic crate using Allis forceps (Figures 2(a)–2(d)). The setup was then placed on top of a table with a pail below it to allow the saline to drain. The GYNECARE VERSAPOINT Bipolar Electrosurgery System (model number 00482, Cardiff, UK) and Olympus VISERA Elite Stack System (model number OTV-S190, Hamburg, Germany) were used to perform endometrial and septal resection.

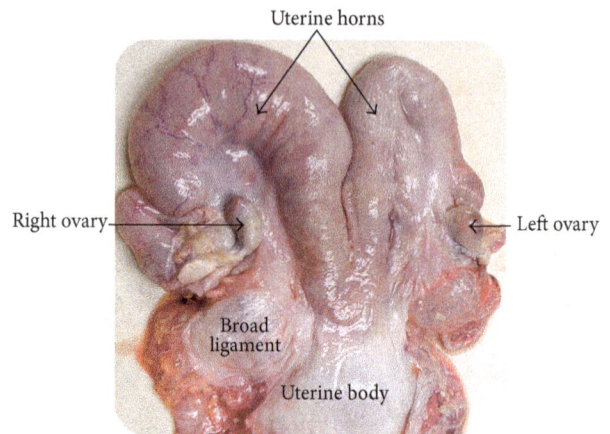

FIGURE 1: The anatomy of the cattle uterus.

3. Results

Candidates attending the course completed feedback questionnaires to provide an overall score (poor, average, good, or excellent) for each station and also to elaborate with free comments. Simulation of endometrial and septal resection using the "Cattle Uterus Model" turned out to be the most popular station and was rated excellent by 13 candidates and good by one. This was markedly better than Virtual Reality Simulator, which was rated as excellent and good by six and eight candidates, respectively. The free comments indicated that the participants favored the model that provided them with "a real feel of how it works."

4. Comment

The "Cattle Uterus Model" offers a realistic platform to develop eye-hand-foot coordination and manual dexterity skills necessary for advanced hysteroscopic surgery. In addition, it offers simulated intraoperative difficulties for real-life events, for example, obscuration of vision due to floating endometrial chips or debris, overhang of the tissue to the wire loop, or saline bubbling. This allows trainees to practice useful manoeuvres to deal with them, for example, to flush out the debris by controlling the output channel and to remove bubbles by placing the scope into the bubble and opening the outflow channel. The only disadvantage of this model, and other animal laboratory models, is that they do not simulate the *in vivo* human condition as regards bleeding [1]. Therefore, we recommend it as a complement to the conventional surgical training and not as a substitute for apprenticeship or experience.

The traditional system of apprenticeship learning offers training under supervision in operating theatres allowing valuable one-to-one practical tuition in real-life situations. However, the implementation of EWTD for junior doctors decreased surgical exposure, which may present risks to the patients when the least experienced surgeon infrequently performs critical procedures using electrosurgery. Furthermore, there is evidence to suggest that teaching trainees in the

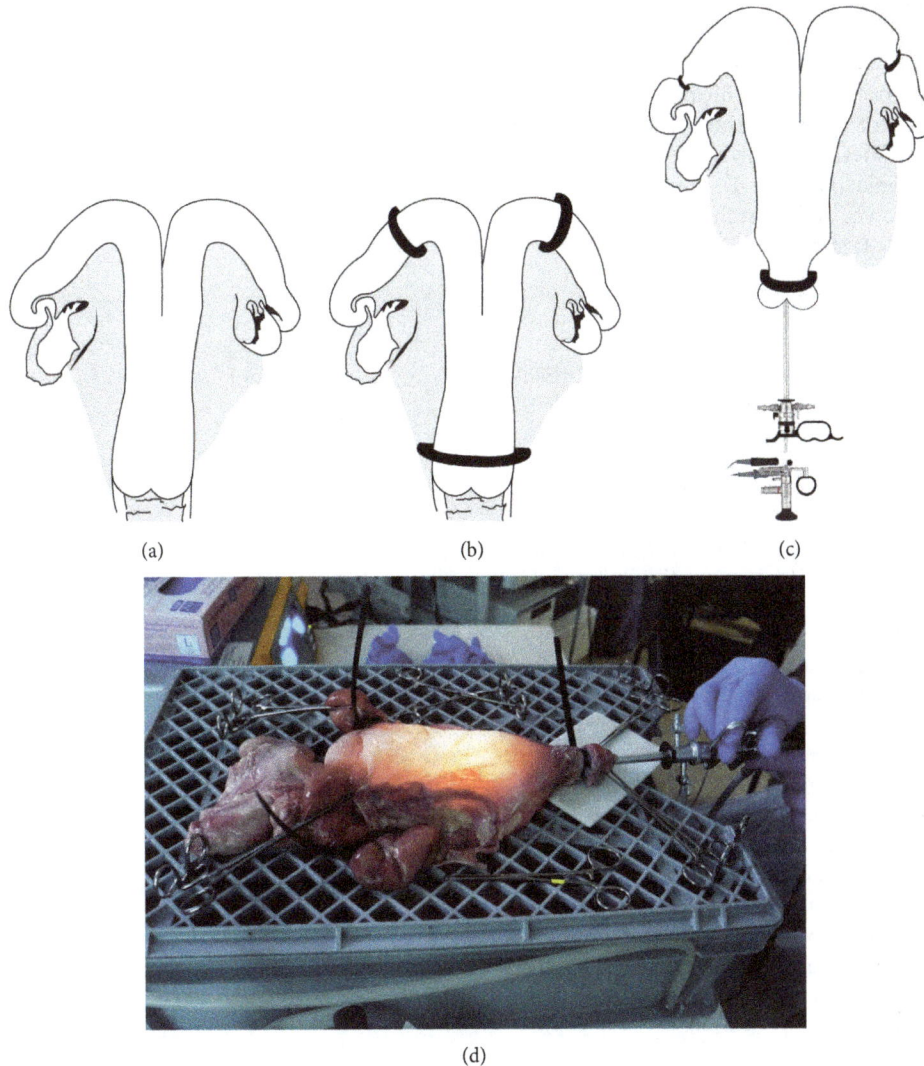

FIGURE 2: A diagram illustrating the shape of the cattle uterus and the site of placement of the 3 adjustable cable ties.

operating room is challenging in terms of operating time and financial cost [1].

Visual Reality Simulators are used by the airline industry and military as well as in many medical specialties to educate, evaluate, and prepare for life-threatening scenarios [1]. They allow the opportunity for repeated practice, feedback, and ability to learn without causing harm. In addition, they are valuable in objectively scoring the trainee and assessing the learning curve with good reliability, validity, and cost-effectiveness [1, 2]. Nonetheless, in hysteroscopic surgery training, it is far from being realistic in terms of the inability to replicate actual tissue elasticity, resistance, and tactile sensation [2].

The Royal College of Obstetricians and Gynaecologists (RCOG) has implemented a structured "Advanced Training Skills Module" in hysteroscopic surgery, which has set several criteria for training and accreditation. It aims for senior trainees who would like to develop special interest in advanced hysteroscopic surgery. Hand-on workshops must

be an integral part of professional development in advanced hysteroscopic surgery, and certainly the RCOG recommends that trainees attend such workshops as part of module completion [8]. We believe that using the "Cattle Uterus Model" will facilitate rapid acquiring of the necessary skills so that the trainees are able to finish the module within the proposed 12-month duration.

Condensation

The "Cattle Uterus Model" offers a realistic platform for hands-on training in advanced hysteroscopic surgery, enabling efficient attainment of high level competency.

Conflict of Interests

The authors declare that there is no conflict of interests regarding the publication of this paper.

Acknowledgments

The authors would like to thank Mr. Jim Ng, Advanced Theatre Practitioner, Sandwell and West Birmingham Hospitals NHS Teaching Trust, for his effort and support to develop this training model. They would like also to thank Mrs. Amie Bebbington, Senior Graphic Designer, The Illustration Department, Sandwell and West Birmingham Hospitals NHS, for producing the first draft of Figures 2(a)–2(c).

References

[1] M. Erian, G. McLaren, and A. Erian, "Advanced hysteroscopic surgery training," *Journal of the Society of Laparoendoscopic Surgeons*, vol. 18, no. 4, pp. 1–7, 2014.

[2] Y. W. Ng and Y. F. Fong, "Get 'real' with hysteroscopy using the pig bladder: a 'uterine' model for hysteroscopy training," *Annals of the Academy of Medicine*, vol. 42, no. 1, pp. 18–23, 2013.

[3] Z. Ramsey-Marcelle, A. Chase, S. Okolo, D. Hamilton-Fairley, and W. Yoong, "Making simulation stimulating: how to set up a simulation workshop," *The Obstetrician & Gynaecologist*, vol. 13, no. 4, pp. 253–257, 2011.

[4] W. J. Mayo, "Medical education for the general practitioner," *The Journal of the American Medical Association*, vol. 88, no. 18, pp. 1377–1379, 1927.

[5] A. Warnick, *Anatomy and Endocrinology of Cow Reproduction*, 2015, http://www.fao.org/Wairdocs/ILRI/x5442E/x5442e04.htm.

[6] W. Singleton and M. Diekman, *Reproductive Physiology and Anatomy of the Sow*, 2015, http://www.ansc.purdue.edu/swine/porkpage/repro/physiol/reppaper.htm.

[7] Wetlab-Medical-Tissue, "Tissue Supply," 2014, http://wetlab.co.uk/instruments_and_supplies/tissue_supply.aspx.

[8] RCOG, *Benign Gynaecological Surgery: Hysteroscopy Advanced Training Skills Module*, 2015, https://www.rcog.org.uk/globalassets/documents/careers-and-training/atsms/atsm_benigngynae-surgery_curriculum.pdf.

23

Fertility and Symptom Relief following Robot-Assisted Laparoscopic Myomectomy

Michael C. Pitter,[1] **Serene S. Srouji,**[2] **Antonio R. Gargiulo,**[2] **Leslie Kardos,**[3]
Usha Seshadri-Kreaden,[4] **Helen B. Hubert,**[5] **and Glenn A. Weitzman**[6]

[1]*Department of Obstetrics & Gynecology, Columbia University Medical Center, New York, NY 10032, USA*
[2]*Department of Obstetrics and Gynecology, Center for Infertility and Reproductive Surgery, Brigham and Women's Hospital,*
 Harvard Medical School, 75 Francis Street, Boston, MA 02115, USA
[3]*Department of Obstetrics and Gynecology, California Pacific Medical Center, 475 Brannan Street, San Francisco, CA 94107, USA*
[4]*Department of Clinical Affairs, Intuitive Surgical Inc., 1266 Kifer Road, Building 101, Sunnyvale, CA 94086, USA*
[5]*Stanford University School of Medicine Emerita, 1043 Oakland Avenue, Menlo Park, CA 94025, USA*
[6]*Nashville Fertility Center, 345 23rd Avenue, Nashville, TN 37203, USA*

Correspondence should be addressed to Michael C. Pitter; mp3422@cumc.columbia.edu

Academic Editor: Gian Carlo Di Renzo

Objective. To examine success of robot-assisted laparoscopic myomectomy (RALM) measured by sustained symptom relief and fertility. *Methods.* This is a retrospective survey of 426 women who underwent RALM for fibroids, symptom relief, or infertility at three practice sites across the US. We examined rates of symptom recurrence and pregnancy and factors associated with these outcomes. *Results.* Overall, 70% of women reported being symptom-free, with 62.9% free of symptoms after three years. At >3 years, 66.7% of women who underwent surgery to treat infertility and 80% who were also symptom-free reported achieving pregnancy. Factors independently associated with symptom recurrence included greater time after surgery, preoperative dyspareunia, multiple fibroid surgeries, smoking after surgery, and preexisting diabetes. Factors positively correlated with achieving pregnancy included desiring pregnancy, prior pregnancy, greater time since surgery, and Caucasian race. Factors negatively correlated with pregnancy were advanced age and symptom recurrence. *Conclusions.* This paper, the first to examine symptom recurrence after RALM, demonstrates both short- and long-term effectiveness in providing symptom relief. Furthermore, RALM may have the potential to improve the chance of conception, even in a population at high risk of subfertility, with greater benefits among those who remain symptom-free. These findings require prospective validation.

1. Introduction

Myomas are benign tumors of the smooth muscle cells of the myometrium. The incidence of myomas increases with age, reaching 40–60% of women by age 35 [1]. Although some myomas are asymptomatic, others can cause bleeding, pain, urinary symptoms, and subfertility, leading women to seek treatment. Myomectomy serves as an effective, fertility-preserving option for the surgical treatment of uterine leiomyomas, although its precise role in enhancing fertility remains controversial [2].

Conventional laparoscopic myomectomy (LM) provides a minimally invasive alternative and results in reduced blood loss, incidence of fever, hospital stay, and convalescence time when compared to abdominal myomectomy (AM); with similar symptom relief and pregnancy outcomes [3, 4] there are surgical challenges associated with LM that have limited patient eligibility and widespread adoption [5].

In 2005, the Food and Drug Administration approved the da Vinci Surgical System for gynecologic indications (Intuitive Surgical, Inc., Sunnyvale, CA, USA). Surgical ergonomics, high definition 3-dimensional vision, and wrist-like flexibility of the instrumentation expanded the range and complexity of cases that could be reliably completed laparoscopically. A recent meta-analysis reported significant short-term benefits with robot-assisted laparoscopic myomectomy

(RALM) when compared to AM, including reduced blood loss, fewer blood transfusions and fevers, and a reduced hospital stay [6].

However, long-term outcomes following RALM, in particular symptom recurrence and pregnancy rates, have received little attention thus far. Fertility following RALM has been reported only in a few small case series [7–9]. Pitter et al. [10] studied outcomes of pregnant women following RALM in a large patient series but made no reference to women who did not achieve pregnancy. Thus, no pregnancy rates or correlates of success could be determined. The objective of this large patient study was to determine the long-term success of myomectomy as measured by rates of symptom relief and pregnancy over time, as well as factors associated with the recurrence of symptoms and the likelihood of achieving pregnancy following RALM.

2. Methods

This multicenter study included investigators and participants from three gynecology practices in the northeast, southeast, and western US. One practice specialized in treating infertility (Nashville Fertility Center, GW) while the other two larger academic centers (Newark Beth Israel Medical Center, MP; California Pacific Medical Center, KL) provided all gynecologic care.

2.1. Ethical Approval. This study was conducted according to the Declaration of Helsinki for Medical Research Involving Human Subjects. The Institutional Review Board at each of the sites approved the study design and execution.

2.2. Participants. All women who had previously undergone RALM under the supervision of any one of the investigators were eligible to participate in the study. Eligible patients with current phone numbers were contacted and given an explanation about the study and what participation would entail. Women who consented were then emailed a link to the structured survey or, if preferred, sent a hard copy of the instrument by post, along with unique subject and site identification numbers. Nonrespondents were contacted a maximum of two more times, either electronically or by phone, and were again asked to participate. The study purpose, maintenance of confidentiality, and consent via questionnaire completion were further discussed on an introductory page of the survey.

2.3. Data Collection. Patients who had RALM between August 2005 and November 2013 were contacted to participate. Surveys were completed during a 9-month period between September 2013 and May 2014. MarketTools (http://www.markettools.com) administered the online survey, and paper forms were later transcribed into the online database. All information was downloaded from the website and stored in a secure, encrypted database. Only deidentified data were collected and investigators and research staff alone were permitted access.

Information was collected on each patient's primary reason for undergoing myomectomy: to treat symptoms with no intention of becoming pregnant, to treat symptoms with the possibility of becoming pregnant in the future, or to improve the current chance of pregnancy. Additional variables of interest included patient information and sociodemographic characteristics at the time of survey completion (months since the myomectomy, age, height, weight, and ethnicity), status prior to myomectomy (smoking status, preexisting medical conditions, pregnancies and their outcomes, attempted pregnancy without success, infertility treatments, symptoms or conditions that caused patients to seek treatment, and prior surgery for fibroids), and postsurgical information (smoking status, time waited before attempting pregnancy, achieved pregnancy and outcomes, time until achieving pregnancy, use of fertility interventions, complications of pregnancy, and symptom or condition recurrence).

2.4. Statistical Analysis. Analyses were performed on completed surveys only, although skipped questions were permissible. Data were stratified into three groups defined by each participant's primary reason for undergoing myomectomy: group 1: to treat symptoms with no intention of becoming pregnant, group 2: to treat symptoms with the possibility of becoming pregnant in the future, and group 3: to improve the current chance of pregnancy. Using this stratification, variables were described by means and standard deviations or percentages, as appropriate. Analyses, further stratified by respondents' time since myomectomy, included rates of symptom remission (groups 1, 2, and 3) and pregnancy (groups 2 and 3 only). Tests for trends in the percentage of women who were symptom-free over time and the percentage of women who achieved pregnancy over time were conducted using a Cochrane-Armitage trend test. Multivariable forward stepwise logistic regression was used to identify patient sociodemographic factors, preexisting conditions, and other pre- and postmyomectomy characteristics significantly associated (two-sided $P < 0.05$) with symptom recurrence and, for groups 2 and 3, achieving pregnancy. Results are described using the odds ratio (OR) and 95% confidence interval (95% CI). All analyses were done using SAS version 9.2.1 (SAS Inc., Cary NC).

3. Results

3.1. Survey Response Rate. Invitations to participate were extended to 852 women who had undergone RALM and had current phone numbers; 59.0% requested to complete the survey online and 41.0% preferred paper forms that were sent and returned by post. The survey response rate was 50%; thus, data were available for analysis from 426 patients with a prior RALM. The average time between myomectomy and survey completion was approximately 2.5 years and ranged from 1 month to 7.5 years.

3.2. Patient Characteristics. Women in group 1, who only wanted symptom treatment and had no intention of becoming pregnant, comprised 19.2% of the cohort. The largest

TABLE 1: Patient characteristics at myomectomy.

Characteristics	Group 1[a]	Group 2[b]	Group 3[c]	Total
Number of patients	$N = 82$	$N = 281$	$N = 63$	$N = 426$
Age at myomectomy, yrs	42.5 ± 5.0[d]	36.5 ± 5.5	38.0 ± 4.9	37.9 ± 5.8
Smoking prior to surgery, n (%)	16 (19.8)	40 (14.3)	13 (20.6)	69 (16.3)
Preexisting conditions, n (%)[e]	36 (45.0)	131 (47.1)	24 (38.1)	191 (45.4)
Anemia	15 (18.8)	65 (23.4)	8 (12.7)	88 (20.9)
Endometriosis	10 (12.5)	38 (13.7)	8 (12.7)	56 (13.3)
Hypertension	13 (16.3)	22 (7.9)	3 (4.8)	38 (9.0)
Diabetes	1 (1.3)	8 (2.9)	1 (1.6)	10 (2.4)
Heart disease	0	0	0	0
Other	6 (7.5)	13 (4.7)	4 (6.3)	23 (5.5)
Reasons for seeking treatment, n (%)[e]				
Fibroids	68 (82.9)	249 (88.6)	52 (82.5)	369 (86.6)
Excessive menstrual bleeding	49 (59.8)	148 (52.7)	23 (36.5)	220 (51.6)
Pain/pressure	40 (48.8)	152 (54.1)	16 (25.4)	208 (48.8)
Frequent urination	22 (26.8)	62 (22.1)	3 (4.8)	87 (20.4)
Infertility	2 (2.4)	40 (14.2)	38 (60.3)	80 (18.8)
Painful intercourse	18 (22.0)	57 (20.3)	5 (7.9)	80 (18.8)
Endometriosis	8 (9.8)	35 (12.5)	7 (11.1)	50 (11.7)
Ovarian cyst	6 (7.3)	21 (7.5)	4 (6.3)	31 (7.3)
Other	1 (1.2)	1 (.4)	0	2 (.5)
Symptoms with fibroids, n (%)[e]				
Excessive menstrual bleeding	39 (57.4)	131 (52.6)	22 (42.3)	192 (52.0)
Pain/pressure	32 (47.1)	130 (52.2)	15 (28.9)	177 (48.0)
Infertility	1 (1.5)	36 (14.5)	31 (59.6)	68 (18.4)
Bleeding and pain	24 (35.3)	84 (33.7)	11 (21.2)	119 (32.2)
Bleeding, pain, and infertility	0	14 (5.6)	7 (14.1)	21 (5.7)
None of these	11 (16.2)	56 (22.5)	12 (23.1)	79 (21.4)
≥ 2 fibroid surgeries, n (%)	11 (13.4)	42 (14.9)	9 (14.3)	62 (14.6)
Prior pregnancy, n (%)	56 (68.3)	143 (50.9)	29 (46.0)	228 (53.5)
Attempted but did not achieve pregnancy, n (%)	12/58 (20.7)	73/163 (44.8)	24/34 (70.6)	109/255 (42.8)
Outcomes of prior pregnancies, n (%)[e]				
Vaginal delivery ≥ 1	29 (51.8)	42 (29.4)	4 (13.8)	75 (32.9)
C-section ≥ 1	14 (25.0)	41 (28.7)	10 (34.5)	65 (28.5)
Miscarriage ≥ 1	8 (14.3)	58 (40.6)	17 (58.6)	83 (36.4)
Ectopic ≥ 1	1 (1.8)	4 (2.8)	2 (6.9)	7 (3.0)
Prior infertility treatments, n (%)	8/56 (14.3)	20/162 (12.3)	9/34 (26.5)	37/252 (14.7)

[a]Group 1 = desire to treat symptoms with no intention of becoming pregnant.
[b]Group 2 = desire to treat symptoms and preserve ability to get pregnant in the future.
[c]Group 3 = desire to improve current chance of pregnancy after myomectomy.
[d]Data are mean ± standard deviation unless stated otherwise.
[e]Data not mutually exclusive.

group was group 2 (66.0%) and included those who wanted symptom treatment with the possibility of becoming pregnant in the future. Group 3, women desiring to improve their current chances of pregnancy, was the smallest (14.8%). At the time of the survey, the average participants' age was 40.4 ± 6.1 years, most women being self-identified as African American (46.5%) or as Caucasian (38.2%). BMI was 27.0 ± 6.0 kg/m^2 and the majority of women (92.9%) were nonsmokers. Among those who possibly or definitely desired pregnancy (groups 2 and 3, resp.), infertility after myomectomy was diagnosed in about 8% overall and 16% in group 3 alone.

Age at the time of myomectomy was 37.9 ± 5.8 years (Table 1). Smoking was prevalent in 16.3%. Preexisting conditions included anemia (20.9%), endometriosis (13.3%), hypertension (9.0%), and diabetes (2.4%). The two most common reasons for seeking treatment included excessive menstrual bleeding (51.6%) and pain/pressure (48.8%). However, 21% did not report either of these symptoms or infertility as reasons for RALM. About 15% of women had undergone two or more prior surgeries for fibroid treatment.

While 53% of women had become pregnant prior to their robotic myomectomy, 43% had attempted but not conceived during this time (Table 1). More than one-third of the women

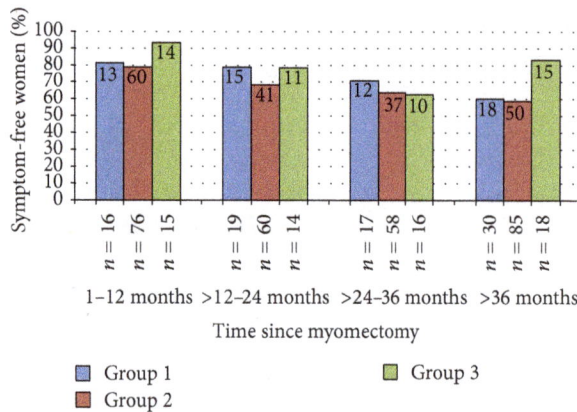

FIGURE 1: Women who were symptom- and condition-free since myomectomy, by group and time since myomectomy. Group 1 (blue bars) desired to treat symptoms with no intention of becoming pregnant; group 2 (red bars) desired to treat symptoms and preserve ability to get pregnant in the future; group 3 (green bars) desired to improve current chance of pregnancy after myomectomy. N in bars is the number of symptom-free women; N below the bars is the total number of women in that group and time period.

who had prior pregnancies experienced miscarriages (36%), with the highest rates in groups 2 and 3. Infertility treatments were obtained by 15% of women overall and 27% in group 3 alone.

3.3. Symptom Relief.

Approximately 70% of participants reported that they were symptom-free at the time of survey completion. The overall proportion of women who were symptom-free decreased as the interval of time since surgery increased: 81.3% were symptom-free up to 12 months, 72% at 12–24 months, 64.8% at 24–36 months, and 62.9% at greater than 3 years from surgery. Symptom recurrences were mostly excessive menstruation (52%) and pain/pressure (48%). One patient (0.3%) reported having received additional treatment after her original RALM. This group 2 patient underwent an AM two years after her robotic myomectomy.

The group 1 patients who sought treatment solely for the purpose of symptom relief best demonstrate the effectiveness of robotic surgery to improve fibroid-related symptoms. The proportion of women who were symptom-free in this group also decreased as the time from surgery increased (Figure 1): 81.3% were symptom-free at 1–12 months, 78.9% at 12–24 months, 70.6% at 24–36 months, and 60% at greater than 3 years (trend test $P = 0.041$).

Women in group 3, who had surgery to improve fertility, had the greatest relief of symptoms and the lowest rate of symptom recurrence over time. While the trend in symptom relief over time for group 2 women who had surgery for symptom relief and fertility preservation was statistically significant ($P = 0.003$), the difference in trends between groups 1 and 2 was not statistically significant ($P = 0.483$), nor were there differences in trends between group 3 and group 2 ($P = 0.576$) or between group 3 and group 1 ($P = 0.161$).

Characteristics that were independently associated with symptom recurrence were identified using stepwise logistic regression (Figure 2).

Variables examined included group status, age at myomectomy, months between surgery and survey, ethnicity, BMI, smoking after myomectomy, preexisting medical conditions, symptoms, and multiple fibroid surgeries. Factors associated with recurrence were longer time between myomectomy and survey (OR = 1.45; 95% CI = 1.19, 1.77), prior symptoms of pain with intercourse (OR = 2.40; 1.40, 4.13), two or more fibroid surgeries (OR = 2.51; 95% CI = 1.37, 4.61), smoking after myomectomy (OR = 3.16; 1.41, 7.11), and preexisting diabetes (OR = 5.50; 1.37, 22.11). Although only 2.4% of women had diabetes at myomectomy, diabetics were over five times more likely to have a recurrence of symptoms. The probability of recurrence increased 45% with each 12-month period after surgery.

3.4. Achieving Pregnancy.

In order to assess the impact of surgery on fertility potential, it was necessary to limit the analysis to groups 2 and 3, those who desired pregnancy in the future or currently. These groups differed somewhat in their *a priori* risk of subfertility. Patients in group 3 were older at surgery (mean 38.0 ± 4.9 years versus 36.5 ± 5.5 years, $P = 0.029$) and had a significantly higher rate of infertility as a reason for treatment (60.3% versus 14.2%, $P < 0.0001$), prior miscarriage (58.6% versus 40.6%, $P = 0.013$), and use of preoperative infertility treatments (26.5% versus 12.3%, $P = 0.006$). Despite these poor prognostic indicators, more than half (50.8%) of group 3 patients achieved pregnancy. The pregnancy rates increased with follow-up time after surgery in both groups (Figure 3(a)) and were even higher when restricted to women who were symptom-free (Figure 3(b)).

For the women who achieved pregnancy, the mean time to pregnancy after starting to attempt was 7.9 ± 9.4 months (Table 2). Women waited an average of 4.3 ± 3.1 months before trying to conceive and, thus, time between myomectomy and pregnancy was 12.3 ± 10.3 months. A larger percentage of women in group 3 used medications to achieve pregnancy compared to group 2 (46.9% versus 20%, $P = 0.007$). Although women in group 3 were two years older than women in group 2, major complications during pregnancy (abnormal placentation, uterine rupture, or premature delivery) were lower in group 3 (3.2% versus 15.6%, $P = 0.103$). Those with complications were two years younger on average than the group as a whole. The proportions that miscarried during pregnancy in groups 2 and 3 were 30.5% and 37.5%, respectively.

Logistic regression was used to examine characteristics independently associated with achieving pregnancy after myomectomy in groups 2 and 3 (Figure 4).

Variables chosen included group status, age at myomectomy, months between surgery and survey, ethnicity, BMI, smoking after myomectomy, preexisting conditions, infertility as a reason for myomectomy, pregnancy prior to myomectomy, symptom recurrence after myomectomy, and multiple fibroid surgeries. Characteristics that were significantly and independently associated with achieving pregnancy included

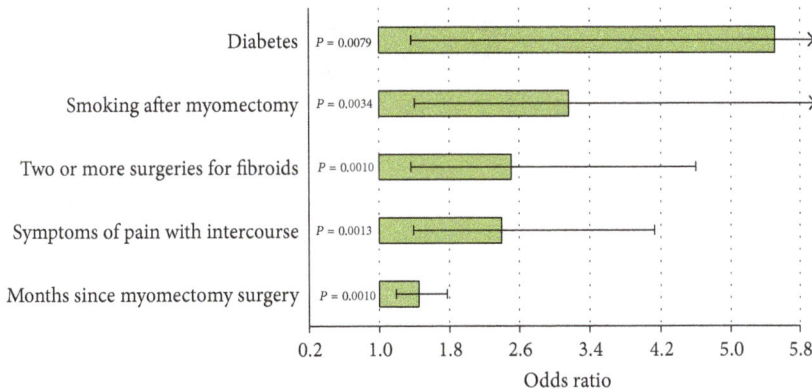

FIGURE 2: Factors independently associated with recurrence of symptoms. Shown are the factors that were statistically significant at $P < 0.05$ in forward stepwise logistic regression.

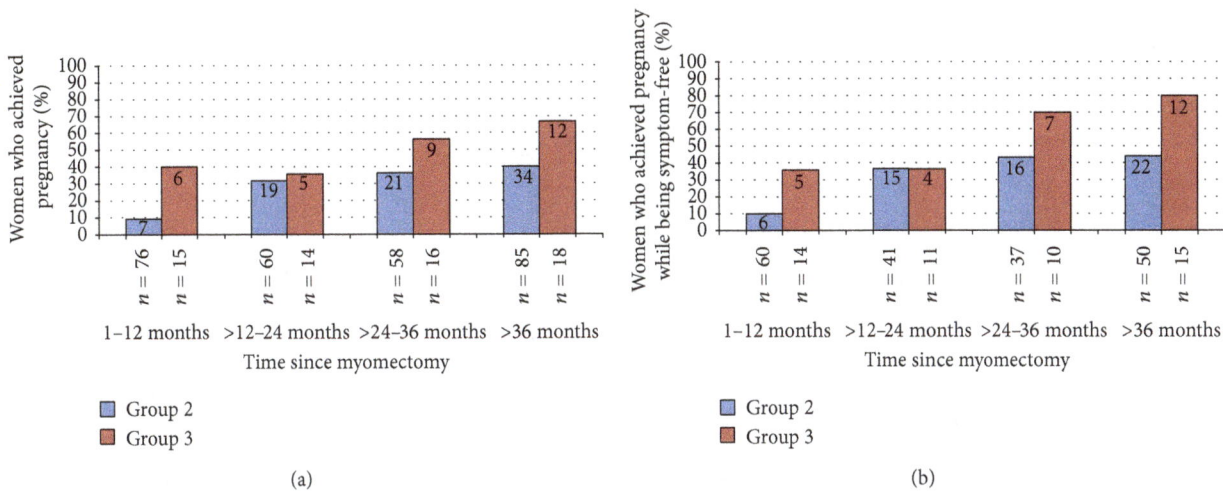

FIGURE 3: Pregnancy status after myomectomy in women who desired pregnancy, by group and time between myomectomy and survey. Group 2 (blue bars) desired to treat symptoms and preserve ability to get pregnant in the future; group 3 (red bars) desired to improve current chance of pregnancy after myomectomy. N in bars is the number of women who became pregnant; N below the bars is the total number of women in that group and time period. (a) All women and (b) women who were symptom-free.

Caucasian race (OR = 1.74; 95% CI = 1.01, 3.02), longer time between myomectomy and survey (OR = 1.92; 95% CI = 1.51, 2.43), prior pregnancy (OR = 2.35; 95% CI = 1.39, 4.00), and group 3 status (actively desiring pregnancy) (OR = 3.50, 95% CI = 1.83, 6.71). Older age at myomectomy (OR = 0.41; 95% CI = 0.26, 0.64) and symptom recurrence (OR = 0.49; 95% CI = 0.27, 0.87) were negatively associated with achieving pregnancy. Each increasing decade of age at myomectomy (20–29, 30–39, 40–49, etc.) decreased the odds of pregnancy by 41%.

4. Discussion

4.1. Principal Findings. We have shown long-term treatment success for the majority of women undergoing RALM. Relief from symptoms was achieved in 70% of all patients, with 62.9% of women still symptom-free more than three years after surgery. Pregnancy rates were high in those actively trying to conceive (50.8% overall and 66.7% after more

than three years postoperatively), despite this group's age and subfertility. Moreover, staying symptom-free increased the chances of conception, with an 80% pregnancy rate for symptom-free patients in group 3 after more than three-year follow-up. These results suggest a sustained benefit of RALM on fertility potential and patient comfort.

4.2. Relation to Other Studies. This multicenter study is among the first to examine the long-term success of RALM. There have been only a few papers examining pregnancy rates following RALM, and no published studies of symptom recurrence were identified in our searches. Cela and colleagues [7] reported an overall pregnancy rate of 13% in 48 patients, with a success rate of 77.8% in 9 women desiring pregnancy. In the study by Lonnerfors and Persson [8], 15 out of 22 (68.2%) women who actively wanted to achieve pregnancy were successful after removal of deep intramural myomas by RALM. Tusheva et al. [9] reported a success rate

TABLE 2: Characteristics of women who achieved pregnancy after myomectomy.

Characteristics	Group 2[a]	Group 3[b]	Total
Months to achieve pregnancy after starting to attempt			
Number of patients	$N = 77$	$N = 31$	$N = 108$
Mean ± SD	8.2 ± 10.1	7.3 ± 7.5	7.9 ± 9.4
Range	(1–60)	(1–32)	(1–60)
Months to achieve pregnancy after myomectomy			
Number of patients	$N = 82$	$N = 32$	$N = 114$
Mean ± SD	13.0 ± 11.1	10.6 ± 8.3	12.3 ± 10.3
Range	(2.5–64.5)	(2.5–33.5)	(2.5–64.5)
Used medications or procedures to achieve pregnancy, n (%)	16/80 (20.0)	15/32 (46.9)	31/112 (27.7)
Age at pregnancy, yrs	35.7 ± 5.0[c]	37.7 ± 5.3	36.3 ± 5.1
Age at pregnancy for women with a complication, yrs	34.5 ± 6.2	33.5 ± 0.0	34.4 ± 5.9
Complications during pregnancy, n (%)[d]	12 (15.6)	1 (3.2)	13 (12.0)
Premature delivery <37 wks	10 (13.0)	1 (3.2)	11 (10.2)
Abnormal placentation	4 (5.2)	0	4 (3.7)
Uterine rupture	1 (1.3)	0	1 (0.9)
Miscarriage during pregnancy, n (%)	25/82 (30.5)	12/32 (37.5)	37/114 (32.5)

[a]Group 2 = desire to treat symptoms and preserve ability to get pregnant in future.
[b]Group 3 = desire to improve current chance of pregnancy after myomectomy.
[c]Data are mean ± standard deviation unless stated otherwise.
[d]Data are not mutually exclusive.

of 75% in 16 RALM patients desiring pregnancy. We have previously reported on pregnancies following RALM in a large, multicenter study [10] and found an overall conception rate of 12.3%, similar to the rate of 13% shown by Cela et al. [7]. However, it is unknown how many women were actively trying to conceive.

In the present study, the pregnancy rate was 26.8% for all women, including those not desiring pregnancy after surgery. This rate is twice that seen in Cela et al.'s study [7] and in our own prior study [10]. The difference may reflect the larger proportion of women in this study who were actively trying to conceive. Our conception rate after three years among women actively trying to conceive (67%) is on par with the rates from studies discussed above, 68%–78% [7–9]. Average time to pregnancy in our study was 10.6 months, comparable to the median time of 10 months observed by Lonnerfors and Persson [8]. Self-reported miscarriage rates in this study (32%) were higher than those reported in the other smaller RALM studies (0–17%) described above.

RALM may result in improved conception rates relative to conventional LM and AM. A weighted average conception rate for women actively desiring pregnancy based on our and the abovementioned published RALM studies is 46/65 or approximately 71%. This rate is at the high end of the range of pregnancy rates (33%–75%) reported in a recent review of LM among patients undergoing the procedure for reasons of infertility [3]. In addition, a recent abstract by Celestine and colleagues [11] showed a higher rate of spontaneous conception (58%) after RALM compared to AM (32%). Prospective comparative studies are needed to examine whether RALM may result in improved pregnancy rates among women actively trying to conceive.

Since we were unable to find published reports of symptom recurrence after RALM, we examined the LM literature. Our definition of recurrence was based on the self-reported reappearance of fibroid-related symptoms. Recurrence during the first postoperative year was 19.7%, 28% the second year, 35.2% the third year, and 37.1% after three years. Radosa et al. [12] reported an overall rate of symptom recurrence at 35.7%, on par with the overall rate of 30% in the present study. Two studies of LM with a stricter definition of recurrence requiring the return of symptoms followed by ultrasound confirmation of fibroids found lower recurrence rates at 24 months (4.9% and 12.7%) and 60 months (16.7% and 21.4%) [12, 13]. LM studies that utilized a definition of recurrence requiring only the presence of fibroids on follow-up sonograms reported intermediary rates of recurrence at 24 months (20% and 20%) and 60 months (51.5% and 52.9%) [14, 15]. We would argue that basing the recurrence rate on appearance of symptoms might be more clinically relevant. All of these studies reported an increase in recurrence rates over time, as in our study, and an increased risk of recurrence with the presence of multiple myomas. In the present study there was an increased risk of recurrence in patients with two or more prior fibroid surgeries. While our findings are in line with what has been previously reported following LM, studies are needed to determine if RALM provides any additional benefit.

We found that, in addition to longer time since myomectomy and prior fibroid surgery, symptom recurrence was higher among patients who complained of painful intercourse preoperatively, smoked, and had diabetes. Painful intercourse may correlate with larger myoma size or greater number of myomas, which have been shown to correlate

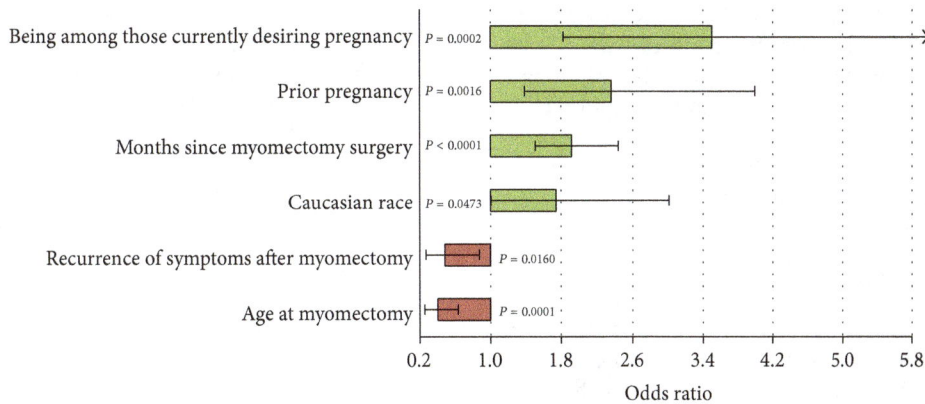

FIGURE 4: Factors independently associated with achieving pregnancy. Shown are the factors that were statistically significant at $P < 0.05$ in forward stepwise logistic regression.

with recurrence [12–15]. To the best of our knowledge, this study is the first to examine the relationships of smoking and diabetes with symptom recurrence following myomectomy. Our findings contradict studies reporting a decreased risk of fibroids with smoking [16–19] thought to be mediated by inducing enzymes that promote estrogen metabolism, thus lowering estrogen levels and impeding myoma development [16]. It is possible that smoking correlated with another, unmeasured factor or that those in pain due to symptom recurrence were more likely to smoke. Findings in one review agree with our results, reporting an increased risk of myomas with diabetes, stating that this is most likely mediated by insulin resistance, increased IGF-1 activity (a growth factor for fibroid cells in vitro), and elevated androgen levels [17]. Other studies have reported a deceased risk of myomas with diabetes [19–21] and suggest that the protective effect comes from the medications taken. For example, insulin and pioglitazone have been shown to have myoma inhibitory effects [20, 22] and IGF-1 levels decrease in treated diabetics [23]. Differences among studies may be due to the complex etiology of diabetes, levels of blood sugar control, and the wide range of diabetes medications and their effects.

We found that, in addition to longer time since surgery and an active desire to conceive (group 3 women), achieving pregnancy was associated with younger age, prior conception success, Caucasian race, and remaining symptom-free. Other RALM [8, 9] and LM [12, 15, 24, 25] studies have reported a negative association between pregnancy and increasing age and a positive association between prior pregnancy and future conception success [1]. The positive effect of Caucasian race may be related to a lower risk of myoma regrowth without symptom recurrence (controlled for in logistic analysis). Epidemiological studies have consistently reported that African American women are at higher risk for myoma development [16, 19]. It is also likely that Caucasian women had greater access to fertility treatments and assisted technologies, improving their chances of conception. Unfortunately, this factor could not be considered in analyses since it was not assessed in all women. The significant negative association between recurrence and achieving pregnancy has

been previously shown in two LM studies in which recurrence was defined by reappearance of fibroids on sonography [13, 15]. It is notable that we found a higher pregnancy rate in symptom-free patients at each time interval postoperatively (compared to rates overall and in those who experienced recurrence), with the highest rate (80%) seen after three years in patients actively attempting to conceive (group 3).

4.3. Strengths and Weaknesses. To our knowledge, this is the first published study on long-term recurrence rates following RALM and one of the largest RALM studies to report on pregnancy success. Caveats regarding the results pertain to the retrospective, cross-sectional nature of the design. Survey responses for each participant were captured at differing time periods following myomectomy. This may have resulted in the introduction of bias if, for example, women who had more recent robotic myomectomies had better recall. However, such limitations would have affected all study groups similarly. Furthermore, the parameter, "time since myomectomy," was adjusted for in all logistic analyses. While our results may not be generalizable to all myomectomy patients, the study included a relatively large number of women from three different US locations and two types of practices and, thus, attempted to introduce greater patient heterogeneity and the potential for generalizability. Although it is possible that data from multiple practices may have introduced unmeasured differences influencing the study findings, there was no impact of "practice site" on symptom recurrence or pregnancy success in the logistic analyses. The impact of fertility interventions, perioperative outcomes, and location, number, or size of myomas could not be assessed since this information was not uniformly collected at all study sites.

5. Conclusions

We found that 50.8% of women desiring pregnancy were able to achieve it, in spite of the fact that 60.3% reported infertility as the reason for undergoing myomectomy and many were also at high risk for reproductive failure due to advanced reproductive age and other independent risk factors. Symptom relief in that group overall was 79.4%. These findings are encouraging for women with symptomatic fibroid uteri who desire a minimally invasive approach to treatment of their disease while maintaining their comfort and fertility potential. More research, particularly prospective study, is needed to confirm or refute these results.

Conflict of Interests

Usha Seshadri-Kreaden owns stock in and is an employee of Intuitive Surgical, the manufacturer of the da Vinci Surgical System. Helen B. Hubert is a consultant for Intuitive Surgical. Michael C. Pitter is on the Speaker's Bureau for Intuitive Surgical. Serene S. Srouji, Antonio R. Gargiulo, Leslie Kardos, and Glenn A. Weitzman do not have any conflict of interests.

Authors' Contribution

Michael C. Pitter, Serene S. Srouji, Antonio R. Gargiulo, Leslie Kardos, and Glenn A. Weitzman were involved in the acquisition and interpretation of data, revised the paper for important intellectual content, and approved the final version of the paper. Usha Seshadri-Kreaden performed the statistical analysis, revised the paper critically for important intellectual content, and approved the final version of the paper. Michael C. Pitter, Serene S. Srouji, Antonio R. Gargiulo, and Helen B. Hubert made substantial contributions to the conception and design, drafted the paper, and approved the final version of the paper.

Acknowledgments

The authors wish to thank Shalini Murkherjee, Ph.D., for her assistance in study implementation. The patient follow-up was funded by Intuitive Surgical, Inc.

References

[1] W. H. Parker, "Etiology, symptomatology, and diagnosis of uterine myomas," *Fertility and Sterility*, vol. 87, no. 4, pp. 725–736, 2007.

[2] P. C. Brady, A. K. Stanic, and A. K. Styer, "Uterine fibroids and subfertility: an update on the role of myomectomy," *Current Opinion in Obstetrics and Gynecology*, vol. 25, no. 3, pp. 255–259, 2013.

[3] V. Buckley, E. M. Nesbitt-Hawes, P. Atkinson et al., "Laparoscopic myomectomy: clinical outcomes and comparative evidence," *Journal of Minimally Invasive Gynecology*, vol. 22, no. 1, pp. 11–25, 2015.

[4] C. Jin, Y. Hu, X. C. Chen et al., "Laparoscopic versus open myomectomy—a meta-analysis of randomized controlled trials," *European Journal of Obstetrics & Gynecology and Reproductive Biology*, vol. 145, pp. 14–21, 2009.

[5] S. M. Walid and R. L. Heaton, "The role of laparoscopic myomectomy in the management of uterine fibroids," *Current Opinion in Obstetrics and Gynecology*, vol. 23, no. 4, pp. 273–277, 2011.

[6] J. Pundir, V. Pundir, R. Walavalkar, K. Omanwa, G. Lancaster, and S. Kayani, "Robotic-assisted laparoscopic vs abdominal and laparoscopic myomectomy: systematic review and meta-analysis," *Journal of Minimally Invasive Gynecology*, vol. 20, no. 3, pp. 335–345, 2013.

[7] V. Cela, L. Freschi, G. Simi et al., "Fertility and endocrine outcome after robot-assisted laparoscopic myomectomy (RALM)," *Gynecological Endocrinology*, vol. 29, no. 1, pp. 79–82, 2013.

[8] C. Lonnerfors and J. Persson, "Pregnancy following robot-assisted laparoscopic myomectomy in women with deep intramural myomas," *Acta Obstetricia et Gynecologica Scandinavica*, vol. 90, no. 9, pp. 972–977, 2011.

[9] O. A. Tusheva, A. Gyang, and S. D. Patel, "Reproductive outcomes following robotic-assisted laparoscopic myomectomy (RALM)," *Journal of Robotic Surgery*, vol. 7, no. 1, pp. 65–69, 2013.

[10] M. C. Pitter, A. R. Gargiulo, L. M. Bonaventura, J. S. Lehman, and S. S. Srouji, "Pregnancy outcomes following robot-assisted myomectomy," *Human Reproduction*, vol. 28, no. 1, pp. 99–108, 2013.

[11] C. Celestine, W. Ziegler, V. Johnson, Y.-H. Kuo, and J. Mann, "Pregnancy after abdominal versus robotically assisted laparoscopic myomectomy," *Fertility and Sterility*, vol. 102, no. 3, supplement, pp. e287–e288, 2014.

[12] M. P. Radosa, Z. Owsianowski, A. Mothes et al., "Long-term risk of fibroid recurrence after laparoscopic myomectomy," *European Journal of Obstetrics & Gynecology and Reproductive Biology*, vol. 180, pp. 35–39, 2014.

[13] V. Doridot, J.-B. Dubuisson, C. Chapron, A. Fauconnier, and K. Babaki-Fard, "Recurrence of leiomyomata after laparoscopic myomectomy," *Journal of the American Association of Gynecologic Laparoscopists*, vol. 8, no. 4, pp. 495–500, 2001.

[14] F. R. Nezhat, M. Roemisch, C. H. Nezhat, D. S. Seidman, and C. R. Nezhat, "Recurrence rate after laparoscopic myomectomy," *The Journal of the American Association of Gynecologic Laparoscopists*, vol. 5, no. 3, pp. 237–240, 1998.

[15] E.-H. Yoo, P. I. Lee, C.-Y. Huh, D.-H. Kim, B.-S. Lee, and J.-K. Lee, "Predictors of leiomyoma recurrence after laparoscopic myomectomy," *Journal of Minimally Invasive Gynecology*, vol. 14, no. 6, pp. 690–697, 2007.

[16] E. Faerstein, M. Szklo, and N. Rosenshein, "Risk factors for uterine leiomyoma: a practice-based case-control study. I. African-American heritage, reproductive history, body size, and smoking," *American Journal of Epidemiology*, vol. 153, no. 1, pp. 1–10, 2001.

[17] S. Okolo, "Incidence, aetiology and epidemiology of uterine fibroids," *Best Practice & Research: Clinical Obstetrics & Gynaecology*, vol. 22, no. 4, pp. 571–588, 2008.

[18] R. K. Ross, M. C. Pike, M. P. Vessey, D. Bull, D. Yeates, and J. T. Casagrande, "Risk factors for uterine fibroids: reduced risk associated with oral contraceptives," *British Medical Journal (Clinical Research ed)*, vol. 293, no. 6543, pp. 359–362, 1986.

[19] C. Templeman, S. F. Marshall, C. A. Clarke et al., "Risk factors for surgically removed fibroids in a large cohort of teachers," *Fertility and Sterility*, vol. 92, no. 4, pp. 1436–1446, 2009.

[20] D. D. Baird, G. Travlos, R. Wilson et al., "Uterine leiomyomata in relation to insulin-like growth factor-I, insulin, and diabetes," *Epidemiology*, vol. 20, no. 4, pp. 604–610, 2009.

[21] L. A. Wise, J. R. Palmer, E. A. Stewart, and L. Rosenberg, "Polycystic ovary syndrome and risk of uterine leiomyomata," *Fertility and Sterility*, vol. 87, no. 5, pp. 1108–1115, 2007.

[22] C. J. Loy, S. Evelyn, F. K. Lim, M. H. Liu, and E. L. Yong, "Growth dynamics of human leiomyoma cells and inhibitory effects of the peroxisome proliferator-activated receptor-gamma ligand, pioglitazone," *Molecular Human Reproduction*, vol. 11, no. 8, pp. 561–566, 2005.

[23] D. R. Clemmons, "Modifying IGF1 activity: an approach to treat endocrine disorders, atherosclerosis and cancer," *Nature Reviews Drug Discovery*, vol. 6, no. 10, pp. 821–833, 2007.

[24] S. Campo, V. Campo, and P. Gambadauro, "Reproductive outcome before and after laparoscopic or abdominal myomectomy for subserous or intramural myomas," *European Journal of Obstetrics & Gynecology and Reproductive Biology*, vol. 110, no. 2, pp. 215–219, 2003.

[25] J. Kumakiri, H. Takeuchi, M. Kitade et al., "Pregnancy and delivery after laparoscopic myomectomy," *Journal of Minimally Invasive Gynecology*, vol. 12, no. 3, pp. 241–246, 2005.

24

Is Risk Malignancy Index a Useful Tool for Predicting Malignant Ovarian Masses in Developing Countries?

Aliya B. Aziz and Nida Najmi

Department of Obstetrics and Gynaecology, Aga Khan University Hospital, Karachi 74800, Pakistan

Correspondence should be addressed to Aliya B. Aziz; azizaliya@hotmail.com

Academic Editor: Enrique Hernandez

Introduction. Risk of Malignancy Index (RMI) is widely studied for prediction of malignant pelvic masses in Western population. However, little is known regarding its implication in the developing countries. The objective of this study is to determine how accurately the RMI can predict the malignant pelvic masses. *Materials and Methods.* The study is a retrospective review of patients attending the gynecological clinic between January 2004 and December 2008 with adnexal masses. Information on demographic characteristics, ultrasound findings, menopausal status, CA125, and histopathology was collected. RMI score for each patient in the study group was calculated. *Results.* The study group included a total of 283 patients. Analysis of the individual parameters of RMI revealed that ultrasound was the best predictor of malignancy with a sensitivity, specificity, and positive likelihood ratio of 78.3%, 81.5%, and 4.2, respectively. At a standard cut-off value of 250, RMI had a positive likelihood ratio of 8.1, while it was 6.8 at a cut-off of 200, albeit with comparable sensitivity and specificity. *Conclusion.* RMI is a sensitive tool in predicting malignant adnexal masses. A cut-off of 200 may be suitable in developing countries for triaging and early referral to tertiary care centers.

1. Introduction

Ovarian masses are a frequent cause of gynecological consults and are often detected during imaging studies or exploratory surgery for evaluation of abdominal or pelvic pain syndromes. They occur across age groups and could result from benign or malignant disease. With more than 250,000 new cases reported every year, ovarian malignancies represent the fourth commonest cause of cancer deaths worldwide [1]. They also have the lowest 5-year survival rate (30–50%) among all gynecological cancers [2]. A recent report indicated an increasing incidence of ovarian cancers in the developing world, compared to the developed countries [3].

Early identification of ovarian carcinomas and referral to a gyneco-oncologist can facilitate accurate staging of the disease and optimal cytoreductive treatment, enhancing patient survival [4, 5]. Histopathology remains the diagnostic gold standard for this cancer, and a definitive biomarker has not been identified yet. Risk of Malignancy Index (RMI), which considers the serum CA125 level, menopausal status, and ultrasonographic findings in predicting malignant pelvic masses, is widely employed in the developed countries [6]. However, its utility in risk prediction in the developing countries is currently unknown.

The present study evaluated how accurately the RMI can predict the risk of malignant pelvic masses, among patients with an ovarian mass.

2. Material and Methods

After the approval of our institutional review board we conducted a retrospective review of the case files of patients with adnexal masses who attended the Gynecological Clinic at the Aga Khan University, Karachi, Pakistan, between January 2004 and December 2008. The International Classification of Diseases, 9th Revision, Clinical Modification (ICD-9-CM) criteria were used to identify adnexal masses. Patients with advanced disease were excluded from the study. We collected information on demographic characteristics, ultrasonographic findings, menopausal status, serum CA125 level, and histopathology. The RMI for each patient was calculated using the standard formula [6].

3. Results

3.1. Demographic Data. The study group consisted of a total of 283 patients. The age of the patients varied from 8 to 85 years (mean, 38.6 years). Premenopausal patients predominated in our study with 227 (80.8%) cases, while 54 (19.2%) of the affected patients were in the postmenopausal group.

3.2. Ultrasonography Findings. Two hundred and seven (73.7%) patients had a transabdominal ultrasonography for diagnosis, while transvaginal ultrasonography detected the disease in 74 (26.3%) cases. Table 1 shows the summary of ultrasound findings in our patients.

3.2.1. Laterality of Lesion. The investigation revealed a unilateral cyst in 252 (89.7%) cases, while 29 (10.3%) had bilateral cysts.

3.2.2. Loculation. The lesions were multilocular in 166 (59%) patients and unilocular in 115 (41%).

3.2.3. Echogenicity. Solid areas were absent in the lesions in 196 (69.8%) patients, while these were detected in 85 (30.2%) patients.

3.2.4. Evidence of Metastasis. The majority of patients (272, 96.8%) had no evidence of metastasis, while 9 (3.2%) had metastatic disease.

3.2.5. Presence of Ascites. Ascites was present in only 19 (6.8%) patients.

3.2.6. Ultrasound Score. We assigned scores of 0 (absence of specific findings), 1 (presence of one finding), or 3 (two or more findings) to the subjects, depending on the ultrasound findings. One hundred and nineteen (42.3%) cases had an ultrasound score of 1, while lesions of 88 (31.3%) and 74 (26.3%) patients were scored 0 and 3, respectively. Of the 207 (73.6%) patients with an ultrasound score 1, 196 (69.7%) had benign disease, while 8 (2.8%) and 3 (1%) had malignant and borderline disease, respectively. Seventy-four (26.3%) patients in our series had an ultrasound score of 3, and among them, 41 (14.5%) had benign, 29 (10.3%) had malignant, and 4 (1.4%) had borderline disease, respectively.

3.2.7. Ovarian Size. Ovarian size varied from 3 to 73 cm (mean, 10.5 cm).

3.3. Histopathology Findings. As shown in Table 2, 237 (84.3%) patients had benign lesions, while 37 (13.2%) had a malignant disease. Seven (2.5%) patients under 60 years of age had borderline lesions. One hundred and thirty-nine (49.4%) of the benign tumours occurred in patients aged 20 to 39 years, and 60 (21.3%) cases were in those aged 41–59 years. Patients aged ≤20 years and ≥60 years reported 24 (8.5%) and 14 (4.9%) cases of benign disease, respectively. Malignant disease peaked in the age group 40–59 years with 21 (7.4%) cases, while 10 (3.5%), 4 (1.4%), and 2 (0.7%) cases occurred among patients aged ≥60 years, 20–39 years, and ≤20 years,

TABLE 1: Summary of ultrasound findings in the study.

	Frequency	Percentage (%)
Transabdominal scan	207	73.7
Transvaginal scan	74	26.3
Unilateral cyst	252	89.7
Bilateral cyst	29	10.3
Unilocular cyst	115	41.0
Multilocular cyst	166	59.0
Presence of solid areas	85	30.2
Absence of solid areas	196	69.8
Evidence of metastasis present	9	3.2
Evidence of metastasis absent	272	96.8
Presence of ascites	19	6.8
Absence of ascites	262	93.2
Ultrasound score 0	88	31.3
Ultrasound score 1	119	42.3
Ultrasound score 3	74	74

TABLE 2: Distribution of cases in the study.

	Benign (%)	Borderline (%)	Malignant (%)	Total (%)
Histopathology	237 (84.3)	7 (2.5)	37 (13.2)	281
Age (years)				
≤20	24 (8.5)	1 (0.3)	2 (0.7)	27 (9.6)
20–39	139 (49.4)	3 (1.0)	4 (1.4)	146 (51.9)
40–59	60 (21.3)	3 (1.0)	21 (7.4)	84 (29.8)
≥60	14 (4.9)	0 (0)	10 (3.5)	24 (8.5)
Premenopausal	203 (72.2)	6 (2.1)	18 (6.4)	227 (80.7)
Postmenopausal	34 (12.0)	1 (0.3)	19 (6.7)	54 (19.2)
Ultrasound score 1	196 (69.7)	3 (1.0)	8 (2.8)	207 (73.6)
Ultrasound score 3	41 (14.5)	4 (1.4)	29 (10.3)	74 (26.3)
CA125 ≥ 35	75 (26.6)	4 (1.4)	26 (9.2)	105 (37.3)
Ca125 < 35	162 (57.6)	3 (1.0)	11 (3.9)	176 (62.6)
RMI groups				
≤25	117 (41.6)	0 (0)	3 (1.0)	120 (42.7)
25.1–249.9	106 (37.7)	5 (1.7)	14 (4.9)	125 (44.4)
≥250	14 (4.9)	2 (0.7)	20 (7.1)	36 (12.8)

respectively. Three cases of borderline disease occurred in the age groups 21–39 and 40–59 years, and one (0.3%) case was in a woman aged ≤20 years, while such lesions were not detected in women ≥60 years. Two hundred and three (72.2%) of the 227 premenopausal patients had benign disease, while 18 (6.4%) had malignant, and 6 (2.1%) had borderline lesions. Among the 54 (19.2%) postmenopausal patients, 34 (12%) had benign disease, while 19 (6.7%) and 1 (0.3%) had malignant and borderline disease, respectively.

3.4. Serum CA125 Levels. The serum CA125 levels in the patients varied from 1.2 to 6803 U/mL (mean, 197 U/mL) (Table 2). One hundred and seventy-six (62.6%) patients had a serum CA125 level less than 35 U/mL, while the levels

TABLE 3: Diagnostic performance of the different RMI cut-offs employed.

RMI cut-off value	Sensitivity	Specificity	PPV	NPV	+LR ratio	−LR ratio
250	54.05 (20/37)	93.4 (228/244)	55.5 (20/36)	93.06 (228/245)	8.1	0.49
200	53.8 (21/39)	92.2 (225/244)	52.5 (21/40)	92.5 (225/243)	6.8	0.50
150	61.5 (24/39)	89.3 (218/244)	48.0 (24/50)	93.5 (218/233)	5.7	0.43
100	66.6 (26/39)	84.0 (205/244)	40.0 (26/65)	94.0 (205/218)	4.1	0.39

TABLE 4: Diagnostic performance of the criteria evaluated.

	Sensitivity %	Specificity %	PPV (%)	NPV (%)	+ve likelihood ratio	−ve likelihood ratio
RMI ≥ 250	54.05 (20/37)	93.4 (228/244)	55.5 (20/36)	93.06 (228/245)	8.1	0.49
CA125 ≥ 35	70.2 (26/37)	67.6 (165/244)	24.7 (26/105)	93.7 (165/176)	2.1	0.44
Ultrasound score 3	78.3 (29/37)	81.5 (199/244)	39.1 (29/74)	96.1 (199/207)	4.2	0.26
Menopause score 3	51.3 (19/37)	85.6 (209/244)	35.1 (19/54)	92.0 (209/227)	3.5	0.56

were higher in 105 (37.3%) patients. Among the patients with CA125 levels greater than 35 U/mL, 75 (26.6%) had benign disease, 26 (9.2%) had malignant, and 4 (1.4%) had borderline lesions. One hundred and sixty-two (57.6%) patients with CA125 levels less than 35 U/mL had benign lesions, while 11 (3.9%) had malignant, and 3 (1%) had borderline disease.

3.5. RMI. The RMI was calculated according to a standard formula (Jacobs et al., 1990). The RMI scores of the patients varied from 1.9 to 32364 (mean, 601.1 ± 3196.3) (Table 2). Two hundred and forty-five (87.1%) patients had an RMI score less than 250, while 36 (12.8%) had scores above 250. Twenty of the patients with RMI scores ≥250 had malignant disease, while 14 had benign and 2 had borderline lesions. Among patients with RMI scores less than 250, 223 (79.3%) had benign disease, while 17 (6%) and 5 (1.7%) had malignant and borderline lesions, respectively.

3.6. Risk Stratification Based on RMI Scores. We assessed the distribution of benign, borderline, and malignant ovarian cancers when the patients were categorized based on their RMI scores.

In order to identify the RMI score that was an effective risk predictor, we studied the sensitivity and specificity of RMI scores at four levels, namely, ≤100, ≤150, ≤200, and ≤250. The sensitivity, specificity, and positive and negative predictive values of RMI score at each of these levels are summarized in Table 3.

One hundred and twenty (42.7%) patients had RMI scores ≤25, among whom 117 (41.6%) had benign disease, 3 (1%) had malignant disease, and none had borderline lesions. The scores ranged from 25.1 to 249 in 125 (42.7%) patients. In this group, 106 (37.7%) patients had benign disease and 5 (1.7%) had borderline disease, while 14 (4.9%) had malignant disease. In the third group with RMI scores ≥ 250, 20 (7.1%) had malignant disease, 2 (0.7%) had borderline disease, and 14 (4.9%) had benign disease.

To find out the RMI score that could most effectively classify the disease, we calculated the sensitivity, specificity, positive predictive value, negative predictive value, and the likelihood ratios at RMI cut-off levels of 100, 150, 200, and 250. A comparison of the diagnostic indices with these cut-offs is shown in Table 3.

As shown in Table 3, an RMI of 250 yielded the ideal combination of sensitivity (54.05), specificity (93.4), positive predictive value (55.5), negative predictive value (93.06), and positive (8.1) and negative (0.49) likelihood ratios. Though cut-offs of 100 and 150 showed higher sensitivity in detecting malignant disease, they had lower specificity, positive predictive value, and likelihood ratios, compared to 250.

We also compared the diagnostic performance of RMI scores >250 against CA125 levels >35 U/mL, ultrasound score of 3 and menopausal score of 3. Table 4 summarizes the findings from this analysis. Among the three criteria, an ultrasound score of 3 had the highest sensitivity (78.3%), while an RMI score ≥250 had the highest specificity (93.4%). The latter also had the highest positive predictive value of 55.5%, while negative predictive value was highest for an ultrasound score of 3 (96.1%). The positive likelihood ratio was highest for RMI score ≥250, while a score of 100 had the least negative likelihood ratio (0.39).

4. Discussion

About 10% of women undergo exploratory surgery for evaluation of ovarian masses during their lifetime [7]. Prompt identification of ovarian malignancies and referral to a gyneco-oncologist can enhance the patient survival rates [8], but a single method which can accurately predict ovarian malignancy is still unavailable. Herein we report that the multiparametric RMI score can be a useful tool in prediction of malignant ovarian disease, in low-resource settings.

The mean age of the patients with ovarian mass in our study was 36.87 years (range, 8 to 85 years). This is slightly higher than that reported in a similar study by Akdeniz et al. in 2009 [9].

In our study, 13.2% of the patients with an ovarian mass had malignant disease. Thirty-five percent of malignancies occurred in postmenopausal patients and 7.9% among the premenopausal patients. The data seem to agree with earlier reports of similar incidence rates and preponderance in postmenopausal patients [9–12].

Ultrasonography is widely appreciated as the best imaging method for evaluation of ovarian pathology. Several groups have reported higher sensitivity, specificity, and positive predictive values for this method (Agarwal et al., 2011, and references therein). In our study, an ultrasound score of 3 had the highest sensitivity (78.3%) and negative predictive value (96.1%) and the least negative likelihood ratio (0.26), among the parameters evaluated.

Several candidate biomarkers and their combinations have been employed in assessing the risk of ovarian malignancies, albeit with varying efficiency [13]. Serum CA125 level is widely appreciated as a useful biomarker for estimating the risk of ovarian cancer, though other gynecological pathology can also increase its levels. Myers et al. [14] have earlier reported sensitivity and specificity of less than 80%, for this marker, in the prediction of ovarian cancers. Simsek et al. (2014) [15] reported a sensitivity of 78.6% and specificity of 63.5% for a CA125 cut-off of 35 U/mL. Another report indicated a sensitivity of 88% and specificity of 97% for CA125 at a higher cut-off of 88 U/mL [12]. In our study, CA125 levels ≥35 U/mL had a sensitivity of 70.2%, specificity of 67.6%, positive predictive value of 24.7%, negative predictive value of 93.7, and positive and negative likelihood ratios of 2.1 and 0.44, respectively. We suggest that a higher prevalence of inflammatory and nonspecific uterine and ovarian pathology might have contributed to elevated CA125 levels in the majority of our patients and thus its low diagnostic performance in the detection of malignant ovarian disease.

Rao (2014) [16] has recently reported higher sensitivity, specificity, and positive and negative predictive values for a postmenopausal score of 3. In our study, this parameter had a higher specificity and negative predictive value, but lower sensitivity and positive predictive values in assessing malignancy risk.

RMI was first proposed by Jacobs et al. and is calculated from the serum CA125 antigen level, menopausal status, and ultrasonographic findings [6]. Several retrospective and prospective studies have reported it to be the best available tool for triage and referral of ovarian malignancies [17, 18]. Its utility as a diagnostic tool depends on the prevalence of malignancy in the study population [15]. We observed a low prevalence of malignancy (13.2%) among our study group, significantly lesser than some of the earlier reports of 30–43% [6, 17, 19].

Jacobs et al. (1990) [6], studying 143 patients, reported a sensitivity of 85.4% and specificity of 96.9% for this method, with a cut-off of 200. Subsequently, several groups have reported its superior sensitivity and specificity in estimating the risk of ovarian malignancy, compared to other parameters [19–25]. The RMI cut-offs in many studies ranged from 25 to 250 (reviewed in Geomini et al., 2009) [18]. Most studies reported an increased diagnostic accuracy and performance with an RMI cut-off of 200 [6, 16, 19, 20, 22, 24, 26–32]. A recent study reported a sensitivity of 89.5%, specificity of 96.2%, positive predictive value of 77.3%, and negative predictive value of 98.4% [11], when a higher RMI cut-off of 238 was used for the screening. Yamamoto et al. (2009) [25] reported a sensitivity and specificity of 75% and 91%, respectively, using a cut-off of 450. The best performance

in the present study was seen with an RMI cut-off of 250, and the low sensitivity (54.5%) and high specificity (93.4%) observed were comparable to the majority of earlier reports that employed a similar cut-off [6, 19, 20, 22, 26, 29–35].

We conclude that, in the absence of a definitive biomarker, the multiparametric Risk of Malignancy Index serves as a very useful tool for identification of malignant ovarian disease and their prompt triage and referral to expert care.

Conflict of Interests

The authors declare that there is no conflict of interests regarding the publication of this paper.

References

[1] A. Jemal, R. Siegel, J. Xu, and E. Ward, "Cancer statistics, 2010," *CA Cancer Journal for Clinicians*, vol. 60, no. 5, pp. 277–300, 2010.

[2] J. Ferlay, I. Soerjomataram, M. Ervik et al., "Cancer incidence and mortality worldwide: IARC Cancer Base No. 11," in *GLOBOCAN 2012 v1.0*, International Agency for Research on Cancer, Lyon, France, 2013, http://globocan.iarc.fr.

[3] *Breakaway: The Global Burden of Cancer-Challenges and Opportunities*, The Economist Intelligence Unit, London, UK, 2009.

[4] L. McGowan, "Patterns of care in carcinoma of the ovary," *Cancer*, vol. 71, no. 2, pp. 628–633, 1993.

[5] R. E. Bristow, R. S. Tomacruz, D. K. Armstrong, E. L. Trimble, and F. J. Montz, "Survival effect of maximal cytoreductive surgery for advanced ovarian carcinoma during the platinum era: a meta-analysis," *Journal of Clinical Oncology*, vol. 20, no. 5, pp. 1248–1259, 2002.

[6] I. Jacobs, D. Oram, J. Fairbanks, J. Turner, C. Frost, and J. G. Grudzinskas, "A risk of malignancy index incorporating CA 125, ultrasound and menopausal status for the accurate preoperative diagnosis of ovarian cancer," *British Journal of Obstetrics and Gynaecology*, vol. 97, no. 10, pp. 922–929, 1990.

[7] Royal College of Obstetricians and Gynaecologists, "Management of suspected ovarian masses in premenopausal women," RCOG/BSGE Joint Guideline, Royal College of Obstetricians and Gynaecologists, 2011, http://bogs.org.in/RCOG_Guideline_Sukumar_Barik.pdf.

[8] A. Agarwal, B. J. D. Rein, S. Gupta, R. Dada, J. Safi, and C. Michener, "Potential markers for detection and monitoring of ovarian cancer," *Journal of Oncology*, vol. 2011, Article ID 475983, 17 pages, 2011.

[9] N. Akdeniz, U. Kuyumcuoğlu, A. Kale, M. Erdemoğlu, and F. Caca, "Risk of malignancy index for adnexal masses," *European Journal of Gynaecological Oncology*, vol. 30, no. 2, pp. 178–180, 2009.

[10] M. A. Roett and P. Evans, "Ovarian cancer: an overview," *American Family Physician*, vol. 80, no. 6, pp. 609–616, 2009.

[11] T. Ashrafgangooei and M. Rezaeezadeh, "Risk of malignancy index in preoperative evaluation of pelvic masses," *Asian Pacific Journal of Cancer Prevention*, vol. 12, no. 7, pp. 1727–1730, 2011.

[12] Z. Bouzari, S. A. Yazdani, M. H. Ahmadi et al., "Comparison of three malignancy risk indices and CA-125 in the preoperative evaluation of patients with pelvic masses," *BMC Research Notes*, vol. 4, article 206, 2011.

[13] J. M. Escudero, J. M. Auge, X. Filella, A. Torne, J. Pahisa, and R. Molina, "Comparison of serum human epididymis protein

4 with cancer antigen 125 as a tumor marker in patients with malignant and nonmalignant diseases," *Clinical Chemistry*, vol. 57, no. 11, pp. 1534–1544, 2011.

[14] E. R. Myers, L. A. Bastian, L. J. Havrilesky et al., "Management of adnexal mass," *Evidence Report/Technology Assessment*, no. 130, pp. 1–145, 2006.

[15] H. S. Simsek, A. Tokmak, E. Ozgu et al., "ole of a risk of malignancy index in clinical approaches to adnexal masses," *Asian Pacific Journal of Cancer Prevention*, vol. 15, no. 18, pp. 7793–7797, 2014.

[16] J. H. Rao, "Risk of malignancy index in assessment of pelvic mass," *International Journal of Biomedical Research*, vol. 5, no. 3, pp. 184–186, 2014.

[17] A. P. Davies, I. Jacobs, R. Woolas, A. Fish, and D. Oram, "The adnexal mass: benign or malignant? Evaluation of a risk of malignancy index," *British Journal of Obstetrics and Gynaecology*, vol. 100, no. 10, pp. 927–931, 1993.

[18] P. Geomini, R. Kruitwagen, G. L. Bremer, J. Cnossen, and B. W. J. Mol, "The accuracy of risk scores in predicting ovarian malignancy: a systematic review," *Obstetrics and Gynecology*, vol. 113, no. 2, pp. 384–394, 2009.

[19] S. Ma, K. Shen, and J. Lang, "A risk of malignancy index in preoperative diagnosis of ovarian cancer," *Chinese Medical Journal*, vol. 116, no. 3, pp. 396–399, 2003.

[20] A. P. Manjunath, K. Sujatha, and R. Vani, "Comparison of three risk of malignancy indices in evaluation of pelvic masses," *Gynecologic Oncology*, vol. 81, no. 2, pp. 225–229, 2001.

[21] N. Asif, A. Sattar, M. M. Dawood, T. Rafi, M. Aamir, and M. Anwar, "Pre-operative evaluation of ovarian mass: risk of malignancy index," *Journal of the College of Physicians and Surgeons Pakistan*, vol. 14, no. 3, pp. 128–131, 2004.

[22] B. R. Obeidat, Z. O. Amarin, J. A. Latimer, and R. A. Crawford, "Risk of malignancy index in the preoperative evaluation of pelvic masses," *International Journal of Gynecology and Obstetrics*, vol. 85, no. 3, pp. 255–258, 2004.

[23] S. Leelahakorn, S. Tangjitgamol, S. Manusirivithaya, P. Thongsuksai, P. Jaroenchainon, and C. Jivangkul, "Comparison of ultrasound score, CA125, menopausal status, and risk of malignancy index in differentiating between benign and borderline or malignant ovarian tumors," *Journal of the Medical Association of Thailand*, vol. 88, no. 2, pp. S22–S30, 2005.

[24] S. Ulusoy, O. Akbayir, C. Numanoglu, N. Ulusoy, E. Odabas, and A. Gulkilik, "The risk of malignancy index in discrimination of adnexal masses," *International Journal of Gynecology and Obstetrics*, vol. 96, no. 3, pp. 186–191, 2007.

[25] Y. Yamamoto, R. Yamada, H. Oguri, N. Maeda, and T. Fukaya, "Comparison of four malignancy risk indices in the preoperative evaluation of patients with pelvic masses," *European Journal of Obstetrics Gynecology and Reproductive Biology*, vol. 144, no. 2, pp. 163–167, 2009.

[26] S. Tingulstad, B. Hagen, F. E. Skjeldestad et al., "Evaluation of a risk of malignancy index based on serum CA125, ultrasound findings and menopausal status in the pre-operative diagnosis of pelvic masses," *BJOG: An International Journal of Obstetrics & Gynaecology*, vol. 103, no. 8, pp. 826–831, 1996.

[27] G. Morgante, A. La Marca, A. Ditto, and V. de Leo, "Comparison of two malignancy risk indices based on serum CA125, ultrasound score and menopausal status in the diagnosis of ovarian masses," *BJOG: An International Journal of Obstetrics & Gynaecology*, vol. 106, no. 6, pp. 524–527, 1999.

[28] J. C. C. Torres, S. F. M. Derchain, A. Faundes, R. C. Gontijo, E. Z. Martinez, and L. A. L. A. Andrade, "Risk-of-malignancy index in preoperative evaluation of clinically restricted ovarian cancer," *Sao Paulo Medical Journal*, vol. 120, no. 3, pp. 72–76, 2002.

[29] E. S. Andersen, A. Knudsen, P. Rix, and B. Johansen, "Risk of malignancy index in the pre-operative evaluation of patients with adnexal masses," *Gynecologic Oncology*, vol. 90, no. 1, pp. 109–112, 2003.

[30] Y. N. Chia, D. E. Marsden, G. Robertson, and N. F. Hacker, "Triage of ovarian masses," *Australian and New Zealand Journal of Obstetrics and Gynaecology*, vol. 48, no. 3, pp. 322–328, 2008.

[31] W. Moolthiya and P. Yuenyao, "The risk of malignancy index (RMI) in diagnosis of ovarian malignancy," *Asian Pacific Journal of Cancer Prevention*, vol. 10, no. 5, pp. 865–868, 2009.

[32] M. Terzić, J. Dotlić, I. L. Ladjević, J. Atanacković, and N. Ladjević, "Evaluation of the risk malignancy index diagnostic value in patients with adnexal masses," *Vojnosanitetski Pregled*, vol. 68, no. 7, pp. 589–593, 2011.

[33] S. Tingulstad, B. Hagen, F. E. Skjeldestad, T. Halvorsen, K. Nustad, and M. Onsrud, "The risk of malignancy index to evaluate potential ovarian cancers in local hospitals," *Obstetrics and Gynecology*, vol. 93, no. 3, pp. 448–452, 1999.

[34] H. A. Tanriverdi, H. Sade, V. Akbulut, A. Barut, and Ü. Bayar, "Clinical and ultrasonographic evaluation of pelvic masses," *Journal of the Turkish German Gynecology Association*, vol. 8, no. 1, pp. 67–70, 2007.

[35] O. Meray, I. Türkçüoğlu, M. M. Meydanlı, and A. Kafkaslı, "Risk of malignancy index is not sensitive in detecting non-epithelial ovarian cancer and borderline ovarian tumor," *Journal of the Turkish German Gynecological Association*, vol. 11, no. 1, pp. 22–26, 2010.

25

Failure Rate of Single Dose Methotrexate in Managment of Ectopic Pregnancy

Feras Sendy,[1] **Eman AlShehri,**[2] **Amani AlAjmi,**[2] **Elham Bamanie,**[3] **Surekha Appani,**[3] **and Taghreed Shams**[4]

[1]*Obstetrics and Gynecology Department, King Fahad Medical City, Riyadh, Saudi Arabia*
[2]*King Khalid University Hospital, King Saud University, Riyadh, Saudi Arabia*
[3]*Obstetrics and Gynecology Department, King Abdualaziz Medical City,*
 King Saud Bin Abdualziz University for Health Science (KSAU-HS), Riyadh, Saudi Arabia
[4]*Obstetrics and Gynecology Department, King Abdualaziz Medical City,*
 King Saud Bin Abdualziz University for Health Science (KSAU-HS), P.O. Box 9515, Jeddah 21423, Saudi Arabia

Correspondence should be addressed to Taghreed Shams; shamsta@ngha.med.sa

Academic Editor: Robert Coleman

Background. One of the treatment modalities for ectopic pregnancy is methotrexate. The purpose of this study is to identify the failure rate of methotrexate in treating patients with ectopic pregnancy as well as the risk factors leading to treatment failure. *Methods.* A retrospective chart review of 225 patients who received methotrexate as a primary management option for ectopic pregnancy. Failure of single dose of methotrexate was defined as drop of BHCG level less than or equal to 14% in the seventh day after administration of methotrexate. *Results.* 225 patients had methotrexate. Most of the patients (151 (67%)) received methotrexate based on the following formula: f 50 mg X body surface area. Single dose of methotrexate was successful in 72% (162/225) of the patients. 28% (63/225) were labeled as failure of single dose of methotrexate because of suboptimal drop in BhCG. 63% (40/63) of failure received a second dose of methotrexate, and 37% (23/63) underwent surgical treatment. Among patient who received initial dose of methotrexate, 71% had moderate or severe pain, and 58% had ectopic mass size of more than 4 cm on ultrasound. *Conclusion.* Liberal use of medical treatment of ectopic pregnancy results in 71% success rate.

1. Introduction

Implantation of a fertilized ovum outside the uterine cavity is known as ectopic pregnancy (EP) [1–3]. It is a medical emergency due to the high morbidity and mortality in the reproductive age [4–7]. The incidence of ectopic pregnancies is 1-2% in the developed countries [8]. Ninety-eight percent of the implants are in the fallopian tube but also can be implanted at various sites such as ampulla, isthmus, ovaries, abdomen, and broad ligament [9, 10].

The etiology is uncertain but there are various risk factors, such as infertility, previous tubal surgery, contraceptive failure, cigarette smoking, and previous ectopic pregnancy [11]. Patients usually come with lower abdominal pain and vaginal bleeding from the 6th to 10th week of gestation [1]. It has been reported that one-third of patients have no clinical symptoms

[12, 13]. If a patient came with syncope and signs of shock with a positive pregnancy test ruptured ectopic pregnancy should be suspected [11].

When the patient is pregnant, the physician should perform a work-up to detect possible ectopic or ruptured EP. Prompt ultrasound evaluation is the key in diagnosing ectopic pregnancy. Equivocal ultrasound results should be combined with quantitative beta subunit of human chorionic gonadotropin (BhCG) levels [14, 15]. If a patient has a BhCG level of 1,500 MIU per mL or greater, but the transvaginal ultrasonography does not show an intrauterine gestational sac, EP should be suspected [16].

While surgical approaches are the mainstay of treatment, advances in early diagnosis facilitated the introduction of medical therapy with methotrexate (MTX) in the 1980 [17–19]. Approximately 35% of women with EP are eligible for medical treatment [20]. The use of methotrexate (MTX) to treat early unruptured EP has been shown to be a safe and effective alternative to surgery in properly selected cases [21–23].

A Cochrane systemic review concluded that MTX treatment of EP had the highest success rate when plasma BhCG levels were below 3,000 IU/mL. It was stated that side effects from multiple-dose MTX treatment impaired quality of life [24]. In addition, MTX treatment was more expensive than laparoscopic salpingotomy when initial plasma-BhCG levels were above 3,000 IU/L [25]. Treatment with a single dose of MTX had fewer side effects, but the success rate was less than following a multiple-dose regimen [26].

Due to the routine use of early ultrasound among infertile patients who conceive, diagnosis of EP can be established early and medical treatment can be administered in most cases. The overall success rate of medical treatment in properly selected women is nearly 90% [27–29].

Our rational in this study was to review the cases that were diagnosed with EP and treated medically with MTX and observe the failure rate among them.

2. Methodology

Medical records of patients admitted to KAMC with a diagnosis of ectopic pregnancy which were retrospectively reviewed in the period between 2005 and 2011 were screened. Patients who had methotrexate as medical treatment of ectopic pregnancy were identified and included in this review. Patients who underwent surgical treatment as the first option of management were excluded.

The primary outcome measure of this review was the failure of first dose of methotrexate. Failure is defined in two ways: firstly, as suboptimal drop in BHCG level to 14% or less that necessitate second dose of methotrexate or surgical treatment; secondly, as the need for emergency laparoscopy or laparotomy in case of hemodynamic instability or severe abdominal pain. The following data were collected: demographic data including age, weight, and height, presenting symptoms, methotrexate dose given, ultrasound finding including ectopic size, fluid in pouch of Douglas, and BhCG level on day one and day 7 of methotrexate administration. BhCG level on the day of 1 at the time of methotrexate administration was called day 1. Some variation might be noted in the numbers of patients and that is due to some missing data. Bivariate associations were evaluated with use of odds ratio (OR) and Pearson's #2. Logistic regression was used to create an explanatory model for MTX failure. All analyses were performed with use of SPSS software (version 17).

3. Results

371 charts were reviewed. 146 subjects were excluded, 140 subjects were excluded because patients had surgery as primary mode of treatment, and 6 subjects were excluded because of the need for emergency surgery due to suspension of ruptured ectopic data after admission. 225 charts were included in the study and analyzed. The diagnosis of EP was

TABLE 1: Baseline characteristics.

Variable	Mean (SD)
Age	30.3 (5.7)
Body weight (in kg)	72.7 (15.7)
Height (in centimeter)	154.2 (12.6)
Methotrexate dose (mg)	85.9 (12.7)
Clinical presentation	
Before starting treatment	
Asymptomatic	65 (28.9%)
Moderate pain	153 (68%)
Severe pain	7 (3.1%)
After receiving the 1st dose of methotrexate	
Asymptomatic	182 (80.8%)
Symptomatic	43 (19.1%)
Ectopic size on U/S	
Less than 4 cm	86 (42%)
More than 4 cm	119 (58%)
BHCG level	
Day 1	Mean 2219
Day 7	Mean 1802

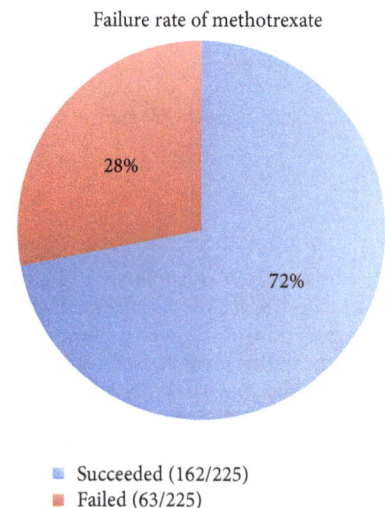

FIGURE 1: Failure rate of the 1st dose of methotrexate.

based on the admitting physician assessment note. Dosing of methotrexate was based on body surface area (50 mg X BSA) in 151/225 (67%) of the patients; the rest received dose based on 1mg per kg body weight.

The average age was 30 years old. Before receiving methotrexate, most of the patients (68%) quantified their pain as moderate, only 29% were asymptomatic (Figure 3). Size of ectopic pregnancy on ultrasound was more than 4 cm in 58% of cases (Table 1).

In 72% of the patients (162/225), single dose of methotrexate was successful; that is, BhCG decreased by more than 15% in the seventh day after administration. 28% (63/225) were labeled as failure of single dose of methotrexate because of suboptimal drop in BhCG (Figure 1).

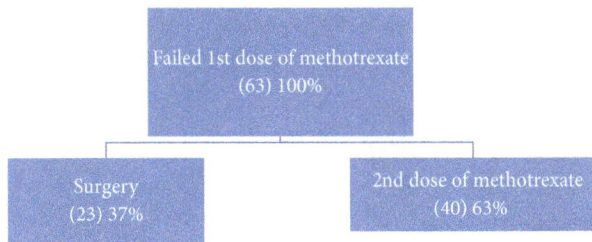

FIGURE 2: Modalities of treatment after failure methotrexate.

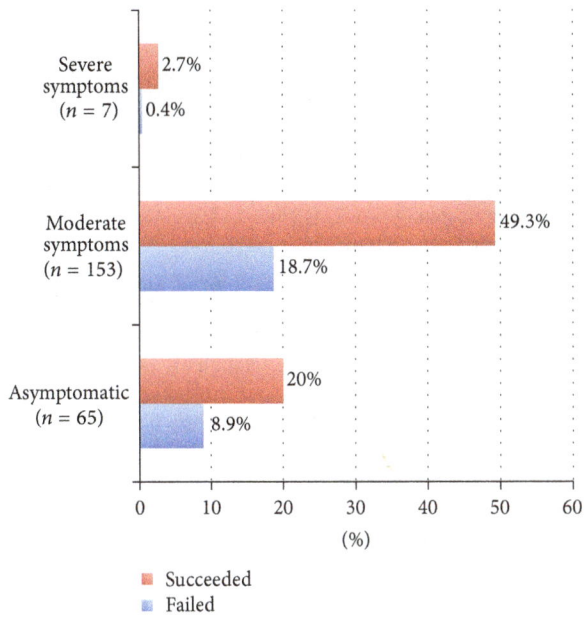

FIGURE 3: Symptomatology and failure of medical treatment.

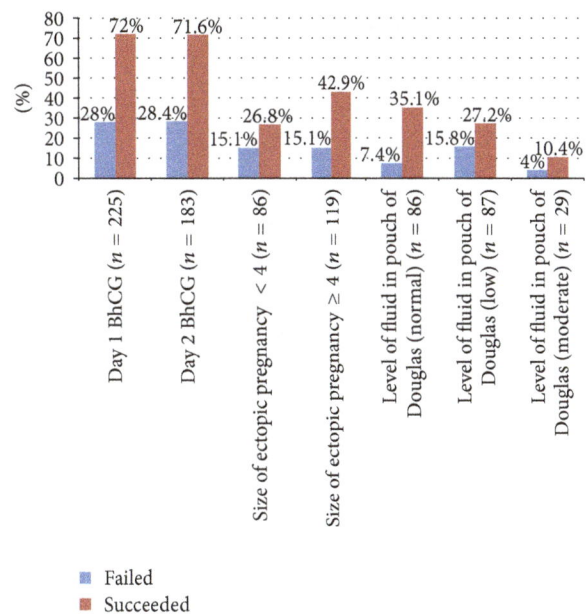

FIGURE 4: Predictors of failure of medical treatment.

TABLE 2: Indications for surgical treatment in patient whom failed first dose of methotrexate.

Indications	Number 23	Percentage
Patient refusal of second dose of MTX	9	39
Presence of pain on day 7 after medical treatment	8	35
Rupture of ectopic	6	26

63% (40/63) of failure received a second dose of methotrexate, and 37% (23/63) underwent surgical treatment (Figure 2).

The indication for surgical treatment were patient choice in 39%. Presence of pain 7 days after medical treatment 35% and rupture of ectopic 26% (Table 2).

Predictors for failure of single dose of methotrexate is Figure 4.

(i) Initial Level of BhCG (Table 3). The higher the BHCG on day one, the lower is the failure rate (odds ratio of failure 0.3 95% CI (0.1–0.7); *P* value 0.004). In another term, with every increase log of beta HCG milli-international units per

milliliter (mIU/mL) on day one, there is 60% chance of reducing likelihood of medical treatment failure.

(ii) BHCG Day 7. The higher is the levels of BhCG on day seven, the higher is the failure rate. (OR 3.66 95% CI 2.0–6.4; *P* value = 0.0001). With every increase log of beta HCG milli-international units per milliliter (mIU/mL) at day 7, there are 3.6 times higher odds of medical treatment failure. Mass size of ectopic pregnancy being ≥4 cm on U/S has not been shown to be statistically significant predictor of failure in our review.

4. Discussion

Methotrexate was first introduced as a successful treatment option for EP in the 1980's by Tanaka et al. [29]. Numerous published literatures have presented different success rates of medical management in resolving an EP; these rates were ranging from 85% to 95% [30, 31]. A study in Scandinavia showed a success rate of medical treatment in EP 76.2% [32]. Nguyen et al., 2010, described an outstandingly success rate of 100% (*n* = 30). In 2013, a similar cohort study presented a success rate of 89% [33]. Another study conducted in Makkah showed that all patients given methotrexate were successfully treated [34].

In this study the success rate of the medical management of ectopic pregnancy with methotrexate was found to be 72%. It appears to be relativity lower than international rates, an average of 90%; however our study had a remarkably higher success rate than a study conducted in Nigeria, which presented a success rate of only 3.8% [35]. This lower success rate in our study compared to the majority of equivalent studies may be attributed to the lack of a careful selection of patients as candidates for medical therapy and confining to a strict selection criterion. Among patient who received

TABLE 3: Association between level of BhCG and failure of medical treatment (multivariate regression analysis).

Variable	OR	95% OR CI	P value
BhCG day 1	0.3	0.1–0.7	0.004
Fluid in pouch of Douglas	0.4	0.1–1.1	0.1
Size of ectopic ≥4 cm	1.3	0.5–3.3	0.4
BhCG day 7	3.66	2.0–6.4	0.0001

medical treatment, 71% had moderate or severe pain, and 58% had ectopic mass size of more than 4 cm.

As it has been established in a similar study conducted in Oman, following strict selection criteria raised the success rate of methotrexate therapy up to 20% more than their previous average success rate 40% [36].

Of those 28% who had failed medical treatment, 63% received a second dose of MTX, which is comparable to around 15–20% of women receiving a single dose of methotrexate who required a repeat dose of this chemotherapeutic agent in related studies [33–38], while the rest (37%) underwent surgical management either due to rupture of the EP, patient preference, or new onset of severe pain.

One of the risk factors of developing EP is being of age 40 years or older [27]. In this study, the mean age was 30 years, which is comparable to former studies [35–37]. Maternal age is not a predictor of MTX treatment in our study. It did however appear in a similar study that an increased maternal age will lead to a decrease in the in the success rate of MTX [36]. There were no mortalities in this study compared to the to a mortality report in the UK (issued in December 2007), showing a total of 10 deaths. These fatalities occurred during the nonsurgical management of an accurately established diagnosis of EP rather than because of an overlooked diagnosis or delayed surgical management, as these were the most common reasons for EP mortality during the previous four years [37, 38].

Conflict of Interests

The authors declare that there is no conflict of interests regarding the publication of this paper.

Acknowledgment

This study was done as part of research summer school program of King Abdullah International Medical Research Center (KAIMRC).

References

[1] J. J. Walker, "Ectopic pregnancy," Clinical Obstetrics and Gynecology, vol. 50, no. 1, pp. 89–99, 2007.

[2] D. Della-Giustina and M. Denny, "Ectopic pregnancy," Emergency Medicine Clinics of North America, vol. 21, no. 3, pp. 565–584, 2003.

[3] R. Varma and J. Gupta, "Tubal ectopic pregnancy," Clinical Evidence, vol. 2009, p. 1406, 2009.

[4] C. J. Berg, J. Chang, W. M. Callaghan, and S. J. Whitehead, "Pregnancy-related mortality in the United States, 1991-1997," Obstetrics and Gynecology, vol. 101, no. 2, pp. 289-296, 2003.

[5] A. K. Majhi, N. Roy, K. S. Karmakar, and P. K. Banerjee, "Ectopic pregnancy—an analysis of 180 cases," Journal of the Indian Medical Association, vol. 105, no. 6, pp. 308–314, 2007.

[6] J. L. V. Shaw, S. K. Dey, H. O. D. Critchley, and A. W. Horne, "Current knowledge of the aetiology of human tubal ectopic pregnancy," Human Reproduction Update, vol. 16, no. 4, Article ID dmp057, pp. 432–444, 2010.

[7] G. O. Udigwe, O. S. Umeonihu, and I. I. Mbachu, "Ectopic pregnancy: a 5 year review of cases at nnamdi azikiwe university teaching hospital (NAUTH) Nnewi," Nigerian Medical Journal, vol. 51, no. 4, pp. 160–163, 2010.

[8] T. E. Goldner, H. W. Lawson, Z. Xia et al., "Surveillance for ectopic pregnancy—United States, 1970-1989," MMWR CDC Surveillance Summaries, vol. 42, pp. 73–85, 1993.

[9] J. A. Wong and J. F. Clark, "Correlation of symptoms with age and location of gestation in tubal pregnancy," Journal of the National Medical Association, vol. 60, no. 3, pp. 221–223, 1968.

[10] A. Kellogg, "Intratubalmethotrexate versus laproscopicsalpingotomy," World Journal of Laparoscopic Surgery, vol. 2, no. 2, pp. 18–21, 2009.

[11] V. Sivalingam, W. Duncan, E. Kirk, L. Shephard, and A. Horne, "Diagnosis and management of ectopic pregnancy," Journal of Family Planning and Reproductive Health Care, vol. 37, pp. 231–240, 2011.

[12] J. I. Tay, J. Moore, and J. J. Walker, "Ectopic pregnancy," British Medical Journal, vol. 320, no. 7239, pp. 916–919, 2000.

[13] B. C. Kaplan, R. G. Dart, M. Moskos et al., "Ectopic pregnancy: prospective study with improved diagnostic accuracy," Annals of Emergency Medicine, vol. 28, no. 1, pp. 10–17, 1996.

[14] K. Barnhart, M. T. Mennuti, I. Benjamin, S. Jacobson, D. Goodman, and C. Coutifaris, "Prompt diagnosis of ectopic pregnancy in an emergency department setting," Obstetrics and Gynecology, vol. 84, no. 6, pp. 1010–1015, 1994.

[15] C. R. Gracia and K. T. Barnhart, "Diagnosing ectopic pregnancy: decision analysis comparing six strategies," Obstetrics and Gynecology, vol. 97, no. 3, pp. 464–470, 2001.

[16] A.-M. Lozeau and B. Potter, "Diagnosis and management of ectopic pregnancy," American Family Physician, vol. 72, no. 9, pp. 1707–1714, 2005.

[17] I. A. Rodi, M. V. Sauer, M. J. Gorrill et al., "The medical treatment of unruptured ectopic pregnancy with methotrexate and citrovorum rescue: preliminary experience," Fertility and Sterility, vol. 46, no. 5, pp. 811–813, 1986.

[18] T. G. Stovall, F. W. Ling, and J. E. Buster, "Outpatient chemotherapy of unruptured ectopic pregnancy," Fertility and Sterility, vol. 51, no. 3, pp. 435–438, 1989.

[19] M. D. Pisarska, S. A. Carson, and J. E. Buster, "Ectopic pregnancy," The Lancet, vol. 351, no. 9109, pp. 1115–1120, 1998.

[20] S. K. van den Eeden, J. Shan, C. Bruce, and M. Glasser, "Ectopic pregnancy rate and treatment utilization in a large managed care organization," Obstetrics & Gynecology, vol. 105, no. 5, part 1, pp. 1052–1057, 2005.

[21] P. J. Hajenius, S. Engelsbel, B. W. J. Mol et al., "Randomised trial of systemic methotrexate versus laparoscopic salpingostomy in tubal pregnancy," *The Lancet*, vol. 350, no. 9080, pp. 774–779, 1997.

[22] S. J. Ory, A. L. Villanueva, P. K. Sand, and R. K. Tamura, "Conservative treatment of ectopic pregnancy with methotrexate," *The American Journal of Obstetrics and Gynecology*, vol. 154, no. 6, pp. 1299–1306, 1986.

[23] T. G. Stovall and F. W. Ling, "Single-dose methotrexate: an expanded clinical trial," *The American Journal of Obstetrics and Gynecology*, vol. 168, no. 6, pp. 1759–1765, 1993.

[24] P. J. Hajenius, F. Mol, B. W. Mol, P. M. Bossuyt, W. M. Ankum, and F. van der Veen, "Interventions for tubal ectopic pregnancy," *Cochrane Database of Systematic Reviews*, no. 1, Article ID CD000324, 2007.

[25] B. W. J. Mol, P. J. Hajenius, S. Engelsbel et al., "Treatment of tubal pregnancy in the Netherlands: an economic comparison of systemic methotrexate administration and laparoscopic salpingostomy," *The American Journal of Obstetrics and Gynecology*, vol. 181, no. 4, pp. 945–951, 1999.

[26] M. C. Sowter, C. M. Farquhar, K. J. Petrie, and G. Gudex, "A randomised trial comparing single dose systemic methotrexate and laparoscopic surgery for the treatment of unruptured tubal pregnancy," *British Journal of Obstetrics and Gynaecology*, vol. 108, no. 2, pp. 192–203, 2001.

[27] K. T. Barnhart, G. Gosman, R. Ashby, and M. Sammel, "The medical management of ectopic pregnancy: a meta-analysis comparing 'single dose' and 'multidose' regimens," *Obstetrics and Gynecology*, vol. 101, no. 4, pp. 778–784, 2003.

[28] C. M. Farquhar, "Ectopic pregnancy," *The Lancet*, vol. 366, no. 9485, pp. 583–591, 2005.

[29] R. J. Morlock, J. E. Lafata, and D. Eisenstein, "Cost-effectiveness of single-dose methotrexate compared with laparoscopic treatment of ectopic pregnancy," *Obstetrics and Gynecology*, vol. 95, no. 3, pp. 407–412, 2000.

[30] T. Tanaka, H. Hayashi, T. Kutsuzawa, S. Fujimoto, and K. Ichinoe, "Treatment of interstitial ectopic pregnancy with methotrexate: report of a successful case," *Fertility and Sterility*, vol. 37, no. 6, pp. 851–852, 1982.

[31] G. H. Lipscomb, V. M. Givens, N. L. Meyer, D. Bran, and S. Zinberg, "Comparison of multidose and single-dose methotrexate protocols for the treatment of ectopic pregnancy," *The American Journal of Obstetrics and Gynecology*, vol. 192, no. 6, pp. 1844–1847, 2005.

[32] M. B. Potter, L. A. Lepine, and D. J. Jamieson, "Predictors of success with methotrexate treatment of tubal ectopic pregnancy at Grady Memorial Hospital," *The American Journal of Obstetrics and Gynecology*, vol. 188, no. 5, pp. 1192–1194, 2003.

[33] D. T. Westaby, O. Wu, W. C. Duncan, H. O. D. Critchley, S. Tong, and A. W. Horne, "Has increased clinical experience with methotrexate reduced the direct costs of medical management of ectopic pregnancy compared to surgery?" *BMC Pregnancy and Childbirth*, vol. 12, article 98, 2012.

[34] M. Skubisz, P. Dutton, W. C. Duncan, A. W. Horne, and S. Tong, "Using a decline in serum hCG between days 0–4 to predict ectopic pregnancy treatment success after single-dose methotrexate: a retrospective cohort study," *BMC Pregnancy and Childbirth*, vol. 13, article 30, 2013.

[35] A. Ayaz, S. Emam, and M. U. Farooq, "Clinical course of ectopic pregnancy: a single-center experience," *Journal of Human Reproductive Sciences*, vol. 6, no. 1, pp. 70–73, 2013.

[36] A. Panti, N. E. Ikechukwu, O. lukman, E. Yakubu, S. Egondu, and B. A. Tanko, "Ectopic pregnancy at Usmanu Danfodiyo University Teaching Hospital Sokoto: a ten year review," *Annals of Nigerian Medicine*, vol. 6, no. 2, pp. 87–91, 2012.

[37] U. Mahboob and S. B. Mazhar, "Management of ectopic pregnancy: a two-year study," *Journal of Ayub Medical College, Abbottabad*, vol. 18, no. 4, pp. 34–37, 2006.

[38] L. C. Edozien, "Non-surgical management of ectopic pregnancy: appropriate risk management must be in place," *Archives of Gynecology and Obstetrics*, vol. 283, no. 5, pp. 925–927, 2011.

26

Circadian System and Melatonin Hormone:
Risk Factors for Complications during Pregnancy

F. J. Valenzuela,[1,2] **J. Vera,**[1,2] **C. Venegas,**[1,2] **F. Pino,**[1] **and C. Lagunas**[1,2]

[1]*Department of Basic Sciences, Universidad del Bío-Bío, Campus Fernando May, Avenida Andres Bello s/n, Chillán, Chile*
[2]*Grupo de Ciencias Biotecnológicas, Basic Sciences Department, Universidad del Bío-Bío, Avenida Andres Bello s/n, Chillán, Chile*

Correspondence should be addressed to F. J. Valenzuela; fvalenzuela@ubiobio.cl

Academic Editor: Enrique Hernandez

Pregnancy is a complex and well-regulated temporal event in which several steps are finely orchestrated including implantation, decidualization, placentation, and partum and any temporary alteration has serious effects on fetal and maternal health. Interestingly, alterations of circadian rhythms (i.e., shiftwork) have been correlated with increased risk of preterm delivery, intrauterine growth restriction, and preeclampsia. In the last few years evidence is accumulating that the placenta may have a functional circadian system and express the clock genes *Bmal1*, *Per1-2*, and *Clock*. On the other hand, there is evidence that the human placenta synthesizes melatonin, hormone involved in the regulation of the circadian system in other tissues. Moreover, is unknown the role of this local production of melatonin and whether this production have a circadian pattern. Available information indicates that melatonin induces in placenta the expression of antioxidant enzymes catalase and superoxide dismutase, prevents the injury produced by oxidative stress, and inhibits the expression of vascular endothelial growth factor (VEGF) a gene that in other tissues is controlled by clock genes. In this review we aim to analyze available information regarding clock genes and clock genes controlled genes such as VEGF and the possible role of melatonin synthesis in the placenta.

1. Introduction

Pregnancy is a complex and well-regulated temporal event in which several steps are finely orchestrated including implantation, decidualization, placentation, and partum [1]. The chronological transitions are critical for a normal pregnancy and any temporary alteration may have detrimental effects for fetal development and/or maternal health [2–4]. The placenta is the unit of communication and exchange between mother and fetus. This organ is in charge of bidirectional transference and metabolism of hormones, nutrients, and gases (oxygen/CO_2) [5]. The major site of complication in pregnancy is the placenta and the main cause of development of obstetric syndrome is the placentation [6]. The impaired placentation causes spontaneous abortion, preeclampsia, preterm birth, and placental abruption [7]. Moreover, placenta mediates the maternal-fetal interaction in the regulation of glucocorticoids, human placental lactogen (hPL), human chorionic gonadotropin (hCG), and progesterone and estriol, among others [5, 8]. In this regard, hormonal production and activity is regulated by a circadian system, which, in fact, is composed by a family of genes named "clock genes" (Bmal1, Clock, Per1-3, and Cry1-2) [9].

2. Circadian Rhythms and Pregnancy

The circadian time-keeping system is actively engaged in the maintenance of normal physiology, not only in adults, but also during development [10]. Within an individual, the peak and trough of the rhythms for different physiological variables occurs at different clock times. For instance, in humans under normal light-dark condition, cortisol peaks at 08 h, while temperature peaks at 14–17 h, and melatonin at 02 h [11]. Similarly, during normal pregnancy different circadian rhythm are observed in the mother such as temperature [12, 13], leukocytes count, blood pressure [13], circadian pattern of weight gain [14], rhythms of uterine contraction, blood flow [15], and intra-amniotic fluid pressure [5, 15]. The final output of the circadian system during pregnancy is the labor. Humans and monkeys (diurnal animals) show a peak in the second middle of the night and early in the morning [3, 16, 17]. The rat and mice (nocturnal animals) show a time birth in the afternoon or final hours of the day [18, 19]. An important factor during the pregnancy is photoperiod, and light exposition during night hours (inhibition of melatonin production) is able to modify the hours of labor in monkeys and rats [18, 20]. At level of fetus, circadian rhythms of fetal heart rate and tachycardia are observed in twin pregnancy, showing a peak during light hours [21], showing that both the mother and the fetus have circadian rhythms.

Placenta during the pregnancy has important function of being in charge of bidirectional transference and metabolism of hormones, nutrients, and gases (oxygen/CO_2) [5]. Some hormones produced by placenta show a circadian rhythm such as human chorionic gonadotropin (hCG) showing a peak at 12–15 h [8, 22, 23]. Progesterone and the products of aromatase from placenta which convert dehydroepiandrosterone sulphate (DHES) to estriol and estradiol [5] and placental lactogen show a circadian pattern in junctional and labyrinthine zones in the rat placenta [24].

The phase relation between the circadian rhythms of different physiological variables in the 24 h cycles generates an internal temporal order [25, 26], and recent data show that alterations of circadian rhythms correlated to increased susceptibility to cancer in humans [27]. In addition, it has been reported that incidence of breast cancer increases significantly in women working in shifts, being higher among individuals who spend more years and hours per week working at night [28]. In this sense, during human pregnancy several reports suggest alterations of circadian rhythms are correlated to increased susceptibility to pregnancy disease and a meta-analysis published by Bonzini et al. (2011) showed the impacts of shiftwork in those women [4]. Thus, shiftwork was associated with an increased risk of small for gestational age (<10th percentile) and low birth weight and reported eleven studies showing elevated risk for preterm birth [4]. In animal, pregnant rats exposed to light-dark cycle that mimics shiftwork showed an increase of fat weight and changes in peak hours of plasmatic glucose and leptine in three-month-old offspring [29].

In mammals, circadian rhythms are commanded by a central clock located in the Suprachiasmatic Nucleus of the Hypothalamus (SCN) acting on peripheral circadian clocks located in almost every tissue of the body, for example, in the adrenal gland [30]. In both the SCN and peripheral tissues, the circadian oscillation depends on a transcription/translation feedback loop of a group of genes collectively named "clock genes." This family of clock genes include the transcription factors BMAL1 and CLOCK; the proteins encoded by genes Per1-3, Cry1-2 and the enzyme casein kinase 1 epsilon (CK1ε) [31] (see Figure 1). The mutation of any of the clock genes causes severe disruptions in circadian rhythms [32]. The heterodimer composed of CLOCK-BMAL1 protein is a positive regulator and binds to the E-box sequences (CACGTG) of the promoters of Per and Cry, inducing their expression. The negative regulator is a complex of the proteins PER and CRY which translocate to the nucleus and by protein-protein interaction with CLOCK-BMAL1 inhibits the transcription of Per and Cry. Translocation to the nucleus

PER and CRY requires the formation of a complex with CK1ε and provides a delay in the system to achieve a period of 24 h [33]. Clock genes are expressed in multiple tissues: heart, liver, kidney, pancreas, muscle, pars tuberalis, adrenal gland, and isolated cells such as fibroblasts and cardiomyocytes [30, 34–41].

Circadian clock genes are expressed in the placenta of rats and mice [42, 43] and in the cell line of human trophoblast [44] previously stimulated by serum shock, a potent stimulator of the circadian system such as what has been described in fibroblast [45], immortalized human breast epithelial cell [46], or hepatoma cells [47]. The circadian expression of two genes potentially controlled by clock genes has been also shown in the placenta, the vascular endothelial growth factor (VEGF), and placental lactogen (PL-II). Thus, in the cell line of human trophoblast stimulated with serum shock, the VEGF is expressed with a circadian pattern [44]. Besides in culture of rat placenta stimulated by serum shock, a circadian rhythm of PL-II expression reaching a peak at 04:00 hrs in the junctional zone and at 16:00 hrs in labyrinth zones has been showed [24].

In humans, alterations in the levels of VEGF and human PL (hPL-II) proteins have been proposed as risk markers for preeclampsia or placental dysfunction [48–50] and we speculate that the chronodisruption might be part of pathophysiological process during pregnancies diseases. The vascular endothelial growth factor A (VEGF-A) has been related with occurrence of pregnancy pathologies such as preeclampsia [48, 51]. VEGF-A is a protein that is under control of the complex CLOCK-BMAL. Thus, the promoter of VEGF has four putative E-box elements (CANNTG) to respond to clock genes, showing a circadian pattern of expression in implanted tumor cell with a peak during light hours [52]. The in vitro transcription of VEGF cotransfected with CLOCK-BMAL increases the level of VEGF protein [52]. On the other hand, the transient expression of Per2 and Cry1 inhibits the expression of VEGF [52]. In vivo experiments have showed that implanted tumor cells in mice are subordinated to SCN of the host animal. These cells show circadian rhythms of expression of clock genes and VEGF, observing a peak for the latter during the light hours, in a pattern similar to that observed for Bmal1 [52]. Considering that both reduced expression and activity of VEGF in the placenta [51] and altered circadian rhythms are associated with pathologies of pregnancy [4, 53], we could speculate that the circadian expression of clock genes would be controlling many placental functions in both normal and pathological placenta. This assumption would be difficult to test in human being; therefore investigation should include culture cell or animal models.

Nevertheless, an important question is whether in the culture of fresh human placenta, the clock gene expression is maintained as in vivo condition (i.e., circadian peripheral oscillator). In regard, we demonstrated the expression of the clock genes Bmal1 and Per2 during 36 hours in explant cultures of the adrenal gland without stimulation of serum shock, suggesting that the adrenal gland is a peripheral oscillator [30]. Whether the placenta contains a peripheral clock able to sustain an oscillation in vitro in absence of

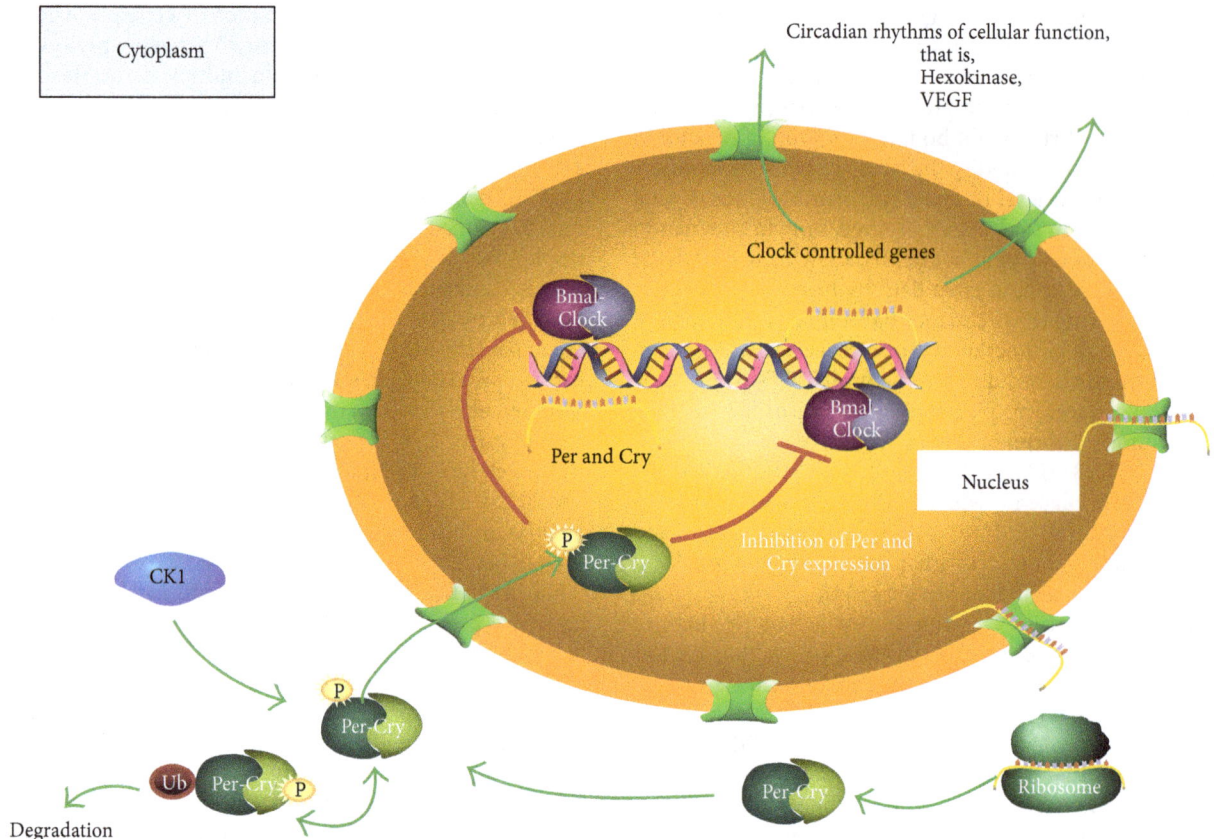

FIGURE 1: Molecular Circuit of Circadian Oscillator. See details in the text. Positive regulation of clock genes Bmal1 and Clock stimulate promoter of negative regulators Per 1-2, Cry 1-2 and controlled clock genes Hexokinase and VEGF.

synchronizing stimuli is unknown. However, Frigato et al. (2009) showed that the circadian expression of Per2 is stimulated by serum shock in culture of trophoblast [44], suggesting that placental cell in culture might maintain the circadian oscillation observed *in vivo*.

In vivo, oscillation of clock genes in some peripheral organs requires the SCN. Guo et al. (2006) demonstrated in hamsters that oscillatory expression of the clock genes Per1, Per2, and Bmal1 in the heart, liver, kidney, renal cortex, adrenal medulla, muscle, and spleen is eliminated by ablating the SCN [54]. Transplantation of SCN restored the circadian oscillation of clock genes only in the liver and kidney, suggesting that the synchronizing signal from the SCN to the other organs involves neural pathways. These could include the autonomic nervous system or corticosterone and melatonin rhythms that are not restored by SCN transplants [54]. Since the placenta is not innervated but expresses melatonin receptors [55], we believe that melatonin could regulate the expression of clock genes in the placenta.

3. Melatonin and the Placenta

The pineal gland synthesizes melatonin, a lipophilic indoleamine hormone, increasing immediately in response to light-off. This increase gives chronobiotic information to the body for its circadian organization [11]. The extension of

melatonin during the night is directly proportional to photoperiod (winter or summer), which in turn may modulate the gonadotropin axis and the time of mating sheep [35, 56]. A second function proposed for melatonin is as homeostatic hormone, regulating several aspects of fetal physiology. For instance, during the pregnancy, maternal melatonin provides a chronobiotic signal for the fetus and also plays a role in the development and maintenance of the fetal adrenal function under conditions suitable for fetal life, an effect that may also involve other fetal systems as shown in fetal sheep [9]. A third function of melatonin in placenta is to modulate the redox status, via both direct scavenger activity for radical species such as hydroxyl, alkoxyl, peroxyl, and nitric oxide (NO) [11, 57, 58], or regulating the expression of antioxidant enzymes such as catalase and manganese superoxide dismutase [59]. Additionally, in adult tissues melatonin has been shown to increase the expression of several genes such as Bax, p53, p21-27, caspases 3, 8, and 9 [60], NeuroD1, Pbef/Nampt, Hif1α [61], SGK, Nfκbia, DNA-damage-inducible transcript 4, C/EBP-δ, pdk4, Ets-1, HSP [62], HOXA4, FOXO1A, GTFIIF1, PPARδ, and TCEB3 [63] or decrease the expression of genes Bax, Bcl-2 [64]; P450 7α (CYP7B) [65]; metalloproteinase 9, 3 (MMP-9, MMP-3) [66]; heat shock proteins HSP [62]; ZNF33A and PHF15 [63]. Moreover, we have found that melatonin inhibited the expression of Per1, Bmal1, and PGC1α in response to

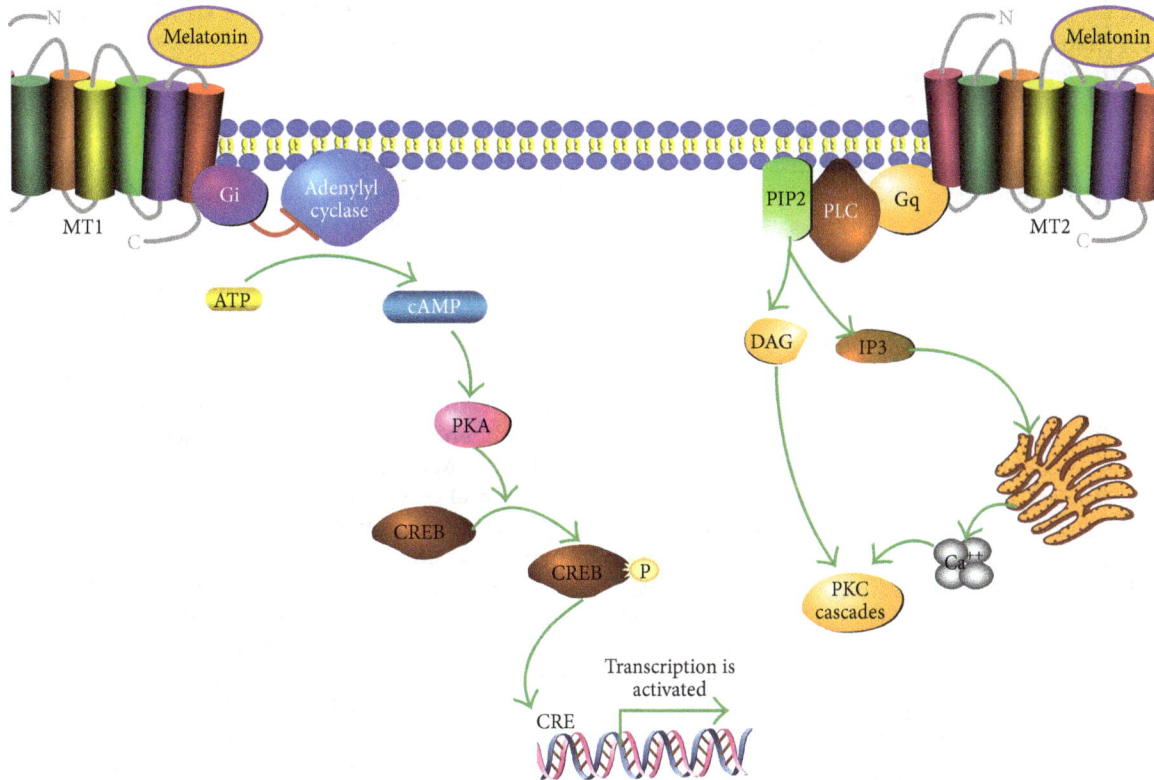

FIGURE 2: Signaling of MT1 and MT2. Both are G protein-coupled receptors. MT1 is associated with Gi protein and inhibition of adenylyl cyclase. MT2 receptor is associated with PKC stimulation and increase of calcium associated with IP3 (for details see Dubocovich et al. [11]).

adrenocorticotropin (ACTH) in humans and sheep [38, 67], strongly suggesting a loop of regulation between melatonin production and clock genes expression.

Melatonin acts through membrane receptors (see Figure 2), although some effects of melatonin could be mediated by binding to endogenous ligand, the orphan nuclear hormone receptor superfamily RZR/ROR [68]. There are two melatonin membrane receptors named MT1 and MT2. Both are G protein-coupled receptors. Thus, MT1 is associated with (i) Gi and inhibition of adenylyl cyclase with decrease of cAMP, (ii) stimulation of potassium channels, and (iii) increase of Ca^{2+} via phospholipase C (PLC), whereas the MT2 receptor is associated with (a) Protein Kinase C (PKC) stimulation or (b) increase of calcium associated with IP_3. Melatonin receptors MT1 and MT2 are present in many tissues [11, 69] although their function is not quite understood. However, their participation has been described in several mechanisms as indicated below.

3.1. Chronobiotic and Homeostatic Effects of Melatonin. In *vivo* treatment (2 hours) with melatonin increases the expression of Cry-2 in rat *pars tuberalis* [36] and decreases in the amplitude of the peak of Per1, suggesting an inhibitory effect of melatonin on this gene expression. In sheep, in which the secretion of melatonin was abolished by exposure to continuous light, expression of the clock genes Per 1-2 and Bmal1 continued in the *pars tuberalis*. However, melatonin

treatment at any point in the day for a period of 3 hours induced mRNA expression of Cry-1 and inhibited the expression of Per 1-2 and Bmal1, effects that were not observed in the SCN [70]. In capuchin monkey, adrenal explants maintain an oscillatory expression of Bmal1 and Per2 for at least 36 hours in culture, and the treatment with melatonin decreased the expression of Bmal1 and Per2 [30]. Similar effects have been shown in the rat fetal adrenal in culture [40] and recently we detected that melatonin inhibit the expression of Per1 and Bmal1 in response to ACTH in newborn sheep and human adrenal gland [38, 67]. Moreover, melatonin via melatonin receptor MT1 and MT2 can modify the levels of pro- or antiapoptotic proteins such as Bax and Bcl-2 in human neuroblastoma cells [64]; similarly in placenta, treatment with 10 μM of melatonin in villous trophoblast cells increases the survival via inhibition of loss of mitochondrial membrane potential and stimulating the formation of complex Bax/Bcl-2 (intrinsic via), expression of caspase-9, and the activation of ROCK1 [71].

3.2. Antioxidant Effects of Melatonin. Melatonin has a potent scavenger activity over hydroxyl, alkoxyl, and peroxyl radicals, as well as over species derived from nitrogen such as nitric oxide (NO) radicals [11, 57, 58]. In this regard, Milczarek et al. (2010) reported in placentas obtained after delivery a potent antioxidant effect of melatonin, specifically preventing the NADPH and iron dependent lipid peroxidation in the mitochondria [72]. Moreover, in studies of fetal growth restriction in animal model by placental ischemia, increased placental level of 8-hydroxy-2-deoxyguanosine has been detected (8-OHdG, i.e., a marker of a marker of oxidative DNA damage) [73] compared with controls. Both growth restriction and DNA damage were reverted when the rats received an oral dose of melatonin. Similarly, in rat undernourished pregnancy at day 20 of gestation, the fetal biometry showed lower values for fetal body weight and fetal body/placental weight ratio; moreover a tendency to a higher value of melatonin in maternal and fetal plasma is observed. Placentas from undernourished pregnancy showed no changes in the expression of antioxidant enzymes Mn-SOD, catalase, and GPx-1. However, the melatonin treatment during the pregnancy restores the placental efficiency at level of fetal body weight and fetal body/placental weight and induces the protein expression of Mn-SOD and catalase [59], suggesting that melatonin could be a candidate for protection/treatment of diseases characterized by placental ischemia such as intrauterine growth restriction, preeclampsia [73], or undernourished pregnancy [59]. Indeed, recent evidences have described that melatonin administration improved fetal-placental hemodynamic [74] and increased umbilical blood flow, an effect associated with "NO-dependent mechanisms" [75], as what occurs in cotyledonary placental arteries, via increased sensitivity to vasorelaxation agents such as bradykinin and lower contractile response to noradrenaline [76]. Additionally, melatonin administration reverted the increment of lipid peroxidation in the placenta and liver of mother and fetus exposed to cholestasis of pregnancy [77]. Interestingly, in human it has been described that oral melatonin administration increased glutathione peroxidase (GSH-Px) in the placenta of Japanese women with pregnancies of 7 and 9 weeks of gestation [78].

Protective effects of other antioxidant agents on fetal growth and development strongly support the protective effects of melatonin in adverse pregnancy being due to its antioxidant rather than antioxidant-independent properties, for example, developmental programming of cardiovascular dysfunction by prenatal hypoxia and oxidative stress.

3.3. Melatonin and Vascular Remodeling. In rats, it has been described that melatonin regulate the levels of NO and VEGF in the nervous system, that is, in the choroid plexus, cerebellum, periventricular white matter, and hippocampus [79–82]. Moreover, melatonin treatment for short or long periods of time inhibits the endogenous expression of VEGF and hypoxia induced factor 1 alpha (HIF-1α) in tumor cells [83]. In addition, melatonin induces the expression of VEGF and matrix metalloproteinase- (MMP-) 2 in extrapineal tissues such as gastric mucosa [66]. Also melatonin increases bone defect repair in rabbits [84]. All these indirect evidences suggest that melatonin may control vessel formation. Nevertheless, other reports have showed reduced tumor angiogenesis in mice treated with melatonin [85], as well as reduced human umbilical vein endothelial cell proliferation/migration induced by VEGF [86, 87].

4. Extrapineal Production of Melatonin: The Placenta

The critical enzymes for the synthesis of melatonin are arylalkylamine N-acetyltransferase (AA-NAT) and hydroxyindole O-methyltransferase (HIOMT). These enzymes are expressed in the major site of synthesis of melatonin, in the pineal gland with a circadian pattern of activity for AA-NAT [11], and in the human placenta [88]. Therefore, the human placenta can be considered as an extrapineal source of melatonin similar to retina [89] and lymphocytes [90]. In this regard, expression (mRNA and protein) of AA-NAT and HIOMT has been detected in both cell line of human placental trophoblasts and human term placentas [71, 88, 91]. In addition, other reports have described the presence of MT1 and MT2 in total human placenta [55] or placental endothelial cells [88]. Interestingly, MT1 is expressed at high levels in the junctional zone during day hours (16:00 hrs) and in the labyrinth during night hours (04:00 hrs) in mice [24].

We do not know whether the production of melatonin in the human placenta changes with the hours of the day. Interestingly, in normal pregnancies, serum levels of melatonin increase progressively until 32 weeks of gestation and decrease prior to delivery reaching the lowest levels at 2 days postpartum [92–95]. Moreover, the level of melatonin is higher in human twins pregnancies [92], as well as it is correlated with the number of pups in animal models [94], suggesting a relationship between placental volume and melatonin level. Nevertheless, in human pregnancies associated with placental alteration, the maternal circadian production of melatonin is lost and it is associated with diminished levels of melatonin. For example, circadian alteration has been observed in humans at the level of diastolic blood pressure, plasma concentration, and circadian production of melatonin during preeclampsia. After pregnancy, these women showed a normal circadian diastolic blood pressure but maintained altered rhythm for melatonin [53]. In contrast to humans, AA-NAT is not expressed in the placenta of rats, and an increase of maternal melatonin is a consequence of placental factor released into the circulation, which would stimulate the maternal pineal gland [94].

Although melatonin has multiple effects on placental function, including induction of the expression in undernourished pregnancy of antioxidant enzymes such as superoxide dismutase (Mn-SOD) and catalase [59], prevention of oxidative stress-mediated injury during placental ischemia [73], inhibition of hCG release in trophoblast cells [91], and inhibition of formation of proapoptotic complex [71], the role of this local production in the human placenta is not well understood and opens the possibility of autocrine, intracrine, or paracrine effects. Although there are no direct evidences, other studies using lymphoid cells, which express the enzymes NAT and HIOMT and produce 5-fold more melatonin than pineal gland, have described that melatonin produced locally has a minor effect on melatonin serum level but has a local role incrementing the IL-2 production [90]. This last effect was inhibited by luzindole and CGP 55644, an antagonist of membrane and nuclear receptors of melatonin [96]. Then, it is feasible that melatonin can be modulating

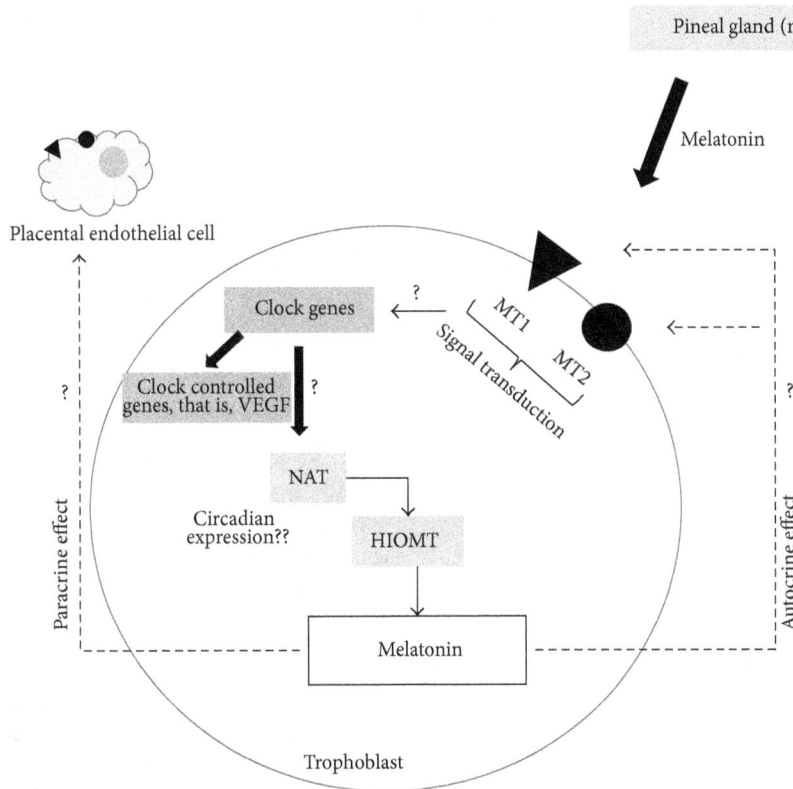

FIGURE 3: Autocrine and paracrine effects of melatonin over circadian system and enzyme of synthesis of melatonin localized in trophoblast and endothelial cells.

the circadian system in the placenta, see Figure 3, producing changes in clock genes that may control VEGF or enzymes NAT and HIOMT. We encourage the scientific community with this idea.

5. Conclusion

Participation of the circadian regulatory system has been described as a feedback regulatory loop where melatonin is downregulating the clock genes. In turn, clock genes upregulate the expression of output genes such as VEGF, SOD, NAT, and HIOMT. Current evidences describe that the placenta is a nonpineal organ, which synthesizes melatonin, and the activity of this organ is regulated by a circadian system. Moreover, an impaired circadian system is associated with an altered production of melatonin; however, the effect of this alteration on clock gene expression or output genes (VEGF) has not been described. We believe that circadian system and melatonin are a keystone molecule in the placental physiology, but more studies are necessary in order to test this idea. In this regard, we propose that melatonin may control clock gene expression (Bmal1, Per1-3, Cry1-2, and Clock) and output genes (VEGF) during normal pregnancies.

Glossary

BMAL1: Aryl hydrocarbon receptor nuclear translocator-like

CLOCK: Circadian locomotor output cycles kaput
PER: Homolog of period, *Drosophila*
E-BOX: Promoter sequence for binding of clock-bmal1 complex (CACGTG)
CREB: cAMP response element-binding protein
PGC1α: Peroxisome proliferator-activated receptor-gamma, coactivator 1α.

Conflict of Interests

None of the authors have a conflict of interests.

Acknowledgment

This paper received funding Conicyt 79112027 (Chile).

References

[1] J. Cha, X. Sun, and S. K. Dey, "Mechanisms of implantation: strategies for successful pregnancy," *Nature Medicine*, vol. 18, no. 12, pp. 1754–1767, 2012.

[2] P. H. Andraweera, G. A. Dekker, and C. T. Roberts, "The vascular endothelial growth factor family in adverse pregnancy outcomes," *Human Reproduction Update*, vol. 18, no. 4, Article ID dms011, pp. 436–457, 2012.

[3] J. Olcese, "Circadian aspects of mammalian parturition: a review," *Molecular and Cellular Endocrinology*, vol. 349, no. 1, pp. 62–67, 2012.

[4] M. Bonzini, K. T. Palmer, D. Coggon, M. Carugno, A. Cromi, and M. M. Ferrario, "Shift work and pregnancy outcomes: a systematic review with meta-analysis of currently available epidemiological studies," *BJOG*, vol. 118, no. 12, pp. 1429–1437, 2011.

[5] M. Serón-Ferré, C. A. Ducsay, and G. J. Valenzuela, "Circadian rhythms during pregnancy," *Endocrine Reviews*, vol. 14, no. 5, pp. 594–609, 1993.

[6] W. P. Mutter and S. A. Karumanchi, "Molecular mechanisms of preeclampsia," *Microvascular Research*, vol. 75, no. 1, pp. 1–8, 2008.

[7] R. Romero, J. P. Kusanovic, T. Chaiworapongsa, and S. S. Hassan, "Placental bed disorders in preterm labor, preterm PROM, spontaneous abortion and abruptio placentae," *Best Practice and Research: Clinical Obstetrics and Gynaecology*, vol. 25, no. 3, pp. 313–327, 2011.

[8] S. Rotmensch, C. Celentano, N. Elliger et al., "Diurnal variation of human chorionic gonadotropin β-core fragment concentrations in urine during second trimester of pregnancy," *Clinical Chemistry*, vol. 47, no. 9, pp. 1715–1717, 2001.

[9] M. Seron-Ferre, G. J. Valenzuela, and C. Torres-Farfan, "Circadian clocks during embryonic and fetal development," *Birth Defects Research Part C: Embryo Today: Reviews*, vol. 81, no. 3, pp. 204–214, 2007.

[10] M. Serón-Ferré, N. Mendez, L. Abarzua-Catalan et al., "Circadian rhythms in the fetus," *Molecular and Cellular Endocrinology*, vol. 349, no. 1, pp. 68–75, 2012.

[11] M. L. Dubocovich, P. Delagrange, D. N. Krause, D. Sugden, D. P. Cardinali, and J. Olcese, "International union of basic and clinical pharmacology. LXXV. Nomenclature, classification, and pharmacology of G protein-coupled melatonin receptors," *Pharmacological Reviews*, vol. 62, no. 3, pp. 343–380, 2010.

[12] M. Serón-Ferré, M. L. Forcelledo, C. Torres-Farfan et al., "Impact of chronodisruption during primate pregnancy on the maternal and newborn temperature rhythms," *PLoS ONE*, vol. 8, no. 2, Article ID e57710, 2013.

[13] J. Malek, K. Suk, M. Brestak, and V. Maly, "Daily rhythm of leukocytes, blood pressure, pulse rate, and temperature during pregnancy.," *Annals of the New York Academy of Sciences*, vol. 98, pp. 1018–1041, 1962.

[14] M. Barr Jr., "Prenatal growth of Wistar rats: circadian periodicity of fetal growth late in gestation," *Teratology*, vol. 7, no. 3, pp. 283–288, 1973.

[15] M. A. Morgan, S. L. Silavin, R. A. Wentworth et al., "Different patterns of myometrial activity and 24-H rhythms in myometrial contractility in the gravid baboon during the second half of pregnancy," *Biology of Reproduction*, vol. 46, no. 6, pp. 1158–1164, 1992.

[16] M. Vatish, P. J. Steer, A. M. Blanks, M. Hon, and S. Thornton, "Diurnal variation is lost in preterm deliveries before 28 weeks of gestation," *BJOG: An International Journal of Obstetrics and Gynaecology*, vol. 117, no. 6, pp. 765–767, 2010.

[17] J. Malek, J. Gleich, and V. Maly, "Characteristics of the daily rhythm of menstruation and labor.," *Annals of the New York Academy of Sciences*, vol. 98, pp. 1042–1055, 1962.

[18] H. Takayama, Y. Nakamura, H. Tamura et al., "Pineal gland (melatonin) affects the parturition time, but not luteal function and fetal growth, in pregnant rats," *Endocrine Journal*, vol. 50, no. 1, pp. 37–43, 2003.

[19] C. K. Ratajczak, M. Asada, G. C. Allen et al., "Generation of myometrium-specific Bmal1 knockout mice for parturition analysis," *Reproduction, Fertility and Development*, vol. 24, no. 5, pp. 759–767, 2012.

[20] C. A. Ducsay and S. M. Yellon, "Photoperiod regulation of uterine activity and melatonin rhythms in the pregnant rhesus macaque," *Biology of Reproduction*, vol. 44, no. 6, pp. 967–974, 1991.

[21] Y. Maeda, M. Muro, M. Shono, H. Shono, and T. Iwasaka, "Diurnal rhythms in fetal heart rate baseline and sustained fetal tachycardia in twin pregnancy," *Early Human Development*, vol. 82, no. 10, pp. 637–644, 2006.

[22] L. Díaz-Cueto, J. P. Méndez, J. Barrios-de-Tomasi et al., "Amplitude regulation of episodic release, in vitro biological to immunological ratio, and median charge of human chorionic gonadotropin in pregnancy," *Journal of Clinical Endocrinology and Metabolism*, vol. 78, no. 4, pp. 890–897, 1994.

[23] S. T. Nakajima, T. Mcauliffe, and M. Gibson, "The 24-hour pattern of the levels of serum progesterone and immunoreactive human chorionic Gonadotropin in Normal Early Pregnancy," *Journal of Clinical Endocrinology and Metabolism*, vol. 71, no. 2, pp. 345–353, 1990.

[24] C. K. Lee, D. H. Moon, C. S. Shin et al., "Circadian expression of Mel_{1a} and PL-II genes in placenta: effects of melatonin on the PL-II gene expression in the rat placenta," *Molecular and Cellular Endocrinology*, vol. 200, no. 1-2, pp. 57–66, 2003.

[25] M. C. Moore-Ede, "Physiology of the circadian timing system: predictive versus reactive homeostasis," *The American Journal of Physiology—Regulatory Integrative and Comparative Physiology*, vol. 250, no. 5, part 2, pp. R737–R752, 1986.

[26] I. Edery, "Circadian rhythms in a nutshell," *Physiol Genomics*, vol. 3, no. 2, pp. 59–74, 2000.

[27] C.-M. Hsu, S.-F. Lin, C.-T. Lu, P.-M. Lin, and M.-Y. Yang, "Altered expression of circadian clock genes in head and neck squamous cell carcinoma," *Tumor Biology*, vol. 33, no. 1, pp. 149–155, 2012.

[28] E. S. Schernhammer, F. Laden, F. E. Speizer et al., "Rotating night shifts and risk of breast cancer in women participating in the nurses' health study," *Journal of the National Cancer Institute*, vol. 93, no. 20, pp. 1563–1568, 2001.

[29] T. J. Varcoe, N. Wight, A. Voultsios, M. D. Salkeld, and D. J. Kennaway, "Chronic phase shifts of the photoperiod throughout pregnancy programs glucose intolerance and insulin resistance in the rat," *PLoS ONE*, vol. 6, no. 4, Article ID e18504, 2011.

[30] F. J. Valenzuela, C. Torres-Farfan, H. G. Richter et al., "Clock gene expression in adult primate suprachiasmatic nuclei and adrenal: is the adrenal a peripheral clock responsive to melatonin?" *Endocrinology*, vol. 149, no. 4, pp. 1454–1461, 2008.

[31] J. C. Dunlap, J. J. Loros, Y. Liu, and S. K. Crosthwaite, "Eukaryotic circadian systems: cycles in common," *Genes to Cells*, vol. 4, no. 1, pp. 1–10, 1999.

[32] K. Bae, X. Jin, E. S. Maywood, M. H. Hastings, S. M. Reppert, and D. R. Weaver, "Differential functions of *mPer1*, *mPer2*, and *mPer3* in the SCN circadian clock," *Neuron*, vol. 30, no. 2, pp. 525–536, 2001.

[33] M. Akashi, Y. Tsuchiya, T. Yoshino, and E. Nishida, "Control of intracellular dynamics of mammalian period proteins by casein kinase I epsilon (CKIepsilon) and CKIdelta in cultured cells," *Molecular and Cellular Biology*, vol. 22, no. 6, pp. 1693–1703, 2002.

[34] M. Stratmann and U. Schibler, "Properties, entrainment, and physiological functions of mammalian peripheral oscillators," *Journal of Biological Rhythms*, vol. 21, no. 6, pp. 494–506, 2006.

[35] G. A. Lincoln, H. Andersson, and D. Hazlerigg, "Clock genes and the long-term regulation of prolactin secretion: evidence for a photoperiod/circannual timer in the pars tuberalis," *Journal of Neuroendocrinology*, vol. 15, no. 4, pp. 390–397, 2003.

[36] H. Dardente, J. S. Menet, V.-J. Poirel et al., "Melatonin induces *Cry1* expression in the pars tuberalis of the rat," *Molecular Brain Research*, vol. 114, no. 2, pp. 101–106, 2003.

[37] D. R. Lemos, J. L. Downs, and H. F. Urbanski, "Twenty-four-hour rhythmic gene expression in the rhesus macaque adrenal gland," *Molecular Endocrinology*, vol. 20, no. 5, pp. 1164–1176, 2006.

[38] C. Campino, F. J. Valenzuela, C. Torres-Farfan et al., "Melatonin exerts direct inhibitory actions on ACTH responses in the human adrenal gland," *Hormone and Metabolic Research*, vol. 43, no. 5, pp. 337–342, 2011.

[39] C. Torres-Farfan, V. Rocco, C. Monsó et al., "Maternal melatonin effects on clock gene expression in a nonhuman primate fetus," *Endocrinology*, vol. 147, no. 10, pp. 4618–4626, 2006.

[40] C. Torres-Farfan, N. Mendez, L. Abarzua-Catalan, N. Vilches, G. J. Valenzuela, and M. Seron-Ferre, "A circadian clock entrained by melatonin is ticking in the rat fetal adrenal," *Endocrinology*, vol. 152, no. 5, pp. 1891–1900, 2011.

[41] H. Oster, S. Damerow, S. Kiessling et al., "The circadian rhythm of glucocorticoids is regulated by a gating mechanism residing in the adrenal cortical clock," *Cell Metabolism*, vol. 4, no. 2, pp. 163–173, 2006.

[42] M. D. Wharfe, P. J. Mark, and B. J. Waddell, "Circadian variation in placental and hepatic clock genes in rat pregnancy," *Endocrinology*, vol. 152, no. 9, pp. 3552–3560, 2011.

[43] S. Akiyama, H. Ohta, S. Watanabe et al., "The uterus sustains stable biological clock during pregnancy," *The Tohoku Journal of Experimental Medicine*, vol. 221, no. 4, pp. 287–298, 2010.

[44] E. Frigato, L. Lunghi, M. E. Ferretti, C. Biondi, and C. Bertolucci, "Evidence for circadian rhythms in human trophoblast cell line that persist in hypoxia," *Biochemical and Biophysical Research Communications*, vol. 378, no. 1, pp. 108–111, 2009.

[45] A. Balsalobre, L. Marcacci, and U. Schibler, "Multiple signaling pathways elicit circadian gene expression in cultured Rat-1 fibroblasts," *Current Biology*, vol. 10, no. 20, pp. 1291–1294, 2000.

[46] S. Xiang, L. Mao, T. Duplessis et al., "Oscillation of clock and clock controlled genes induced by serum shock in human breast epithelial and breast cancer cells: regulation by melatonin," *Breast Cancer: Basic and Clinical Research*, vol. 6, no. 1, pp. 137–150, 2012.

[47] A. Balsalobre, F. Damiola, and U. Schibler, "A serum shock induces circadian gene expression in mammalian tissue culture cells," *Cell*, vol. 93, no. 6, pp. 929–937, 1998.

[48] F. J. Valenzuela, A. Pérez-Sepúlveda, M. J. Torres, P. Correa, G. M. Repetto, and S. E. Illanes, "Pathogenesis of preeclampsia: the genetic component," *Journal of Pregnancy*, vol. 2012, Article ID 632732, 8 pages, 2012.

[49] P. J. Dutton, L. K. Warrander, S. A. Roberts et al., "Predictors of poor perinatal outcome following maternal perception of reduced fetal movements—a prospective cohort study," *PLoS ONE*, vol. 7, no. 7, Article ID e39784, 2012.

[50] R. V. Anthony, S. L. Pratt, R. Liang, and M. D. Holland, "Placental-fetal hormonal interactions: impact on fetal growth," *Journal of Animal Science*, vol. 73, no. 6, pp. 1861–1871, 1995.

[51] Y. Wang and S. Zhao, *Vascular Biology of the Placenta*, Morgan & Claypool Life Sciences, San Rafael, Calif, USA, 2010.

[52] S. Koyanagi, Y. Kuramoto, H. Nakagawa et al., "A molecular mechanism regulating circadian expression of vascular endothelial growth factor in tumor cells," *Cancer Research*, vol. 63, no. 21, pp. 7277–7283, 2003.

[53] A. L. Tranquilli, A. Turi, S. R. Giannubilo, and E. Garbati, "Circadian melatonin concentration rhythm is lost in pregnant women with altered blood pressure rhythm," *Gynecological Endocrinology*, vol. 18, no. 3, pp. 124–129, 2004.

[54] H. Guo, J. M. Brewer, M. N. Lehman, and E. L. Bittman, "Suprachiasmatic regulation of circadian rhythms of gene expression in hamster peripheral organs: effects of transplanting the pacemaker," *The Journal of Neuroscience*, vol. 26, no. 24, pp. 6406–6412, 2006.

[55] D. Lanoix, R. Ouellette, and C. Vaillancourt, "Expression of melatoninergic receptors in human placental choriocarcinoma cell lines," *Human Reproduction*, vol. 21, no. 8, pp. 1981–1989, 2006.

[56] S. R. Pandi-Perumal, V. Srinivasan, G. J. M. Maestroni, D. P. Cardinali, B. Poeggeler, and R. Hardeland, "Melatonin: nature's most versatile biological signal?" *FEBS Journal*, vol. 273, no. 13, pp. 2813–2838, 2006.

[57] A. Galano, D. X. Tan, and R. J. Reiter, "Melatonin as a natural ally against oxidative stress: a physicochemical examination," *Journal of Pineal Research*, vol. 51, no. 1, pp. 1–16, 2011.

[58] R. J. Reiter, D.-X. Tan, L. C. Manchester, S. D. Paredes, J. C. Mayo, and R. M. Sainz, "Melatonin and reproduction revisited," *Biology of Reproduction*, vol. 81, no. 3, pp. 445–456, 2009.

[59] H. G. Richter, J. A. Hansell, S. Raut, and D. A. Giussani, "Melatonin improves placental efficiency and birth weight and increases the placental expression of antioxidant enzymes in undernourished pregnancy," *Journal of Pineal Research*, vol. 46, no. 4, pp. 357–364, 2009.

[60] C. H. Kim and Y.-M. Yoo, "Melatonin induces apoptotic cell death via p53 in LNCaP cells," *Korean Journal of Physiology and Pharmacology*, vol. 14, no. 6, pp. 365–369, 2010.

[61] S. M. Dupré, D. W. Burt, R. Talbot et al., "Identification of melatonin-regulated genes in the ovine pituitary pars tuberalis, a target site for seasonal hormone control," *Endocrinology*, vol. 149, no. 11, pp. 5527–5539, 2008.

[62] E. H. Sharman, S. C. Bondy, K. G. Sharman, D. Lahiri, C. W. Cotman, and V. M. Perreau, "Effects of melatonin and age on gene expression in mouse CNS using microarray analysis," *Neurochemistry International*, vol. 50, no. 2, pp. 336–344, 2007.

[63] E. Ha, E. Han, H. J. Park et al., "Microarray analysis of transcription factor gene expression in melatonin-treated human peripheral blood mononuclear cells," *Journal of Pineal Research*, vol. 40, no. 4, pp. 305–311, 2006.

[64] W. Wisessmith, P. Phansuwan-Pujito, P. Govitrapong, and B. Chetsawang, "Melatonin reduces induction of Bax, caspase and cell death in methamphetamine-treated human neuroblastoma SH-SY5Y cultured cells," *Journal of Pineal Research*, vol. 46, no. 4, pp. 433–440, 2009.

[65] K. Tsutsui, S. Haraguchi, K. Inoue et al., "Identification, biosynthesis, and function of 7α-hydroxypregnenolone, a new key neurosteroid controlling locomotor activity, in nonmammalian vertebrates," *Annals of the New York Academy of Sciences*, vol. 1163, pp. 308–315, 2009.

[66] K. Ganguly and S. Swarnakar, "Induction of matrix metal-loproteinase-9 and -3 in nonsteroidal anti-inflammatory drug-induced acute gastric ulcers in mice: regulation by melatonin," *Journal of Pineal Research*, vol. 47, no. 1, pp. 43–55, 2009.

[67] F. J. Valenzuela, H. E. Reynolds, C. Torres-Farfán, G. J. Valenzuela, and M. Serón-Ferré, "Melatonin inhibition of the cortisol response to aCth may be exerted through period circadian protein homolog 1 (Per1)," *Revista Chilena de Endocrinología y Diabetes*, vol. 5, no. 1, pp. 6–12, 2012.

[68] B. Claustrat, J. Brun, and G. Chazot, "The basic physiology and pathophysiology of melatonin," *Sleep Medicine Reviews*, vol. 9, no. 1, pp. 11–24, 2005.

[69] C. Ekmekcioglu, "Melatonin receptors in humans: biological role and clinical relevance," *Biomedicine and Pharmacotherapy*, vol. 60, no. 3, pp. 97–108, 2006.

[70] J. D. Johnston, B. B. Tournier, H. Andersson, M. Masson-Pévet, G. A. Lincoln, and D. G. Hazlerigg, "Multiple effects of melatonin on rhythmic clock gene expression in the mammalian pars tuberalis," *Endocrinology*, vol. 147, no. 2, pp. 959–965, 2006.

[71] D. Lanoix, P. Guérin, and C. Vaillancourt, "Placental melatonin production and melatonin receptor expression are altered in preeclampsia: new insights into the role of this hormone in pregnancy," *Journal of Pineal Research*, vol. 53, no. 4, pp. 417–425, 2012.

[72] R. Milczarek, A. Hallmann, E. Sokołowska, K. Kaletha, and J. Klimek, "Melatonin enhances antioxidant action of α-tocopherol and ascorbate against NADPH- and iron-dependent lipid peroxidation in human placental mitochondria," *Journal of Pineal Research*, vol. 49, no. 2, pp. 149–155, 2010.

[73] R. Nagai, K. Watanabe, A. Wakatsuki et al., "Melatonin preserves fetal growth in rats by protecting against ischemia/reperfusion-induced oxidative/nitrosative mitochondrial damage in the placenta," *Journal of Pineal Research*, vol. 45, no. 3, pp. 271–276, 2008.

[74] C. O. Lemley, A. M. Meyer, L. E. Camacho et al., "Melatonin supplementation alters uteroplacental hemodynamics and fetal development in an ovine model of intrauterine growth restriction," *The American Journal of Physiology—Regulatory Integrative and Comparative Physiology*, vol. 302, no. 4, pp. R454–R467, 2012.

[75] A. S. Thakor, E. A. Herrera, M. Serón-Ferré, and D. A. Giussani, "Melatonin and vitamin C increase umbilical blood flow via nitric oxide-dependent mechanisms," *Journal of Pineal Research*, vol. 49, no. 4, pp. 399–406, 2010.

[76] P. Shukla, C. O. Lemley, N. Dubey, A. M. Meyer, S. T. O'Rourke, and K. A. Vonnahme, "Effect of maternal nutrient restriction and melatonin supplementation from mid to late gestation on vascular reactivity of maternal and fetal placental arteries," *Placenta*, vol. 35, no. 7, pp. 461–466, 2014.

[77] M. J. Perez, B. Castaño, J. M. Gonzalez-Buitrago, and J. J. G. Marin, "Multiple protective effects of melatonin against maternal cholestasis-induced oxidative stress and apoptosis in the rat fetal liver-placenta-maternal liver trio," *Journal of Pineal Research*, vol. 43, no. 2, pp. 130–139, 2007.

[78] Y. Okatani, A. Wakatsuki, K. Shinohara, C. Kaneda, and T. Fukaya, "Melatonin stimulates glutathione peroxidase activity in human chorion," *Journal of Pineal Research*, vol. 30, no. 4, pp. 199–205, 2001.

[79] V. Sivakumar, J. Lu, E. A. Ling, and C. Kaur, "Vascular endothelial growth factor and nitric oxide production in response to hypoxia in the choroid plexus in neonatal brain," *Brain Pathology*, vol. 18, no. 1, pp. 71–85, 2008.

[80] C. Kaur, V. Sivakumar, Y. Zhang, and E. A. Ling, "Hypoxia-induced astrocytic reaction and increased vascular permeability in the rat cerebellum," *Glia*, vol. 54, no. 8, pp. 826–839, 2006.

[81] C. Kaur, V. Sivakumar, J. Lu, F. R. Tang, and E. A. Ling, "Melatonin attenuates hypoxia-induced ultrastructural changes and increased vascular permeability in the developing hippocampus," *Brain Pathology*, vol. 18, no. 4, pp. 533–547, 2008.

[82] C. Kaur, V. Sivakumar, and E. A. Ling, "Melatonin protects periventricular white matter from damage due to hypoxia," *Journal of Pineal Research*, vol. 48, no. 3, pp. 185–193, 2010.

[83] M. Dai, P. Cui, M. Yu, J. Han, H. Li, and R. Xiu, "Melatonin modulates the expression of VEGF and HIF-1α induced by $CoCl_2$ in cultured cancer cells," *Journal of Pineal Research*, vol. 44, no. 2, pp. 121–126, 2008.

[84] M. P. Ramírez-Fernández, J. L. Calvo-Guirado, J. E.-M. S. de-Val et al., "Melatonin promotes angiogenesis during repair of bone defects: a radiological and histomorphometric study in rabbit tibiae," *Clinical Oral Investigations*, vol. 17, no. 1, pp. 147–158, 2013.

[85] K.-J. Kim, J.-S. Choi, I. Kang, K.-W. Kim, C.-H. Jeong, and J.-W. Jeong, "Melatonin suppresses tumor progression by reducing angiogenesis stimulated by HIF-1 in a mouse tumor model," *Journal of Pineal Research*, vol. 54, no. 3, pp. 264–270, 2013.

[86] V. Alvarez-García, A. González, C. Martínez-Campa, C. Alonso-González, and S. Cos, "Melatonin modulates aromatase activity and expression in endothelial cells," *Oncology Reports*, vol. 29, no. 5, pp. 2058–2064, 2013.

[87] V. Alvarez-García, A. González, C. Alonso-González, C. Martínez-Campa, and S. Cos, "Regulation of vascular endothelial growth factor by melatonin in human breast cancer cells," *Journal of Pineal Research*, vol. 54, no. 4, pp. 373–380, 2013.

[88] D. Lanoix, H. Beghdadi, J. Lafond, and C. Vaillancourt, "Human placental trophoblasts synthesize melatonin and express its receptors," *Journal of Pineal Research*, vol. 45, no. 1, pp. 50–60, 2008.

[89] P. M. Iuvone, G. Tosini, N. Pozdeyev, R. Haque, D. C. Klein, and S. S. Chaurasia, "Circadian clocks, clock networks, arylalkylamine N-acetyltransferase, and melatonin in the retina," *Progress in Retinal and Eye Research*, vol. 24, no. 4, pp. 433–456, 2005.

[90] A. Carrillo-Vico, J. R. Calvo, P. Abreu et al., "Evidence of melatonin synthesis by human lymphocytes and its physiological significance: possible role as intracrine, autocrine, and/or paracrine substance." *The FASEB Journal*, vol. 18, no. 3, pp. 537–539, 2004.

[91] S. Iwasaki, K. Nakazawa, J. Sakai et al., "Melatonin as a local regulator of human placental function," *Journal of Pineal Research*, vol. 39, no. 3, pp. 261–265, 2005.

[92] Y. Nakamura, H. Tamura, S. Kashida et al., "Changes of serum melatonin level and its relationship to feto-placental unit during pregnancy," *Journal of Pineal Research*, vol. 30, no. 1, pp. 29–33, 2001.

[93] H. Tamura, Y. Nakamura, M. P. Terron et al., "Melatonin and pregnancy in the human," *Reproductive Toxicology (Elmsford, N.Y.)*, vol. 25, no. 3, pp. 291–303, 2008.

[94] H. Tamura, H. Takayama, Y. Nakamura, R. J. Reiter, and N. Sugino, "Fetal/placental regulation of maternal melatonin in rats," *Journal of Pineal Research*, vol. 44, no. 3, pp. 335–340, 2008.

[95] F. Wierrani, W. Grin, B. Hlawka, A. Kroiss, and W. Grünberger, "Elevated serum melatonin levels during human late pregnancy and labour," *Journal of Obstetrics and Gynaecology*, vol. 17, no. 5, pp. 449–451, 1997.

[96] A. Carrillo-Vico, P. J. Lardone, J. M. Fernández-Santos et al., "Human lymphocyte-synthesized melatonin is involved in the regulation of the interleukin-2/interleukin-2 receptor system," *The Journal of Clinical Endocrinology & Metabolism*, vol. 90, no. 2, pp. 992–1000, 2005.

27

N-Acetylcysteine for Polycystic Ovary Syndrome: A Systematic Review and Meta-Analysis of Randomized Controlled Clinical Trials

Divyesh Thakker,[1] Amit Raval,[2] Isha Patel,[3] and Rama Walia[4]

[1]Department of Pharmacology, SAL Institute of Pharmacy, Ahmadabad, Gujarat 380060, India
[2]Department of Pharmaceutical Systems and Policy, School of Pharmacy, West Virginia University, Morgantown, WV 26506, USA
[3]Department of Biopharmaceutical Sciences, Bernard J. Dunn School of Pharmacy, Shenandoah University, Winchester, VA 22601, USA
[4]Department of Endocrinology, Post-Graduate Medical Education and Research Institute (PGIMER), Chandigarh 160012, India

Correspondence should be addressed to Amit Raval; amitravalwaves@gmail.com

Academic Editor: Curt W. Burger

Objective. To review the benefits and harms of N-acetylcysteine (NAC) in women with polycystic ovary syndrome (PCOS). *Method.* Literature search was conducted using the bibliographic databases, MEDLINE (Ovid), CINAHL, EMBASE, Scopus, PsyInfo, and PROQUEST (from inception to September 2013) for the studies on women with PCOS receiving NAC. *Results.* Eight studies with a total of 910 women with PCOS were randomized to NAC or other treatments/placebo. There were high risk of selection, performance, and attrition bias in two studies and high risk of reporting bias in four studies. Women with NAC had higher odds of having a live birth, getting pregnant, and ovulation as compared to placebo. However, women with NAC were less likely to have pregnancy or ovulation as compared to metformin. There was no significant difference in rates of the miscarriage, menstrual regulation, acne, hirsutism, and adverse events, or change in body mass index, testosterone, and insulin levels with NAC as compared to placebo. *Conclusions.* NAC showed significant improvement in pregnancy and ovulation rate as compared to placebo. The findings need further confirmation in well-designed randomized controlled trials to examine clinical outcomes such as live birth rate in longer follow-up periods. Systematic review registration number is CRD42012001902.

1. Introduction

Polycystic ovary syndrome (PCOS) is one of the most common endocrine disorders, affecting approximately 5% to 15% of women of reproductive age [1–3]. PCOS is mainly associated with anovulation, infertility, insulin resistance, and hyperandrogenism leading to metabolic disorders such as diabetes and cardiovascular diseases [4–6]. Treatment remains a challenge for women with PCOS. Although clomiphene citrate (CC) is the first-line of treatment for chronic anovulation among women with PCOS, failure to ovulate after receiving 150 mg/day is common and occurs in approximately 15% to 40% of women [7]. For those who do not respond to CC, there are very few therapies that can be tried before moving on to gonadotropin therapy or laparoscopic ovarian drilling (LOD). CC treatment has shown discrepancy between ovulation rates (75% to 80%) and conception rates (30% to 40%) unlike LOD treatment used in women with CC resistant PCOS [8]. The discrepancy might persist to a certain extent with gonadotropin treatment as well [9]. Insulin-sensitizing agents have been explored for treating the underlying cause of disorders associated with insulin resistance. Metformin, a widely used oral biguanide for treating type 2 diabetes, decreases the levels of insulin and androgens and increases the level of sex-hormone-binding globulin, thereby improving the endocrine parameters such as glucose tolerance and ovulation rates in women with PCOS [10]. However, a recent Cochrane review revealed that even though metformin was associated with improved clinical pregnancy and ovulation rate, it did not improve live birth rates when used alone or in combination with clomiphene or when compared with clomiphene [11]. Therefore, there is need for developing therapeutic options for treating the women with PCOS.

N-Acetyl cysteine (NAC) is a commonly used safe mucolytic drug, In addition, NAC increases the cellular levels of antioxidant and reduces glutathione at higher doses. Therefore, NAC has a potential to improve insulin receptor activity in human erythrocytes and improve insulin secretion in response to glucose [13]. Improvement in insulin receptor activity in hyperinsulinemic subjects can lead to a secondary decrease in the β-cell responsiveness to the oral glucose tolerance test. Decreased levels of circulating insulin can lead to significant reduction in Testosterone levels and free androgen index in women responding to the treatment [13, 14]. Advantages resulting from administration of NAC include prevention of endothelial damage resulting from oxidants in noninsulin-dependent adult diabetic subjects and biological effects such as, protection against focal ischemia, inhibition of phospholipid metabolism inhibition, proinflammatory cytokine release, and protease activity [14]. Therefore, it was suggested that the above effects exerted by NAC at the ovarian level may be as beneficial as its insulin-enhancing effects in inducing ovulation. In the absence of effective treatment options for PCOS, establishment of data on new options like NAC as monotherapy or supportive therapy may provide valuable information. There is no systematic review assessing effectiveness of NAC in PCOS. The present systematic review aims to assess the benefits and harms of NAC therapy in women with PCOS.

2. Objective

The purpose of this study was to determine if NAC therapy was more effective and safe in women with PCOS compared to placebo/metformin.

3. Materials and Methods

3.1. Types of Studies, Interventions, Inclusion, and Exclusion Criteria. We included randomized studies in which NAC was compared to placebo or other agent(s) or NAC in combination with another drug to another class of drug alone. We excluded quasi- or pseudorandomized controlled trials or if the trails did not have a control group. In case of cross-over trials, we used data only from the first phase, that is, before cross-over of women with PCOS. Polycystic ovary syndrome had to be diagnosed according to the European Society for Human Reproduction and Embryology (ESHRE) and American Society for Reproductive Medicine (ASRM) sponsored PCOS Consensus Workshop criteria (the Rotterdam criteria) [15] or the National Institutes of Health (NIH) consensus criteria [16]. If the diagnostic criteria were not clearly stated in the trial, we contacted the trial authors for clarification. If clarification was not available, we excluded the trial.

The primary outcomes of this study were live birth rate per woman randomized and clinical pregnancy rate per woman randomized. Clinical pregnancy was defined as the presence of a gestational sac on ultrasound, as confirmed by the presence of a fetal heart rate or number of follicles produced per treatment cycle. Secondary outcomes were related to the safety. They included the following: ovarian hyperstimulation syndrome (OHSS) rate per woman randomized, defined according to the definition adopted by the reporting authors; miscarriage rate per woman randomized, where miscarriage was defined as the involuntary loss of a pregnancy before 20 weeks of gestation; and multiple pregnancy rate per woman randomized, where multiple pregnancy was defined as more than one intrauterine pregnancy. Other outcomes assessed in the study were resumption of menstrual regularity and spontaneous ovulation. Resumption of menstrual regularity was defined as initiation of menses or significant shortening of cycles. Number of women with resumption of normal menstrual cycle was defined as being between 21 and 34 days. Resumption of spontaneous ovulation was documented by biochemical methods, that is, measuring progesterone, where ovulation was defined as the evidence of serum progesterone in the luteal range of the reference laboratory, or a basal body temperature rise by $>0.4°C$ for 10 days or more, as measured on a basal body temperature chart. Further, we also assessed other outcomes like improvement in body mass index (BMI), testosterone level, fasting glucose, fasting insulin, glucose/insulin ratio, and homeostatic model assessment-insulin resistance (HOMA-IR).

3.2. Search Strategy and Data Extraction. Two authors independently (DT, AR) ran electronic search strategy. It involved conducting a literature search for all pertinent published studies on the use of NAC for PCOS in terms of restoration of menstruation, induction of ovulation, and pregnancy using the bibliographic databases like the Cochrane Central Register of Controlled Trials (CENTRAL) in the Cochrane Library (from inception to September 2013), MEDLINE (Ovid) (from inception to September 2013), Scopus (from inception to September 2013), CINAHL (from inception to September 2013), and PsycINFO (from inception to September 2013). The references provided in selected articles identified were hand-searched to find additional studies. We also used ProQuest and ISI-Web of Science database for additional relevant citations. We contacted known experts and personal contacts regarding any unpublished materials.

Search terms included were: "Polycystic ovary syndrome" and "N-acetylcysteine" or "NAC" and "Hyperandrogaenemia". The details of complete search strategies and results on number of hits are presented in Appendix 1 (in Supplementary Material available online at http://dx.doi.org/10.1155/2014/817849).

3.3. Data Extraction and Management. The PRISMA (preferred reporting items for systematic reviews and meta-analyses) flowchart was used for study selection [23]. Two authors independently appraised the methodological quality of the studies using the Cochrane Collaboration's tool for assessing risk of bias, a six-item quality assessment instrument. This tool evaluates the following areas: method of randomization, concealment of allocation, blinding, completeness of follow-up, selective outcome reporting, and other sources of bias [24]. As per the Cochrane Handbook for Systematic Reviews of Interventions [16], we stated any important concerns about bias that were not addressed in the other domains, that is, any baseline imbalance in factors strongly related to outcome measures. We rated the studies as "high," "low," or "unclear" risk of bias in each domain. An "unclear" judgment was made if insufficient detail on what happened in the study was reported; if what happened in the study was known but the risk of bias is unknown; or if an entry was not relevant to the study at hand (particularly for assessing blinding and incomplete outcome data, when the outcome being assessed had not been measured in the study report). Two authors (AR, DT) independently entered data into a data extraction form about the study characteristics including methods, participants, interventions, and outcomes. Any disagreement was resolved by referring to the trial report and through discussion and consultation with a third author (RW). If data from the trial reports were insufficient or missing, we contacted the investigators of the studies for additional information. Where possible, we extracted data to allow an intention-to-treat analysis. If the number randomized and the analyzed were inconsistent, we calculated the percentage loss to follow-up and reported this information in an additional table.

3.4. Data Analysis. We calculated a summary statistic for each outcome with respect to the interventions using a fixed-effect model in RevMan 5.2 software. We used the Peto odds ratio (OR) as a measure of effect for each dichotomous outcome and the mean difference (MD) for each continuous outcome. If the data were reported using geometric means, we extracted standard deviations on the log scale. We contacted study authors for missing data. If missing data were not available from the authors, we did not use the data in the analysis. Heterogeneity was assessed using Chi-square statistic. A low P value or large Chi-sqaure statistic relative to the degree of freedom indicates heterogeneity. The I^2 statistic was used to quantify the heterogeneity [25]. Subgroup analyses were performed based on type of comparison, duration of intervention, and ethnicity of participants, to investigate source of heterogeneity. Publication bias was assessed using funnel plot. We also performed sensitivity analyses to examine the impact on the results in relation to a number of factors including comedication, quality of allocation concealment, blinding, intention-to-treat analysis, source of funding, and different diagnostic criteria of PCOS or obesity [26].

4. Results

We retrieved 191 articles (MEDLINE: 9, The Cochrane library: 7, PsycINFO: 0, Scopus: 90; CINAHL: 26; ISO-Web of Science: 18; ProQuest: 38, and 3 citations using conference proceedings and hand-searching of journals). Two studies were excluded due to lack of a control group and had a prepost study design for evaluating treatment [13, 27]. After excluding

narrative reviews, nonrandomized studies, intervention studies on agents other than NAC, and duplicate publications, we included eight studies (eight articles) [14, 17–22, 28]. Figure 1 describes the selection procedures for eight studies using the PRISMA flow diagram.

Figure 2 describes the summary of risk of bias among the included studies. The methods for randomization were unclear in six studies. Only two studies described the use of computer generated randomization list for sequence allocation [21, 22]. Treatment allocation was concealed by administration of third party (nurse) using opaque sealed envelopes in four studies [14, 20–22], unclear in three studies [18, 19], and not done in one study [28]. Only four studies had low-risk of performance bias due to proper blinding [14, 17, 20, 22], and two studies [21, 28] were open-label with high risk of performance bias, while in remaining two studies blinding was unclear. Four studies [14, 17, 19, 20] had high risk of selective reporting bias especially on primary outcomes and safety outcomes. Three studies reported outcomes, which were not specified in the protocol. Those outcomes were homeostasis model assessment for insulin resistance (HOMA-IR) and Ferriman-Gallwey scale, fasting glucose, fasting insulin and glucose/insulin ratio, lipid profile and TNF-alpha, acne, infertility, and weight gain and testosterone level. Two studies had high risk of attrition bias with attrition rate of more than 20% [17, 18].

Characteristics of included studies are provided in Table 1. All the studies except Rizk et al. provided the diagnostic criteria, modified Rotterdam criteria, for PCOS. In Rizk et al., PCOS was diagnosed only by a finding of bilaterally normal or enlarged ovaries (ovarian volume < 12 cm^3) with the presence of at least 7 to 10 peripheral cysts per ovary [20]. All the studies confirmed absence of the following diseases: hyperprolactinaemia, Cushing's disease, and androgen-secreting tumors. Three studies included women with PCOS ($n = 261$) as main inclusion criteria, while five studies included women with clomiphene-resistant PCOS ($n = 649$) as main inclusion criteria. Clomiphene resistance was identified as 100 mg CC daily for 5 days per cycle for at least three cycles for persistent anovulation, in one study and 150 mg CC daily for 5 days per cycle for at least three cycles for persistent anovulation, in other three studies. All the studies included women with only reproductive age ranging from 18 to 39 years. Presence of diabetes, thyroid disorders, and use of medications affecting glucose metabolism were main exclusion criteria in all the included studies. One study had used treatment following laparoscopy.

Eight studies with a total of 910 women with PCOS were randomized to NAC and placebo or metformin. Four studies randomized 441 women to NAC and placebo in 1 : 1 randomization ratio, while remaining four randomized 469 women to NAC or metformin in 1 : 1 randomization ratio. All the included studies were published in English and carried out at single academic medical center associated with university in Middle East (Egypt, Iran, and Turkey) and one in Asia (India). The number of women participating in each trial varied from 60 to 192 with an average of 113 women

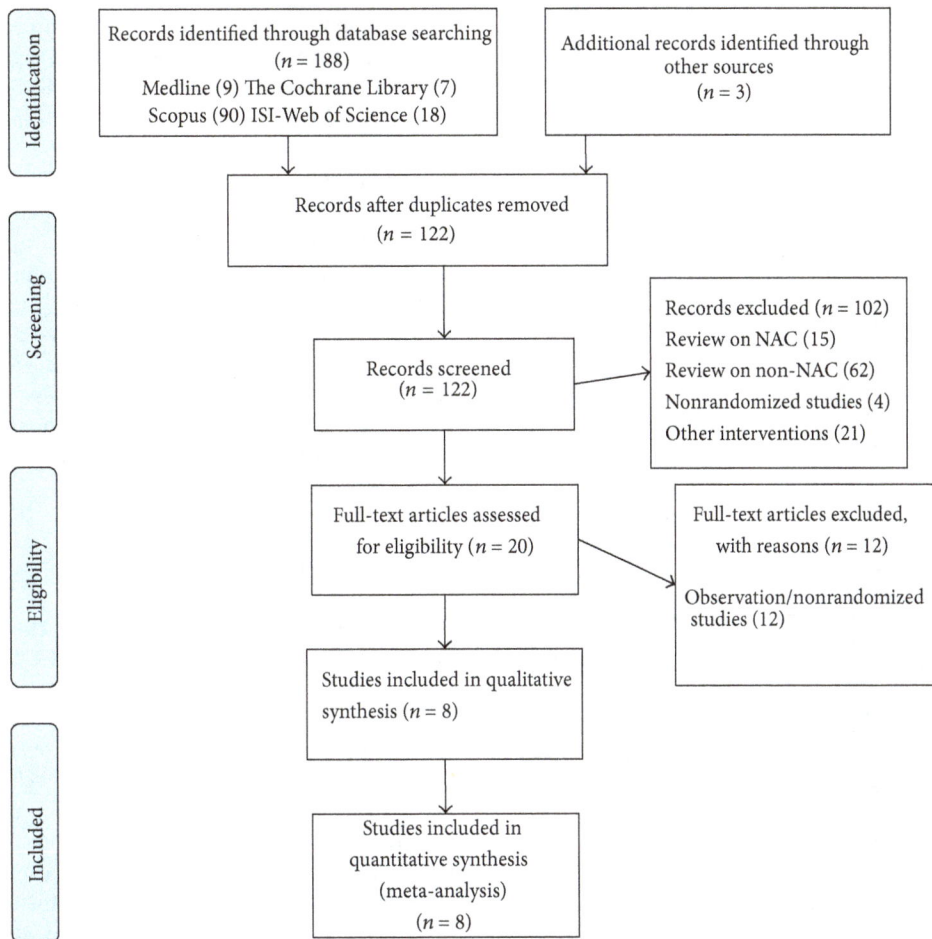

FIGURE 1: PRISMA flow diagram for selection of studies for the systematic review. Flow diagram style adapted from Moher et al. [12].

per study. The study duration ranged from 2 to 12 months. Overall, a total of 842 women completed the studies with overall attrition rate of 9.3% in all the studies.

In studies of women with PCOS, two studies reported concurrent use of clomiphene citrate. All the studies asked to use normal diet and maintain normal lifestyle habit during studies. Baseline characteristics of included studies are shown in Table 2. The mean age of included studies ranged from 20 years to 33 years. One study had obese women (BMI > 30 kg/m^2) [20], six studies had moderately obese women (BMI: 25–30 kg/m^2) [14, 17–19, 21, 22], and one study had nonobese women (BMI: 20–25 kg/m^2) [28]. Only four studies reported rate of menstrual irregularity and amenorrhea or oligomenorrhea, which ranged from 6% [21] to 17% [22] and from 23% [14] to 93.7% [21], respectively. Three studies reported hirsutism with prevalence ranging from 4% to 61.1% [17, 22, 28] while two studies reported problems with acne, ranging from 2% to 27.8% [17, 28]. Six studies reported duration of infertility, of which the four studies reported mean duration of infertility around 4 to 5 years [14, 17, 19, 20] while for one study it was as high as 10 years of infertility [28]. Women had normal fasting glucose level in all the included studies.

Primary outcome of this review was live-birth rate which was assessed in a single study [22]. The odds of live birth with NAC was nearly three times higher in women with PCOS as compared to placebo (Peto odds ratio, pOR: 3.00; 95% CI: 1.05, 8.60; $P = 0.04$; 1 trial; 60 women) (Figure 3). Five studies assessed pregnancy rate per woman. Compared to placebo, women with NAC were around three and half times more likely to have pregnancy (pOR: 3.58; 95% CI: 2.05, 6.25; $P < 0.0001$; $I^2 = 56\%$; 3 trials; 377 women) (see Figure 4). In subgroup based on PCOS status, CC resistant PCOS, or PCOS, it was found that, in women with CC resistant PCOS, NAC increased likelihood, around five times, of pregnancy compared to placebo (pOR: 4.83; 95% CI: 2.30–10.13; $P < 0.0001$; $I^2 = 68\%$; 2 trials; 210 women). In contrast, compared to metformin, women on NAC were 60% less likely to have pregnancy (pOR: 0.40; 95% CI: 0.23, 0.71; $I^2 = 70$; 2 trials; 290 women) without considerable heterogeneity among the studies (see Figure 5). Only three studies reported normal semen analysis of partner while assessing pregnancy outcomes.

In terms of secondary outcomes, there was no significant difference in the miscarriage per woman compared to placebo (Peto OR: 1.28; 95% CI: 0.35, 4.70; $P = 0.71$; $I^2 = 82\%$; 2 trials,

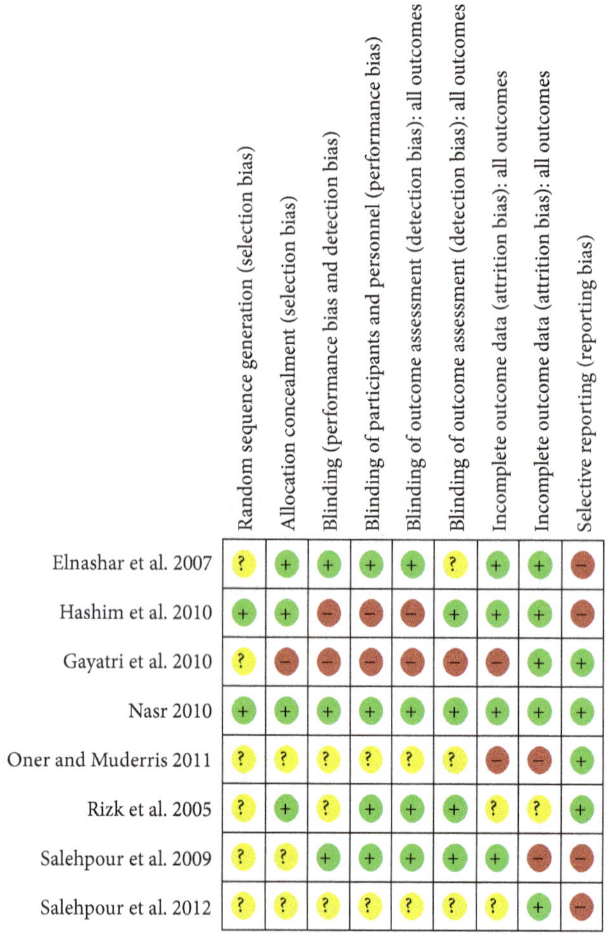

FIGURE 2: Cochrane risk of bias tool summary for included studies.

hirsutism rate/severity of hirsutism following NAC treatment compared to placebo, or metformin. Further, compared to metformin, NAC significantly reduced BMI (MD: −1.00; 95% CI: −1.49, −0.52; $P < 0.0001$; $I^2 = 0\%$, 3 studies; 236 women), while there was no significant change in BMI following NAC treatment compared to placebo (see Figure 7). Addressing the hyperandrogenism, NAC reduced total testosterone level (MD: −0.19; 95% CI: −0.29, −0.10; $P = 0.0001$; $I^2 = 0\%$; 2 trials; 175 women) compared to metformin but did not show any difference in testosterone level (MD: −0.83; 95% CI: −1.79, 0.13; $P = 0.09$; 1 trial, 36 women) compared to placebo (see Figure 8). Compared to metformin or placebo, NAC significantly reduced fasting glucose levels in women with PCOS (see Figure 9). In addition, compared to placebo or metformin, NAC did not significantly improve fasting insulin or HOMA-IR.

5. Discussion

This review was conducted to assess clinical benefits and harms of NAC among women with PCOS. A total of eight randomized controlled trials with 910 women compared effects of NAC with placebo or metformin in women with PCOS. NAC significantly improved rates of live births and spontaneous ovulation compared to placebo in women with PCOS. However, we found no evidence of effects of NAC on improving menstrual regularity, acne, hirsutism, BMI, fasting insulin, fasting glucose, or HOMA-IR. NAC was not associated with greater benefits to metformin for improving pregnancy rate, spontaneous ovulations, and menstrual regularity. Metformin also improved the BMI, total testosterone, insulin level, and lipid levels compared to NAC. The side effect profiles were mild to moderate with no serious adverse drug events reported. Minor side effects were not reported in detail. All the studies were of short duration (three months) and long-term data on the comparative effects of NAC are lacking for important clinical outcomes such as resumption of menstrual regularity.

We aimed to minimize the risk of bias to provide good quality of systematic review. Therefore, we included only randomized controlled clinical trials, ideally with proper randomization, allocation concealment, blinding, and free from selective reporting. However, not all the studies fulfilled all these criteria. The methods used for randomization, allocation concealment, and blinding were not clearly reported by seven out of eight studies. None of the studies has adjusted for baseline difference in characteristics. Two studies had attrition rate of more than 20% [17, 18]. Four studies did not report testing on semen quality of partner which would be a critical factor for pregnancy rates and live birth rates [14, 17, 18, 28]. The studies assessing the pregnancy rate should assess the semen analysis of the partner. Only three studies assessed for normal semen analysis [14, 17, 18]. Five studies did not mention the restriction on the use of body hair removal methods while assessing hirsutism as an outcome. In addition, there is a need to have proper blinding of participants and investigators to prevent observation biases while assessing subjective outcomes such as hirsutism and

190 women) with considerable heterogeneity. Six studies reported ovulation rate. Compared to placebo, women on NAC were three times as likely to have ovulation (pOR: 3.13; 95% CI: 1.54, 6.36; $P = 0.002$; $I^2 = 0\%$; 2 trials, 200 women) in women PCOS, and, for CC-resistant PCOS, women on NAC were nine times as likely to have ovulation (pOR: 8.40; 95% CI: 4.50, 15.67; $P = 0.04$; $I^2 = 77.5\%$; 2 trials, 210 women) with considerable heterogeneity (see Figure 6). However, this association was in opposite direction for the comparison between NAC and metformin. Compared to metformin, women on NAC were 87% less likely to have ovulation (pOR: 0.13; 95% CI: 0.08, 0.22; $P < 0.001$; $I^2 = 0$; 2 trials, 253 women). All the studies reported mild adverse events, however, did not describe the nature of adverse event in details. Two studies reported no incidence of OHSS in any of the groups. No cases of OHSS were reported. There was no significant difference in rate of menstrual regulation with NAC compared to placebo (pOR: 3.00; 95% CI: 0.92, 9.83; $P = 0.07$; 1 trial; 60 women) or metformin (Peto OR: 1.20; 95% CI: 0.58, 2.45; $P = 0.63$; $I^2 = 0\%$; 2 trials, 136 women). Due to difference in the reporting and measurement of acne and hirsutism across the studies, meta-analysis was not feasible; however studies showed that there was no difference in acne/acne severity,

TABLE 1: Characteristics of included studies: study information, treatments, inclusion and exclusion criteria systematic reviews of randomized controlled trials.

Study ID	Study period	Country	Treatment arms	Study duration	Diagnosis criteria	Inclusion criteria	Exclusion criteria
Among women with polycystic ovary syndrome							
Salehpour et al. 2009 [17]	Feb 2007–February 2008	Iran	NAC: 1800 mg/day, divided into three daily doses; placebo: ORS, divided into three daily doses	6 months	Rotterdam criteria, ESHRE/ASRM 2003	Presence of PCOS; spontaneous onset of maturation; and normal sexual development	Diabetes mellitus; use of medications affecting glucose metabolism Use hormonal analogues other than progesterone Severe hepatic or kidney diseases; active peptic ulcer
Gayatri et al. 2010 [28]	June 2006–December 2007	India	NAC: 1800 mg/day, orally divided in three doses; metformin: 500 mg/day for week 1; 500 mg twice daily for week 2 and 500 mg thrice daily afterwards	3 months	Rotterdam criteria, ESHRE/ASRM 2003	Presence of PCOS	Diabetes mellitus; use of medications affecting glucose metabolism Use hormonal analogues other than progesterone Severe hepatic or kidney diseases; active peptic ulcer
Oner and Muderris 2011 [18]	March 2008–April 2009	Turkey	NAC: 1800 mg/day, orally divided in three doses; metformin: 1500 mg/day, orally divided in three doses	6 months	Rotterdam criteria, ESHRE/ASRM 2004	Presence of PCOS	Diabetes mellitus; thyroid disease Use of any drugs that could interfere with the normal function of the hypothalamic-pituitary-gonadal axis
Salehpour et al. 2012 [19]	Jan 2008–Dec 2009	Iran	NAC: 1200 mg/day, divided into two daily doses; Placebo: ORS, divided into two daily doses	3 months	Rotterdam criteria, ESHRE/ASRM 2004	Presence of PCOS; Age 20–35 years; Infertility duration less than 10 years; BMI <35 kg/m²; Normal semen analysis	Thyroid dysfunction; History of large ovarian cyst formation (>6 cm); History of visual disturbance caused by CC; History of asthma and or allergy to medications; Use of medications affecting glucose metabolism; Use hormonal analogues other than progesterone;
Among women with clomiphene resistant polycystic ovary syndrome							
Rizk et al. 2005 [20]	March 2002–Nov 2003	Egypt	NAC:		Other	Presence of CC resistant PCOS; Age 18–39 years	Thyroid disfunction; Allergy to medications; Use of medications affecting glucose metabolism; Use hormonal analogues other than progesterone;
Elnashar et al. 2007 [14]	Dec 2004–Dec 2005	Egypt	NAC: 1800 mg/day, orally divided in three doses; Metformin: 1500 mg/day, orally divided in three doses	2 months	Rotterdam criteria, ESHRE/ASRM 2003	Presence of CC resistant PCOS; Age 18–39 years; Period of infertility >2 years	History of pelvic surgery or infertility factor other than anovulation; Patients with hyperglycemia (fasting blood sugar of <100 mg/dL)

TABLE 1: Continued.

Study ID	Study period	Country	Treatment arms	Study duration	Diagnosis criteria	Inclusion criteria	Exclusion criteria
Hashim et al. 2010 [21]	Jan 2005–June 2009	Egypt	NAC: 1800 mg/day, orally divided in three doses; Metformin: 1500 mg/day, orally divided in three doses	3 Months	Rotterdam criteria, ESHRE/ASRM 2003	Presence of CC resistant PCOS	Diabetes mellitus; Use of medications affecting glucose metabolism; Use hormonal analogues other than progesterone; Smoking & alcohol use; Age more than 40 years
Nasr 2010 [22]	April 2007–June 2009	Egypt	NAC: 1200 mg/day, divided into two daily doses; Placebo: ORS, divided into two daily doses	12 months	Rotterdam criteria, ESHRE/ASRM 2003	Presence of CC resistant PCOS; Age 18–38 years; >2 years with infertility; Patent fallopian tubes & Normal semen analysis	Use hormonal analogues other than progesterone; contraindications to laparoscopy or general anaesthesia

Note: All the studies were carried out in single center within academic medical centers. Rotterdam European Society for Human Reproduction and Embryology/American Society for Reproductive Medicine-sponsored PCOS Consensus Workshop, that is, the presence of at least two of the following three criteria: (1) oligo- or anovulation, (2) clinical and/or chemical signs of hyperandrogenism, and/or (3) polycystic ovaries; and exclusion of other aetiologies such as congenital adrenal hyperplasia, Cushing's syndrome or androgen-secreting tumours. Clomiphene Citrate (CC) resistant was defined as 100 mg CC daily for 5 days per cycle for at least three cycles for persistent anovulation in Rizk et al. 2005 [20] and 150 mg CC daily for 5 days per cycle for at least three cycles for persistent anovulation in other studies. Gayatri et al. 2010 [28] used 50 mg/day of CC from day 2 to 6 and gradual increment in next cycle by 50 mg/day with maximum up to 150 mg/day. None of the included studies were funded by commercial funding agencies like Pharmaceutical Industries. However, drugs for the studies were provided by the Pharmaceutical Companies. All the women were asked to have normal life-style and eating habit during the study.

TABLE 2: Characteristics of included studies: baseline characteristics systematic reviews of randomized controlled trials.

Characteristics	Among women with PCOS					Among women with clomiphene resistant PCOS		
	Salehpour et al. 2009 [17]	Gayatri et al. 2010 [28]	Oner and Muderris 2011 [18]	Salehpour et al. 2012 [19]	Rizk et al. 2005 [20]	Elnashar et al. 2007 [14]	Hashim et al. 2010 [21]	Nasr 2010 [22]
	NAC/placebo	NAC/metformin	NAC/metformin	NAC/placebo	NAC/placebo	NAC/metformin	NAC/metformin	NAC/placebo
Total randomized, n	46	115	100	180	153	64	192	60
Randomised, n	46	56/59	50/50	90/90	NA	32/32	95/97	30/30
Completed, n	36	50/50	45/31	82/85	75/75	30/31	97/95	30/30
Total, n	36	100	76	167	150	61	192	60
Attrition rate	21.7%	13%	24%	7%	2%	4.7%	0%	0%
Baseline Characteristics								
Age, years	27.2 (5.4); 27.8 (6.1)	22.6 (3.8); 23.2 (4.1)	23.7 (4.4); 22.6 (4.8)	27.22 (3.32); 27.41 (3.41)	28.9 (4.7); 28.4 (5.7)	27.33 (3.35); 26.73 (5.36)	27.3 (2.6); 26.8 (2.2)	28.4 (4.2); 29.2 (3.7)
Weight, kg	74.1 (11.7); 74.1 (13.2)	70.5 (3.45); 69.8 (8.32)	NA	NA	101.3 (12.4); 99.2 (12.3)	NA	NA	NA
BMI, kg/m^2	29.5 (4.1); 29.5 (4.4)	26.54 (2.35); 27.28 (3.25)	23 (4.6); 24.3 (6.2)	26.78 (2.24); 26.67 (2.01)	30.5 (2.6); 30.1 (3.1)	25.8 (0.94); 26.8 (1.52)	26.6 (2.2); 26.3 (2.3)	28.6 (3.7); 29.1 (4.2)
Amenorrhea patients (%)	2 (11.1%); 2 (11.1%)	4 (8%); 4 (8%)	NA	NA	NA	NA	6 (6.3%); 7 (7.2%)	5 (17%); 6 (20%)
Oligomenorrhea, n (%)	NA	29 (58%); 30 (60%)	NA	NA	NA	76.7 (23); 77.4 (24)	89 (93.7%); 90 (92.8%)	NA
Hirsutism, n (%)	11 (61.1%); 10 (55.6%)	2 (4%); 3 (6%)	NA	NA	NA	NA	NA	16 (53%); 18 (60%)
Acne, n (%)	5 (27.8%); 5 (27.8%)	1 (2); 2 (4)	NA	NA	NA	NA	NA	NA
Duration of Infertility, mean (SD)	4.5 (2.2); 4.2 (3.3)	10 (20); 8 (16)	NA	4.39 (1.96); 4.45 (1.94)	5 (2.9); 4.4 (2.6)	NA	4.5 (1.2); 4.7 (1.3)	5.3 (1.9); 4.9 (2.1)
Testosterone level, nmol/dL, mean (SD)	0.91 (0.48); 1.01 (0.45)	1.55 (0.29); 1.65 (0.24)	80.8 (41.1); 86.1 (48.4)	NA	NA	98.27 (31.5); 106.5 (44.6)	1.06 (0.27); 1.03 (0.31)	NA
FPG, mg/dL, mean (SD)	95.6 (10.9); 96.8 (27.7)	88.53 (5.14); 87.65 (4.34)	88.5 (6.8); 88.9 (7.4)	NA	81.9 (12.6); 85.9 (14.1)	83.3 (8.8); 85.9 (9.4)	91.3 (1.5); 89.6 (1.4)	NA
HOMA-IR	5.22 (5.58); 4.9 (4.2)	5.52 (1.35); 5.42 (1.36)	4.5 (1.2); 4.3 (0.9)	NA	NA	NA	NA	NA

Study or subgroup	NAC Events	NAC Total	Placebo Events	Placebo Total	Weight	Odds ratio M-H, fixed, 95% CI	Odds ratio M-H, fixed, 95% CI
Nasr 2010	20	30	12	30	100.0%	3.00 [1.05, 8.60]	
Total (95% CI)		**30**		**30**	**100.0%**	**3.00 [1.05, 8.60]**	
Total events	20		12				
Heterogeneity: not applicable							
Test for overall effect: $Z = 2.04$ ($P = 0.04$)							

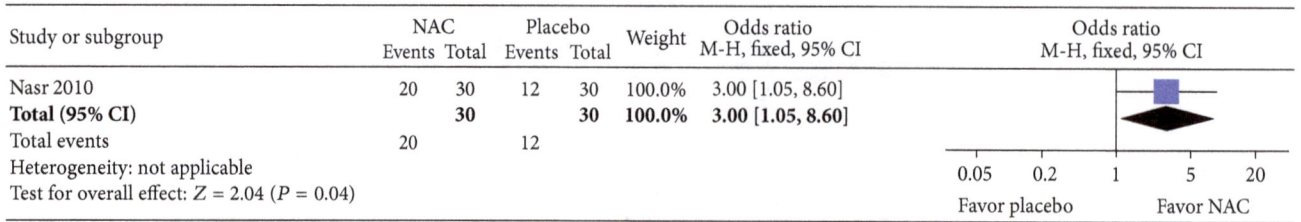

FIGURE 3: Forest plot: outcome: live birth rate in women with PCOS comparing NAC with placebo.

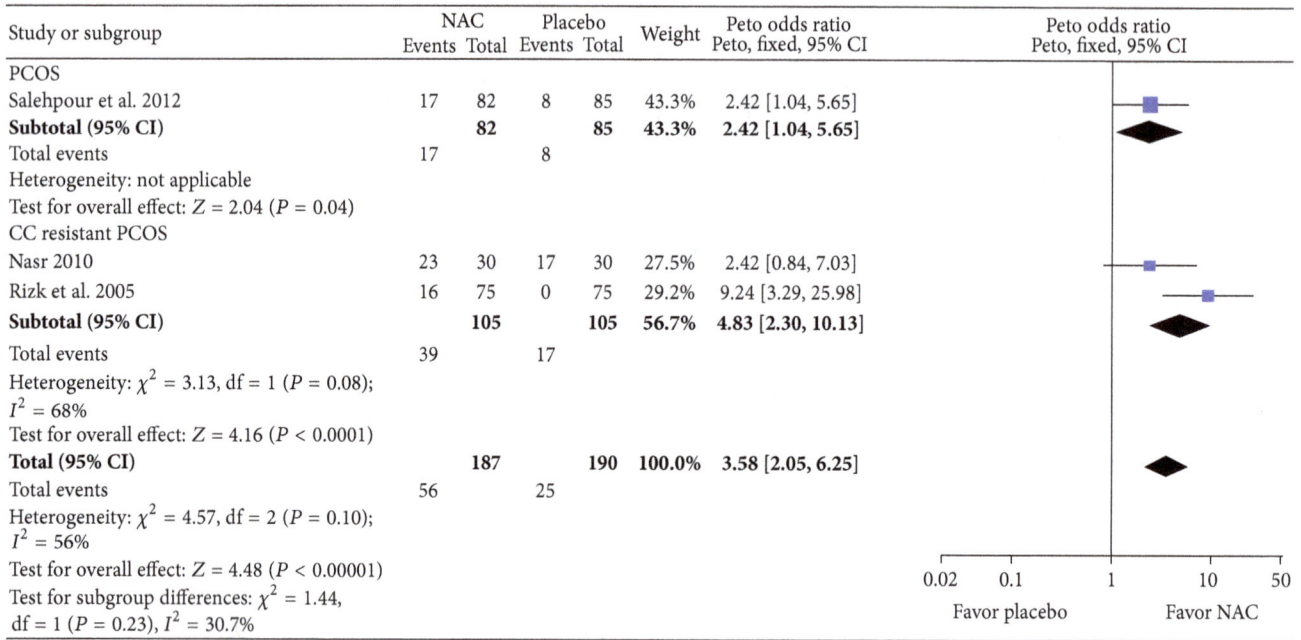

Study or subgroup	NAC Events	NAC Total	Placebo Events	Placebo Total	Weight	Peto odds ratio Peto, fixed, 95% CI	Peto odds ratio Peto, fixed, 95% CI
PCOS							
Salehpour et al. 2012	17	82	8	85	43.3%	2.42 [1.04, 5.65]	
Subtotal (95% CI)		**82**		**85**	**43.3%**	**2.42 [1.04, 5.65]**	
Total events	17		8				
Heterogeneity: not applicable							
Test for overall effect: $Z = 2.04$ ($P = 0.04$)							
CC resistant PCOS							
Nasr 2010	23	30	17	30	27.5%	2.42 [0.84, 7.03]	
Rizk et al. 2005	16	75	0	75	29.2%	9.24 [3.29, 25.98]	
Subtotal (95% CI)		**105**		**105**	**56.7%**	**4.83 [2.30, 10.13]**	
Total events	39		17				
Heterogeneity: $\chi^2 = 3.13$, df = 1 ($P = 0.08$); $I^2 = 68\%$							
Test for overall effect: $Z = 4.16$ ($P < 0.0001$)							
Total (95% CI)		**187**		**190**	**100.0%**	**3.58 [2.05, 6.25]**	
Total events	56		25				
Heterogeneity: $\chi^2 = 4.57$, df = 2 ($P = 0.10$); $I^2 = 56\%$							
Test for overall effect: $Z = 4.48$ ($P < 0.00001$)							
Test for subgroup differences: $\chi^2 = 1.44$, df = 1 ($P = 0.23$), $I^2 = 30.7\%$							

FIGURE 4: Forest plot: outcome: pregnancy rate in women with PCOS comparing NAC with placebo.

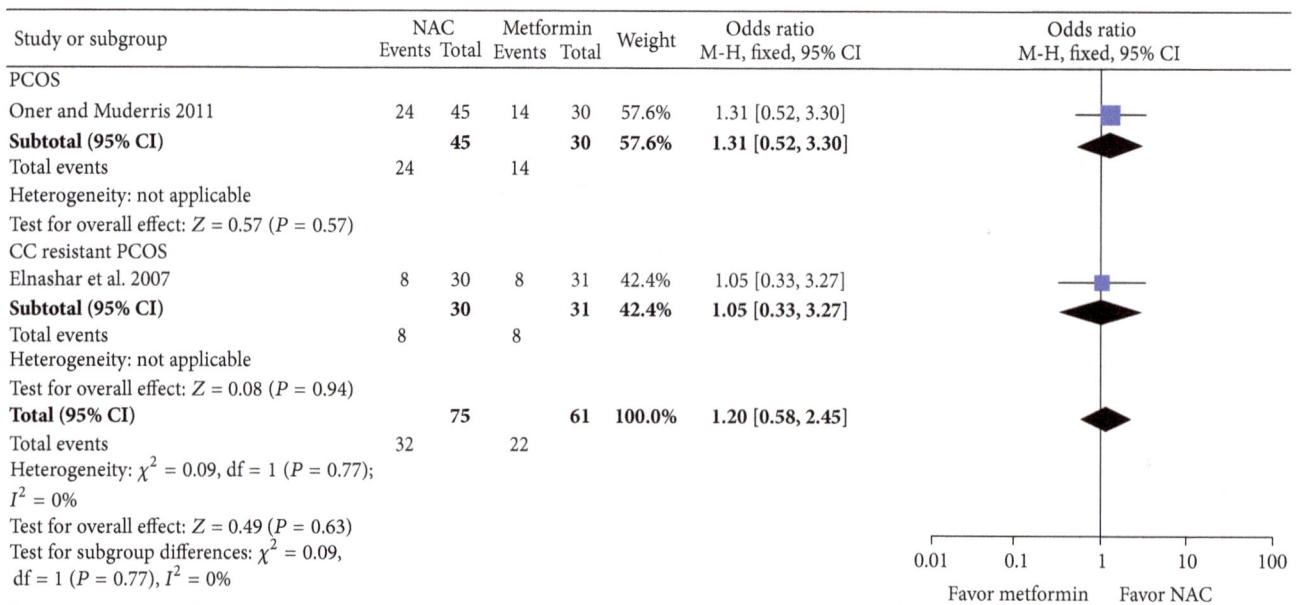

Study or subgroup	NAC Events	NAC Total	Metformin Events	Metformin Total	Weight	Odds ratio M-H, fixed, 95% CI	Odds ratio M-H, fixed, 95% CI
PCOS							
Oner and Muderris 2011	24	45	14	30	57.6%	1.31 [0.52, 3.30]	
Subtotal (95% CI)		**45**		**30**	**57.6%**	**1.31 [0.52, 3.30]**	
Total events	24		14				
Heterogeneity: not applicable							
Test for overall effect: $Z = 0.57$ ($P = 0.57$)							
CC resistant PCOS							
Elnashar et al. 2007	8	30	8	31	42.4%	1.05 [0.33, 3.27]	
Subtotal (95% CI)		**30**		**31**	**42.4%**	**1.05 [0.33, 3.27]**	
Total events	8		8				
Heterogeneity: not applicable							
Test for overall effect: $Z = 0.08$ ($P = 0.94$)							
Total (95% CI)		**75**		**61**	**100.0%**	**1.20 [0.58, 2.45]**	
Total events	32		22				
Heterogeneity: $\chi^2 = 0.09$, df = 1 ($P = 0.77$); $I^2 = 0\%$							
Test for overall effect: $Z = 0.49$ ($P = 0.63$)							
Test for subgroup differences: $\chi^2 = 0.09$, df = 1 ($P = 0.77$), $I^2 = 0\%$							

FIGURE 5: Forest plot: outcome: pregnancy rate in women with PCOS comparing NAC with metformin.

Study or subgroup	NAC Events	Total	Placebo Events	Total	Weight	Peto odds ratio Peto, fixed, 95% CI	Peto odds ratio Peto, fixed, 95% CI
PCOS							
Salehpour 2009	10	18	3	18	12.2%	5.15 [1.35, 19.69]	
Salehpour 2012	18	82	8	85	31.5%	2.58 [1.12, 5.94]	
Subtotal (95% CI)		**100**		**103**	**43.7%**	**3.13 [1.54, 6.36]**	
Total events	28		11				

Heterogeneity: $\chi^2 = 0.73$, df = 1 ($P = 0.39$); $I^2 = 0\%$
Test for overall effect: $Z = 3.16$ ($P = 0.002$)

CC Resistant PCOS							
Nasr 2010	26	30	20	30	15.6%	3.00 [0.92, 9.83]	
Rizk 2005	37	75	1	75	40.7%	12.44 [5.97, 25.90]	
Subtotal (95% CI)		**105**		**105**	**56.3%**	**8.40 [4.50, 15.67]**	
Total events	63		21				

Heterogeneity: $\chi^2 = 3.99$, df = 1 ($P = 0.05$); $I^2 = 75\%$
Test for overall effect: $Z = 6.68$ ($P < 0.00001$)

Total (95% CI)		**205**		**208**	**100.0%**	**5.46 [3.42, 8.71]**	
Total events	91		32				

Heterogeneity: $\chi^2 = 8.92$, df = 3 ($P = 0.03$); $I^2 = 66\%$
Test for overall effect: $Z = 7.10$ ($P < 0.00001$)
Test for subgroup differences: $\chi^2 = 4.20$, df = 1 ($P < 0.04$), $I^2 = 76.2\%$

0.01 0.1 1 10 100
Favor placebo   Favor NAC

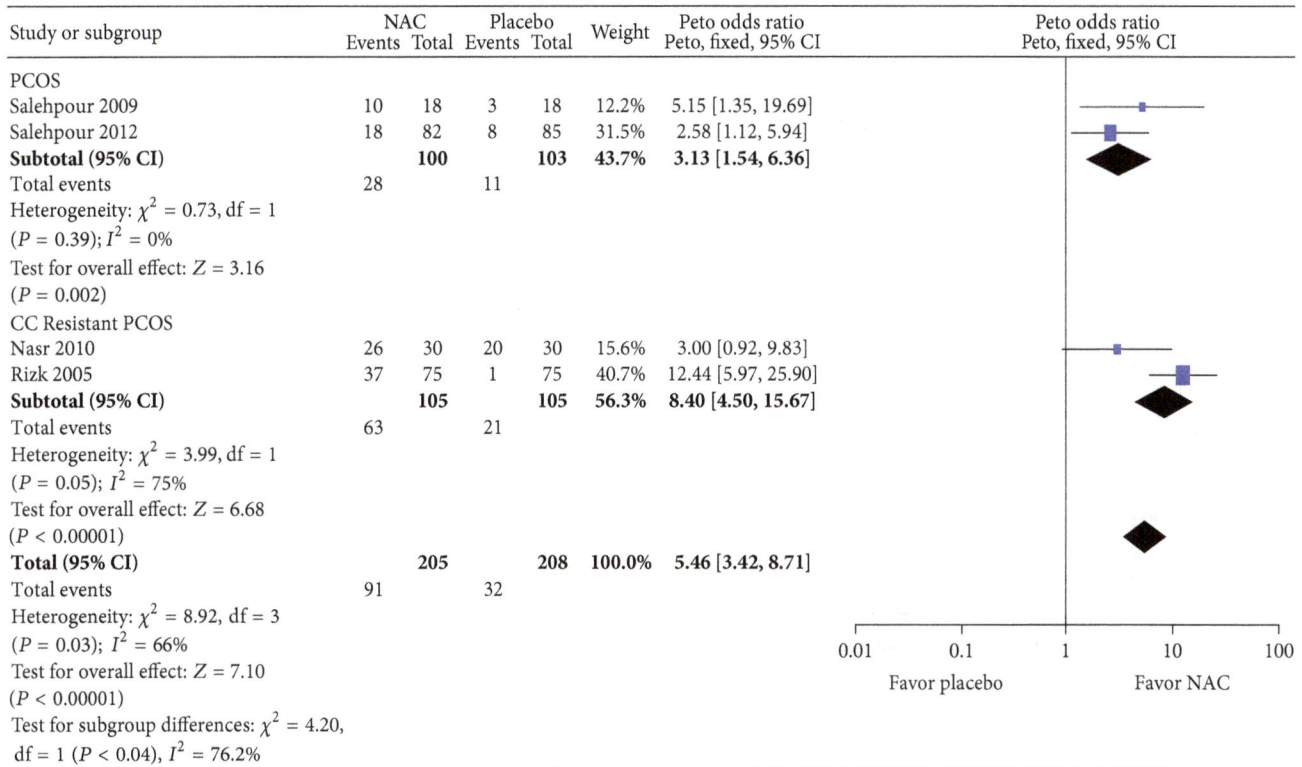

FIGURE 6: Forest plot: outcome: ovulation rate in women with PCOS comparing NAC with placebo.

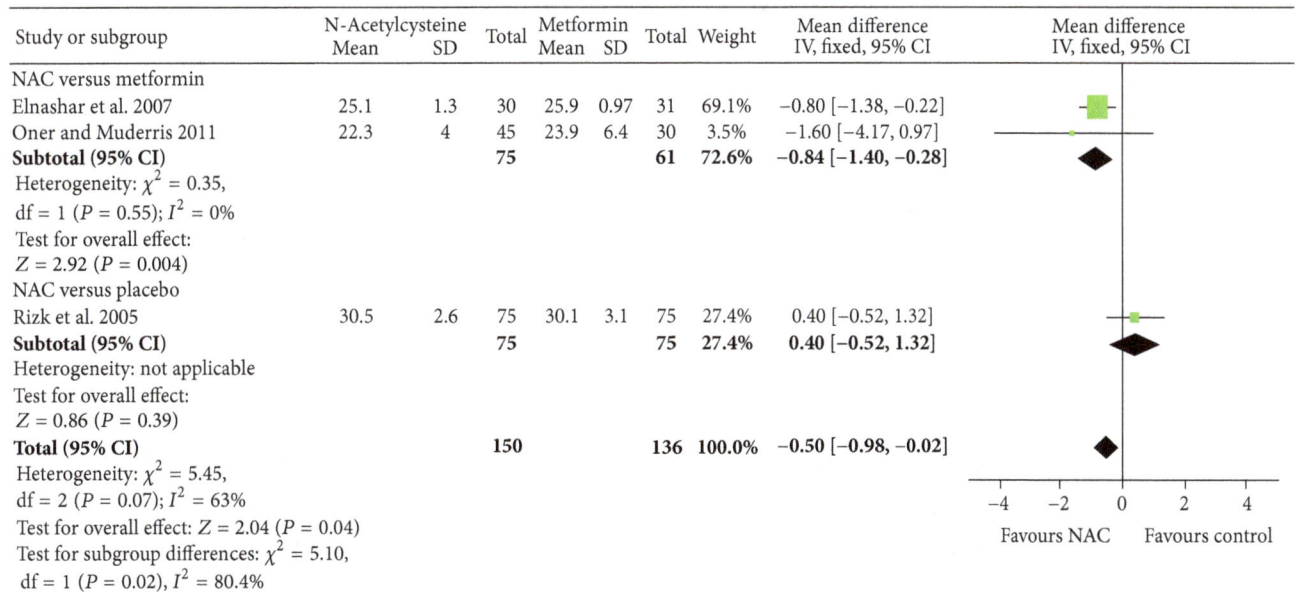

Study or subgroup	N-Acetylcysteine Mean	SD	Total	Metformin Mean	SD	Total	Weight	Mean difference IV, fixed, 95% CI	Mean difference IV, fixed, 95% CI
NAC versus metformin									
Elnashar et al. 2007	25.1	1.3	30	25.9	0.97	31	69.1%	−0.80 [−1.38, −0.22]	
Oner and Muderris 2011	22.3	4	45	23.9	6.4	30	3.5%	−1.60 [−4.17, 0.97]	
Subtotal (95% CI)			**75**			**61**	**72.6%**	**−0.84 [−1.40, −0.28]**	

Heterogeneity: $\chi^2 = 0.35$, df = 1 ($P = 0.55$); $I^2 = 0\%$
Test for overall effect: $Z = 2.92$ ($P = 0.004$)

NAC versus placebo									
Rizk et al. 2005	30.5	2.6	75	30.1	3.1	75	27.4%	0.40 [−0.52, 1.32]	
Subtotal (95% CI)			**75**			**75**	**27.4%**	**0.40 [−0.52, 1.32]**	

Heterogeneity: not applicable
Test for overall effect: $Z = 0.86$ ($P = 0.39$)

Total (95% CI)			**150**			**136**	**100.0%**	**−0.50 [−0.98, −0.02]**	

Heterogeneity: $\chi^2 = 5.45$, df = 2 ($P = 0.07$); $I^2 = 63\%$
Test for overall effect: $Z = 2.04$ ($P = 0.04$)
Test for subgroup differences: $\chi^2 = 5.10$, df = 1 ($P = 0.02$), $I^2 = 80.4\%$

−4 −2 0 2 4
Favours NAC   Favours control

FIGURE 7: Forest plot: outcome: body-mass index (BMI) (kg/m^2) in women with PCOS comparing NAC with placebo/metformin.

acne [17, 18, 20, 22, 28]. Theoretically, studies of a relatively short duration could demonstrate a significant impact on clinical outcomes such as menstrual regularity or ovulation rate, although this is somewhat unlikely, even with regards to important adverse events. Only one study evaluated the long-term efficacy and safety of NAC in women with PCOS and live birth rate as an outcome [22].

There are no other systematic reviews on NAC for women with PCOS. This review is the first to generate the hypothesis on the use of NAC for PCOS. In order to limit bias in the review process, the search strategies exclusively performed to get both formal and nonformal sources of information without any restrictions on language of the search. The study selection, risk of bias assessment, and data collection were

Study or subgroup	N-Acetylcysteine Mean	SD	Total	Metformin Mean	SD	Total	Weight	Mean difference IV, fixed, 95% CI
NAC versus metformin								
Elnashar et al. 2007	0.26	0.6	30	0.27	0.1	31	85.9%	−0.01 [−0.23, 0.21]
Oner and Muderris 2011	2.36	1.35	45	2.31	1.28	30	11.1%	0.05 [−0.55, 0.65]
Subtotal (95% CI)			75			61	97.0%	−0.00 [−0.21, 0.20]

Heterogeneity: $\chi^2 = 0.03$, df = 1 (P = 0.85); $I^2 = 0\%$
Test for overall effect: Z = 0.03 (P = 0.98)

NAC versus placebo								
Fulghesu et al. 2002	1.91	1.04	31	2.43	1.39	6	3.0%	−0.52 [−1.69, 0.65]
Subtotal (95% CI)			31			6	3.0%	−0.52 [−1.69, 0.65]

Heterogeneity: not applicable
Test for overall effect: Z = 0.87 (P = 0.38)

| **Total (95% CI)** | | | 106 | | | 67 | 100.0% | −0.02 [−0.22, 0.18] |

Heterogeneity: $\chi^2 = 0.76$, df = 2 (P = 0.68); $I^2 = 0\%$
Test for overall effect: Z = 0.18 (P = 0.86)
Test for subgroup differences: $\chi^2 = 0.73$, df = 1 (P = 0.39), $I^2 = 0\%$

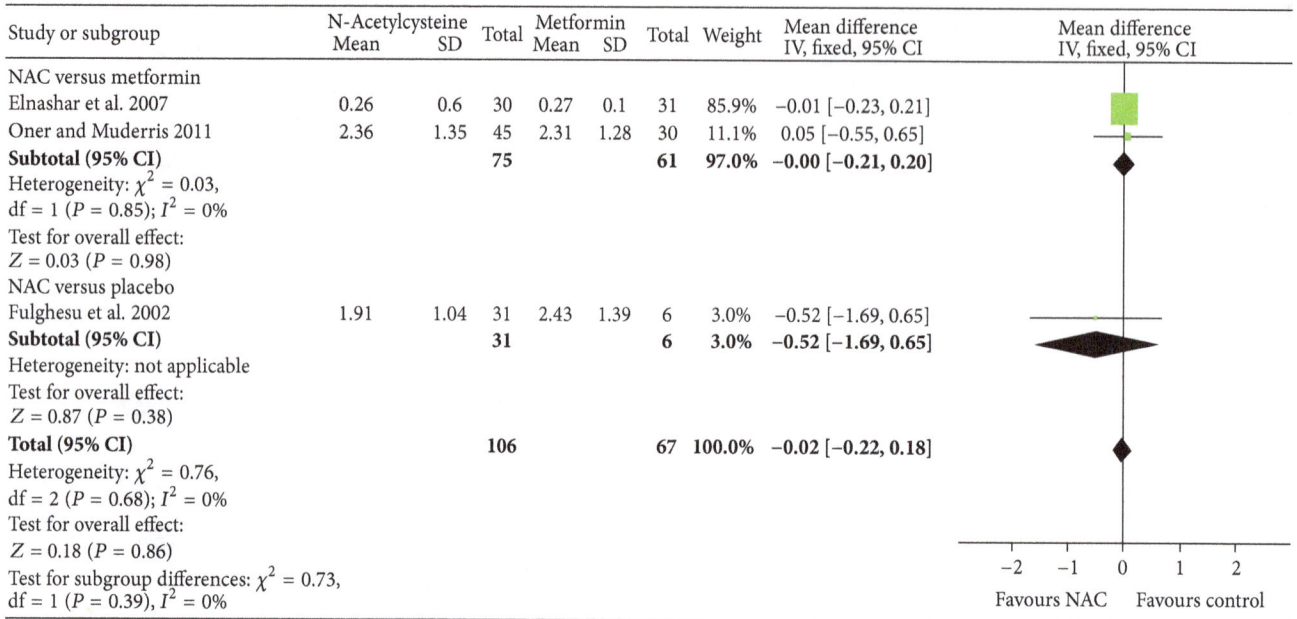

FIGURE 8: Forest plot: outcome: testosterone level (nmol/L) in women with PCOS comparing NAC with placebo/metformin.

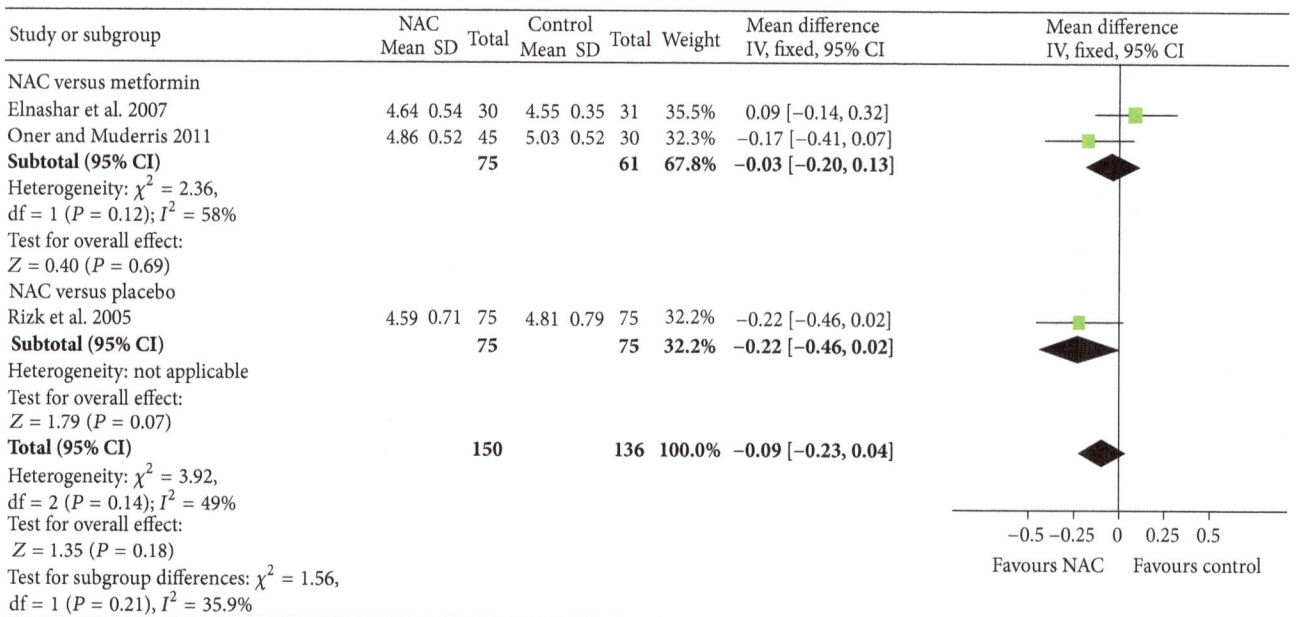

Study or subgroup	NAC Mean	SD	Total	Control Mean	SD	Total	Weight	Mean difference IV, fixed, 95% CI
NAC versus metformin								
Elnashar et al. 2007	4.64	0.54	30	4.55	0.35	31	35.5%	0.09 [−0.14, 0.32]
Oner and Muderris 2011	4.86	0.52	45	5.03	0.52	30	32.3%	−0.17 [−0.41, 0.07]
Subtotal (95% CI)			75			61	67.8%	−0.03 [−0.20, 0.13]

Heterogeneity: $\chi^2 = 2.36$, df = 1 (P = 0.12); $I^2 = 58\%$
Test for overall effect: Z = 0.40 (P = 0.69)

NAC versus placebo								
Rizk et al. 2005	4.59	0.71	75	4.81	0.79	75	32.2%	−0.22 [−0.46, 0.02]
Subtotal (95% CI)			75			75	32.2%	−0.22 [−0.46, 0.02]

Heterogeneity: not applicable
Test for overall effect: Z = 1.79 (P = 0.07)

| **Total (95% CI)** | | | 150 | | | 136 | 100.0% | −0.09 [−0.23, 0.04] |

Heterogeneity: $\chi^2 = 3.92$, df = 2 (P = 0.14); $I^2 = 49\%$
Test for overall effect: Z = 1.35 (P = 0.18)
Test for subgroup differences: $\chi^2 = 1.56$, df = 1 (P = 0.21), $I^2 = 35.9\%$

FIGURE 9: Forest plot: outcome: fasting glucose (mg/dL) in women with PCOS comparing NAC with placebo/metformin.

conducted independently by two review authors but without blinding. Any disagreement was resolved by discussion with the third review author. We did not exclude any study due to lack of additional information. Failure to obtain the primary study data in analyzable format was the main limitation of the review. It was not feasible to perform sensitivity analyses to determine whether there was an effect on outcome from allocation concealment, blinding, or obesity due to insufficient data. In addition due to limited studies, we were

not able to see publication bias. A number of the results were constrained by small numbers of participants and wide confidence intervals, which limited the precision and confidence of the conclusions. Meta-analysis was not possible for a number of primary and secondary outcomes, comparing NAC to placebo due to either an absence of trials or the presence of a single trial only. In the future, well-designed RCTs with large sample sizes are warranted to confirm or refute the current evidence.

6. Conclusion

NAC showed significant improvement in pregnancy and ovulation rate in the studies with short-term outcomes compared to placebo. However, the given the limitations of existing studies such as poor quality, less studies assessing live-birth rates, in future, well-designed randomized-controlled trials should conducted.

Disclosure

Amit Raval, Divyesh Thakker, Isha Patel, Rama Walia N-acetylcysteine for women with polycystic ovary syndrome. PROSPERO 2012: CRD42012001902 Available from http://www.crd.york.ac.uk/PROSPERO/display_record.asp?ID=CRD42012001902.

Conflict of Interests

All authors have completed and submitted the ICMJE form for disclosure of potential conflicts of interest and none were reported.

Authors' Contribution

Mr. Amit Raval had full access to all of the data in the study and takes responsibility for the integrity of the data and the accuracy of the data analysis. Study concept and design were performed by Amit Raval and Rama Walia. Acquisition of data was done by Divyesh Thakker, Amit Raval, and Isha Patel. Analysis and interpretation of data were performed by Divyesh Thakker, Amit Raval, Isha Patel, and Rama Walia. Drafting the paper was done by Divyesh Thakker, Amit Raval, Isha Patel, and Rama Walia. Critical revision of the paper for important intellectual content was done by Divyesh Thakker, Amit Raval, Isha Patel, and Rama Walia. Statistical analysis was performed by Divyesh Thakker, Amit Raval, and Isha Patel. Obtained funding: None Administrative, technical, or material support: Amit Raval. Study was supervised by Amit Raval and Rama Walia.

References

[1] M. Shannon and Y. Wang, "Polycystic ovary syndrome: a common but often unrecognized condition," *Journal of Midwifery & Women's Health*, vol. 57, no. 3, pp. 221–230, 2012.

[2] B. O. Yildiz, G. Bozdag, Z. Yapici, I. Esinler, and H. Yarali, "Prevalence, phenotype and cardiometabolic risk of polycystic ovary syndrome under different diagnostic criteria," *Human Reproduction*, vol. 27, no. 10, pp. 3067–3073, 2012.

[3] C. Christakou and E. Diamanti-Kandarakis, "Role of androgen excess on metabolic aberrations and cardiovascular risk in women with polycystic ovary syndrome," *Women's Health*, vol. 4, no. 6, pp. 583–594, 2008.

[4] A. Huang, K. Brennan, and R. Azziz, "Prevalence of hyperandrogenemia in the polycystic ovary syndrome diagnosed by the National Institutes of Health 1990 criteria," *Fertility and Sterility*, vol. 93, no. 6, pp. 1938–1941, 2010.

[5] American Association of Clinical Endocrinologists Polycystic Ovary Syndrome Writing Committee, "American association of clinical endocrinologists position statement on metabolic and cardiovascular consequences of polycystic ovary syndrome," *Endocrine Practice*, vol. 11, no. 2, pp. 126–134, 2005.

[6] B. Pangaribuan, I. Yusuf, M. Mansyur, and A. Wijaya, "Serum adiponectin and resistin in relation to insulin resistance and markers of hyperandrogenism in lean and obese women with polycystic ovary syndrome," *Therapeutic Advances in Endocrinology and Metabolism*, vol. 2, no. 6, pp. 235–245, 2011.

[7] J. Brown, C. Farquhar, J. Beck, C. Boothroyd, and E. Hughes, "Clomiphene and anti-oestrogens for ovulation induction in PCOS," *The Cochrane Database of Systematic Reviews*, no. 4, Article ID CD002249, 2009.

[8] C. M. Farquhar, Y. A. Wang, and E. A. Sullivan, "A comparative analysis of assisted reproductive technology cycles in Australia and New Zealand 2004–2007," *Human Reproduction*, vol. 25, no. 9, pp. 2281–2289, 2010.

[9] C. Farquhar, J. Brown, and J. Marjoribanks, "Laparoscopic drilling by diathermy or laser for ovulation induction in anovulatory polycystic ovary syndrome," *Cochrane Database of Systematic Reviews*, vol. 6, Article ID CD001122, 2012.

[10] K. A. Awartani and A. P. Cheung, "Metformin and polycystic ovary syndrome: a literature review," *Journal of Obstetrics and Gynaecology Canada*, vol. 24, no. 5, pp. 393–401, 2002.

[11] T. Tang, J. M. Lord, R. J. Norman, E. Yasmin, and A. H. Balen, "Insulin-sensitising drugs (metformin, rosiglitazone, pioglitazone, D-chiro-inositol) for women with polycystic ovary syndrome, oligo amenorrhoea and subfertility," *Cochrane Database of Systematic Reviews*, no. 5, Article ID CD003053, 2012.

[12] D. Moher, A. Liberati, J. Tetzlaff, D. G. Altman, and The PRISMA Group, "Preferred reporting items for systematic reviews and meta-analyses: the PRISMA statement," *PLoS Medicine*, vol. 6, no. 6, Article ID e1000097, 2009.

[13] A. M. Fulghesu, M. Ciampelli, G. Muzj et al., "N-acetyl-cysteine treatment improves insulin sensitivity in women with polycystic ovary syndrome," *Fertility and Sterility*, vol. 77, no. 6, pp. 1128–1135, 2002.

[14] A. Elnashar, M. Fahmy, A. Mansour, and K. Ibrahim, "N-acetyl cysteine vs. metformin in treatment of clomiphene citrate-resistant polycystic ovary syndrome: a prospective randomized controlled study," *Fertility and Sterility*, vol. 88, no. 2, pp. 406–409, 2007.

[15] The Rotterdam ESHRE/ASRM-Sponsored PCOS Consensus Workshop Group, "Revised 2003 consensus on diagnostic criteria and long-term health risks related to polycystic ovary syndrome," *Fertility and Sterility*, vol. 81, no. 1, pp. 19–25, 2004.

[16] J. Zawadzki and A. Dunaif, "A. diagnostic criteria for polycystic ovary syndrome: towards a rational approach," in *Polycystic Ovarian Syndrome*, A. Dunaif, J. Givens, F. Haseltine, and G. Merriam, Eds., pp. 377–84, Blackwell Scientific, Boston, Mass, USA, 1992.

[17] S. Salehpour, M. Tohidi, M. R. Akhound, and N. Amirzargar, "N acetyl cysteine, a novel remedy for poly cystic ovarian syndrome," *International Journal of Fertility and Sterility*, vol. 3, no. 2, pp. 66–73, 2009.

[18] G. Oner and I. I. Muderris, "Clinical, endocrine and metabolic effects of metformin vs N-acetyl-cysteine in women with polycystic ovary syndrome," *European Journal of Obstetrics Gynecology and Reproductive Biology*, vol. 159, no. 1, pp. 127–131, 2011.

[19] S. Salehpour, A. A. Sene, N. Saharkhiz, M. R. Sohrabi, and F. Moghimian, "N-acetylcysteine as an adjuvant to clomiphene citrate for successful induction of ovulation in infertile patients with polycystic ovary syndrome," *Journal of Obstetrics and Gynaecology Research*, vol. 38, no. 9, pp. 1182–1186, 2012.

[20] A. Y. Rizk, M. A. Bedaiwy, and H. G. Al-Inany, "N-acetyl-cysteine is a novel adjuvant to clomiphene citrate in clomiphene citrate-resistant patients with polycystic ovary syndrome," *Fertility and Sterility*, vol. 83, no. 2, pp. 367–370, 2005.

[21] H. A. Hashim, K. Anwar, and R. A. El-Fatah, "N-acetyl cysteine plus clomiphene citrate versus metformin and clomiphene citrate in treatment of clomiphene-resistant polycystic ovary syndrome: a randomized controlled trial," *Journal of Women's Health*, vol. 19, no. 11, pp. 2043–2048, 2010.

[22] A. Nasr, "Effect of N-acetyl-cysteine after ovarian drilling in clomiphene citrate-resistant PCOS women: a pilot study," *Reproductive BioMedicine Online*, vol. 20, no. 3, pp. 403–409, 2010.

[23] A. Liberati, D. G. Altman, J. Tetzlaff et al., "The PRISMA statement for reporting systematic reviews and meta-analyses of studies that evaluate health care interventions: explanation and elaboration," *PLoS Medicine*, vol. 6, no. 7, Article ID e1000100, 2009.

[24] J. P. T. Higgins and S. Green, Eds., *Cochrane Handbook for Systematic Reviews of Interventions Version 5.1.0*, The Cochrane Collaboration, 2011, http://handbook.cochrane.org.

[25] J. P. T. Higgins, S. G. Thompson, J. J. Deeks, and D. G. Altman, "Measuring inconsistency in meta-analyses," *British Medical Journal*, vol. 327, no. 7414, pp. 557–560, 2003.

[26] R. D. Riley, J. P. Higgins, and J. J. Deeks, "Interpretation of random effects meta-analyses," *British Medical Journal*, vol. 342, article d549, 2011.

[27] T. Kilic-Okman and M. Kucuk, "N-acetyl-cysteine treatment for polycystic ovary syndrome," *International Journal of Gynecology & Obstetrics*, vol. 85, no. 3, pp. 296–297, 2004.

[28] K. Gayatri, J. S. Kumar, and B. B. Kumar, "Metformin and N-acetyl cysteine in polycystic ovarian syndrome—a comparative study," *Indian Journal of Clinical Medicine*, vol. 1, no. 1, pp. 7–13, 2010.

28

Cervical Cancer Screening Program by Visual Inspection: Acceptability and Feasibility in Health Insurance Companies

Apollinaire G. Horo,[1] **Judith Didi-Kouko Coulibaly,**[2] **Abdoul Koffi,**[1] **Boris Tchounga,**[3] **Konan Seni,**[1] **Kacou Edèle Aka,**[1] **and Mamourou Kone**[1]

[1]*Department of Gynaecology and Obstetrics, Teaching Hospital of Yopougon, Félix Houphouët Boigny (FHB) University, Abidjan, Côte d'Ivoire*
[2]*Oncology Department, Félix Houphouët Boigny (FHB) University, Teaching Hospital of Treichville, Abidjan, Côte d'Ivoire*
[3]*PACCI Program, IeDEA West Africa Collaboration, Abidjan, Côte d'Ivoire*

Correspondence should be addressed to Apollinaire G. Horo; horoapollinaire@yahoo.fr

Academic Editor: Enrique Hernandez

Objective. To assess willingness to participate and diagnostic accuracy of visual inspection for early detection of cervical neoplasia among women in a health insurance company. *Patients and Method.* Cervical cancer screening was systematically proposed to 800 women after consecutive information and awareness sessions. The screening method was visual inspection with acetic acid (VIA) or Lugol's iodine (VILI). *Results.* Among the 800 identified women, 640 (82%) have accepted the screening, their mean age was 39 years, and 12.0% of them were involved in a polygamist couple. 28.2% of women had prior cervical screening. VIA has been detected positive in 5.9% of women versus 8.6% for VILI. The sensitivity was 72.9% and specificity was 95.2% for VIA versus 71.2% and 97.3% for VILI respectively. The histological examination highlighted a nonspecific chronic cervicitis in 4.6%, CIN1 lesions in 5.91%, and CIN2/3 in 1.2% of the cases. *Conclusion.* Cervical cancer screening by visual inspection showed appropriate diagnostic accuracy when used to detect early cervical lesions. It is a simple and easy to perform method that could be introduced progressively in the health insurance policy while waiting for a national screening program.

1. Introduction

Each year, about 490 000 new cases of cervical cancer occurred worldwide, mainly in developing countries (80%) [1]. In these countries, cervical cancer is the second most common cancer among women after breast cancer and the leading cause of cancer deaths [1, 2]. In developed countries, the incidence and mortality of cervical cancer decreased significantly, due to implementation of organized cervical cancer screening programs [2]. Such programs are not yet implemented in many resources constrained settings, where access to early detection of cervical neoplasia is still challenging and most patients are diagnosed at an advanced stage [3]. In Côte d'Ivoire, cervical cancer screening is based only on cytology and is not organized in a subsidized program; the cost is then supported by women themselves. Since 2005 the World Health Organization (WHO) recommended visual inspection of cervix with acetic acid (VIA) or Lugol's iodine (VILI) as alternative screening techniques for the detection of cervical precancerous lesions. Many field evaluation surveys reported that visual inspection demonstrated diagnostic accuracy close to cytology and was more affordable and easy to perform for nonmedical health workers in developing countries [2, 4]. Côte d'Ivoire is now planning to implement a national cervical cancer screening program and the screening technic as well as the entry point to screen a maximum of women that are questions of interest.

In order to propose solutions to national cancer control program, we assess the willingness to participate in a screening program among women working in a health insurance company and the diagnostic accuracy of visual inspection as screening method in Côte d'Ivoire (West Africa).

2. Method

2.1. Study Design. A cross-sectional survey was conducted among women working in health insurance companies from January to December 2010.

2.2. Study Population. During this period, cervical screening by VIA and VILI was proposed to all the 800 identified women working in health insurance companies in Abidjan.

2.3. Visual Inspection with Acetic Acid (VIA). VIA was done with 5% freshly prepared dilute acetic acid. The color changes were observed one minute after the application of the acetic acid. The results of the VIA were recorded as suspect cancer, positive (for acetic white lesion at the squamocolumnar junction), negative (no acetowhite lesion), or squamocolumnar junction not visible.

2.4. Visual Inspection with Lugol's Iodine. Following VIA, visual inspection with Lugol's iodine (VILI) was also performed. A positive VILI test was characterized by a dense, thick, bright, mustard-yellow, or saffron-yellow iodine non-uptake area seen in the transformation zone.

Results of VIA and VILI were both classified as negative, positive, or indicative only of ICC according to the WHO Guidelines for Screening and Treatment of Precancerous Lesions [5].

2.5. Colposcopy. Patients who were positive at either of the screening tests underwent a colposcopy exam. Cervical biopsy was performed to positives women. Histopathological findings were categorized into five classes: normal or non-neoplastic changes, cervical intraepithelial neoplasia grade 1 (CIN1) including HPV changes, CIN2, CIN3, and ICC (invasive cervical cancer).

2.6. Data Collection and Analysis. A structured survey form was used to collect data on the willingness to participate and the results of screening when it was performed. The analysis was performed using Epi info software, and qualitative variables were presented in rough values and in percentage while quantitative variables were presented in means and standard deviation.

2.7. Patient's Outcomes. When visual inspection was negative, the patient was reassured and called for a new test within a period of 3 years. For CIN2/3 lesions (cervical intraepithelial neoplasia grade 2/3) a cryotherapy or a loop electrosurgical excision (LEE) procedure was performed the same day or delayed for 24 hours. CIN1 benefited from annual monitoring, and ICCs were treated by Wertheim's hysterectomy when the patient agreed.

2.8. Ethical Statements. This study was approved by the Ethics Committee of the University Hospital of Yopougon, and all the participants gave a written consent before being included in the study.

TABLE 1: Demographic characteristics of participants of the screening.

	Frequency (n)	Percentage (%)
Age (years)		
20–29	69	6.6
30–39	266	25.8
40–49	216	20.9
≥50	90	8.7
Parity		
0–2 (pauciparous)	236	22.9
3-4 (multiparous)	331	51.7
5 (high multiparous)	73	7.1
Polygamy		
Yes	77	12.0
No	401	62.7
Does not know	125	19.5
Separate	37	5.8
Delay screening		
0–3 years	66	10.3
3 years	71	11.1
Never detected	503	78.6

3. Results

3.1. Demographics Characteristics. Among the 800 women identified in health insurance companies, 640 (80%) accepted to participate in the study and to have a cervical cancer screening by visual inspection.

The median age of the participant was 39 [21–59] years, 603 (94.2%) were married, and 12.0% were in a polygamist couple. The average number of childbirth per woman was 2.2 and 28.2% of women had already a cervical cancer screening (Table 1).

3.2. Results of Cervical Cancer Screening. Among the 640 women tested, VIA remains positive in 5.9% of cases while VILI was positive in 8.6% and colposcopy was abnormal in 9.3%. VIA showed 72.9% sensitivity and 95.2% specificity, while VILI showed 71.2% and 97.3%, respectively (Table 2). Histological examination of biopsy showed non-specific chronic cervicitis in 4.6% (26 cases), CIN1 (5.9%), and CIN2/3 lesions: 1.2% (Table 3).

4. Discussion

This study reports the results of a cervical cancer screening among 640 women working in health insurance companies. Globally the willingness to participate was 80%, and less than 10% of the tests performed remain abnormal, principally due to nonspecific chronic cervicitis and CIN1.

Most of the participants were aged 30 to 49 years and the youngest was 21 years old. In Côte d'Ivoire, like in many other African countries there is no recommendation concerning the beginning age for cervical cancer screening. In France, the High Authority for Health (HAS) recommends starting pap smear at 25 years because of the high proportion of transient HPV infections, while the American Gynecologist Association leans toward a first smear at 21 years

Table 2: Diagnostic performances of visual inspection.

	Sensitivity (%)	Specificity (%)
VIA (visual inspection with acetic acid)	72.9	95.2
VILI (visual inspection with Lugol's iodine)	71.2	97.3

Table 3: Histological results.

Lesions	Frequency (n)	Percentage (%)
Nonspecific chronic cervicitis	26	4.6
CIN1	33	5.9
CIN2/3	7	1.2
Total	66	11.7

(or 3 years after first sexual intercourse) based therefore on a period of 36 months to see lesions CIN3 [6, 7]. All gynecologist societies agree that performing cervical cancer screening on teenager age 21 leads to anxiety, increased costs, and inappropriate treatments [8, 9].

Furthermore, we investigated the determinants of cervical cancer in our population. Regarding obstetric history, participants were pauciparous in 22.9% of cases like Blumenthal found in Ghana [1]. However in Cameroon in a rural area, Tebeu et al. [10] reported an average rate of 5.6 children during a one-time screening campaign. It is established that the multiparous and the precocity of sexual intercourse are risk factors for cervical cancer [11]. But in our study, there were mainly young, active, and literate pauciparous women who participated in the screening program. Moreover, 7.5% of women were involved in a polygamist couple, and this factor is often underestimated because there is a form of polygamy not formalized in most African countries. In Thailand, Cameroon, and Ghana, the partner was widely polygamist [1, 6, 10] with at least two sexual partners.

In our survey only 21.4% of women had performed a cervical cancer screening prior to the study with a delay of several years. This is related to the absence of national policies for early detection of cervical neoplasia. So far only a few hospitals offer cervical cancer screening by visual inspection. However an extensive provincial health workers training program is underway for cervical screening and treatment of cervical lesions.

4.1. Coverage Rates.
Women's participation was 80%, and it is the minimum threshold for cervical cancer screening to impact on cervical cancer mortality. This result seems to be unsatisfactory considering the awareness campaign, before the study, and can predict the low interest in the general population.

4.2. Performance of Visual Inspection.
Our study showed a positive VIA in 5.8% and 8.6% for the VILI. In Angola, Muwonge [9] did the same study on a population of 8851 women. The VIA and VILI were, respectively, positive in 6.6% and 5.2% of the cases. In Ghana, the test was positive in 13.2% of women [1]. The figures of precancerous lesions vary across the authors around 10%.

The sensitivity of the VIA was 72.9% and its specificity was 95.2% in our survey. These values are close to those found by many authors [1, 4, 12–14]. Acetic acid is cheaper and available while Lugol's iodine is more expensive. Because of the limited resources, some countries such as Ghana, Angola, China, and India fail to realize combined screening with acetic acid and Lugol's iodine. Thus they showed that VIA alone is sufficient for the detection of cervical precancerous lesions. Its sensitivity and specificity vary, respectively, between 66 and 96% and 64 and 98% according to Basu et al. and JHPIEGO (Johns Hopkins Program for International Education in Gynecology and Obstetrics) [15]. Several authors have conducted surveys in low resource countries, performing visual inspection with acetic acid compared to cytology.

Arbyn et al. [13] realized multicentric studies in a low setting population in 2008 using only acetic acid for cervical screening. They noted 79% for sensibility and 85% for specificity.

Fifteen studies in total were reviewed by Gafirikin et al. [14]; they reported sensitivity ranged between 66% and 96% and specificity between 64% and 98%. Finally, they suggested that VIA has the potential to be a cervical cancer screening tool, especially in low resource settings. Besides, Basu et al. [15] presented a comparison between VIA and cytology. The sensitivity of VIA to detect CIN 2-3 lesions was 55.7%, and the specificity was 82.1%. The sensitivity and specificity of cytology were 29.5% and 92.3%, respectively. Ardahan and Temel [16] in Turkey reported 85.29% sensitivity and 68.75% specificity when comparing colposcopy and VIA.

Furthermore we observed for VILI 71.2% sensitivity and a specificity of 97.3%. These results are consistent with others found in the literature, showing the superiority of Lugol's compared to acetic acid [2, 7]. However, using Lugol's is still challenging due to its cost and accessibility. In some remote parts of India repeated shortages have imposed the single use of acetic acid [4].

Regarding treatment, according to WHO recommendations cryotherapy should be used for CIN1 and conization or LEE for CIN2/3 [4, 16]. Treatment of CIN2 by LEE is still discussed due to obstetric complications when these lesions are found in young women between 25 and 35 years [6, 7, 17]. The authors argue that the risk of cancer is very low in this age group where CIN is frequent. Monitoring is recommended, but the treatment is acceptable. We systematically treated lesions due to strong possibility of being lost to follow-up (36% in a similar study in an HIV clinic) [18].

5. Conclusion

Cervical cancer screening by visual inspection showed appropriate diagnostic accuracy when used to detect early cervical lesions. It is a simple and easy to perform method that could be introduced progressively in the health insurance policy while waiting for a national screening program.

Conflict of Interests

The authors declare that there is no conflict of interests regarding the publication of this paper.

References

[1] P. D. Blumenthal, L. Gaffikin, S. Deganus, R. Lewis, M. Emerson, and S. Adadevoh, "Cervical cancer prevention: safety, acceptability, and feasibility of a single-visit approach in Accra, Ghana," *American Journal of Obstetrics and Gynecology*, vol. 196, no. 4, pp. 407.e1–407.e9, 2007.

[2] R. Sankaranarayanan and R. S. Wesley, "Guide pratique pour le dépistage visuel des néoplasies cervicales," Publication Technique du Centre International de Recherche sur le Cancer Lyon 41, CIRC, Lyon, France, 2004.

[3] K. Seni, A. Horo, M. Diakité, G. Quenum, and M. Fanny, "Evaluation de la prise en charge du cancer invasif du col de l'utérus au CHU de Yopougon (Abidjan) de 1991–2002," *Annals of the SOGGO*, vol. 7, no. 18, pp. 37–41, 2012.

[4] L. Gaffikin, P. D. Blumenthal, M. Emerson, and K. Limpaphayom, "Safety, acceptability, and feasibility of a single-visit approach to cervical-cancer prevention in rural Thailand: a demonstration project," *The lancet*, vol. 361, pp. 814–820, 2003.

[5] World Health Organization, *WHO Guidelines for Screening and Treatment of Precancerous Lesions for Cervical Cancer Prevention*, World Health Organization, Geneva, Switzerland, 2013.

[6] M. C. Voltzenlogel, J. P. Harlicot, J. Coiffic, E. Bauville, F. Foucher, and J. Levêque, "Quand faut-il commencer le dépistage du cancer du col utérin?" in *Mises à jour en gynécologie médicale*, J. Lansac, D. Luton, and E. Daraï, Eds., pp. 539–554, Collège National des Gynécologues et Obstétriciens Français (CNGOF), Paris, France, 2009.

[7] R. P. Insinga, A. G. Glass, and B. B. Rush, "Diagnoses and outcomes in cervical cancer screening: a population-based study," *American Journal of Obstetrics and Gynecology*, vol. 191, no. 1, pp. 105–113, 2004.

[8] T. S. Pandey, "Age appropriate screening for cancer: evidence-based practice in the United States of America," *Journal of Postgraduate Medicine*, vol. 60, no. 3, pp. 318–321, 2014.

[9] Haute Autorité de Santé (HAS), *État des Lieux et Recommandations pour le Dépistage du Cancer du Col de l'Utérus en France*, edited by: S. R. L. Mozzon, Haute Autorité de Santé (HAS), Florence, Italie, 2010.

[10] P. M. Tebeu, I. Sandjong, N. Nkele et al., "Lésions précancéreuses du col utérin en zone rurale: etude transversale," *Medicine d'Afrique Noire*, vol. 52, no. 1, pp. 27–31, 2005.

[11] M. Touré, I. Adoubi, C. J. Didi-kouko, A. Toowlis, and K. A. Echimane, "Aspects épidémiologiques, anatomocliniques et thérapeutiques du cancer du col dans le service de cancérologie du CHU de Treichville à Abidjan," *Médecine d'Afrique Noire*, no. 5810, pp. 474–478, 2011.

[12] R. Muwonge, M. D. G. Manuel, A. P. Filipe, J. B. Dumas, M. R. Frank, and R. Sankaranarayanan, "Visual screening for early detection of cervical neoplasia in Angola," *International Journal of Gynecology and Obstetrics*, vol. 111, no. 1, pp. 68–72, 2010.

[13] M. Arbyn, R. Sankaranarayanan, R. Muwonge et al., "Pooled analysis of the accuracy of five cervical cancer screening tests assessed in eleven studies in Africa and India," *International Journal of Cancer*, vol. 123, no. 1, pp. 153–160, 2008.

[14] L. Gafirikin, M. Lauterbach, and P. D. Blumenthal, "Performance of visual inspection with acetic acid for cervical cancer screening: a qualitative summary of evidence to date," *Obstetrical and Gynecological Survey*, vol. 58, no. 8, pp. 543–550, 2003.

[15] P. S. Basu, R. Sankaranarayanan, R. Mandal et al., "Visual inspection with acetic acid and cytology in the early detection of cervical neoplasia in Kolkata, India," *International Journal of Gynecological Cancer*, vol. 13, no. 5, pp. 626–632, 2003.

[16] M. Ardahan and A. B. Temel, "Visual inspection with acetic acid in cervical cancer screening," *Cancer Nursing*, vol. 34, no. 2, pp. 158–163, 2011.

[17] Y. Z. Zhang, J. F. Ma, F. H. Zhao et al., "Three-year follow-up results of visual inspection with acetic acid/Lugol's iodine (VIA/VILI) used as an alternative screening method for cervical cancer in rural areas," *Chinese Journal of Cancer*, vol. 29, no. 1, pp. 4–8, 2010.

[18] A. Horo, A. Jaquet, D. K. Ekouevi et al., "Cervical cancer screening by visual inspection in Côte d'Ivoire, operational and clinical aspects according to HIV status," *BMC Public Health*, vol. 12, article 237, 2012.

29

The Extracellular Matrix Contributes to Mechanotransduction in Uterine Fibroids

Phyllis C. Leppert,[1] Friederike L. Jayes,[1] and James H. Segars[2]

[1] Duke University School of Medicine, Durham, NC 27710, USA
[2] Unit on Reproductive Endocrinology and Infertility, Program on Pediatric and Adult Endocrinology, NICHD, NIH, Bethesda, MD 20892-1109, USA

Correspondence should be addressed to Phyllis C. Leppert; phyllis.leppert@duke.edu

Academic Editor: Peter E. Schwartz

The role of the extracellular matrix (ECM) and mechanotransduction as an important signaling factor in the human uterus is just beginning to be appreciated. The ECM is not only the substance that surrounds cells, but ECM stiffness will either compress cells or stretch them resulting in signals converted into chemical changes within the cell, depending on the amount of collagen, cross-linking, and hydration, as well as other ECM components. In this review we present evidence that the stiffness of fibroid tissue has a direct effect on the growth of the tumor through the induction of fibrosis. Fibrosis has two characteristics: (1) resistance to apoptosis leading to the persistence of cells and (2) secretion of collagen and other components of the ECM such a proteoglycans by those cells leading to abundant disposition of highly cross-linked, disoriented, and often widely dispersed collagen fibrils. Fibrosis affects cell growth by mechanotransduction, the dynamic signaling system whereby mechanical forces initiate chemical signaling in cells. Data indicate that the structurally disordered and abnormally formed ECM of uterine fibroids contributes to fibroid formation and growth. An appreciation of the critical role of ECM stiffness to fibroid growth may lead to new strategies for treatment of this common disease.

1. Introduction

Uterine fibroids are firm, stiff nodular tumors, a fact understood by all clinicians and confirmed by biomechanical studies (as discussed in [1–3]). The proteins of the extracellular matrix (ECM), particularly the interstitial collagens are responsible for this property of "firmness" and for the mechanical strength of the tissue. In biomechanical terms this property is referred to as stiffness. Fibroids feature an accumulation of altered collagen and differing amounts of glycosaminoglycans along with proliferation of cells, which is by definition fibrosis. A complete understanding of the role of the ECM proteins, especially collagen, and their effect on growth and development of fibroids must take into account the process of mechanotransduction, a dynamic system whereby mechanical forces initiate chemical signaling within cells. This bidirectional process is promoted by the stiffness of the ECM and initiates cell-matrix interactions in a progressive, ever changing process leading to activation of signaling cascades. While soluble signaling molecules have long been recognized as important factors in fibroid growth, development, differentiation, and function, mechanical signaling has only more recently been shown to play a critical role.

Here we focus on the ECM and the properties of cell and tissue *stiffness* that lead to signal transduction and then review current knowledge regarding the ECM of uterine fibroids. This information is placed in the context of the modern appreciation of how the ECM functions in other tissues and organs and the contemporary understanding of mechanotransduction. It is universally accepted that a myriad of chemical signaling molecules has been identified in fibroids and that reproductive tract hormones regulate the complex systems leading to fibroid development and growth. These chemical and hormonal signals are part of the biological mechanism of the development of these tumors, but these signals alone do not fully account for fibroid development and growth. We provide evidence in this review to suggest that mechanical force contributes to the triggering of these signaling pathways and plays a major role in the pathobiology of uterine fibroids.

2. Mechanotransduction: A Mechanism of Disease

Individual cells are capable of translating mechanical stimuli such as stretch or compression from their environment into biochemical signals through a complex system of cytoskeletal ECM receptors and transmembrane molecules that interconnect with integrin subunits and cell surface proteoglycans (as discussed in [4]). The highly dynamic mechanotransduction process is defined as cooperative signaling between the cell and the ECM. It has been suggested that this mechanotransduction system would be able to transfer signals through the entire cell and therefore would be more rapid than the diffusion based system (discussed in [4]). In response to mechanical force in living tissue there is a reciprocal or "back and forth" activity where extracellular remodeling, rapid transient cell-cell, and cell-matrix interactions all have essential functions (as discussed in [5, 6]). This interaction occurs between one cell and its extracellular matrix as well as between many cells and the matrix within tissues. Mechanical force is an upstream signal and will initiate physiological processes such as those in development and disease states. Recent studies show that ECM collagen provides a dynamic role in the breast cell microenvironment and is actually active in the promotion of tumor progression (as discussed by [7]). Increased ECM stiffness generated by collagen regulates breast epithelial signaling through integrin activation of β-catenin and MYC (a transcription factor persistently expressed in cancers, so named because it is similar to the myelocytomatosis viral oncogene) to activate the microRNA-18a expression that drives breast tumor progression (as discussed by [8]). This tumor progression is induced by MiRna reduction of tumor suppressor phosphatase and tensin homolog (PTEN) by the reduction of homoebox A9 (HOXA9) (as discussed by [8]). Mechanotransduction can be altered by mutations in downstream signaling cascades. Abnormal mechanical signaling as a result of modifications in these interactions or cellular sensitivity to mechanical stress contributes to disease development (as discussed in [6]). The molecules in the cell-ECM network appear to be linked mechanically from the ECM to the cytoskeleton (Figure 1). Intriguingly, recent work has indicated a system linked from the ECM through the cytoskeleton to the nucleus (as reported in [9]).

While the cell's membrane receptors, especially integrins, allow the transmission of mechanical signals across the cell surface, change in the ECM structure and the amount within the microenvironment are the sources of the mechanical forces. This dynamic relationship is noted in the disease process of fibrosis. The formation of fibrosis correlates with new collagen deposition and TGF-beta-induced myofibroblast differentiation, as well as elastin gene expression, WNT-1

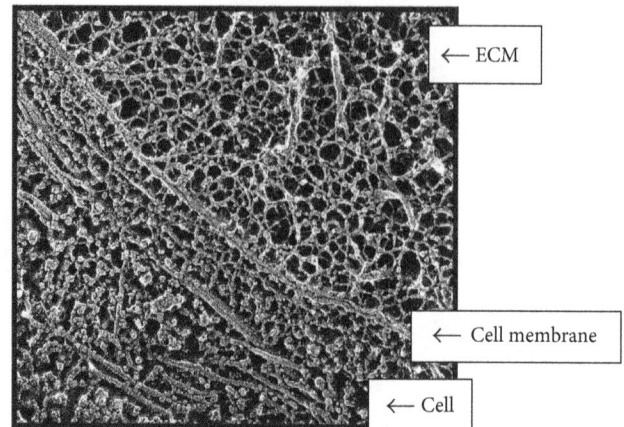

FIGURE 1: Interconnected structural components of cells and ECM. Quick freeze, deep etch electron micrograph of a fetal ear cartilage chondrocyte cell to illustrate the integration of structures inside and outside the cell. The ECM (containing a meshwork of proteoglycans, collagen, fibronectin, and laminin), the cell membrane (integrins receptors), and the cell (containing microtubules) are visualized. In the ECM the thinnest fibrils in the meshwork are $4 \pm I$ nm and are presumed to be proteoglycans. The larger thicker fibrils are collagen. Micrograph courtesy of Robert Mecham and John Heuser, Washington University, St. Louis, MO, USA. This figure illustrates that mechanical forces can be transmitted across the cell surface and into the cell by means of interconnected structural components (as discussed in [4]).

inducible signaling pathway protein-1, lysyl oxidase, and type V collagen gene expression (as discussed in [10]). In addition there is often the accumulation of glycosaminoglycans as well as resistance to apoptosis in fibrotic tissue (discussed in [11] and references therein). Fibrosis occurs when there is a hyperproduction of collagen and lack of appropriate remodeling and degradation. The increased accumulation of the ECM observed in fibrotic tissue causes stiffness in the microenvironment of the individual cells in tissues and organs and contributes to mechanotransduction (as discussed in [4, 8]). While the individual cell contributes in this dynamic process and changes within it cause signals to the ECM, this review is focused on the ECM and its functions. As the ECM accumulates additional mechanical force is produced by the ECM. To complete the picture, the role of extracellular fluid (ECF) in the generation of intrinsic mechanical force is now accepted (as discussed in [11]). Conformational changes in proteins that are mechanosensitive are sensed by the cells and open membrane channels, alter binding affinities, and increase phosphorylation thus activating downstream signaling pathways. Although the specific pathways of mechanotransduction have not been completely elucidated in uterine myometrial or fibroid cells, it is reasonable to suggest that mechanical signaling pathways exist in these cells as they do in the cells of tissues studied so far.

The ECM is able to initiate the mechanotransduction process and actually serves as a reservoir for matricellular proteins, growth factors, and cytokines. Often, activation of these factors occurs in the ECM. For example, TGF is activated in the ECM by a very complex mechanism.

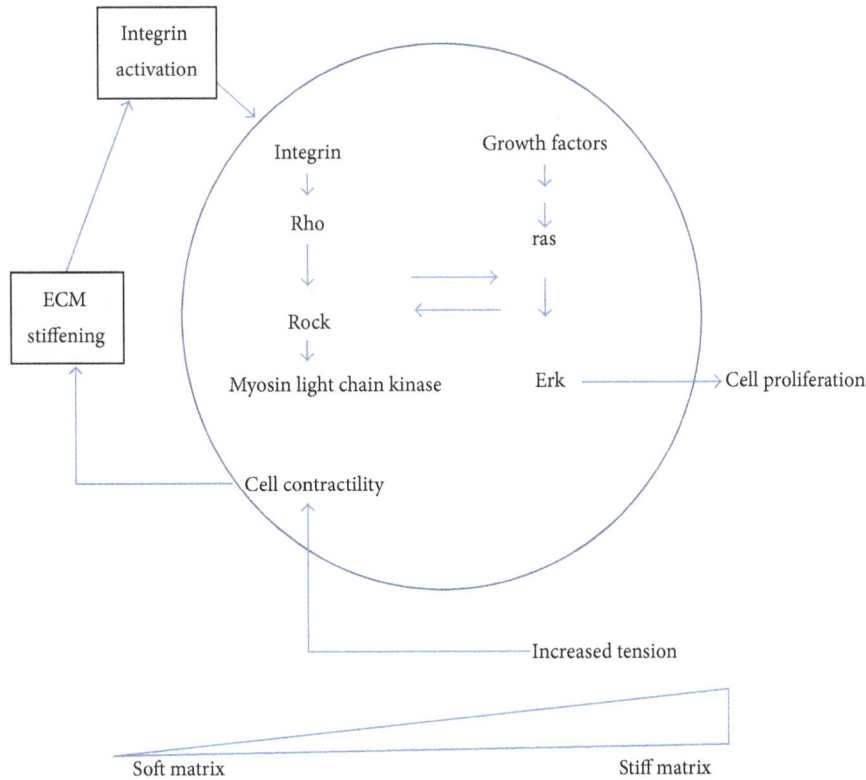

FIGURE 2: Elements of mechanical signaling. A simplified pathway of mechanical signaling in cells is depicted. As the cell cytoskeleton contracts (a process called cell contractility) and ECM accumulates in the cell microenvironment, integrin activation occurs leading to activation of Rho (as discussed in [1]). Rho in turn activates ROCK leading to activation of ras. In fibroid cells obtained either at the time of hysterectomy or myomectomy, RhoA activity is attenuated. This adaptation of the fibroid cell is not ROCK dependent (as discussed in [2]). These findings suggest that fibroid cells in symptomatic tumors where treatment was needed are fundamentally adapted to their stiff microenvironment and thus become insensitive to moderate mechanical cues. It is not certain when in the natural history of fibroid development that this adaptive response to mechanotransduction occurs. Nevertheless, mechanical sensing does occur in fibroid cells.

The ECM is able to transmit physical and chemical signals to the cell membrane leading to signal propagation and amplification via a multiplex array of intracellular signals. Specifically, the Rho/ROCK/MAPK signaling pathway is one important pathway in mechanotransduction (Figure 2). RhoA belongs to a family of small GTP-binding proteins. Both RhoA and Rho-kinase (ROCK), a downstream target of Rho, are involved in the regulation of a wide variety of cellular processes, including changes in cell motility and morphology, focal adhesion formation, and light chain phosphorylation (as discussed in [12]). An important concept is that reciprocity is an indispensable quality of mechanosensitive cells. Cells respond to biophysical and biochemical cues from the ECM, but cells also help maintain and remodel the ECM through secretion of various ECM components and the molecules that degrade the ECM. Thus, ECM remodeling will produce a matrix that can be either flexible or stiff depending on protein cross-links, content of glycoproteins, hydration, and other components of the ECM.

Mechanotransduction has long been viewed as a mechanism of disease (as discussed in [13]).

Mechanical signaling has been well described in dermal wounds and has also been studied in other tissues such as blood vessels, stem cells, respiratory epithelium, and musculoskeletal tissues. Notably, the reproductive system is dynamic and constantly undergoes extensive structural remodeling throughout each reproductive cycle—featuring a remarkable plasticity of the ECM. This remodeling is achieved, in part, by changes in the ECM, which are regulated by cyclic hormonal cues as well as cytokines and growth factors. Mechanotransduction is highly reciprocal and involves extensive bidirectional signals from the ECM to and from the cell (as presented and discussed in [14]).

3. Extracellular Matrix in the Human Uterus

Appreciation of the complexities of the ECM is essential to the understanding of the fibrotic process and its role in mechanotransduction in the human uterus. The uterine myometrium consists mainly of smooth muscle cells that stain positive for α smooth muscle actin and desmin and are interspersed with interstitial collagens. These collagens are large rigid molecules that are responsible for the mechanical strength of uterine tissue as well as all other tissues in the body. Histological examination demonstrates a basketweave pattern of the smooth muscle cells and the interstitial collagens (as discussed in [15, 16]). Notably, myometrium is a complex tissue and heterogeneous in the proportion of tissue stained by Masson Trichrome, a collagen stain (as discussed in [17]). Trichrome staining of tissue, however, will not differentiate between the numerous types of human interstitial collagens. At the ultrastructural level the interstitial collagen fibrils are observed in parallel to the smooth muscle cells, a feature which allows the uterus to maintain its strength as it expands during pregnancy (as discussed in [18]). The collagen superfamily of proteins is complex in molecular organization and is distributed widely in tissues and diverse in function (as discussed by [19]). Twenty-nine types of collagens encoded by numerous genes located on different chromosomes are known in humans.

The predominate collagens found in the interstitial areas of the myometrium are Type I, Type III, and Type V, although types IV and VI are also present in the uterus (as discussed in [20–24]). Type IV collagen is membrane collagen, arrayed as a meshwork (as discussed in [25]). All collagens have three polypeptide chains and have tandem repeated Gly-Xaa-Yaa sequences, where X is proline and Y is hydroxyproline. These peptide chains are able to assemble into stable triple helical structures. Glycine is the smallest amino acid and its location in the collagen molecule allows for a tightly coiled helix as glycine is easily "packed" into the center of the assembled helix. The hydroxyprolines are located on the outside of the triple helix stabilizing the molecule. Three alpha chains make up a collagen molecule. As examples, Type I, the most abundant collagen type in the human body is made up of chains encoded by the genes COL1A1 and COL1A2. COL1A1 gene produces the pro-alpha 1 (I) chain and the COL1A2 gene produces the pro-alpha 2(I) chain. Two pro-alpha 1 chains and one pro-alpha 2 chain form type 1 procollagen. Type III collagen consists of three alpha 1(III) chains encoded by COL3A1. Type IV collagen consists of two alpha 1 IV chains and one alpha 2 IV chain and is the type of collagen found in membranes, blood vessels, and nerves (as discussed in [26]).

The biosynthesis of collagen is complicated. Therefore, gene expression studies alone do not reflect the abundance of native, cross-linked collagen in tissue. In general, collagen synthesis includes extensive co- and posttranslational modifications that stabilize the helix and assist with higher order molecular assembly (shown below) (as discussed in [26]).

Synthesis of Type I Collagen: An Interstitial Collagen.

(1) COL1A1 gene → pro-alpha1 (I) chain,
    COL1A2 gene → pro-alpha2 (I) chain,

(2) in ER → preprocollagen,

(3) ER Lumen → signal peptides cleaved; proline and lysine hydroxylation, 2 pro-alpha1 and 1 pro-alpha2 chains → Type I procollagen, triple helix formed →

(4) in Golgi packaged and secreted →

(5) outside cell propeptides cleaved → tropocollagen

    fibrils formed,

(6) lysyl oxidase creates intramolecular and intermolecular cross-links.

In the above list synthesis of Type I collagen is described. Other interstitial collagens, such as Type III and Type V, are synthesized in a similar manner.

Briefly, the genes are transcribed and their mRNAs are processed similarly to other molecules. Then the peptide chains are translated in the rough endoplasmic reticulum (RER). These peptide chains are known as preprocollagen and have a signal peptide and propeptides on each end. The signal peptide is cleaved to form pro-alpha chains. In the lumen of the RER, hydroxylation of the proline and lysine amino acids occurs, a step dependent on ascorbic acid (vitamin C) (as discussed in [26]). Specific hydroxylysine residues are glycosylated and the triple helical structure as noted is formed from two alpha-1 chains and one alpha-2 chain. This assembly is assisted by disulfide bonding between the chains (as discussed in [27]). The procollagen molecule has an N-terminal propeptide, the central helix, and a C-propeptide region (as discussed in [28]). This tight triple helix ensures that this part of the molecule is inaccessible to modifying enzymes and the propeptides prevent fibril formation inside the cell. Next, the procollagen moves to the Golgi where it is packaged and secreted (as discussed in [26]).

Once outside the cell, the collagen propeptides are cleaved in the extracellular space and tropocollagen is formed by the enzymatic action of procollagen peptidase (as discussed in [29]). In the case of Types I and III collagens, the tropocollagen molecules spontaneously form fibrils by the alignment of charged and hydrophobic amino acid clusters (as discussed in [30]). These fibrils are laid down in a staggered fashion such that a d-band of alternating regions of protein density in the fibril produces a characteristic gap and overlap appearance of negatively contrasted fibrils observed in transmission electron microscopy (as discussed in [31]). Finally in the extracellular space copper-dependent lysyl oxidase (LOX) enzymatically creates the intramolecular and intermolecular cross-links that form the mature collagen fibrils (as discussed in [32, 33]). These covalent cross-links are di-, tri-, and tetrafunctional and further stabilize the collagen helix (as discussed in [34]). The more lysine derived cross-links in collagenous tissue, the stiffer the tissue. In some tissues Type I and Type III collagen molecules are present within the same collagen fibril, covalently bound between the N-terminal regions (as discussed in [35]). In liver fibrosis Types I and III collagens colocalize in collagen fibers (as discussed in [36]) and while this has not been studied in the uterine fibrosis this type of fiber could be a possibility in that situation. However, in most tissues the collagen fibrils consist of all Type I collagen molecules or all Type III collagen molecules with tissues characterized by specific Type I/Type III ratios. In pathological situations cells are capable of altering this ratio. For instance, in healing wounds there is an increase in Type III collagen and in some situations an increase in Type V collagen as well.

Other major components of the uterine ECM are proteoglycans which are glycoproteins that contain a core protein with covalently attached high negatively charged glycosaminoglycan (GAG) side chains. GAGs are sulfated polysaccharides that contain repeating disaccharides (as discussed in [26]). There is one exception and that is hyaluronic acid. It is not attached to a protein core and it is not sulfated (as discussed in [26, 37]). The disaccharides are unique to each proteoglycan. Glucuronic acid-N-acetylgalactosamines are components of chondroitin sulfate; iduronic acid-N-acetylgalactosamines are units of dermatan sulfate; heparin contains glucuronic acid-N-acetylglucosamines and heparan sulfate contains glucuronic acid-N-acetylglucosamines. Keratan sulfate is the one glycosaminoglycan that does not contain uronic acid; it contains N-acetylglucosamine-galactose (as discussed in [26]). Proteoglycan synthesis begins with the core protein which is then modified in the RER. After this monosaccharides and sulfate, the building blocks for the GAGs are taken up by the cell through specialized transporters in the plasma membrane (as discussed in [36]). These molecules are activated in the cytosol to form UDP-sugars and $5'$-phosphosulfate (PAPS) and transported to the Golgi (as discussed in [37]). In the Golgi, the monosaccharides (xylosyl-, galactosyl-galactosyl-uronic acid) and the linker tetrasaccharide are attached to the core protein at selected serine residues, and additional disaccharides are attached to the proteoglycan. The addition of a fifth saccharide then determines if the GAG chain will become chondroitin sulfate, dermatan sulfate, or heparan sulfate or heparin (as discussed in [37]). Heparan sulfate and heparin undergo even more complex modification. When polymerization is finished, O-sulfation occurs. This modification is different depending on the proteoglycan (as discussed in [37]). Proteoglycans attract cations and bind water enabling tissues to accommodate to pressure changes. Proteoglycans also play important roles in the control of cell growth and differentiation. The small dermatan sulfate proteoglycan decorin, a member of the small leucine-rich repeat class of proteins (SLRP) through its interaction with collagen, may aid in the adaption of tissue to increased mechanical loads (force) (as discussed in [38]). Decorin interacts with specific regions of the collagen fibrils and regulates their formation (as discussed by [39–42]). Decorin and collagen colocalize in both myometrium and fibroids indicating this interaction may be present in the uterus (as discussed in [43]). Larger and longer GAGs of the side chains on the decorin molecule most likely exert higher osmotic pressure and thus affect both ECM organization and matrix-cell interaction. Decorin has been studied in the uterine cervix and appears to have a role in the cervical changes of gestation and parturition by interaction with collagen fibers (as discussed by [44–46]). Hyaluronan becomes dominant at term cervix in mice and women and contributes to the loss of tensile strength of the cervix during parturition (as discussed in [47, 48]). Hyalectans, another family of ECM proteoglycans, interact with hyaluronic acid and are very important in the regulation of water retention and distribution in tissue. One member of this family is versican, a protein glycosylated with galactosaminoglycan side chains and which is increased in tumors compared to normal tissue (as discussed in [49, 50]).

In addition to collagen and glycosaminoglycans, elastin, a hydrophobic ECM protein is an important component of the uterus. Elastin is responsible for the ability of tissue to stretch and recoil and is a hydrophobic protein with a complex synthesis (as discussed in [51]). Elastin is found in the uterus

in fibrils and thin sheets from 0.1 to 0.4 microns in thickness that are capable of multidimensional stretch, in contrast to the elastin lamellae found in the aorta which are 1 to 2.5 microns in thickness and stretch in one dimension (as discussed in [52]). The uterine elastin is so thin that elastic fibers are often not seen in histological sections of nonpathological conditions (as discussed in [52]). During pregnancy, elastin allows the uterus to achieve its remarkable increase in size, to stretch, and to accommodate the growing fetus.

Mechanical force is transmitted across the cell membrane by integrins, transmembrane receptors expressed in all cells. These surface molecules are important in both cell to matrix (inside out) and ECM to cell signaling (outside in) and act as mechanosensors generating signals that affect cell physiology and pathology by complex mechanisms (as discussed in [53, 54]). Integrins are heterodimers consisting of an alpha subunit and a beta subunit and are involved in numerous processes such as adhesion, ECM organization, signaling, cell survival, proliferation, and in mechanotransduction (as discussed in [55]). Although there are multiple integrins that bind to many proteins, only those pertinent to this review are mentioned here. The references cited discuss many additional integrins and their functions. There are four collagen-binding integrins in the $\beta1$ subfamily, namely, $\alpha1\beta1$, $\alpha2\beta1$, $\alpha10\beta1$, and $\alpha11\beta1$ (as discussed in [53]). Three of these collagen binding integrins have been demonstrated to be present in fibroids as well as in the myometrium and in the cervix (as discussed in [56–59]). Integrins binding to fibronectin, $\alpha3\beta1$, $\alpha4\beta1$, $\alpha5\beta1$, $\alpha v\beta1$, and $\alpha v\beta3$ and to laminin, $\alpha1\beta1$, $\alpha3\beta1$, $\alpha6\beta1$, and $\alpha v\beta3$ are also expressed in myometrium (as described by [57]). The integrin subunit $\beta1$ is expressed in myometrium and in uterine fibroids (as discussed in [57, 60]). Fibronectin, an ECM molecule with multiple functions mediates the assembly of the matrix binding collagen, integrins, and other ECM molecules by undergoing a series of conformational changes that expose cryptic binding sites (as discussed in [61]). Mechanical forces are capable of inducing further conformational changes in fibronectin thus mediating multiple effects on ECM and cell and tissue functions (as discussed in [62]). Thus fibronectin is an organizer of matrix assembly (as discussed by [53, 60]).

The turnover and degradation of the ECM is also complex. Humans are considered to have 23, or as some suggest, up to 28 matrix metalloproteinases (MMPs) that degrade both matrix and nonmatrix proteins and are important in tissue repair and remodeling (as discussed in [63–65]). These enzymes break down cell-surface and ECM molecules that alter cell-matrix or cell-cell interactions and also release growth factors not related to the degradation of collagen or other matrix molecules including proteoglycans (as discussed in [64]). MMPs play roles also in cell migration, growth, differentiation, apoptosis, and inflammatory responses (as discussed in [65]). All MMPs utilize Zn^{2+} ion linked to their catalytic site to hydrolyze specific peptide substrates. After secretion MMPs must be activated by protein cleavage. For example, ProMMP-1 is activated by cleavage of its propeptide by MMP-3 (as discussed in [66]). MMP-1 binds to and locally unwinds the triple helix before it hydrolyses the collagen molecule into 2 fragments (as discussed in [67]). MMPs are

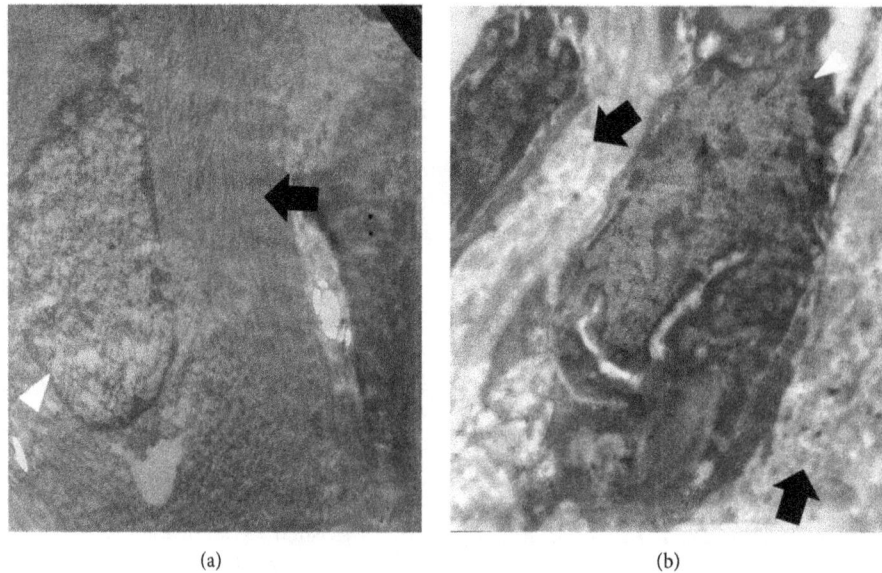

(a)   (b)

FIGURE 3: Collagen fibrils in myometrium and fibroids. Comparison of collagen fibril organization in the extracellular matrix of myometrium or uterine fibroid using electron microscopy. (a) Myometrium. Collagen fibrils are tightly packed and well-aligned, as shown by the black arrow. The nucleus is denoted by the white arrowhead. Magnification = 11,500x. (b) Fibroid. The collagen fibrils are randomly aligned and widely spaced, as shown by black arrows. The nucleus is notched and denoted by the white arrowhead. Magnification = 15,500x. Representative sections on samples harvested from a single uterus.

inhibited by tissue inhibitors of matrix metalloproteinases (TIMPs) and α_2-macroglobulin. Thus MMPs are regulated in several ways: during gene expression, by the need for activation of latent proenzymes and by being bound to inhibitory molecules. This equilibrium between activation and inhibition is delicate and results in situations where a particular signal may regulate an MMP in the direction of activation but will regulate another MMP by inhibition (as discussed by [68]). The regulation of TIMPs in some situations can be hormone-dependent (as discussed by [68]). Demonstration of the presence of MMP mRNA or protein in a particular tissue, however, does not prove how MMP is functioning in that tissue (as discussed by [64, 68]). Recent compelling studies demonstrate that vitamin D inhibits the nuclear factor-$\kappa\beta$ (NF-$\kappa\beta$) pathway directly regulating genes that contribute to cell proliferation, inflammation, fibrogenesis, increased oxidative stress, and decreased MMP-9 (as discussed by [69]). Experiments in rats showed that vitamin D reduced ECM deposition in induced liver fibrosis and lowered the fibrotic score in the animals (as discussed by [70]).

4. Extracellular Matrix of Uterine Fibroids

Compared to myometrium, in fibroids not only is the expression of collagen genes increased (as discussed by [71]), but also the amount of mature cross-linked collagen protein is increased and most importantly is altered (discussed in [18]) (Figure 3). The collagen fibrils are shorter and are disordered compared to normal myometrium (discussed by [18, 72]). Furthermore, the ratio of Type I/III collagen is altered. Several investigators demonstrated that Type V collagen, a type thought to be found in fibrotic tissue was a noticeable

component of fibroids (as discussed by [73, 74]). Studies have also shown that fibroids and myometrium possess different percentages of the glycosaminoglycans chondroitin sulfate and dermatan sulfate as there is 78% in myometrium and 95% in fibroids (as discussed in [75]). The main glycosaminoglycan is decorin whose presence correlates with fibroid size (as discussed in [76]) and as noted previously interacts with specific regions on the surface of the interstitial collagens and is involved in the organization and assembly of collagen fibrils. Interestingly, decorin exists in fibroids in a higher molecular weight form compared to normal myometrium, as it is glycosylated with longer dermatan sulfate side chains but has unaltered core proteins (as discussed by [55]). These modifications in decorin structure could increase osmotic pressure within the fibroid tissue. Distribution patterns of decorin and collagen were completely different in fibroids compared to normal myometrium when observed by immunofluorescence, and the ratio of decorin to Type I collagen was increased in fibroids (as discussed by [76]). These changes most likely affect the ECM organization of fibroids and would affect its stiffness.

Fibroids have increased fluid content relative to myometrium which could contribute to their mechanical properties and response to certain GnRH analogue therapies (as discussed by [77, 78]). One GnRH analogue, leuprolide acetate, will cause a regression of fibroid size; however, the tumors regrow rapidly after treatment is discontinued (as discussed by [79]). Since fibroids have a low mitotic index this regrowth is thought to be due to changes in the regulation of ECM component of the tumors rather than cell proliferation. A recent study demonstrated that leuprolide acetate may act directly on fibroids by an increase in the ECM genes, COL1A1, fibronectin, and veriscan variant 0, followed by return to normal after five days of treatment (as discussed by [80]). These findings were supported by the presence of GnRH receptors in uterine fibroid and subject-matched myometrium (as discussed by [81]). Similar to the concept of reciprocity for mechanical stress, hydration of the ECM requires an osmotic response regulated by the transcription factor, nuclear factor of activated T cells-5 (NFAT5) that coordinates expression of hyperosmolarity response genes, such as aldose reductase and sodium myoinositol transporter 1 (SMIT), all of which were increased in fibroid cells, compared to myometrial cells (as discussed by [82]). The contribution of hydration to the stiffness of fibroids was supported by viscoelastic measurements of fibroid tumors that took into account the contribution of water to ECM stiffness (as discussed by [2]).

Evidence is accumulating that it is the fibrotic process that contributes to the greater stiffness of fibroids compared to adjacent myometrium (as discussed in [1–3]). Fibrosis was detected by Masson Trichrome staining of collagen in uterine fibroids >1 cm. (as discussed by [83]). Fibrosis was found in 21% of 159 small "seedling" fibroids in premenopausal women and was increased to 50% in the same size tumors in postmenopausal women [84]. Substantial fibrosis, analyzed by morphometry, was noted in 23% of fibroids 2–4 mm in size, while 40% of the 5–9 mm tumors contained fibrotic tissue, a statistically significant increase. Cells were smaller in postmenopausal small fibroids compared to premenopausal fibroids matched within one degree of fibrosis or "fibrous degeneration" (as discussed in [83, 84]). Clearly, cells that could become larger uterine fibroids secreted collagen even before the fibroid was detected clinically. Interestingly, as early as 1983, investigators using electron microscopy observed cells in central regions of fibroids less than 3 mm in size that closely resembled myofibroblasts-cells capable of secreting collagen (as discussed in [85]).

Fibrosis has several components, namely, proliferation and persistence of cells due to resistance of apoptosis and the secretion of collagen by cells and the disposition of abundant highly cross-linked and disoriented collagen fibrils as well as the secretion of proteoglycans and other matrix components (as discussed in [6]). Not only a component of fibrosis is cell proliferation and the formation of new collagen and secretion of proteoglycans, but also an important part of the process is modification of cell proliferation and the correlation of a wide number of genes involved in ECM production including TGF induced myofibroblast differentiation (as discussed in [6]). The stiffness of the ECM that surrounds cells depends on the amount of cross-linking of the newly secreted altered collagen. We have found that LOX is over expressed in fibroids compared to myometrium (unpublished data) which suggests that collagen cross-linking is increased in fibroids. Thus, fibroids meet all of these characteristics of fibrosis. Although some pathologists have traditionally considered fibrosis to be a sign of fibroid senescence, the concept of mechanotransduction challenges this assumption. The changes in the surrounding ECM outlined in the preceding paragraphs would necessarily be accompanied by changes in the mechanical force exerted on resident fibroidal cells, thus leading to changes in cell signaling which

would either enhance or inhibit tumor growth, including ECM secretion. Since fibrotic tissue contains abundant collagen, a stiff protein, these findings underscore the role of mechanotransduction in fibroid growth. Even a small amount of increased collagen and other components of the ECM in a cells microenvironment could increase the mechanical force on individual cells and alter cell signaling. Thus, it is not the altered ECM constitution alone but ECM stiffness that has a direct effect on fibroid formation and growth.

Fibrosis is initiated by many triggers which injure a cell, such as extravasation of blood into tissues, oxidative stress, infection, and chronic inflammation. The exact trigger that initiates the fibrotic process in fibroids remains unclear. It is possible that there is not one trigger but several causes, acting either alone, or in concert. For example, resident uterine stem cells might be triggered to undergo altered morphogenesis featuring fibrosis and hypoxia may play a role. The clonality of uterine fibroids (as discussed by [86] and references therein) supports the hypothesis that fibroids arise from a stem-like cell. The nascent fibroid milieu is certainly hypoxic, due in large part to altered angiogenesis, and this observation suggests a role for oxidative stress as a likely trigger for fibroid development and growth (as reviewed in [87]) We and others (as discussed in [88]) have noted that hypoxia might trigger stem cell proliferation giving rise to fibroids. Thus, hypoxia appears to be one underlying pathophysiologic mechanism promoting development of fibroids and a genetic predisposition might be another. Altered expression of Frizzled-related protein 1 was detected on early microarray studies of fibroids (as discussed in [89]), and altered Wingless-type (WNT)/β-catenin signaling has recently been reported to promote growth of leiomyoma side-population cells (as discussed in [90]). Thus, current evidence suggests that a specialized myometrial side population of cells (as discussed in [88, 91]) is induced to embark on a fibrotic differentiation, a predilection that is very common. To our thinking, the underlying etiology may be due to the remarkable plasticity and capacity of the uterus to respond to pregnancy-related myometrial growth, with ECM stiffness playing a critical role in expansion of that cell population leading to fibroid growth.

Intriguingly, fibroids are more common than expected in myometrium, immediately adjacent to endometrium compared to other area of the uterus (as discussed in [92]). Thus, it is equally plausible that extravasation of menstrual blood into the myometrium with its accompanying cytokines and growth factors might cause cell injury leading to fibrosis. Consistent with a location-dependent trigger, fibroids are not observed in equal distribution throughout the uterus. Fibroids are more common in the fundus than in the corpus and isthmus and even less common in the cervix as reported by a detailed morphometric study (as discussed in [92]). It has been hypothesized that ECM stiffness may contribute to tumor development in other systems (as discussed in [93, 94]), most likely through the RhoA pathway (as discussed in [95, 96]). Several studies implicate a role for activation of the mammalian target of rapamycin (mTOR) in the pathogenesis of fibroids (as discussed in [97, 98]). Intriguingly, mechanical signaling through P13 K/AKT induces mTOR (as discussed in [99]). Thus, evidence from direct physical measurements, assessment of ECM structural organization, ECM constitution, microscopic analysis, and *in vitro* studies all support the critical role of ECM stiffness in fibroid growth.

5. New Directions for Fibroid Treatment

Given that uterine fibroids are primarily composed of an abnormally formed matrix, degradation of the ECM is critical for the resolution of the bulk symptoms caused by these tumors. Thus, the concept of mechanical signaling provides rationale for dissolution of the ECM as a treatment of fibroids. A change in mechanical force and signaling to myofibroblasts within the tumor would thus occur. In theory, the decreased force exerted against the cells would decrease signals that cause matrix deposition and then favor apoptosis of the fibroid cells. Consistent with this tenet, we found that degradation of uterine fibroid collagen by a bacterial (clostridium histolyticum) collagenase significantly reduced the tissue stiffness as measured by rheometry. This collagenase, first isolated over sixty years ago (as described by [100]), only degrades the interstitial collagens and it does not degrade Type IV collagen, the collagen found in blood vessels and nerves (discussed by [101]). Furthermore, this collagenase is inhibited by serum proteins (as discussed by [102]).

The altered mechanical properties of uterine fibroids provide support for the dissolution of ECM as a therapy. Fibroids occur in an environment of increased mechanical stress, but their response to the cues from this environment is paradoxically decreased (as discussed by [1, 2]). Myometrial cells reorient their actin cytoskeleton perpendicular to the axis of applied strain, but fibroid cells do not do so to the same degree (as discussed by [2]). Application of mechanical stress to fibroid cells *in vitro* led to diminished activation of RhoA, in contrast to myometrial cells, suggesting that myofibroblasts have an attenuated response to mechanical cues. Additionally, fibroid tumors exhibited increased stiffness in unconfined compression, compared to adjacent myometrium (discussed in [2]). Treatment of fibroid tissue with purified collagenase derived from clostridium demonstrated collagenolysis and reduced stiffness (as discussed in [3]), confirming the critical role of collagen in the ECM stiffness of fibroids. Likewise, the mechanisms of FUS (or HIFU) and uterine artery embolization (UAE/UFE) in reducing fibroid size are due to necrosis, which also decreases fibroid stiffness by destroying ECM-producing cells, either from heat degradation or coagulation necrosis, respectively.

In keeping with investigations of Vitamin D effects on the ECM in other tissues, a recent study found that Vitamin D inhibits the expression and activities of both MMP2 and MMP9 in fibroid cells (as discussed in [103]). The substrates for MMP2 are numerous and include gelatin; collagen Types I, IV, V, VII, and X; and fibronectin, lamin, aggrecan, tenascin C, and vitronectin, while those of MMP-9 include gelatin; collagen Types IV, V, and XVI; aggrecan; and elastin (as discussed by [104]). Thus low vitamin D serum levels might affect numerous ECM proteins and vitamin D therapy might reduce the fibrotic process in the uterus, similar to the reduction of fibrosis in other tissues. It is very provocative that evidence from epidemiology points to low serum vitamin D as a factor in fibroid formation (as discussed by [105]) and may be one mechanism leading to the differences in fibroid growth in African American compared to Caucasian women (as discussed in [106]). In this study, women with sufficient levels of serum vitamin D had an estimated 32% lower risk of having fibroids.

Uterine fibroids do not grow in a consistently linear pattern, an observation consistent with modulation of growth by an altered ECM. In the same woman, as documented by careful MRI studies, some fibroids grew over six months of time and others were static, while others tended to regress in size. This same clinical investigation reported that women of African American ancestry continued to increase the size of their fibroids after age 35 until menopause. However, women who were identified as white tended to have nongrowing tumors during those ages (as discussed by [107]). When the fibroid tissues of women in this study who underwent surgery were studied for gene expression, dermatopontin was consistently downregulated as reported by others (discussed by [72]). Rho and RAC genes involved in mechanotransduction were elevated in growing tumors. Furthermore it appeared that growing fibroids cells accumulated because there is an absence of cell death signals. These investigators stated that growth of the tumors was also due to the mass accumulation of ECM (discussed by [108]). Recently, *in vitro* studies have shown that fibroid smooth muscle cells grown on different (nonpolymerized versus polymerized) collagen matrices exhibit differences in cell morphology, proliferation, and signaling pathways (as discussed by [109]). Consistent with an increase in ECM stiffness, *in vivo* measurement of fibroid elastography revealed heterogeneity between fibroids and supported an increased stiffness in fibroids in six patients (as discussed by [110]). Collectively, these seminal investigations provide strong evidence for a role of ECM and mechanotransduction in the growth of uterine fibroids. The role of integrins as mechanosensors is important to explore more fully. An important question to be answered is how they are involved in the activation stage of the accumulation of altered ECM (as discussed in [111]). Additional studies are needed to quantify ECM stiffness in growing compared to regressing fibroids as such studies may provide a missing piece to the enigmatic puzzle of fibroid growth.

6. Summary

The ECM, especially the interstitial collagens, exert mechanical forces on surrounding cells leading to transmittal of mechanical signals on the cell surface and the initiation of chemical cascades. Uterine fibroids are composed of abundant interstitial collagens (I, III, and V) with fibrils that exhibit a disordered pattern that is increased in amount compared to the adjacent myometrium. Other ECM proteins, especially fibronectin, are also increased relative to myometrium. Proteoglycans especially decorin and versican play roles in the alterations of the ECM organization within fibroids and contribute to the mechanical forces as well and thus to altered mechanical sensing by the cells leading to enhanced accumulation of ECM proteins. The nonlinear growth of fibroids over time and the various patterns of growth and regression of fibroids in the same uterus suggest a local effect of the ECM on mechanical signaling. Therefore, to fully understand uterine fibroids and to elucidate new therapeutic modalities it is essential to investigate further mechanisms of the role the ECM in these common benign tumors.

Conflict of Interests

The authors declare that there is no conflict of interests regarding the publication of this paper.

References

[1] R. Rogers, J. Norian, M. Malik et al., "Mechanical homeostasis is altered in uterine leiomyoma," *The American Journal of Obstetrics and Gynecology*, vol. 198, no. 4, pp. 474.e1–474.e11, 2008.

[2] J. M. Norian, C. M. Owen, J. Taboas et al., "Characterization of tissue biomechanics and mechanical signaling in uterine leiomyoma," *Matrix Biology*, vol. 31, no. 1, pp. 57–65, 2012.

[3] F. L. Jayes, X. Ma, E. M. Flannery, F. T. Moutos, F. Guilak, and P. C. Leppert, *Biomechanical Evaluation of Human Uterine Fibroids after Exposure to Purified Clostridial Collagenase*, Society for the Study of Reproduction, Montreal, Canada, 2013.

[4] N. Wang, J. P. Butler, and D. E. Ingber, "Mechanotransduction across the cell surface and through the cytoskeleton," *Science*, vol. 260, no. 5111, pp. 1124–1127, 1993.

[5] D. E. Jaalouk and J. Lammerding, "Mechanotransduction gone awry," *Nature Reviews Molecular Cell Biology*, vol. 10, no. 1, pp. 63–73, 2009.

[6] N. Boudreau and M. J. Bissell, "Extracellular matrix signaling: integration of form and function in normal and malignant cells," *Current Opinion in Cell Biology*, vol. 10, no. 5, pp. 640–646, 1998.

[7] P. Lu, V. M. Weaver, and Z. J. Werb, "The extracellular matrix: a dynamic niche in cancer progression," *The Journal of Cell Biology*, vol. 196, no. 4, pp. 395–406, 2012.

[8] J. K, Y. Mouw, L. Damiano et al., "Tissue mechanics modulate microRNA-dependent PTEN expression to regulate malignant progression," *Nature Medicine*, vol. 20, no. 4, pp. 360–367, 2014.

[9] Z. Jahed, H. Shams, M. Mehrbod, and M. R. K. Mofrad, "Pathways linking the extracellular matrix to the nucleus," *International Review of Cell and Molecular Biology*, vol. 310, pp. 171–220, 2014.

[10] M. E. Blaauboer, C. L. Emson, L. Verschuren et al., "Novel combination of collagen dynamics analysis and transcriptional profiling reveals fibrosis-relevant genes and pathways," *Matrix Biology*, vol. 3215, no. 7-8, pp. 424–431, 2013.

[11] R. Agha, R. Ogawa, G. Pietramaggiori, and D. P. Orgill, "A review of the role of mechanical forces in cutaneous wound healing," *Journal of Surgical Research*, vol. 171, no. 2, pp. 700–708, 2011.

[12] M. Amano, K. Chihara, K. Kimura et al., "Formation of actin stress fibers and focal adhesions enhanced by Rho- kinase," *Science*, vol. 275, no. 5304, pp. 1308–1311, 1997.

[13] D. E. Ingber, "Mechanobiology and diseases of mechanotransduction," *Annals of Medicine*, vol. 35, no. 8, pp. 564–577, 2003.

[14] P. C. Leppert, "Tissue remodeling in the female reproductive tract: a complex process becomes more complex: the Role of Hox genes," *Biology of Reproduction*, vol. 86, no. 4, article 98, 2012.

[15] R. C. Bentley, G. L. Mutter, and S. J. Robboy, "Normal structure of the uterus," in *Pathology of the Female Genital Tract*, G. S. Mutter, J. Prat, P. Russell, and M. C. Anderson, Eds., p. 297, Elsevier, Churchill Livingstone, London, UK, 2nd edition, 2008.

[16] H. A. Roeder, S. F. Cramer, and P. C. Leppert, "A look at uterine wound healing through a histopathological study of uterine scars," *Reproductive Sciences*, vol. 19, no. 5, pp. 463–473, 2012.

[17] H. Schwalm and V. Dubrauszky, "The structure of the musculature of the human uterus—muscles and connective tissue," *American Journal of Obstetrics and Gynecology*, vol. 94, no. 3, pp. 391–404, 1966.

[18] P. C. Leppert, T. Baginski, C. Prupas, W. H. Catherino, S. Pletcher, and J. H. Segars, "Comparative ultrastructure of collagen fibrils in uterine leiomyomas and normal myometrium," *Fertility and Sterility*, vol. 82, supplement 3, pp. 1182–1187, 2004.

[19] S. Ricard-Blum and F. Ruggiero, "The collagen superfamily: From the extracellular matrix to the cell membrane," *Pathologie Biologie*, vol. 53, no. 7, pp. 430–442, 2005.

[20] K. Y. T. Kao and J. G. Leslie, "Polymorphism in human uterine collagen," *Connective Tissue Research*, vol. 5, no. 2, pp. 127–129, 1977.

[21] M. Z. Abedin, S. Ayad, and J. B. Weiss, "Type v collagen: the presence of appreciable amounts of α3(V) chain in uterus," *Biochemical and Biophysical Research Communications*, vol. 102, no. 4, pp. 1237–1245, 1981.

[22] M. O. Pulkkinen, M. Lehto, M. Jalkanen, and K. Näntö-Salonen, "Collagen types and fibronectin in the uterine muscle of normal and hypertensive pregnant patients," *The American Journal of Obstetrics and Gynecology*, vol. 149, no. 7, pp. 711–717, 1984.

[23] B. Trüeb and P. Bornstein, "Characterization of the precursor form of type VI collagen," *Journal of Biological Chemistry*, vol. 259, no. 13, pp. 8597–8604, 1984.

[24] J. P. Borel, "Uterine Collagen: general review," *Revue Françoise de Gynécologie et d' Obstétriques*, vol. 86, no. 12, pp. 712–715, 1991.

[25] R. Timpl, H. Wiedemann, V. van Delden, H. Furthmayr, and K. Kühn, "A network model for the organization of type IV collagen molecules in basement membranes," *European Journal of Biochemistry*, vol. 120, no. 2, pp. 203–211, 1981.

[26] R. Kokenyesi, "Collagens and proteoglycans," in *The Extracellular Matrix of the Uterus, Cervix and Fetal Membranes: Synthesis, Degradation and Hormonal Regulation*, P. C. Leppert and J. F. Woessner, Eds., pp. 15–28, Perinatology Press, Ithaca, NY, USA, 1991.

[27] R. Myllyla, J. Koivu, T. Pihlajaniemi, and K. I. Kivirikko, "Protein disulphide-isomerase activity in various cells synthesizing collagen," *European Journal of Biochemistry*, vol. 134, no. 1, pp. 7–11, 1983.

[28] D. J. Prockop, K. I. Kivirikko, L. Tuderman, and N. A. Guzman, "The biosynthesis of collagen and its disorders (first of two parts)," *The New England Journal of Medicine*, vol. 301, no. 1, pp. 13 23, 1979.

[29] D. J. Prockop and L. Tuderman, "Posttranslational enzymes in the biosynthesis of collagen: extracellular enzymes," *Methods in Enzymology*, vol. 82, pp. 305–319, 1982.

[30] H. Hofmann, P. P. Fietzek, and K. Kühn, "The role of polar and hydrophobic interactions for the molecular packing of type

I collagen: a three-dimensional evaluation of the amino acid sequence," *Journal of Molecular Biology*, vol. 125, no. 2, pp. 137–165, 1978.

[31] D. F. Holmes, C. J. Gilpin, C. Baldock, U. Ziese, A. J. Koster, and K. E. Kadler, "Corneal collagen fibril structure in three dimensions: Structural insights into fibril assembly, mechanical properties, and tissue organization," *Proceedings of the National Academy of Sciences of the United States of America*, vol. 98, no. 13, pp. 7307–7312, 2001.

[32] R. B. Rücker, N. Romero-Chapman, T. Wong et al., "Modulation of lysyl oxidase by dietary copper in rats," *Journal of Nutrition*, vol. 126, no. 1, pp. 51–60, 1996.

[33] M. Saito, K. Marumo, K. Fujii, and N. Ishioka, "Single-column high-performance liquid chromatographic-fluorescence detection of immature, mature, and senescent cross-links of collagen," *Analytical Biochemistry*, vol. 253, no. 1, pp. 26–32, 1997.

[34] H. A. Lucero and H. M. Kagan, "Lysyl oxidase: an oxidative enzyme and effector of cell function," *Cellular and Molecular Life Sciences*, vol. 63, no. 19-20, pp. 2304–2316, 2006.

[35] W. Henkel and R. W. Glanville, "Covalent crosslinking between molecules of type I and type III collagen," *European Journal of Biochemistry*, vol. 122, no. 1, pp. 205–213, 1982.

[36] K. M. Mak, E. Chu, K. H. V. Lau, and A. J. Kwong, "Liver fibrosis in elderly cadavers: localization of type I, III, and IV, α-smooth muscle actin, and elastic fibers," *The Anatomical Record*, vol. 295, no. 7, pp. 1159–1167, 2012.

[37] K. Prydz and K. T. Dalen, "Synthesis and sorting of proteoglycans," *Journal of Cell Science*, vol. 113, no. 2, pp. 193–205, 2000.

[38] N. A. Visser, G. P. J. Vankampen, M. H. M. T. Dekoning, and J. K. Vanderkorst, "The effects of loading on the synthesis of biglycan and decorin in intact mature articular cartilage in vitro," *Connective Tissue Research*, vol. 30, no. 4, pp. 241–250, 1994.

[39] J. E. Scott and C. R. Orford, "Dermatan sulphate-rich proteoglycan associates with rat tail-tendon collagen at the d band in the gap region," *Biochemical Journal*, vol. 197, no. 1, pp. 213–216, 1981.

[40] E. Schonherr, H. Hausser, L. Beavan, and H. Kresse, "Decorin-type I collagen interaction. Presence of separate core protein-binding domains," *The Journal of Biological Chemistry*, vol. 270, no. 15, pp. 8877–8883, 1995.

[41] H. Kresse, H. Hausser, and E. Schonherr, "Small proteoglycans," *Experientia*, vol. 49, no. 5, pp. 403–416, 1993.

[42] R. V. Iozzo, "The biology of the small leucine-rich proteoglycans. Functional network of interactive proteins," *The Journal of Biological Chemistry*, vol. 274, no. 27, pp. 18843–18846, 1999.

[43] A. G. A. Berto, S. M. Oba, Y. M. Michelacci, and L. O. Sampaio, "Galactosaminoglycans from normal myometrium and leiomyoma," *Brazilian Journal of Medical and Biological Research*, vol. 34, no. 5, pp. 633–637, 2001.

[44] P. C. Leppert, R. Kokenyesi, C. A. Klemenich, and J. Fisher, "Further evidence of a decorin-collagen interaction in the disruption of cervical collagen fibers during rat gestation," *American Journal of Obstetrics and Gynecology*, vol. 182, no. 4, pp. 805–812, 2000.

[45] R. Kokenyesi and J. F. Woessner Jr., "Effects of hormonal perturbations on the small dermatan sulfate proteoglycan and mechanical properties of the uterine cervix of late pregnant rats.," *Connective Tissue Research*, vol. 26, no. 3, pp. 199–205, 1991.

[46] R. Kokenyesi and J. F. Woessner Jr., "Relationship between dilatation of the rat uterine cervix and a small dermatan sulfate proteoglycan," *Biology of Reproduction*, vol. 42, no. 1, pp. 87–97, 1990.

[47] M. Ruscheinsky, C. de la Motte, and M. Mahendroo, "Hyaluronan and its binding proteins during cervical ripening and parturition: dynamic changes in size, distribution and temporal sequence," *Matrix Biology*, vol. 27, no. 5, pp. 487–497, 2008.

[48] Y. Akgul, R. Holt, M. Mummert, A. Word, and M. Mahendroo, "Dynamic changes in cervical glycosaminoglycan composition during normal pregnancy and preterm birth," *Endocrinology*, vol. 153, no. 7, pp. 3493–3503, 2012.

[49] D. A. Carrino, S. Mesiano, N. M. Barker, W. W. Hurd, and A. I. Caplan, "Proteoglycans of uterine fibroids and keloid scars: similarity in their proteoglycan composition," *Biochemical Journal*, vol. 443, no. 2, pp. 361–368, 2012.

[50] C. R. de Lima, J. D. A. dos Santos Jr., A. C. P. Nazário, and Y. M. Michelacci, "Changes in glycosaminoglycans and proteoglycans of normal breast and fibroadenoma during the menstrual cycle," *Biochimica et Biophysica Acta: General Subjects*, vol. 1820, no. 7, pp. 1009–1019, 2012.

[51] J. T. Cirulis, C. M. Bellingham, E. C. Davis et al., "Fibrillins, fibulins, and matrix-associated glycoprotein modulate the kinetics and morphology of *in vitro* self-assembly of a recombinant elastin-like polypeptide," *Biochemistry*, vol. 47, no. 47, pp. 12601–12613, 2008.

[52] P. C. Leppert and S. Y. Yu, "Three-dimensional structures of uterine elastic fibers: scanning electron microscopic studies," *Connective Tissue Research*, vol. 27, no. 1, pp. 15–31, 1991.

[53] M. Barczyk, A. I. Bolstad, and D. Gullberg, "Role of integrins in the periodontal ligament: organizers and facilitators," *Periodontology 2000*, vol. 63, no. 1, pp. 29–47, 2013.

[54] A. Elosegui-Artola, E. Bazellières, M. D. Allen et al., "Rigidity sensing and adaption through regulation of integrin types," *Nature Materials*, vol. 13, no. 6, pp. 631–637, 2014.

[55] S. Israeli-Rosenberg, A. M. Manso, H. Okada, and R. S. Ross, "Integrins and integrins-associated proteins in the cardiac myoctye," *Circulation Research*, vol. 114, no. 3, pp. 572–586, 2014.

[56] G. Mechtersheimer, T. Barth, A. Quentmeier, and P. Möller, "Differential expression of β1 integrins in nonneoplastic smooth and striated muscle cells and in tumors derived from these cells," *American Journal of Pathology*, vol. 144, no. 6, pp. 1172–1182, 1994.

[57] C. V. Taylor, M. Letarte, and S. J. Lye, "The expression of integrins and cadherins in normal human uterus and uterine leiomyomas," *The American Journal of Obstetrics and Gynecology*, vol. 175, no. 2, pp. 411–419, 1996.

[58] M. Peavey, N. Salleh, and P. C. Leppert, "Collagen-binding α11 integrin expression in human myometrium and fibroids utilizing a novel RNA in situ probe," *Reproductive Sciences*, 2014.

[59] H. Ji, V. Long, V. Briody, and E. K. Chien, "Progesterone modulates integrin α2 (ITGA2) and α11 (ITGA11) in the pregnant cervix," *Reproductive Sciences*, vol. 18, no. 2, pp. 156–163, 2011.

[60] M. Malik, J. Segars, and W. H. Catherino, "Integrin β1 regulates leiomyoma cytoskeletal integrity and growth," *Matrix Biology*, vol. 31, no. 7-8, pp. 389–397, 2012.

[61] P. Singh, C. Carraher, and J. E. Schwarzbauer, "Assembly of fibronectin extracellular matrix," *Annual Review of Cell and Developmental Biology*, vol. 26, pp. 397–419, 2010.

[62] D. C. Hocking, P. A. Titus, R. Sumagin, and I. H. Sarelius, "Extracellular matrix fibronectin mechanically couples skeletal muscle contraction with local vasodilation," *Circulation Research*, vol. 102, no. 3, pp. 372–379, 2008.

[63] J. Lohi, C. L. Wilson, J. D. Roby, and W. C. Parks, "Epilysin, a novel human matrix metalloproteinase (MMP-28) expressed in testis and keratinocytes and in response to injury," *The Journal of Biological Chemistry*, vol. 276, no. 13, pp. 10134–10144, 2001.

[64] H. Nagase, R. Visse, and G. Murphy, "Structure and function of matrix metalloproteinases and TIMPs," *Cardiovascular Research*, vol. 69, no. 3, pp. 562–573, 2006.

[65] A. Page-McCaw, A. J. Ewald, and Z. Werb, "Matrix metalloproteinases and the regulation of tissue remodelling," *Nature Reviews Molecular Cell Biology*, vol. 8, no. 3, pp. 221–233, 2007.

[66] K. Suzuki, J. J. Enghild, T. Morodomi, G. Salvesen, and H. Nagase, "Mechanisms of activation of tissue procollagenase by matrix metalloproteinase 3 (stromelysin)," *Biochemistry*, vol. 29, no. 44, pp. 10261–10270, 1990.

[67] L. Chung, D. Dinakarpandian, N. Yoshida et al., "Collagenase unwinds triple-helical collagen prior to peptide bond hydrolysis," *The EMBO Journal*, vol. 23, no. 15, pp. 3020–3030, 2004.

[68] T. E. Curry Jr. and K. G. Osteen, "The matrix metalloproteinase system: changes, regulation, and impact throughout the ovarian and uterine reproductive cycle," *Endocrine Reviews*, vol. 24, no. 4, pp. 428–465, 2003.

[69] H. Khalili, A. H. Talasaz, and M. Salarifar, "Serum vitamin D concentration status and its correlation with early biomarkers of remodeling following acute myocardial infarction," *Clinical Research in Cardiology*, vol. 101, no. 5, pp. 321–327, 2012.

[70] S. Abramovitch, L. Dahan-Bachar, E. Sharvit et al., "Vitamin D inhibits proliferation and profibrotic marker expression in hepatic stellate cells and decreases thioacetamide-induced liver fibrosis in rats," *Gut*, vol. 60, no. 12, pp. 1728–1737, 2011.

[71] E. A. Stewart, A. J. Friedman, K. Peck, and R. A. Nowak, "Relative overexpression of collagen type I and collagen type III messenger ribonucleic acids by uterine leiomyomas during the proliferative phase of the menstrual cycle," *Journal of Clinical Endocrinology and Metabolism*, vol. 79, no. 3, pp. 900–906, 1994.

[72] W. H. Catherino, P. C. Leppert, M. H. Stenmark et al., "Reduced dermatopontin expression is a molecular link between uterine leiomyomas and keloids," *Genes Chromosomes and Cancer*, vol. 40, no. 3, pp. 204–217, 2004.

[73] L. Feng, N. Aviles, S. Leikin, and P. Leppert, "Pattern of collagen types in uterine fibroids," *Reproductive Sciences*, vol. 17, article 270A, 2010.

[74] M. Iwahashi and Y. Muragaki, "Increased type I and V collagen expression in uterine leiomyomas during the menstrual cycle," *Fertility and Sterility*, vol. 95, no. 6, pp. 2137–2139, 2011.

[75] L. O. Sampaio, C. P. Dietrich, and O. Giannotti Filho, "Changes in sulfated mucopolysaccharide composition of mammalian tissues during growth and in cancer tissues," *Biochimica et Biophysica Acta*, vol. 498, no. 1, pp. 123–131, 1977.

[76] A. G. Berto, L. O. Sampaio, C. R. Franco, R. M. Cesar Jr., and Y. M. Michelacci, "A comparative analysis of structure and spatial distribution of decorin in human leiomyoma and normal myometrium," *Biochimica et Biophysica Acta: General Subjects*, vol. 1619, no. 1, pp. 98–112, 2003.

[77] F. A. Aleem and M. Predanic, "The hemodynamic effect of GnRH agonist therapy on uterine leiomyoma vascularity: a prospective study using transvaginal color Doppler sonography," *Gynecological Endocrinology*, vol. 9, no. 3, pp. 253–258, 1995.

[78] S. Okuda, K. Oshio, H. Shinmoto et al., "Semiquantitative assessment of MR imaging in prediction of efficacy of gonadotropin-releasing hormone agonist for volume reduction of uterine leiomyoma: initial experience," *Radiology*, vol. 248, no. 3, pp. 917–924, 2008.

[79] C. P. West, M. A. Lumsden, S. Lawson, J. Williamson, and D. D. Baird, "Shrinkage of uterine fibroids during therapy with goserelin (Zoladex): a luteinizing hormone-releasing hormone agonist administered as a monthly subcutaneous depot," *Fertility and Sterility*, vol. 48, no. 1, pp. 45–51, 1987.

[80] J. L. Britten, M. Malik, G. Levy, M. Mendoza, and W. H. Catherino, "Gonadotropin-releasing hormone (GnRH) agonist leuprolide acetate and GnRH antagonist cetrorelix acetate directly inhibit leiomyoma extracellular matrix production," *Fertility and Sterility*, vol. 98, no. 5, pp. 1299–1307, 2012.

[81] J. D. Parker, M. Malik, and W. H. Catherino, "Human myometrium and leiomyomas express gonadotropin-releasing hormone 2 and gonadotropin-releasing hormone 2 receptor," *Fertility and Sterility*, vol. 88, no. 1, pp. 39–46, 2007.

[82] D. M. McCarthy-Keith, M. Malik, J. Britten, J. Segars, and W. H. Catherino, "Gonadotropin-releasing hormone agonist increases expression of osmotic response genes in leiomyoma cells," *Fertility and Sterility*, vol. 95, no. 7, pp. 2383–2387, 2011.

[83] S. F. Cramer, J. Horiszny, A. Patel, and S. Sigrist, "The relation of fibrous degeneration to menopausal status in small uterine leiomyomas with evidence for postmenopausal origin of seedling myomas," *Modern Pathology*, vol. 9, no. 7, pp. 774–780, 1996.

[84] S. F. Cramer, C. Marchetti, J. Freedman, and A. Padela, "Relationship of myoma cell size and menopausal status in small uterine leiomyomas," *Archives of Pathology & Laboratory Medicine*, vol. 124, no. 10, pp. 1448–1453, 2000.

[85] I. Konishi, S. Fujii, C. Ban, Y. Okuda, H. Okamura, and S. Tojo, "Ultrastructural study of minute uterine leiomyomas," *International Journal of Gynecological Pathology*, vol. 2, no. 2, pp. 113–120, 1983.

[86] J. T. Holdsworth-Carson, M. Zaitseva, B. J. Vollenhoven, and P. A. Rogers, "Clonality of smooth muscle and fibroid cells populations isolated from human fibroid and myometrial tissues," *Molecular Human Reproduction*, vol. 20, no. 3, pp. 250–259, 2014.

[87] R. Tal and J. H. Segars, "The role of angiogenic factors in fibroid pathogenesis: potential implications for future therapy," *Human Reproduction Update*, vol. 20, no. 2, pp. 149–216, 2014.

[88] T. Maruyama, M. Ono, and Y. Yoshimura, "Somatic stem cells in the myometrium and in myomas," *Seminars in Reproductive Medicine*, vol. 31, no. 1, pp. 77–81, 2013.

[89] J. C. M. Tsibris, J. Segars, D. Coppola et al., "Insights from gene arrays on the development and growth regulation of uterine leiomyomata," *Fertility and Sterility*, vol. 78, no. 1, pp. 114–121, 2002.

[90] M. Ono, P. Yin, A. Navarro et al., "Paracrine activation of WNT/β catenin pathway in uterine leiomyoma stem cells promotes tumor growth," *Proceedings of the National Academy of Sciences of the United States of America*, vol. 110, no. 24, pp. 17053–17058, 2013.

[91] M. Ono, T. Maruyama, H. Masuda et al., "Side population in human uterine myometrium displays phenotypic and functional characteristics of myometrial stem cells," *Proceedings of the National Academy of Sciences of the United States of America*, vol. 104, no. 47, pp. 18700–18705, 2007.

[92] S. F. Cramer and A. Patel, "The nonrandom regional distribution of uterine leiomyomas: a clue to histogenesis?" *Human Pathology*, vol. 23, no. 6, pp. 635–638, 1992.

[93] D. E. Ingber, "Can cancer be reversed by engineering the tumor microenvironment?" *Seminars in Cancer Biology*, vol. 18, no. 5, pp. 356–364, 2008.

[94] D. T. Butcher, T. Alliston, and V. M. Weaver, "A tense situation: forcing tumour progression," *Nature Reviews Cancer*, vol. 9, no. 2, pp. 108–122, 2009.

[95] M. J. Paszek and V. M. Weaver, "The tension mounts: mechanics meets morphogenesis and malignancy," *Journal of Mammary Gland Biology and Neoplasia*, vol. 9, no. 4, pp. 325–342, 2004.

[96] M. J. Paszek, N. Zahir, K. R. Johnson et al., "Tensional homeostasis and the malignant phenotype," *Cancer Cell*, vol. 8, no. 3, pp. 241–254, 2005.

[97] J. S. Crabtree, S. A. Jelinsky, H. A. Harris et al., "Comparison of human and rat uterine leiomyomata: identification of a dysregulated mammalian target of rapamycin pathway," *Cancer Research*, vol. 69, no. 15, pp. 6171–6178, 2009.

[98] B. V. Varghese, F. Koohestani, M. McWilliams et al., "Loss of the repressor REST in uterine fibroids promotes aberrant G protein-coupled receptor 10 expression and activates mammalian target of rapamycin pathway," *Proceedings of the National Academy of Sciences of the United States of America*, vol. 110, no. 6, pp. 2187–2192, 2013.

[99] N. E. Zanchi and A. H. Lancha Jr., "Mechanical stimuli of skeletal muscle: Implications on mTOR/p70s6k and protein synthesis," *European Journal of Applied Physiology*, vol. 102, no. 3, pp. 253–263, 2008.

[100] I. Mandl, J. D. MacLennan, and E. L. Howes, "Isolation and characteristics of proteinase and collagenase from Cl histolyticum," *Journal of Clinical Investigation*, vol. 32, no. 12, pp. 1323–1329, 1953.

[101] T. Toyoshima, O. Matsushita, J. Minami, N. Nishi, A. Okabe, and T. Itano, "Collagen-binding domain of a Clostridium histolyticum collagenase exhibits a broad substrate spectrum both in vitro and in vivo," *Connective Tissue Research*, vol. 42, no. 4, pp. 281–290, 2001.

[102] W. Borth, E. J. Menzel, M. Salzer, and C. Steffen, "Human serum inhibitors of collagenase as revealed by preparative isoelectric focusing," *Clinica Chimica Acta*, vol. 117, no. 2, pp. 219–225, 1981.

[103] S. K. Halder, K. G. Osteen, and A. Al-Hendy, "Vitamin D3 inhibits expression and activities of matrix metalloproteinase-2 and -9 in human uterine fibroid cells," *Human Reproduction*, vol. 28, no. 9, pp. 2407–2416, 2013.

[104] B. R. Heaps, M. House, S. Socrate, P. Leppert, and J. F. Strauss III, "Matrix biology and preterm birth," in *Preterm Birth Mechanisms, Mediators, Prediction, Prevention and Interventions*, F. Petraglia, J. F. Strauss III, S. G. Gabbe, and G. Weiss, Eds., chapter 8, pp. 70–93, Oxon, Informa Healthcare, Abington, Ill, USA, 2007.

[105] D. D. Baird, M. C. Hill, J. M. Schectman, and B. W. Hollis, "Vitamin D and the risk of uterine fibroids," *Epidemiology*, vol. 24, no. 3, pp. 447–453, 2013.

[106] D. D. Baird, D. B. Dunson, M. C. Hill, D. Cousins, and J. M. Schectman, "High cumulative incidence of uterine leiomyoma in black and white women: Ultrasound evidence," *American Journal of Obstetrics and Gynecology*, vol. 188, no. 1, pp. 100–107, 2003.

[107] S. D. Peddada, S. K. Laughlin, K. Miner et al., "Growth of uterine leiomyomata among premenopausal black and white women," *Proceedings of the National Academy of Sciences of the United States of America*, vol. 105, no. 50, pp. 19887–19892, 2008.

[108] B. J. Davis, J. I. Risinger, G. V. R. Chandramouli, P. R. Bushel, D. D. Baird, and S. D. Peddada, "Gene Expression in Uterine Leiomyoma from Tumors Likely to Be Growing (from Black Women over 35) and Tumors Likely to Be Non-Growing (from White Women over 35)," *PLoS ONE*, vol. 8, no. 6, Article ID e63909, 2013.

[109] F. Koohestani, A. G. Braudmeier, A. Mahdian et al., "Extracellular matrix collagen alters cell proliferation and cell cycle progression of human uterine smooth muscle cells," *PLoS ONE*, vol. 10, Article ID 0075844, 2013.

[110] E. A. Stewart, F. A. Taran, J. Chen et al., "Magnetic resonance elastography of uterine leiomyomas: a feasibility study," *Fertility and Sterility*, vol. 95, no. 1, pp. 281–284, 2011.

[111] D. Gullberg, "Shift happens—a paradigm shift for the role of integrins in fibrosis," *Matrix Biology*, vol. 28, no. 7, p. 383, 2009.

30

Community Awareness of HPV Screening and Vaccination in Odisha

Niharika Khanna,[1] **Aparna Ramaseshan,**[2] **Stephanie Arnold,**[1]
Kalpana Panigrahi,[3] **Mark D. Macek,**[4] **Bijaya K. Padhi,**[5] **Diptirani Samanta,**[6]
Surendra N. Senapati,[7] **and Pinaki Panigrahi**[3,8]

[1]*Department of Family & Community Medicine, University of Maryland, MD, USA*

[2]*Department of Obstetrics and Gynecology, University of Maryland School of Medicine, Baltimore, MD 21201, USA*

[3]*Department of Epidemiology, Center for Global Health & Development, College of Public Health,*
 University of Nebraska Medical Center, Omaha, NE, USA

[4]*Department of Dental Public Health, University of Maryland School of Dentistry, Baltimore, MD, USA*

[5]*Asian Institute of Public Health, Bhubaneswar, Odisha, India*

[6]*Department of Medical Oncology, Acharya Harihar Regional Cancer Center, Cuttack, Odisha, India*

[7]*Department of Radiation Oncology, Acharya Harihar Regional Cancer Center, Cuttack, Odisha, India*

[8]*Department of Pediatrics, University of Nebraska Medical Center, Omaha, NE, USA*

Correspondence should be addressed to Niharika Khanna; nkhanna@som.umaryland.edu

Academic Editor: Wiebren A. A. Tjalma

Introduction. A number of new technologies including cervical cancer screening and vaccination have introduced new tools in the fight against cervical cancer. *Methods.* This study was set in Odisha, India, at the Acharya Harihar Regional Cancer Center and study research infrastructure at the Asian Institute of Public Health. IRB approvals were obtained and a research assistant recruited 286 women aged 18–49 years, who provided informed consent and completed a survey tool. Data were entered into EpiData software and statistical analysis was conducted. *Results.* 76.3% women participants were married, 45.5% had sexual debut at age 21 or greater, 60.5% used contraception, 12.2% reported having a Pap smear in the past, and 4.9% reported having prior genital warts. Most, 68.8% had never heard of HPV and 11.9% were aware that HPV is the main cause of cervical cancer. 82.9% women thought that vaccinations prevent disease, and 74.8% said they make the decision to vaccinate their children. *Conclusion.* The Odisha community demonstrated a low level of knowledge about cervical cancer prevention, accepted vaccinations in the prevention of disease and screening, and identified mothers/guardians as the key family contacts.

1. Introduction

Cervical cancer continues to be a major health problem in India where 132,000 women are diagnosed each year and 74,000 deaths are observed [1]. The majority, 70% of cervical cancers, is detected at Stage III or higher, leading to high mortality rates [2]. Despite an annual cervical cancer incidence rate of 25/100,000 in India, there are no large scale public health surveillance programs in cervical cytological screening and human papillomavirus (HPV) typing in India. Human

papillomavirus prophylactic vaccine has been available in the Western world since 2006 due to which there is a real possibility of primary prevention of cervical cancer caused by HPV types 16 and 18.

We designed a study to explore community awareness of HPV and cervical cancer among women in Odisha, India. In addition, we explored the acceptance and understanding of primary and secondary prevention methods for cervical cancer control by adult women who are potential recipients of HPV screening and gatekeepers to their families health. We also explored the perception by women in Odisha to identify the health decision maker for vaccination for young girls in their family. Lastly, we explored possible acceptance of the HPV vaccine and cervical cancer screening in the Odisha community.

This information will inform implementation and dissemination research in cervical cancer prevention including cervical HPV screening and HPV vaccine acceptance.

2. Methods

2.1. Site. Odisha is a site where organized maternal and child health research has been conducted successfully over the last several years by our collaborating team at the Asian Institute of Public Health [3]. Odisha has a population of 36.8 million inhabitants of which 15% are urban populations [4]. There is access to reproductive age women and organizational capacity for the ethical conduct of human research. In addition, there are 6.1 million inhabitants with less than primary school or no education. There have been no organized government sponsored educational campaigns in this area to increase awareness of HPV and cervical cancer control.

2.2. Research Team. There is an existing collaboration arrangement between University of Nebraska Medical Center, College of Public Health, the University of Maryland, the Asian Institute of Public Health (AIPH), and the Acharya Harihar Regional Cancer Center in Cuttack, Odisha. These groups have engaged in collaborative maternal and child health research in these areas and have demonstrated the ability to conduct NIH funded research consistently over the last 12 years. The AIPH utilizes an organized network of 212 villages where there is capability for responsibly conducting research which complies with International Standards of Clinical Research and Harmonization at three levels. There are community health workers known as Anganwadi workers, who are supervised by field supervisors. The field supervisors report directly to the research team at the AIPH. There is capability to ensure that Good Clinical Practices are followed and each Anganwadi worker is trained and retrained in the ethical conduct of human research. Population outreach has been primarily to maternal and child populations over the last 12 years in urban, rural, and tribal settings. In preparation for a future HPV vaccine implementation project, we proposed formative research to sample urban, urban slum, and rural populations in Odisha to approach women and mothers aged 18–49 years to educate and inform them about cervical cancer prevention strategies including cervical cancer screening and the HPV vaccine. We propose to assess their understanding and acceptance of cervical cancer screening and HPV vaccine in the future.

2.3. Patient Recruitment. Following Institutional Review Board approvals at both University of Maryland and the Acharya Harihar Regional Cancer Center (AHRCC), we included a total of 286 women aged 18–49 years, who provided informed consent to participate in the study. We excluded those women who had a previous diagnosis of cervical cancer. Women between 18 and 49 years of age

who were willing to provide informed consent were included in this study. Women who had a previous diagnosis of cervical cancer were excluded from the study. Women were recruited from urban, rural, and tribal areas to capture the knowledge and attitudes of women in different sociocultural and economic strata. The urban surveys were collected at various local women's colleges, malls, and open markets in Bhubaneswar, the capital city of Odisha. The rural surveys were obtained from the villages in the outskirts of Bhubaneswar. The tribal surveys were collected from the tribal sites in Rourkela, Odisha. A significant number of surveys were obtained from patients visiting the Regional Cancer Center which contained a mixture of women from both urban and rural areas. The participants from the cancer center site included women who were patients, employees, and bystanders at the facility.

2.4. Enrollment and Survey Administration. US and AIPH researchers worked together to approach women presenting to the Acharya Harihar Regional Cancer Center, in the urban slums surrounding the AHRCC and the AIPH. Rural women were recruited when presenting to the organized clinical centers and also from the marketplace. Each participant underwent informed consent procedures followed by enrollment procedures including Unique Identifier number assignment. Confidentiality was maintained and each participant was reassured about their anonymity prior to implementing the sensitive research survey tool. The survey was administered by research personnel in the native Oriya language or English and was read to those participants who were illiterate. Answers were recorded in paper format followed by data entry by an assistant into an EpiData database. Data gathering was done with US researchers and AIPH researchers working together to approach women presenting to the Acharya Harihar Regional Cancer Center, in the urban slums surrounding the AHRCC and the AIPH. Rural women were recruited when presenting to the organized clinical centers and also from the marketplace. Each participant underwent informed consent procedures followed by enrollment procedures including Unique Identifier number assignment. Confidentiality was maintained and each participant was reassured about their anonymity prior to implementing the sensitive research survey tool. The survey was administered by research personnel in the native Oriya language or English and was read to those participants who were illiterate.

2.5. Data Gathering. It was done by US researchers and AIPH researchers working together to approach women presenting to the Acharya Harihar Regional Cancer Center, in the urban slums surrounding the AHRCC and the AIPH. Rural women were recruited when presenting to the organized clinical centers and also from the marketplace. Each participant underwent informed consent procedures followed by enrollment procedures including Unique Identifier number assignment. Confidentiality was maintained and each participant was reassured about their anonymity prior to implementing the sensitive research survey tool. The survey was administered by research personnel in the native Oriya language or English and was read to those participants who were illiterate. Data gathering was done with US researchers and AIPH researchers working together to approach women presenting to the Acharya Harihar Regional Cancer Center, in the urban slums surrounding the AHRCC and the AIPH. Rural women were recruited when presenting to the organized clinical centers and also from the marketplace. Each participant underwent informed consent procedures followed by enrollment procedures including Unique Identifier number assignment. Confidentiality was maintained and each participant was reassured about their anonymity prior to implementing the sensitive research survey tool. The survey was administered by research personnel in the native Oriya language or English and was read to those participants who were illiterate. When the survey was conducted orally, the answers were recorded on paper by the survey administrator, which was later transferred into EpiData database (version 3.1). Dual database entry and standard data fidelity procedures were followed to ensure accuracy of the data entry and database cleaning. Database access was password protected and access was restricted to key personnel in the Odisha and US team.

2.6. Survey Details. The survey was administered by a research assistant who provided translation and helped with completion to those women who requested help. Women were queried in the following domains: demographics, patient knowledge, attitudes and self-efficacy outcomes around vaccination, health care for themselves and their families, HPV knowledge, and acceptability of cervical cancer screening methods and HPV vaccination.

3. Statistical Methods

3.1. Survey Tool. It is approved by University of Maryland and Local Odisha IRB, administered by a research assistant using the local language and vernacular data management and analysis.

Responses were manually entered into an EpiData software followed by Unique Identifier number assignment to all participants. Data was deidentified and statistical analysis was conducted. Data was systematically analyzed using univariate and bivariate statistical analyses that were conducted using SAS software (Version 9.1) for Windows. Data was analyzed using the following variable groupings: general information, self-efficacy, social supports, and attitudes towards HPV screening and HPV vaccination. Cross-cutting themes and variables were identified and adjusted for cell frequency, percentages, and odds ratios that were calculated by exact procedures available in SAS. All *p* values were computed by Chi-square test for large samples and by Fisher's exact test for small samples. Factors that may influence the acceptance of HPV screening and HPV vaccination included age, marital status, education, smoking status, self-efficacy, social supports, whether prior Pap received, HPV status, and attitudes towards HPV screening and HPV vaccination.

Data were entered into an EpiData database using dual data entry, and over 10% of the database was further audited to ensure accuracy and completeness. Each participant was

TABLE 1: Sample characteristics, Odisha, India (*n* = 286).

Characteristic	Sample size	Percentage
Age		
20–29 years	98	34.3
30–39 years	104	36.3
≥40 years	80	28.0
Refused/missing	4	1.4
Marital status		
Single (never married)	67	23.4
Married/formerly married	218	76.3
Refused/missing	1	0.3
Sexual history		
Never had sex	52	18.2
First sex at <21 years	85	29.7
First sex at ≥21 years	130	45.5
Refused/missing	19	6.6
Ever used contraception		
Yes	173	60.5
No	113	39.5
Ever used tobacco products		
Yes	39	13.6
No	241	84.3
Refused/missing	6	2.1
Ever had genital warts		
Yes	14	4.9
No	240	83.9
Do not know	19	6.6
Refused/missing	13	4.6
Ever had a Pap smear		
Yes	35	12.2
No	204	71.3
Do not know	24	8.4
Refused/missing	23	8.1

assigned a unique study identifier number to ensure confidentiality, and the database with names was kept in locked room to which only selected study staff had access. Data were analyzed using SAS (Release 9.1, SAS Institute Inc., Cary, North Carolina, USA). Univariate and multivariate statistical analyses were conducted using SAS software.

4. Results

4.1. Demographics. This data was gathered in 2009 in the state of Odisha in 286 urban and rural women presenting to the Acharya Harihar Regional Cancer Center for care, from a public marketplace and from a community college for women. There were 286 women who were willing to participate in the survey and demographics are presented in Table 1. We recruited women between the ages of 18 and 49 years and the majority 76.3% were married or formerly married. The majority, 45.5%, had sexual debut at age 21 or greater and 60.5% used contraception. Tobacco use was reported in 13.6% women and 12.2% reported having a Pap

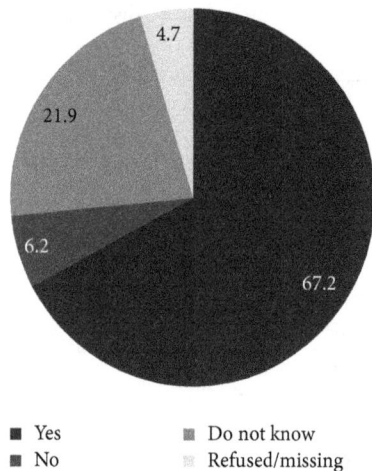

FIGURE 1: Aware that HPV results from sex with infected partner, among those who have heard of HPV, Odisha, India (*n* = 64).

smear in the past and 4.9% reported having prior genital warts (Table 1). Most women participants, 68.8%, had never heard of HPV and 11.9% were aware that HPV is the main cause of cervical cancer. Although 46.9% of women know that you might die from cervical cancer only 15% believed that their current physician would take care of their cervical cancer needs. The understanding that vaccinations prevent disease was widely prevalent and 82.9% of women thought that vaccinations prevent disease, and 74.8% thought that they would be the person in their family to make the decision to vaccinate their children. There was less clarity on whether their community would resist the HPV vaccine and 9.1% of women clearly thought there would be resistance, whereas 29.7% did not know and 7.3% did not answer this question (Table 2).

Among the women who had heard of HPV, women aged 20–29 years were most likely to have heard of HPV and those older than 40 years were least likely to have heard of HPV. In addition, those who had heard of HPV were more likely to be single and to have never had sex (Table 3). Among the 64 women who were aware of HPV, 67.2% stated awareness of the sexual transmission of HPV through an infected partner (Figure 1), 43.7% had the knowledge that HPV is the main cause of cervical cancer (Figure 2). Among these 64 women, only 42.2% were aware that cervical cancer prevention is feasible with the novel HPV vaccine and 37.5% women stated that they were unaware that vaccine mediated prevention was feasible (Figure 3).

5. Discussion

Cervical cancer is an important disease in Odisha and public health campaigns have not occurred to increase community awareness. Recent developments linking HPV to cervical cancer are not known in the community and there is no existing concerted effort to develop public health campaigns to increase this awareness. Community awareness and buy-in is critical to the introduction of newer strategies for cervical

TABLE 2: Knowledge, attitudes, and self-efficacy outcomes, Odisha, India (*n* = 286).

Characteristic	Sample size	Percentage
Believe cervical cancer will lead to death		
Yes	134	46.9
No	37	12.9
Never heard of cervical cancer	64	22.4
Do not know	48	16.8
Refused/missing	3	1.0
Believe your current doctor would also treat cervical cancer needs		
Yes	43	15.0
No	199	69.6
Do not know	28	9.8
Refused/missing	16	5.6
Believe vaccinations prevent disease		
Yes	237	82.9
No	13	4.5
Do not know	31	10.8
Refused/missing	5	1.8
"Very likely" or "likely" to be the person who makes decisions to vaccinate your child		
Yes	214	74.8
No	53	18.6
Refused/missing	19	6.6
Ever heard of HPV		
Yes	64	22.4
No	197	68.8
Do not know	20	7.0
Refused/missing	5	1.8
Know that HPV is main cause of cervical cancer		
Yes	34	11.9
No	61	21.3
Do not know	183	64.0
Refused/missing	8	2.8
Believe that your community might resist HPV vaccinations		
Yes	26	9.1
No	154	53.9
Do not know	85	29.7
Refused/missing	21	7.3

cancer prevention [5]. Recent events in India have led to governmental review of policies surrounding HPV vaccine clinical trials in India [6–8]. A key point raised by activists and others is the vulnerability of the targeted population and the need for review of the ethical mandates by governmental agencies. There is no doubt that affordable, safe vaccination could significantly impact the incidence and mortality from

TABLE 3: Crude odds of having ever heard of HPV, Odisha, India ($n = 286$).

Characteristic	Crude odds ratio (95% confidence interval)
Age	
20–29 years	5.8 (2.4, 14.3)**
30–39 years	3.0 (1.2, 7.5)*
≥40 years	Reference
Marital status (single versus married/formerly married)	3.0 (1.6, 5.6)**
Sexual history	
Never had sex	1.5 (0.8, 3.1)^{NS}
First sex at <21 years	0.1 (0.0, 0.3)**
First sex at ≥21 years	Reference

$*$ = <0.05; $**$ = <0.01; NS = not significant.

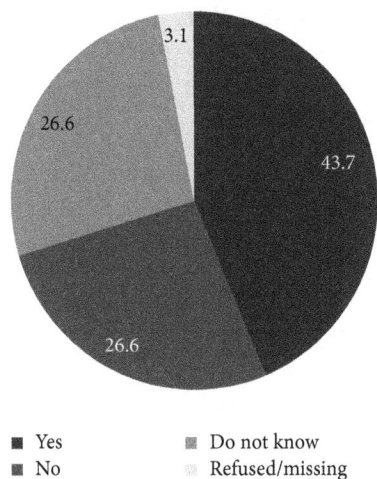

FIGURE 2: Aware that HPV is the main cause of cervical cancer, among those have heard of HPV, Odisha, India ($n = 64$).

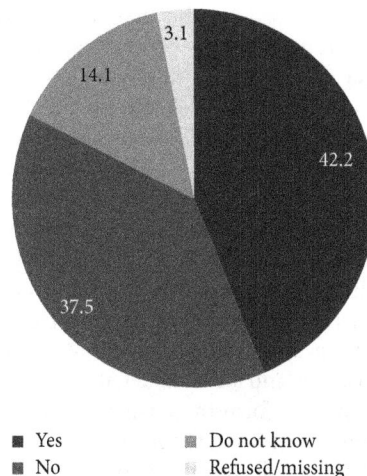

FIGURE 3: Aware that cervical cancer can be prevented by an HPV vaccine, among those who have heard of HPV, Odisha, India ($n = 64$).

cervical cancer in India. However, community awareness, health education, HPV vaccine, and a complementary robust screening program are essential for appropriate cervical cancer impact. Introduction of the HPV vaccine in exploratory studies of acceptance, safety, and immunogenicity in the Indian population are necessary before any consideration for government policy and development of cervical cancer prevention programs. Evaluation of acceptance by the community is necessary prior to the consideration of such clinical implementation studies [9].

The implementation of the HPV vaccine in Western countries has been surrounded by sociocultural issues raised by communities and in several countries, there has been no inclusion in government sponsored and mandated vaccination programs [10]. By extension of this concept, it is expected that there will be significant challenges to the introduction of the HPV vaccine in India where there is low awareness of human papillomavirus and link to cervical cancer. Further, there are challenges with the introduction of a sexually charged discussion with mothers of girls aged 10–14 years. In

addition to cultural issues, religion and the impact of public opinion are critical to the understanding of future methods of HPV vaccine implementation in India.

In developed countries, cervical cancer incidence and mortality have been significantly reduced following the introduction of screening and early detection using cytology. In the US, cytological screening was introduced using public health campaigns led by the American Cancer Society in the 1950s and steady decline in incidence has been observed [11]. Methods for screening were further refined using HPV typing which was introduced to practicing physicians in 1999 in the US. These introductions of new screening and early detection methodologies are accompanied by multimedia campaigns and grassroots advocacy to achieve universal acceptance by the physician and patient communities. Similarly, the introduction of the novel HPV vaccine is accompanied by multimedia campaigns, government policy supporting primary prevention, and the implementation of clinical procedures which allow for increased penetration of primary prevention into the developed world. Newer cervical cancer prevention strategies in the US are based on the potential for primary and secondary prevention using screening and treatment for women who are already infected with HPV and primary prevention using the HPV vaccine for girls in these same communities. This is the first cancer prevention strategy that utilizes robust interventions at the primary and secondary prevention levels and these strategies have enormous potential to reduce the burden of cervical cancer in areas with high incidence [12].

Utilizing the Western experience to extrapolate the understanding of cervical disease prevention to a medium resource country such as India, selecting a strategy that is universally accepted and has high effectiveness will demonstrate the greatest success in the reduction of cervical cancer. Thus, both cervical cancer screening and vaccination have the potential for success in decreasing the incidence, the morbidity, and mortality from cervical cancer. Further, these combined strategies will for the first time allow a shift in detection of advanced stages of cervical cancer to early detection of cervical precancer and reduce the development of cervical disease in girls who receive the HPV vaccine. Considering the advantages and disadvantages of both these strategies individually and collectively will lead to the highest likelihood of success. It is critically important to assess community awareness and sensibilities, combined with good science to guide the development of advocacy and policy which determines the most efficient methods applicable to India. Further, it is important to develop rigorous clinical implementation projects which are limited to a selected region of the country and focus on detailed information gathering which can then form the basis for informed decision making for communities and for governmental agencies [13].

Our Odisha data effectively produced a window into the selected community. Odisha is a site where there have been no government or industry sponsored campaigns to increase community level awareness of cervical cancer prevention and HPV. Thus, our project has the advantage of assessing a community prior to the introduction of educational processes to enhance community awareness and buy-in to cervical cancer prevention methods. Our project included a wide spectrum of women, from those presenting to the regional cancer center, and thus an already aware population, and women from the marketplace who formed a less targeted population. We also recruited women at the local government college where we were interested in the views of young educated women. Thus, the data presented here represents the opinions of a wide variety of women from the State of Odisha.

There was very low awareness of cervical cancer, of cervical cancer prevention, and of HPV and the link to cervical cancer. Interestingly, 12.2% of women had received the Pap smear and clearly there is scope in the rest of the interviewed women to increase the number of women screened by either cytology or HPV typing to ensure cervical cancer secondary prevention. There appeared great interest in disease prevention and our team assessed and were impressed by the proactive stance presented by women as an indicator of future receptivity to education strategies to enhance community awareness leading ultimately to acceptance of dual primary and secondary cervical cancer prevention strategies. There was high awareness of the value of vaccines in preventing disease and women interviewed were confident that they would make the decision for their families to vaccinate against disease. This is borne out in prior research, where women are known gatekeepers of the health of their families and make health related decisions for their family units. This also suggests that future educational campaigns for cervical cancer prevention should target women as recipients of health education and the development of decision support tools for women regarding cervical cancer screening and vaccination [14]. Cervical cancer reduction in India will reduce one quarter of the global burden of disease and impact the global community. It is encouraging that GAVI (The Vaccine Alliance) is considering the HPV vaccine for delivery to underserved populations globally and that discussions are ongoing. In order to decrease the incidence and ultimately to eliminate cervical cancer, new innovations such as the HPV vaccine have enormous potential for success in reducing global burden of disease.

6. Conclusion

The Odisha community surveyed demonstrated an acceptance of screening and vaccinations in the prevention of disease and identified mothers/guardians as the key family contacts. There is an opportunity to increase their knowledge of human papillomavirus, its link to cervical cancer, and the ability of the HPV screening and vaccine to prevent cervical cancer. This opportunity should be utilized to outreach and develop community awareness and encourage acceptance and adherence to three doses of the HPV vaccine and HPV screening to reduce cervical cancer.

Conflict of Interests

The authors declare that there is no conflict of interests regarding the publication of this paper.

Acknowledgment

Arnold P. Gold Foundation supported Aparna Ramaseshan to participate in this study.

References

[1] N. Bhatla, L. Dar, A. R. Patro et al., "Can human papillomavirus DNA testing of self-collected vaginal samples compare with physician-collected cervical samples and cytology for cervical cancer screening in developing countries?" *Cancer Epidemiology*, vol. 33, no. 6, pp. 446–450, 2009.

[2] P. Basu and D. Chowdhury, "Cervical cancer screening & HPV vaccination: a comprehensive approach to cervical cancer control," *Indian Journal of Medical Research*, vol. 130, no. 3, pp. 241–246, 2009.

[3] 2011, http://www.aiph.ac.in/.

[4] 2010, http://censusindia.net/.

[5] http://globocan.iarc.fr/Pages/fact_sheets_cancer.aspx.

[6] June 2011, http://ipsnews.net/news.asp?idnews=55833.

[7] 2011, http://samawomenshealth.wordpress.com/2011/05/26/the-hpv-vaccine-'demonstration-projects'/.

[8] H. J. Larson, P. Brocard, and G. Garnett, "The India HPV-vaccine suspension," *The Lancet*, vol. 376, no. 9741, pp. 572–573, 2010.

[9] R. Biellik, C. Levin, E. Mugisha et al., "Health systems and immunization financing for human papillomavirus vaccine introduction in low-resource settings," *Vaccine*, vol. 27, no. 44, pp. 6203–6209, 2009.

[10] J. W. Fisher and S. I. Brundage, "The challenge of eliminating cervical cancer in the United States: a story of politics, prudishness, and prevention," *Women and Health*, vol. 49, no. 2-3, pp. 246–261, 2009.

[11] A. Jemal, F. Bray, M. M. Center, J. Ferlay, E. Ward, and D. Forman, "Global cancer statistics," *CA— A Cancer Journal for Clinicians*, vol. 61, no. 2, pp. 69–90, 2011.

[12] S. Franceschi, L. Denny, K. L. Irwin et al., "Eurogin 2010 roadmap on cervical cancer prevention," *International Journal of Cancer*, vol. 128, no. 12, pp. 2765–2774, 2011.

[13] E. K. Proctor, J. Landsverk, G. Aarons, D. Chambers, C. Glisson, and B. Mittman, "Implementation research in mental health services: am emerging science with conceptual, methodological, and training challenges," *Administration and Policy in Mental Health and Mental Health Services Research*, vol. 36, no. 1, pp. 24–34, 2009.

[14] A. Shafer, J. R. Cates, S. J. Diehl, and M. Hartmann, "Asking mom: formative research for an HPV vaccine campaign targeting mothers of adolescent girls," *Journal of Health Communication*, vol. 16, no. 9, pp. 988–1005, 2011.

31

Birth Weight Ratio as an Alternative to Birth Weight Percentile to Express Infant Weight in Research and Clinical Practice: A Nationwide Cohort Study

Bart Jan Voskamp,[1] Brenda M. Kazemier,[1] Ewoud Schuit,[1,2] Ben Willem J. Mol,[3] Maarten Buimer,[4] Eva Pajkrt,[1] and Wessel Ganzevoort[1]

[1] *Department of Obstetrics and Gynecology, Room H4-232, Meibergdreef 9, Academic Medical Center, 1105 AZ Amsterdam, The Netherlands*
[2] *Julius Center for Health Sciences and Primary Care, University Medical Center Utrecht, Universiteitsweg 100, 3584 CG Utrecht, The Netherlands*
[3] *The Robinson Institute, School of Paediatrics and Reproductive Health, University of Adelaide, Adelaide, SA 5005, Australia*
[4] *Department of Obstetrics and Gynecology, Skaraborgs Sjukhus, Skövde, 541 85 Västra Götaland, Sweden*

Correspondence should be addressed to Bart Jan Voskamp; b.voskamp@amc.nl

Academic Editor: Gian Carlo Di Renzo

Objective. To compare birth weight ratio and birth weight percentile to express infant weight when assessing pregnancy outcome. *Study Design.* We performed a national cohort study. Birth weight ratio was calculated as the observed birth weight divided by the median birth weight for gestational age. The discriminative ability of birth weight ratio and birth weight percentile to identify infants at risk of perinatal death (fetal death and neonatal death) or adverse pregnancy outcome (perinatal death + severe neonatal morbidity) was compared using the area under the curve. Outcomes were expressed stratified by gestational age at delivery separate for birth weight ratio and birth weight percentile. *Results.* We studied 1,299,244 pregnant women, with an overall perinatal death rate of 0.62%. Birth weight ratio and birth weight percentile have equivalent overall discriminative performance for perinatal death and adverse perinatal outcome. In late preterm infants (33^{+0}–36^{+6} weeks), birth weight ratio has better discriminative ability than birth weight percentile for perinatal death (0.68 versus 0.63, P 0.01) or adverse pregnancy outcome (0.67 versus 0.60, $P < 0.001$). *Conclusion.* Birth weight ratio is a potentially valuable instrument to identify infants at risk of perinatal death and adverse pregnancy outcome and provides several advantages for use in research and clinical practice. Moreover, it allows comparison of groups with different average birth weights.

1. Introduction

Gestational age at delivery and birth weight are considered important predictors of adverse pregnancy outcome [1, 2]. Accurate assessment of fetal growth in relation to gestational age is therefore an important tool for risk assessment in antenatal care.

Fetal growth is usually expressed in percentiles. Birth weight percentile curves are calculated from cross-sectional data of newborns [3]. Thus, birth weight percentiles (BWpercentiles) indicate the value (e.g., 10%) below which a certain percentage of the observations in a group of newborns (10%) can be found. BWpercentiles are often dichotomized, and small for gestational age (SGA) is commonly defined as birth weight below the 10th, 5th, or 2.3th percentile for gestational age in a population-specific reference growth curve [4, 5]. The BWpercentile tells us if an infant belongs to a certain part of the percentile distribution but does not contain any information about the absolute deviation of infant weight from the median birth weight for gestation. As a result, percentiles do not allow comparison of growth between groups with different growth characteristics (e.g., different sexes or ethnicities). Moreover, at the tails of the normal distribution (e.g., at the 2nd percentile), a percentile contains a much wider range of absolute birth weights than close to the median (e.g., at the 50th percentile). Consequently, the use of percentiles and their dichotomization may lead to loss of information that may be useful for patient care and parental counseling.

Birth weight ratio (BWratio) is an alternative method to express growth of an individual with respect to the median. It is defined as the ratio of observed birth weight divided by the median birth weight of the population-specific reference growth curve. Values above 1 indicate "larger for gestational age than the median" and values below 1 indicate "smaller for gestational age than the median." It may offer a solution to the limitations associated with BWpercentiles.

Our objective was to compare BWratio and BWpercentile to express infant growth when assessing pregnancy outcome.

2. Materials and Methods

2.1. Dataset. This study was performed using a nationwide cohort using data from The Netherlands Perinatal Registry (PRN). The PRN consists of population-based data on pregnancies, deliveries, neonatal characteristics, and readmissions until 28 days after birth. The PRN database is obtained by a validated linkage of three different registries, the midwifery registry, the obstetrics registry, and the neonatology registry of hospital admissions of newborn neonates [6, 7]. Records are entered in the PRN registry at the child's level. The coverage of the PRN registry is approximately 96% of all deliveries in The Netherlands. It contains pregnancies of ≥ 22 weeks' gestation and a birth weight of ≥ 500 g and is used primarily for an annual assessment of the quality indicators of obstetric care.

2.2. Ethical Approval. The data in the perinatal registry are anonymous; therefore ethical approval was not needed. The Dutch Perinatal Registry gave their approval to use their data for this study (approval number 13.72).

2.3. Inclusion and Exclusion Criteria. We included all white women who delivered a singleton between 25^{+0} and 42^{+6} weeks gestation in The Netherlands between January 1, 1999, and December 31, 2007. All cases with congenital anomalies were excluded [8].

2.4. Outcome Measures. Outcome measures were perinatal death and a composite of perinatal death and neonatal morbidity. Perinatal death was defined as the sum of intrauterine fetal death (diagnosed after 25^{+0} weeks GA) and neonatal death (until 28 days after birth). The composite of adverse pregnancy outcome consisted of perinatal death, respiratory distress syndrome (RDS), sepsis, necrotizing enterocolitis (NEC), meconium aspiration, and intraventricular hemorrhage (IVH) within the first month of birth. If an infant suffered from neonatal morbidity and died within 28 days after birth, it was only considered as perinatal death in the analyses.

The Dutch reference curves for birth weight by gestational age stratified for parity, sex, and ethnic background were used [9]. Pregnancy dating was performed using last menstrual period (LMP) or by ultrasound measurements before 20 weeks of gestation (crown-rump-length (CRL) or head-circumference (HC) measurement).

We defined SGA as birth weight below the 10th or 5th percentile for gestation. To obtain the best possible comparability with SGA, low BWratio cut-off values of 0.85 and 0.80 were chosen such that (after rounding them to the closest 0.05 value) they resulted in equally large groups of low BWratio infants in the whole population as with the 10th and 5th birth weight percentiles.

We defined LGA as birth weight above the 90th or 95th percentile for gestation. To obtain the best possible comparability with LGA, high BWratio cut-off values 1.25 and 1.30 were chosen such that (after rounding them to the closest 0.05 value) they resulted in groups of high BWratio infants in the whole population that corresponds best with the 90th and 95th birth weight percentiles.

2.5. Population Characteristic and Clinical Characteristics. We registered demographic and obstetric characteristics including maternal age, parity, and socioeconomic status (SES) [10]. Parity was categorized into 0 (first birth), 1 (second birth), and 2+ (third or higher birth).

2.6. Statistics. Baseline characteristics were described and presented as means with standard deviations (SD), median with range, or percentages as appropriate.

We tested for interaction between BWratio and GA at delivery as well as BWpercentile and GA at delivery. These tests were performed separately for the two outcome measures. If statistically significant ($P < 0.05$), analyses were performed stratified for gestational age at delivery in four categories according to the WHO criteria, extremely preterm ($24^{+0}-27^{+6}$ weeks' gestation), very preterm ($28^{+0}-32^{+6}$ weeks' gestation), moderate to late preterm ($33^{+0}-36^{+6}$ weeks' gestation), and term delivery ($37^{+0}-42^{+6}$ weeks' gestation) [11].

We plotted distributions of perinatal death and adverse pregnancy outcome for BWratio and BWpercentile. In addition distributions of perinatal death and adverse pregnancy outcome stratified for gestational age at delivery for BWratio and BWpercentile were plotted.

We also calculated—separate for BWratio and BWpercentile and four strata of gestational age at birth—the population-attributable risk (PAR) of abnormal fetal growth for perinatal death and adverse pregnancy outcome. PAR was based on the prevalence (P) of abnormal growth and the relative risk (RR) of perinatal death and adverse pregnancy outcome in abnormally grown (low BWratio, SGA) and normally grown infants: PAR% = $[P * (RR - 1)/(P * (RR - 1) + 1)] * 100$ [12].

Finally, receiver operator characteristics (ROC) curves were constructed for the whole cohort and for abnormally grown infants only, to compare discriminative ability of birth weight ratio and birth weight percentile for our outcome

TABLE 1: Characteristics of the 1,299,244 pregnancies in the Netherlands, 1999–2007.

	Total ($n = 1,299,244$)
Maternal characteristics	
Maternal age, mean, (SD)	30.7 (4.58)
Nulliparous, %	47.5
Low socioeconomic status, %	18.9
Boys	51.3
Pregnancy and delivery	
Induction of labor, %	35.3
Cesarean section	14.3
Elective cesarean section %	6.2
Emergency cesarean section %	11.3
Vaginal instrumental delivery	12.4
Neonatal characteristics	
Gestational age at delivery (weeks), median (IQR)	39,2 (1.86)
Extremely premature (GA < 29^{+0} weeks), n (%)	4,048 (0.3)
Very premature (GA < 33^{+0} weeks), n (%)	13,885 (1.1)
Mild premature (GA < 37^{+0} weeks), n (%)	75,429 (5.81)

SD, standard deviation.

measures (perinatal death and adverse pregnancy outcome) in the four gestational categories. All statistical tests were 2-sided; a probability value of 0.05 was chosen as the threshold for statistical significance.

The data were analyzed with the SAS statistical software package (version 9.2; SAS Institute Inc., Cary, NC).

3. Results

From January 1, 1999 until December 31, 2007 a total of 1,636,565 pregnancies were registered in the PRN database. We excluded cases that were nonwhite (n = 258,908 (15.82%)), multiple pregnancies (n = 63,857 (3.90%)), infants with congenital anomalies (n = 22,043 (1.35%)), and infants born before 25^{+0} weeks or after 42^{+6} weeks GA (n = 6,967 (0.43%)). After application of the inclusion and exclusion criteria the study population consisted of 1,299,244 pregnancies. Baseline characteristics of the population are shown in Table 1.

3.1. Distribution of Cases. The distribution of birth weight ratios and birth weight percentiles for four strata of gestational age at birth is shown in Figures 1(a) and 1(b). Figure 1(a) shows that most infants are born with a BWratio around one and that both higher and lower BWratios are less common. Moreover, 80% of cases had a BWratio between 0.85 and 1.25. These infants occupy approximately one-third of the width of the graph, while the low BWratio and high BWratio infants occupy the remaining two-thirds. Hence, the spread in BWratio is much larger in the extremes of the birth weight ratio distribution than when using birth weight percentiles.

These characteristics of BWratio distributions make it possible to better distinguish between different degrees of low BWratios and high BWratios.

Figure 1(b) contains the distribution of birth weight percentiles and shows that the population is cut into 100 (approximately) equal parts. As a result, any given percentile always contains about 1% of the population. Consequently, the central 80% of the graph represents 80% of the population, while this only corresponds to approximately one-third of the BWratio distribution. Whereas SGA and LGA infants (20% of the population) logically cover 20% of the percentile distribution, while this group represents the remaining two-thirds of the BWratio distribution.

Figure 1(a) also shows that the BWratio of late premature (33^{+0}–36^{+6} weeks' gestation) and term (37^{+0}–42^{+6} weeks) infants is normally distributed. Distribution of the birth weight ratio of extremely premature (25^{+0}–28^{+6} weeks' gestation) or very premature infants (29^{+0}–32^{+6} weeks gestation) is negatively skewed.

3.2. Incidence of Abnormal Growth. The lines in Figure 1(a) suggest higher rates of low BWratios and high BWratios among infants that are born preterm. At term (37–42 weeks GA), 9.67% [118,331/1,223,815] of infants are born with a BWratio < 0.85. In the preterm period the incidences are significantly higher (P < 0.001) than in the term group, 17.04% [10,487/61,544] (33–36 weeks), 25.73% [2,531/9,837] (29–32 weeks), and 37.8% [1,530/4,084] (25–28 weeks), respectively.

At term (37–42 weeks GA), 6.64% [81,312/1,223,815] of infants are born with a high BWratio (>1.25). In the preterm period, the incidences are significantly higher (P < 0.001) than in the term group, 8.43% [5,188/61,544] (33–36 weeks), 18.39% [1,809/9,837] (29–32 weeks) and 16.48% [667/4,084] (25–28 weeks), respectively.

These findings confirm the presence of an association between prematurity and the incidence of abnormal growth (BWratio < 0.85 as well as BWratio > 1.25) [13–15].

3.3. Perinatal Death and Composite Morbidity. Incidences of perinatal death and adverse pregnancy outcome are shown in Figures 2 and 3. Incidences are shown separate for four strata of gestational age at birth, by birth weight ratios (Figures 2(a) and 3(a)), and birth weight percentiles (Figures 2(b) and 3(b)).

Comparison of mortality rates in Figures 2(a) and 2(b) shows that especially in the late preterm period (33–36 weeks) and at term (37–42 weeks) birth weight ratio allows more accurate differentiation between different SGA grades than birth weight percentiles. This is illustrated by Figure 2. Although it seems in Figure 2(b) that perinatal death between 33 and 36 weeks gestation does not rise above 10% in infants with a birth weight at the 1st percentile, Figure 2(a) shows that perinatal death rate rises until over 40%, depending on the severity of growth restriction.

On the other side of the growth spectrum, birth weight ratio also allows more precise differentiation between different severities of LGA.

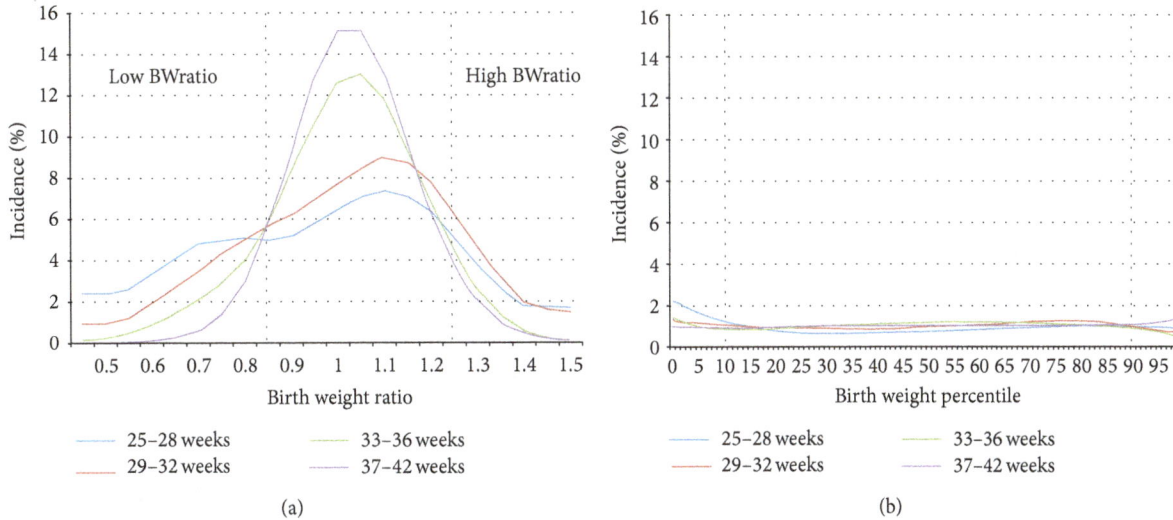

FIGURE 1: The incidence of birth weight ratios and birth weight percentiles for four strata of gestational age at birth separate for birth weight ratio (a) and birth weight percentiles (b).

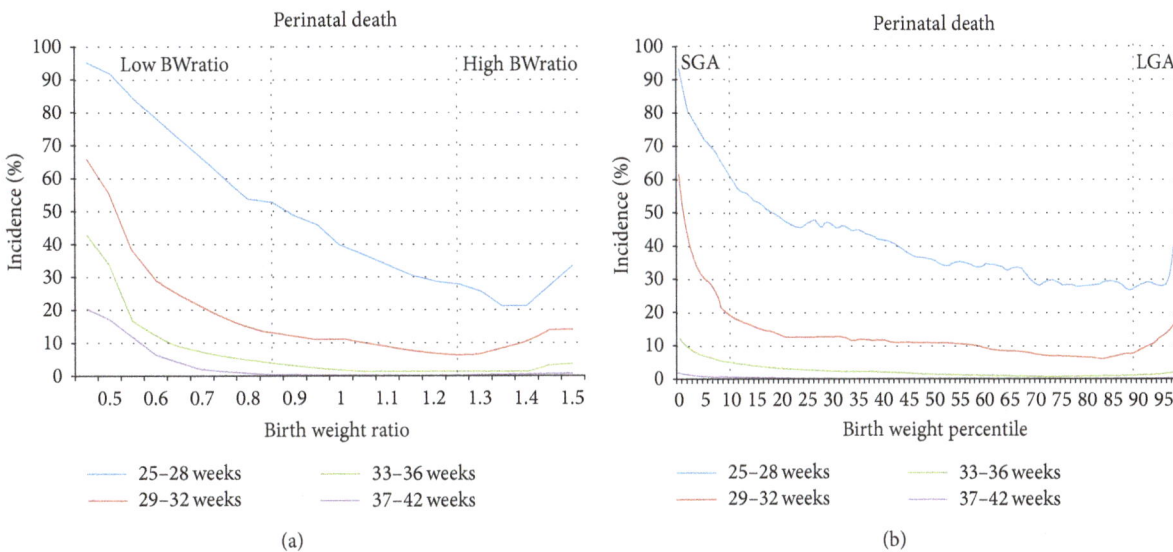

FIGURE 2: Incidences of perinatal death stratified by gestational age at delivery separate for birth weight ratio (a) and birth weight percentiles (b).

Both birth weight ratio and birth weight percentile show a gestation related death rate in the normal range (BWratio 0.85–1.25 and p10–p90, resp.) with higher death rates towards both ends of the growth spectrum. The same effects at the ends of the growth spectrum were found for adverse pregnancy outcome (Figures 3(a) and 3(b)).

3.4. Population-Attributive Risk of Abnormal Growth for Death and Adverse Pregnancy Outcome. The percentage of perinatal death and adverse pregnancy outcome that can be attributed to abnormal growth depends on gestational age at delivery, on whether abnormal growth is defined by BWratio (low/high BWratio) or BWpercentile (SGA/LGA), and on

the cut-off value that is used. PAR of abnormal fetal growth for perinatal death at different gestational ages is shown in Table 2. Depending on gestation and on the definition of abnormal growth, 14–35% of perinatal death and 2–13% of adverse pregnancy outcome can be attributed to abnormal growth.

The population-attributive risk of abnormal growth is higher for death than for adverse pregnancy outcome, which means that a larger percentage of perinatal deaths than adverse pregnancy outcome can be attributed to abnormal growth. PAR of suboptimal growth for perinatal death is small in extremely premature infants, increases with advancing gestational age with a peak in late preterm infants (33–36 weeks), and decrease at term.

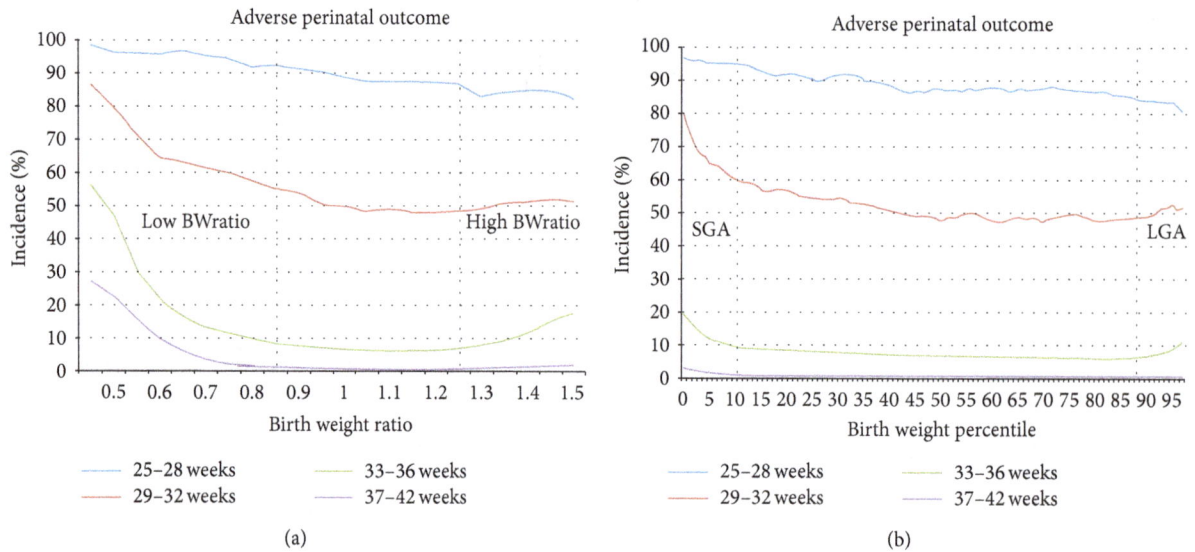

FIGURE 3: Incidences of adverse perinatal outcome stratified by gestational age at delivery separate for birth weight ratio (a) and birth weight percentiles (b).

TABLE 2: Population-attributive risk of abnormal fetal growth, for four definitions of abnormal growth by birth weight ratio and birth weight percentile.

	Population-attributive risk percentage (PAR%)			
	Birth weight ratio		Birth weight percentile	
	<0.80	<0.85	<p5	<p10
25–28 weeks				
Perinatal death	26	28	18	23
Composite adverse outcome	3	3	2	2
29–32 weeks				
Perinatal death	24	27	14	20
Composite adverse outcome	5	6	3	4
33–36 weeks				
Perinatal death	29	35	19	25
Composite adverse outcome	11	12	10	13
37–42 weeks				
Perinatal death	18	24	17	22
Composite adverse outcome	9	11	7	8

Also, PAR of abnormal growth, for example, for perinatal death at term, is higher if less stringent cut-off values to define abnormal growth are chosen (e.g., the 10th percentile instead of the 5th percentile, 22% versus 17%).

3.5. *Discriminative Ability of Birth Weight Ratio and Birth Weight Percentile.* The areas under the receiver operator characteristics curves are shown in Table 3. When assessing the complete growth spectrum, there were no differences in areas under the curve (AUC) between birth weight ratio and birth weight percentile to distinguish between those with and without perinatal death in extremely preterm, very preterm, late preterm, and term infants. Accordingly, the discriminative ability of birth weight ratio and birth weight

percentile for our composite adverse pregnancy outcome did not differ at any gestational age either. The discriminative ability of both methods for death was poor to fair (range 0.64–0.73), and the discriminative ability for adverse pregnancy outcome was bad to poor (range 0.55–0.65) [16].

When we assessed SGA cases only (birth weight below the 10th percentile), the discriminative ability of BWratio was better than that of BWpercentile for death in the late preterm period (33^{+0}–36^{+6} weeks) (0.68 versus 0.63, P 0.01) and at term (0.69 versus 0.67, P 0.05) (Table 4). The discriminative ability of BWratio was also better than that of BWpercentile for adverse pregnancy outcome in the late preterm period (33^{+0}–36^{+6} weeks) (0.67 versus 0.60, P < 0.001).

TABLE 3: Discriminative ability to predict perinatal death or adverse outcome of birth weight ratio and birth weight percentile.

	Area under the curve		P value
	Birth weight ratio	Birth weight percentile	
25–28 weeks			
Perinatal death	0.73	0.73	0.78
Composite adverse outcome	0.65	0.65	1.00
29–32 weeks			
Perinatal death	0.65	0.65	0.88
Composite adverse outcome	0.56	0.56	0.82
33–36 weeks			
Perinatal death	0.70	0.69	0.69
Composite adverse outcome	0.56	0.56	1.00
37–42 weeks			
Perinatal death	0.64	0.64	0.77
Composite adverse outcome	0.55	0.55	0.22

TABLE 4: Discriminative ability of birth weight ratio and birth weight percentile in case of birth weight below the 10th percentile for gestational age.

	Area under the curve		P value
	Birth weight ratio	Birth weight percentile	
25–28 weeks			
Perinatal death	0.70	0.76	0.09
Composite adverse outcome	0.61	0.63	0.75
29–32 weeks			
Perinatal death	0.69	0.68	0.67
Composite adverse outcome	0.61	0.58	0.43
33–36 weeks			
Perinatal death	0.68	0.63	**0.01**
Composite adverse outcome	0.67	0.60	**<0.001**
37–42 weeks			
Perinatal death	0.69	0.67	0.05
Composite adverse outcome	0.65	0.64	0.15

4. Discussion

Discriminative ability of BWratio for perinatal death or adverse pregnancy outcome is comparable to that of birth weight percentile. Birth weight ratio is—for smaller and larger than average infants—a more discriminative instrument for perinatal death and adverse pregnancy outcome than birth weight percentile.

Our findings confirm an association between abnormal fetal growth and premature delivery [13–15], and our data show that approximately one out of five perinatal deaths can be attributed to being SGA.

4.1. Limitations. Some limitations need to be addressed. First, a possible limitation is related to the use population-based birth weight percentiles. Although there exists no unanimity about the question whether references should be based on population birth weight characteristics or on individual growth potential, the latter might have better discriminative ability for adverse outcome [13, 17–23], both with BWratios and BWpercentiles. We were not able to use customized

growth curves because of maternal length and weight, and placental weight and pathology are not registered in the Dutch Perinatal Registry. Therefore the Dutch reference curves for birth weight by gestational age separate for parity, sex, and ethnic background were used [9]. We think however that not being able to use customized growth curves was only a minor limitation, because the concepts put forward in this paper can also be applied if growth is expressed using customized charts.

A second potential limitation is the use of preterm birth weight as standards for preterm BWratio. This might have led to an underestimation of the effect of prematurity on pregnancy outcome because—as this study shows—prematurity is associated with abnormal growth.

Finally, the PRN database does not contain data on how pregnancy dating is performed. Until 2011, no uniform pregnancy dating was performed in The Netherlands. Historically, it was common practice to date pregnancies based on LMP. Since the 1980's the use of ultrasound was gradually introduced in obstetric care. During our study period crown rump length and head circumference measurements had already increasingly replaced LMP for dating, but no quantitative data are available on how pregnancy was dated in individual cases. Inaccurate pregnancy dating might be partially responsible for the wider birth weight spread in the preterm period. However, this wider spread in the preterm period might also be the result of higher incidences of pathologically small or large growth, leading to preterm delivery.

4.2. Strengths. The main strength of this study is the size (1,299,244 pregnancies) and composition (only white women with a singleton without congenital anomalies) of the cohort. The incidence of fetal deaths, neonatal deaths, perinatal deaths, and composite morbidity that we found in this study is in accordance with previous research [24–29]. There is no reason to suspect a systematical gender or parity based bias. The concepts discussed in this paper can be used to assess distribution of growth and risk of abnormal growth and its relation to pregnancy outcome in other populations.

Data are derived from a large, well-maintained population-based national perinatal registry (1999–2007). The vast majority of the caregivers contribute to the PRN registry; therefore, it comprises approximately 96% of all pregnancy and birth characteristics in The Netherlands. The 4% missing birth data are due to 1-2% nonreporting general practitioners and 2-3% nonreporting midwives. The use of population-based growth curves for white mothers, separate for gender and parity, minimizes risk of systematic bias caused by one of these factors.

Finally, this is to our knowledge the first study that compared birth weight ratio and birth weight percentiles using ROC curves. This allowed us to statistically substantiate our findings.

4.3. Interpretation of the Results. As shown in Figure 1(b), only a distribution based on BWratio tells us how growth is distributed within a population. It shows that most infants are born with a birth weight ratio of around one, and incidences of BWratios decrease towards both ends of the distribution.

This study confirms that preterm delivery is associated with increased SGA and LGA rates as compared to term delivery [14, 15] and that the relation between fetal growth and the risk of adverse pregnancy outcome also depends on gestational age at delivery. This means that the relative risk of adverse outcome for an infant with a certain BWratio or BWpercentile at 30 weeks gestation is not the same as that at 40 weeks' gestation.

The results also show that birth weight ratios are not normally distributed in infants that are delivered extremely— or very preterm (25^{+0}–32^{+6} weeks) (Figure 1(a)). Percentiles are only suitable for use in a normally distributed population and are therefore less suitable to express growth in premature and extremely premature infants.

Finally, birth weight ratio allows comparison of groups with different average weights and weight distributions, for example, male infants and female infants or infants of different ethnic origins. Percentiles and ratios both allow comparison of groups, but—as explained before—information on distance from the mean and the incidence of different ratios within a population is lost when percentiles are used.

The different representation of growth with BWratio and BWpercentile that is explained above has two effects that result in better interpretability of infant growth when BWratio is used.

First, the use of BWpercentile causes a loss of discriminative power, especially among SGA and LGA infants. For example, all infants with birthweight <1st percentile (1% of the population and BWpercentile distribution) cover about 10% of the BWratio distribution, thus allowing better differentiation within this group of small infants with BWratio.

Second, birth weight percentiles suggest that an infant (born at term) with a birth weight at the 25th percentile is much lighter than an infant at the 75th percentile. However, this is not the case. The birth weight ratios in this example are 0.9 (25th percentile) and 1.1 (75th percentile) and are both very close to 1.0. The seemingly large difference if growth is expressed in percentiles is caused by the fact that a population is by definition divided into 100 equally large groups instead of groups based on birth weight in relation to the median and that most infants have a birth weight close to the median.

There are two reasons for the fact that neither BWpercentile nor BWratio has high sensitivity and specificity for death and adverse outcome and that only a limited proportion of death and adverse outcome can be attributed to fetal growth below the 10th percentile.

First, unlike other tests, increased risk of death (or adverse outcome) is not associated with a one-directional change in the risk factor (birth weight ratio or percentile). Both low and high birth weight ratios (or percentiles) are associated with increased risk of death (or adverse outcome).

Second, both death and adverse outcome occur at all gestational ages and across the whole growth spectrum. There seems to be a gestational age related basic risk (horizontal part of the line) with increased death and adverse outcome rates at both ends of the growth spectrum.

5. Conclusions

In view of the results we think that BWratio could complement BWpercentiles in clinical practice and can play a role in scientific research. It allows differentiation of SGA infants that is not possible with BWpercentile; it is easy to understand and therefore useful for patient counseling. This study provides in our opinion sufficient evidence for clinicians to use birth weight ratios when assessing risks of adverse outcome when an infant is suspected to be extremely small or large for gestation. Finally, birth weight ratio enables comparison of populations with different baseline characteristics.

This study shows the need to redefine cut-off values that define abnormal fetal growth. Historically, these cut-off values have been set at the 2.5th, 5th, and 10th percentile. However, this study shows that the relation between fetal growth and the risk of adverse pregnancy outcome differs depending on gestational age at delivery. Therefore, future research should focus on defining cut-off values to identify infants at risk of clinically relevant poor growth. To do this, consequences of abnormal growth should be weighed against potential treatment benefit of early detection and intervention, also taking into account costs of follow-up and potential adverse effects of interventions. Given the potentially better associations with adverse pregnancy outcome, such research should be performed using customized weight percentiles.

Conflict of Interests

The authors report no conflict of interests.

Acknowledgments

The authors thank all Dutch midwives, obstetricians, neonatologists, and other perinatal health care providers for the registration of perinatal information and the Foundation of The Netherlands Perinatal Registry (http://www.perinatreg.nl/) for permission to use the registry data.

References

[1] "Acog practice bulletin—clinical management guidelines for obstetrician-gynecologists-number 55, September 2004," *Obstetrics and Gynecology*, vol. 104, no. 3, pp. 639–645, 2004.

[2] S. M. Kady and J. Gardosi, "Perinatal mortality and fetal growth restriction," *Best Practice and Research: Clinical Obstetrics and Gynaecology*, vol. 18, no. 3, pp. 397–410, 2004.

[3] L. O. Lubchenco, C. Hansman, M. Dressler, and E. Boyd, "Intrauterine growth as estimated from liveborn birth-weight data at 24 to 42 weeks of gestation," *Pediatrics*, vol. 32, pp. 793–800, 1963.

[4] D. D. Mcintire, S. L. Bloom, B. M. Casey, and K. J. Leveno, "Birth weight in relation to morbidity and mortality among newborn infants," *The New England Journal of Medicine*, vol. 340, no. 16, pp. 1234–1238, 1999.

[5] H. Xu, F. Simonet, and Z.-C. Luo, "Optimal birth weight percentile cut-offs in defining small-or large-for-gestational-age," *Acta Paediatrica*, vol. 99, no. 4, pp. 550–555, 2010.

[6] N. Méray, J. B. Reitsma, A. C. J. Ravelli, and G. J. Bonsel, "Probabilistic record linkage is a valid and transparent tool to combine databases without a patient identification number," *Journal of Clinical Epidemiology*, vol. 60, no. 9, pp. 883–891, 2007.

[7] M. Tromp, A. C. J. Ravelli, N. Méray, J. B. Reitsma, and G. J. Bonsel, "An efficient validation method of probabilistic record linkage including readmissions and twins," *Methods of Information in Medicine*, vol. 47, no. 4, pp. 356–363, 2008.

[8] M. Tromp, M. Eskes, J. B. Reitsma et al., "Regional perinatal mortality differences in the Netherlands; care is the question," *BMC Public Health*, vol. 9, article 102, 2009.

[9] G. H. A. Visser, P. H. C. Eilers, P. M. Elferink-Stinkens, H. M. W. M. Merkus, and J. M. Wit, "New Dutch reference curves for birthweight by gestational age," *Early Human Development*, vol. 85, no. 12, pp. 737–744, 2009.

[10] Sociaal en Cultureel Planbureau, *Van Hoog Naar Laag; Van Laag Naar Hoog*, Sociaal en Cultureel Planbureau, 1998.

[11] "WHO: recommended definitions, terminology and format for statistical tables related to the perinatal period and use of a new certificate for cause of perinatal deaths. Modifications recommended by FIGO as amended October 14, 1976," *Acta Obstetricia et Gynecologica Scandinavica*, vol. 56, no. 3, pp. 247–253, 1977.

[12] O. S. Miettinen, "Proportion of disease caused or prevented by a given exposure, trait or intervention," *The American Journal of Epidemiology*, vol. 99, no. 5, pp. 325–332, 1974.

[13] J. Gardosi, "New definition of small for gestational age based on fetal growth potential," *Hormone Research*, vol. 65, no. 3, pp. 15–18, 2006.

[14] R. K. Tamura, R. E. Sabbagha, R. Depp, N. Vaisrub, S. L. Dooley, and M. L. Socol, "Diminished growth in fetuses born preterm after spontaneous labor or rupture of membranes," *The American Journal of Obstetrics and Gynecology*, vol. 148, no. 8, pp. 1105–1110, 1984.

[15] J. O. Gardosi, "Prematurity and fetal growth restriction," *Early Human Development*, vol. 81, no. 1, pp. 43–49, 2005.

[16] C. E. Metz, "Basic principles of Roc analysis," *Seminars in Nuclear Medicine*, vol. 8, no. 4, pp. 283–298, 1978.

[17] J. A. Hutcheon, H. McNamara, R. W. Platt, A. Benjamin, and M. S. Kramer, "Placental weight for gestational age and adverse perinatal outcomes," *Obstetrics and Gynecology*, vol. 119, no. 6, pp. 1251–1258, 2012.

[18] A. Ego, D. Subtil, G. Grange et al., "Customized versus population-based birth weight standards for identifying growth restricted infants: a French multicenter study," *The American Journal of Obstetrics and Gynecology*, vol. 194, no. 4, pp. 1042–1049, 2006.

[19] J. Gardosi and A. Francis, "Adverse pregnancy outcome and association with small for gestational age birthweight by customized and population-based percentiles," *The American Journal of Obstetrics and Gynecology*, vol. 201, no. 1, pp. 28.e1–28.e8, 2009.

[20] J. Gardosi, B. Clausson, and A. Francis, "The value of customised centiles in assessing perinatal mortality risk associated with parity and maternal size," *BJOG*, vol. 116, no. 10, pp. 1356–1363, 2009.

[21] C. L. D. De Jong, J. Gardosi, G. A. Dekker, G. J. Colenbrander, and H. P. Van Geijn, "Application of a customised birthweight standard in the assessment of perinatal outcome in a high risk population," *British Journal of Obstetrics and Gynaecology*, vol. 105, no. 5, pp. 531–535, 1998.

[22] L. M. E. McCowan, J. E. Harding, and A. W. Stewart, "Customised birthweight centiles predict SGA pregnancies with perinatal morbidity," *BJOG*, vol. 112, no. 8, pp. 1026–1033, 2005.

[23] F. Figueras, J. Figueras, E. Meler et al., "Customised birthweight standards accurately predict perinatal morbidity," *Archives of Disease in Childhood: fetal and Neonatal Edition*, vol. 92, no. 4, pp. F277–F280, 2007.

[24] R. Chibber, "Unexplained antepartum fetal deaths: What are the determinants?" *Archives of Gynecology and Obstetrics*, vol. 271, no. 4, pp. 286–291, 2005.

[25] B. L. Harlow, F. D. Frigoletto, D. W. Cramer et al., "Determinants of preterm delivery in low-risk pregnancies," *Journal of Clinical Epidemiology*, vol. 49, no. 4, pp. 441–448, 1996.

[26] A. Jakobovits, A. A. Jakobovits, and A. Viski, "Sex ratio of the stillborn fetuses and neonates dying in the first week," *Early Human Development*, vol. 15, no. 3, pp. 131–135, 1987.

[27] J. N. Quiñones, D. M. Stamilio, K. M. Coassolo, G. A. Macones, and A. O. Odibo, "Is fetal gender associated with adverse perinatal outcome in intrauterine growth restriction (IUGR)?" *The American Journal of Obstetrics and Gynecology*, vol. 193, no. 3, pp. 1233–1237, 2005.

[28] G. C. S. Smith, "Sex, birth weight, and the risk of stillbirth in Scotland, 1980–1996," *The American Journal of Epidemiology*, vol. 151, no. 6, pp. 614–619, 2000.

[29] H. I. J. Wildschut, V. Wiedijk, J. Oosting, W. Voorn, J. Huber, and P. E. Treffers, "Predictors of foetal and neonatal mortality in Curacao, Netherlands Antilles. A multivariate analysis," *Social Science and Medicine*, vol. 28, no. 8, pp. 837–842, 1989.

32

Safety and Efficacy of Ferric Carboxymaltose in Anemic Pregnant Women: A Retrospective Case Control Study

Anouk Pels and Wessel Ganzevoort

Department of Obstetrics and Gynecology, Academisch Medisch Centrum, Meibergdreef 9, 1105 AZ Amsterdam, Netherlands

Correspondence should be addressed to Anouk Pels; a.pels@amc.uva.nl

Academic Editor: Enrique Hernandez

Background. Anemia during pregnancy is commonly caused by iron deficiency and can have severe consequences for both the mother and the developing fetus. The aim of this retrospective study was to assess the safety and efficacy of intravenous ferric carboxymaltose (FCM) in pregnant women. *Methods*. All women treated with FCM for anemia during pregnancy between 2010 and 2012 at our institution were included. A matched control group was selected, including women who either were nonanemic or had anemia but were not considered for intravenous iron. Main outcome measures were maternal safety and pregnancy outcomes. *Results*. The study included 128 patients (FCM: 64; control: 64). Median FCM dose was 1000 mg and median gestational age at the time of first treatment was 34 weeks and 6 days. Median Hb increased from 8.4 g/dL (interquartile range 7.7; 8.9 g/dL) at the first FCM administration to 10.7 g/dL (9.8; 11.5 g/dL; $n = 46$ with available Hb at delivery) at the time of delivery, achieving levels similar to those in the control group (10.8 g/dL [9.8; 11.8 g/dL; $n = 48$]). No treatment-related adverse events were reported and no statistically significant differences in pregnancy outcomes were observed between groups. *Conclusions*. Within the limitations of this case control study, FCM was a safe and efficient treatment of anemia during pregnancy.

1. Introduction

Iron deficiency anemia is a prevalent condition during pregnancy and may result from different factors [1]. Many women have low or empty iron stores already at the start of pregnancy. A large French study, which included a total of 6648 women, showed depleted iron stores (serum ferritin <15 μg/L) in one out of five women (22.7%) of childbearing age [2]. During pregnancy, the physiological need for absorbed iron increases from 0.8 mg/day in the first trimester to 7.5 mg/day in the third trimester [3]. Dietary iron intake does not compensate for this strongly increased iron demand. Consequently, the risk of iron deficiency and, ultimately, iron deficient anemia increases during pregnancy.

General symptoms of anemia are fatigue, dizziness, and impaired immune response predisposing to infections [4]. Anemia during pregnancy is associated with increased morbidity and mortality of pregnant women and their developing fetuses [5]. Iron deficiency anemia has been shown to be associated with an increased risk of premature birth and low birth weight [6], preeclampsia [7], placental abruption, and increased peripartum blood loss [8] as well as cardiac failure and related death [9–11].

In pregnant women, oral iron is often used for prophylaxis of iron deficiency and is recommended as first-line treatment for pregnant women with iron deficiency anemia [12]. However, oral iron substitution has shown to be insufficient for the treatment of severe iron deficiency anemia and is often associated with gastrointestinal side effects [13]. Therefore, guidelines recommend that physicians consider intravenous (i.v.) iron administration in pregnant women with severe iron deficiency anemia (Hb < 9.0 g/dL), and in case of intolerability to oral iron as well, insufficient Hb increase after oral iron treatment or if there is a need for rapid Hb reconstitution [12–14]. Intravenous (i.v.) iron preparations provide greater and more rapid repletion of iron stores than oral iron therapy without the gastrointestinal side effects associated with oral substitution [13].

Ferric carboxymaltose (FCM) is an i.v. iron formulation which can be used at high doses and allows rapid administration (up to 1000 mg in a single dose infused in 15 min). Because it is free of dextran and its derivatives, FCM does not cross-react with dextran antibodies [15, 16] and never needed the administration of a test dose. More recently, the European Medicines Agency (EMA) concluded that no test dose should apply to i.v. iron products authorized in the European Union; yet staff and facilities to evaluate and manage anaphylactic or anaphylactoid reactions should be immediately available [17]. The FCM molecules consist of an iron-hydroxide core chelated in a carbohydrate shell and this complex is taken up as a whole by macrophages, leading to very low levels of non-transferrin bound iron, avoiding iron toxicity and oxidative stress [16]. FCM's clinical efficacy and safety have been proven in several large clinical studies across different indications with up to one-year follow-up in severe disease types such as chronic kidney disease and chronic heart failure [18–28]. At least four postpartum studies compared the safety and efficacy of FCM versus oral iron [26–29]. Faster and greater Hb-responses were achieved in FCM-treated patients compared to those receiving oral iron and FCM replenished iron stores efficiently. Rather few studies or cases with limited numbers of FCM-treated pregnant women have been reported [30–33]. A recently completed study comparing FCM and oral iron in pregnant women with iron deficiency anemia (ClinicalTrials.gov NCT01131624) has not been reported yet.

The aim of this retrospective case control study was to assess the efficacy of i.v. FCM in pregnant women.

2. Materials and Methods

2.1. Study Design and Patients. Data for this retrospective case control study were obtained from the electronic patient charts of the Department of Obstetrics and Gynecology of the Academisch Medisch Centrum in Amsterdam, Netherlands. The study design has been reviewed by the Medical Ethical Committee of the Academisch Medisch Centrum and it was confirmed that an official approval of this study by the committee is not required, since the Medical Research Involving Human Subjects Act (WMO) does not apply.

Patients were identified by searching the digital records of the Department of Obstetrics and Gynecology for women who received FCM (Ferinject, Vifor Pharma Ltd., Switzerland) treatment and/or delivered a baby between 2010 and 2012. All women who received at least one administration of FCM during their pregnancy were eligible for the case group. Women who were treated with FCM in the postpartum period were excluded from the analysis group, but safety data were collected. The control group was formed by an equal number of pregnant women who either were nonanemic or had anemia to a lesser degree not necessitating i.v. iron treatment. The women in the control group were matched to the case group for delivery period, type of comorbidity, age, parity, and number of fetuses.

2.2. Treatment Characteristics. Pregnant patients with anemia were treated according to the local protocol. The institutional anemia cutoff value throughout advanced gestation is approximately 9.7 g/dL (1.0 g/dL = 0.62 mmol/L). According to the local protocol, pregnant women with anemia are treated with oral iron (ferrous fumarate, one 200 mg tablet per day) and switched to i.v. iron, if Hb remains <9.7 g/dL despite oral medication. FCM is the institution's first choice i.v. iron agent since 2010, regardless of iron status. The local protocol does not describe the time frame in which the Hb should increase to above 9.7 g/dL. The maximum weekly dose of FCM is 1000 mg (up to 20 mg/kg body weight) in a single infusion given over at least 15 minutes.

2.3. Outcome Measures. Demographic characteristics and baseline data included maternal age, gestational age, educational level, and results from peripheral blood counts. Outcome data were collected on adverse events and pregnancy outcomes. Adverse events (AEs) in FCM-treated patients were defined as allergic or hypersensitivity reactions during or after the infusion of FCM. Assessed pregnancy outcomes were hospital admission (before delivery, for other reasons than FCM administration), intensive care unit admission, intrauterine growth restriction (IUGR), hypertension/preeclampsia, placental abruption, major adverse outcomes (maternal or fetal), minor maternal adverse outcomes, Hb at delivery (g/dL), need for red blood cell transfusion, gestational age at delivery, mode of delivery, estimated blood loss during delivery, fetal weight (g), and neonatal Apgar score.

Major maternal adverse outcomes were defined as death, stroke, neurological symptoms, severe preeclampsia, HELLP (Hemolysis Elevated Liver enzymes Low Platelets) syndrome, and delivery before 34 weeks of gestation. Major adverse fetal outcomes were defined as death, respiratory problems (requiring intubation), neonatal intensive care unit admission, pneumonia, morbidity requiring surgery, birth problems, and Apgar score <7.

The charts were liberally screened for minor adverse outcomes with an inclusive strategy, to include a variety of nonprespecified events.

The local protocol for iron treatment requires minimal diagnostics and follow-up assessment of hematologic iron status parameters. For this reason, Hb measurements and Mean Corpuscular Volume (MCV) were recorded at FCM treatment (in the case group) and Hb measurements at delivery (in case and control group).

2.4. Statistical Analysis. No formal sample size calculation was made, since all FCM-treated women who fulfilled the inclusion criteria were included. Statistical analysis was performed using IBM SPSS Statistics. Safety and efficacy were analyzed using descriptive statistics, comparing the case group to the control group. For the case group, medians have been calculated for the dose, the gestational age at treatment, and Hb at treatment with FCM. For statistical comparison,

t-test and Chi-Square test were used, where appropriate. p values < 0.05 were considered statistically significant.

3. Results

We identified 85 women who received FCM between 2010 and 2012 at our institution. Three women were excluded from the study, since they were not pregnant during the treatment with FCM, and 18 women received FCM postpartum. Sixty-four women received at least one FCM administration during pregnancy and were included in the case group. These patients were matched with 64 controls.

Demographic characteristics such as age (median: 27 years versus 28 years), parity (median 1 versus 1), number of fetuses (singleton pregnancies: 92% versus 92%), percentage of patients with lower educations (20% versus 16%), and prevalence of comorbidities (20% versus 19%) were similar between case and control groups (Table 1). Individual comorbidities were present at low frequency and none of the comorbidities was dominant (1-2 patients per comorbidity). Of note, there were significantly more women of Caucasian origin in the control group (34% versus 7.8%) and more patients were affected by a familial disease in the case group (59% versus 38%). The most frequent familial disease was concomitant hypertension and diabetes (28% in the case group and 20% in the control group). No information about dietary habits or other lifestyle interventions was recorded.

The median FCM dose in the case group was 1000 mg (interquartile range [IQR]: 1000; 1500) and most women (51/64) received only one dose of FCM (Table 2). The maximum number of administered FCM treatments was three (in 3 out of 64 patients) due to persistent anemia. Median gestational age at the time of the first treatment was 244 days (IQR 224; 256 days). Median Hb at first FCM administration was 8.4 g/dL (IQR: 7.7; 8.9 g/dL) and increased to 10.7 g/dL (IQR: 9.8; 11.5 g/dL) at the time of delivery, achieving a similar level as in the control group (10.8 g/dL [IQR: 9.8; 11.8 g/dL]) (Table 3).

No treatment-related adverse events were reported in the case group. Of note, FCM was also used by 18 women in the postpartum period, mostly after postpartum hemorrhage. These women were not included in the case group but their charts were reviewed for adverse events related to the treatment with FCM. In the women who used FCM postpartum no serious adverse events (allergic or hypersensitivity reactions) were reported.

No statistically significant differences were seen in the pregnancy outcomes between groups (Table 3). Major adverse outcomes in the case group were delivery before 34 weeks of gestation ($n = 5$), death of the fetus ($n = 3$), atrioventricular septal defect ($n = 1$), respiratory problems ($n = 1$), pneumonia and skin abnormalities ($n = 1$), and Apgar score <7 ($n - 1$). Major adverse outcomes in the control group were severe preeclampsia ($n = 1$), HELLP syndrome ($n = 3$), encephalopathy with hepatic dysfunction ($n = 1$), delivery before 34 weeks of gestation ($n = 5$), death of the fetus ($n = 3$), neonatal intensive care unit admission ($n = 2$), respiratory problems ($n = 1$), jejunum resection ($n = 1$),

TABLE 1: Demographics.

Characteristics*	Case group ($n = 64$)	Control group ($n = 64$)	p value
Age, years	27 [17–39]	28 [17–40]	0.71
Parity, n	1 [0–4]	1 [0–4]	0.87
Ethnicity			
Caucasian	5 (8%)	22 (34%)	
African descent	38 (59%)	15 (23%)	0.00
Other	11 (17%)	16 (25%)	
Unknown	10 (16%)	11 (17%)	
Education level			
Lower education	13 (20%)	10 (16%)	
Middle education	21 (33%)	12 (19%)	0.18
Higher education	7 (11%)	12 (19%)	
Unknown	23 (36%)	29 (46%)	
Comorbidities†			
Overall	13 (20%)	12 (19%)	
Preexisting hypertension	1 (2%)	2 (3%)	
Preexisting diabetes	1 (2%)	2 (3%)	
Renal/liver transplant	1 (2%)	0	
Renal malignancy in the past	1 (2%)	1 (2%)	
Irritable bowel syndrome	0	1 (2%)	
Uterus myomatosus	2 (3%)	1 (2%)	
Primary hyperoxaluria type 1	1 (2%)	0	0.12
Asthma	1 (2%)	1 (2%)	
Hypothyroidism	2 (3%)	1 (2%)	
Sickle cell anemia	2 (3%)	1 (2%)	
Rheumatoid arthritis	1 (2%)	0	
Ehlers-Danlos type III	0	1 (2%)	
Alpha thalassemia	0	1 (2%)	
HIV infection	1 (2%)	1 (2%)	
IL-12 receptor deficiency	0	1 (2%)	
Unknown	4	0	
Familial diseases			
None	14 (22%)	36 (56%)	
Hypertension	14 (22%)	8 (13%)	
Diabetes	6 (9%)	3 (5%)	0.00
Hypertension and diabetes	18 (28%)	13 (20%)	
Unknown	12 (19%)	4 (6%)	
Number of fetuses			
Singleton pregnancy	59 (92%)	59 (92%)	1.00
Twin pregnancy	5 (8%)	5 (8%)	

*Data shown as median [range] or n (%); †patients could have more than one comorbidity.

severe shoulder dystocia ($n = 1$), tachycardia, low saturation and hepatomegaly ($n = 1$), and Apgar score <7 ($n = 2$).

TABLE 2: Treatment characteristics of the case group ($n = 64$) treated with FCM.

Treatment characteristics[*]	
Hb at 1st FCM treatment, g/dL ($n = 62$)[†]	8.4 [7.7; 8.9]
Hb at 1st FCM treatment, mmol/L ($n = 62$)[†]	5.2 [4.8; 5.5]
MCV at 1st FCM treatment, fL ($n = 49$)[†]	69 [62; 76]
Gestational age at 1st treatment, weeks ($n = 64$)[‡]	34 + 6 [32; 36 + 4]
Gestational age at 2nd treatment, weeks ($n = 13$)[‡]	35 + 2 [32 + 6; 37 + 3]
Gestational age at 3rd treatment, weeks ($n = 3$)[‡]	32 [N/E]
Total dose received, mg	1000 [1000; 1500]
Treatment-related adverse outcomes reported	0 (0%)
Treatment-related serious adverse outcomes	0 (0%)

[*]Data shown as median [IQR] or n (%); [†]patients with available data (for remainder of study population not reported); [‡]total number of patients receiving treatment; Hb: hemoglobin; MCV: mean corpuscular volume; IQR: interquartile range.

TABLE 3: Pregnancy outcomes in cases and controls.

Pregnancy outcome[*]	Case group ($n = 64$)	Control group ($n = 64$)	p value
Hospital admission ($n = 126$)[†]	27 (42%)	20 (31%)	0.13
ICU admission ($n = 127$)[†]	1 (2%)	2 (3%)	0.51
IUGR ($n = 127$)[†]	2 (3%)	5 (8%)	0.30
Hypertension/preeclampsia ($n = 126$)[†]	8 (13%)	9 (14%)	0.36
Placental abruption ($n = 126$)[†]	1 (2%)	0 (0%)	0.22
Median Hb at delivery, g/dL ($n = 94$)[†]	10.7 [9.8; 11.5]	10.8 [9.8; 11.8]	0.76
Median Hb at delivery, mmol/L ($n = 94$)[†]	6.7 [6.1; 7.1]	6.7 [6.1; 7.3]	0.76
Unknown Hb at delivery	18 (28%)	16 (25%)	
Major adverse outcome ($n = 128$)[†]			
Maternal only	3 (5%)	4 (6%)	
Fetal only	5 (8%)	5 (8%)	0.50
Maternal and fetal	2 (3%)	6 (9%)	
Minor maternal outcome[‡] ($n = 127$)[†]	23 (36%)	18 (28%)	0.36
Need for transfusion of blood products ($n = 125$)[†]	2 (3%)	3 (5%)	0.20
Gestational age at delivery, weeks ($n = 124$)[†]	39.2 [38.0; 40.3]	39.1 [36.7; 39.9]	0.18
Mode of delivery ($n = 126$)[†]			
Spontaneous vaginal	46 (72%)	39 (61%)	
Assisted vaginal	2 (3%)	5 (8%)	0.29
Primary Caesarean	9 (14%)	12 (19%)	
Secondary Caesarean	5 (8%)	8 (13%)	
Blood loss during delivery, mL ($n = 124$)[†]	300 [200; 400]	300 [200; 538]	0.64
Fetal weight, g ($n = 128$)[†]			
Singleton babies	3235 [3025; 3565]	3210 [2710; 3500]	0.64
Twin babies	2400 [1872; 2721]	2343 [1675; 2618]	0.33
Apgar score ($n = 125$)[†]			
Singleton babies	10 [10; 10]	10 [9; 10]	0.73
Twin babies	9 [7; 10]	9 [7; 10]	0.92

[*]Data shown as median [IQR] or n (%); [†]patients with available data (for remainder of study population not reported/unknown).

[‡]Minor maternal outcomes: malaise (2 in case group), abdominal pain (3 in case group, 2 in control group), nausea and vomiting of pregnancy (NVP) (3 in case group, 3 in control group), premature contractions (3 in case group), Preterm Premature Rupture Of Membranes (PPROM) (4 in case group, 5 in control group), impaired renal function (1 in case group), meconium amniotic (1 in case group), vaginal blood loss (1 in case group, 1 in control group), preeclampsia (3 in case group), hypertension (2 in case group, 3 in control group), severe hypertension (1 in case group), postpartum hypertension (1 in control group), fever (2 in case group), postpartum fever (2 in control group), urinary tract infection (2 in case group), trauma (1 in case group), reduced signs of fetal life (2 in case group), back pain (1 in case group), tachycardia (1 in case group), gestational diabetes (2 in case group, 1 in control group), herpes gestationis (1 in case group), gestational pyelitis (1 in control group), pulmonary embolism (1 in control group), and positive discongruence (1 in control group).

Hb: hemoglobin; IQR: interquartile range; ICU: intensive care unit; IUGR: intrauterine growth retardation.

4. Discussion

This case control study investigated the efficacy and safety of FCM during pregnancy. FCM treatment efficiently increased Hb in the case group from baseline to delivery to similar levels as were present in the control group. There were no hypersensitivity reactions, anaphylactic reactions, or other adverse events reported with FCM treatment, neither in the case group nor in the group who received FCM postpartum. Maternal and fetal outcomes were similar between the case and the control group.

Most women received only a single dose of 1000 mg iron which is in line with the institution's protocol. Only a minority of women required more than one FCM administration due to persistent anemia (maximum of three iron administrations in three women). This practice of single dose administration is facilitated by the greater stability of the FCM complex compared to less stable i.v. iron compounds such as ferric gluconate and iron sucrose that require multiple administrations of lower doses.

Our results are in line with a number of randomized controlled studies which have shown the safe and efficient use of FCM in the field of gynecology during the postpartum period [26–29] and in heavy uterine bleeding [22]. Randomized controlled studies on the use of FCM during pregnancy are, to date, lacking. In a retrospective study, Christoph et al. [30] showed that, in the second and third trimester, FCM was equally well tolerated as i.v. iron sucrose and demonstrated comparable rates of adverse events (8% FCM; 11% iron sucrose). All adverse events were classified as mild and quickly reversible and included local reactions (such as pain and rash at the injection site) and systemic effects (such as transient hypotension, dizziness, heart palpitation, nausea, and headache). However, the two groups of pregnant women were heterogeneous in i.v. iron treatment indication and therefore not really comparable, regarding pregnancy complications. A study by Myers et al. [31] comparing FCM to iron hydroxide dextran treatment showed similar results regarding adverse events and treatment effect but no pregnancy outcomes were reported. Froessler et al. [32] performed a prospective observational study including 65 anemic pregnant women who received FCM. In this patient group, Hb levels significantly increased after FCM treatment and 66% of women reported an improvement of their well-being after the infusion. No serious adverse effects were reported. Minor side effects occurred in 13 (20%) patients and were self-limiting except for one case of nausea and vomiting which required medication. Froessler et al. also published two case reports of anemia successfully treated using ferric carboxymaltose in the peripartum period [33].

There were some noteworthy differences in the baseline characteristics between the case and the control group in our study. Firstly, the case group contained more women of ethnic minorities which generally have a lower socioeconomic status and worse general health than women of Caucasian ethnicity in our population. Secondly, the case group contained more women with familial hypertension/diabetes than the control group. In addition, women in the control group either were nonanemic or had anemia to a lesser degree than the case group. The expected direction of bias caused by these described differences between case and control group would be to the disadvantage of the case group. In spite of these apparent disadvantages in the case group, we found that pregnancy outcomes were similar in case and control group.

Due to the retrospective case control design, our study has some limitations. Choosing adequate controls in a case control design is difficult. For the control group, we could also have chosen women with a similar degree of anemia as the case group, receiving either no or alternative medication, but these groups are not easily identified and comparisons are subject to indication bias. Due to the retrospective data collection, not all of the assessed parameters were available for all patients and consequently, numbers/medians of certain parameters were based on less than 128 patients (e.g., ethnicity, level of education, familial diseases, and Hb at delivery). Data on additional iron status parameters such as serum ferritin (indicating stored iron) or transferring saturation (indicating iron available for erythropoiesis) would have been useful but these were not required by the local protocol.

While we would not expect any serious events in our case group due to the low patient number ($n = 64$) and the rarity of such events (life threatening adverse events related to i.v. iron preparations generally occur at a rate of 0.6–11 per million patients depending on the i.v. iron compound [31]), we suspect that mild and transient adverse events were underreported in the analyzed patient charts.

5. Conclusions

In conclusion, FCM was effective in treating anemia in this population of pregnant women in the 3rd trimester and appears to be safe for mother and child, although no definite conclusion about safety can be drawn from the results of this small case group. A prospective randomized controlled trial is warranted for a more detailed analysis on pregnancy outcomes.

Conflict of Interests

The conduct of the study was supported by an unrestricted grant from Vifor Pharma Ltd., Netherlands, to Wessel Ganzevoort. No competing interests exist.

Acknowledgments

Thierry Barten (Vifor Pharma Ltd., Netherlands) reviewed and commented on the paper. Editorial support was provided by Bettina Barton (SFL Regulatory Affairs & Scientific Communications, Switzerland). This did not alter the author's adherence to all the policies on sharing data and materials.

References

[1] R. L. Bergmann, J. W. Dudenhausen, J. C. Ennen et al., "Diagnosis and treatment of iron deficiency and anaemia during pregnancy and post partum," *Geburtshilfe und Frauenheilkunde*, vol. 69, no. 8, pp. 682–686, 2009.

[2] P. Galan, H. C. Yoon, P. Preziosi et al., "Determining factors in the iron status of adult women in the SU.VI.MAX study. SUpplementation en VItamines et Minéraux AntioXydants," *European Journal of Clinical Nutrition*, vol. 52, no. 6, pp. 383–388, 1998.

[3] N. Milman, T. Bergholt, K.-E. Byg, L. Eriksen, and N. Graudal, "Iron status and iron balance during pregnancy. A critical reappraisal of iron supplementation," *Acta Obstetricia et Gynecologica Scandinavica*, vol. 78, no. 9, pp. 749–757, 1999.

[4] L. H. Allen, "Anemia and iron deficiency: effects on pregnancy outcome," *The American Journal of Clinical Nutrition*, vol. 71, no. 5, pp. 1280s–1284s, 2000.

[5] J. F. Murphy, R. G. Newcombe, J. O'Riordan, E. C. Coles, and J. F. Pearson, "Relation of haemoglobin levels in first and second trimesters to outcome of pregnancy," *The Lancet*, vol. 327, no. 8488, pp. 992–995, 1986.

[6] T. O. Scholl, "Iron status during pregnancy: setting the stage for mother and infant," *The American Journal of Clinical Nutrition*, vol. 81, no. 5, pp. 1218s–1222s, 2005.

[7] N. Milman, A. O. Agger, and O. J. Nielsen, "Iron status markers and serum erythropoietin in 120 mothers and newborn infants. Effect of iron supplementation in normal pregnancy," *Acta Obstetricia et Gynecologica Scandinavica*, vol. 73, no. 3, pp. 200–204, 1994.

[8] D. L. Arnold, M. A. Williams, R. S. Miller, C. Qiu, and T. K. Sorensen, "Iron deficiency anemia, cigarette smoking and risk of abruptio placentae," *Journal of Obstetrics and Gynaecology Research*, vol. 35, no. 3, pp. 446–452, 2009.

[9] L. Reveiz, G. M. Gyte, L. G. Cuervo, and A. Casasbuenas, "Treatments for iron-deficiency anaemia in pregnancy," *Cochrane Database of Systematic Reviews*, no. 10, Article ID CD003094, 2011.

[10] F. E. Viteri, "The consequences of iron deficiency and anaemia in pregnancy on maternal health, the foetus and the infant," *SCN News*, no. 11, pp. 14–18, 1994.

[11] J. Villar, M. Merialdi, A. M. Gülmezoglu et al., "Nutritional interventions during pregnancy for the prevention or treatment of maternal morbidity and preterm delivery: an overview of randomized controlled trials," *The Journal of Nutrition*, vol. 133, no. 5, supplement 2, pp. 1606s–1625s, 2003.

[12] C. Breymann, C. Honegger, W. Holzgreve, and D. Surbek, "Diagnosis and treatment of iron-deficiency anaemia during pregnancy and postpartum," *Archives of Gynecology and Obstetrics*, vol. 282, no. 5, pp. 577–580, 2010.

[13] N. Milman, "Prepartum anaemia: prevention and treatment," *Annals of Hematology*, vol. 87, no. 12, pp. 949–959, 2008.

[14] P. Beris and A. Maniatis, "Guidelines on intravenous iron supplementation in surgery and obstetrics/gynecology," *Transfusion Alternatives in Transfusion Medicine*, vol. 9, pp. 29–30, 2007.

[15] S. Neiser, M. Wilhelm, K. Schwarz, F. Funk, P. Geisser, and S. Burckhardt, "Assessment of dextran antigenicity of intravenous iron products by an immunodiffusion assay," *Portuguese Journal of Nephrology and Hypertension*, vol. 25, no. 3, pp. 219–224, 2011.

[16] P. Geisser, "The pharmacology and safety profile of ferric carboxymaltose (Ferinject): structure/reactivity relationships of iron preparations," *Portuguese Journal of Nephrology and Hypertension*, vol. 23, no. 1, pp. 11–16, 2009.

[17] European Medicines Agency (EMA), *Assessment Report for: Iron Containing Intravenous (IV) Medicinal Products*, 2013, http://www.ema.europa.eu/docs/en_GB/document_library/Referrals_document/IV_iron_31/WC500150771.pdf.

[18] S. Kulnigg, S. Stoinov, V. Simanenkov et al., "A novel intravenous iron formulation for treatment of anemia in inflammatory bowel disease: the ferric carboxymaltose (FERINJECT) randomized controlled trial," *American Journal of Gastroenterology*, vol. 103, no. 5, pp. 1182–1192, 2008.

[19] T. Steinmetz, B. Tschechne, O. Harlin et al., "Clinical experience with ferric carboxymaltose in the treatment of cancer- and chemotherapy-associated anaemia," *Annals of Oncology*, vol. 24, no. 2, Article ID mds338, pp. 475–482, 2013.

[20] R. Evstatiev, P. Marteau, T. Iqbal et al., "FERGIcor, a randomized controlled trial on ferric carboxymaltose for iron deficiency anemia in inflammatory bowel disease," *Gastroenterology*, vol. 141, no. 3, pp. 846–853.e2, 2011.

[21] S. D. Anker, J. C. Colet, G. Filippatos et al., "Ferric carboxymaltose in patients with heart failure and iron deficiency," *The New England Journal of Medicine*, vol. 361, no. 25, pp. 2436–2448, 2009.

[22] D. B. Van Wyck, A. Mangione, J. Morrison, P. E. Hadley, J. A. Jehle, and L. T. Goodnough, "Large-dose intravenous ferric carboxymaltose injection for iron deficiency anemia in heavy uterine bleeding: a randomized, controlled trial," *Transfusion*, vol. 49, no. 12, pp. 2719–2728, 2009.

[23] W. Y. Qunibi, C. Martinez, M. Smith, J. Benjamin, A. Mangione, and S. D. Roger, "A randomized controlled trial comparing intravenous ferric carboxymaltose with oral iron for treatment of iron deficiency anaemia of non-dialysis-dependent chronic kidney disease patients," *Nephrology Dialysis Transplantation*, vol. 26, no. 5, pp. 1599–1607, 2011.

[24] A. Covic and G. Mircescu, "The safety and efficacy of intravenous ferric carboxymaltose in anaemic patients undergoing haemodialysis: a multi-centre, open-label, clinical study," *Nephrology Dialysis Transplantation*, vol. 25, no. 8, pp. 2722–2730, 2010.

[25] G. R. Bailie, N. A. Mason, and T. G. Valaoras, "Safety and tolerability of intravenous ferric carboxymaltose in patients with iron deficiency anemia," *Hemodialysis International*, vol. 14, no. 1, pp. 47–54, 2010.

[26] M. H. Seid, R. J. Derman, J. B. Baker, W. Banach, C. Goldberg, and R. Rogers, "Ferric carboxymaltose injection in the treatment of postpartum iron deficiency anemia: a randomized controlled clinical trial," *American Journal of Obstetrics and Gynecology*, vol. 199, no. 4, pp. 435.e7–437.e7, 2008.

[27] D. B. Van Wyck, M. G. Martens, M. H. Seid, J. B. Baker, and A. Mangione, "Intravenous ferric carboxymaltose compared with oral iron in the treatment of postpartum anemia: a randomized controlled trial," *Obstetrics and Gynecology*, vol. 110, no. 2, part 1, pp. 267–278, 2007.

[28] C. Breymann, F. Gliga, C. Bejenariu, and N. Strizhova, "Comparative efficacy and safety of intravenous ferric carboxymaltose in the treatment of postpartum iron deficiency anemia," *International Journal of Gynecology and Obstetrics*, vol. 101, no. 1, pp. 67–73, 2008.

[29] A. Pfenniger, C. Schuller, P. Christoph, and D. Surbek, "Safety and efficacy of high-dose intravenous iron carboxymaltose vs. iron sucrose for treatment of postpartum anemia," *Journal of Perinatal Medicine*, vol. 40, no. 4, pp. 397–402, 2012.

[30] P. Christoph, C. Schuller, H. Studer, O. Irion, B. M. De Tejada, and D. Surbek, "Intravenous iron treatment in pregnancy: comparison of high-dose ferric carboxymaltose vs. iron sucrose," *Journal of Perinatal Medicine*, vol. 40, no. 5, pp. 469–474, 2012.

[31] B. Myers, O. Myers, and J. Moore, "Comparative efficacy and safety of intravenous ferric carboxymaltose (Ferinject) and

iron(III) hydroxide dextran (Cosmofer) in pregnancy," *Obstetric Medicine*, vol. 5, no. 3, pp. 105–107, 2012.

[32] B. Froessler, J. Collingwood, N. A. Hodyl, and G. Dekker, "Intravenous ferric carboxymaltose for anaemia in pregnancy," *BMC Pregnancy and Childbirth*, vol. 14, article 115, 2014.

[33] B. Froessler, G. Dekker, and G. McAuliffe, "To the rescue: the role of intravenous iron in the management of severe anaemia in the peri-partum setting," *Blood Transfusion*, vol. 13, no. 1, pp. 150–152, 2015.

33

A Comparison of Pattern of Pregnancy Loss in Women with Infertility Undergoing IVF and Women with Unexplained Recurrent Miscarriages Who Conceive Spontaneously

Vidya A. Tamhankar,[1] **Beiyu Liu,**[2] **Junhao Yan,**[1] **and Tin-Chiu Li**[3]

[1]*Department of Reproductive Medicine, University of Sheffield, Sheffield Teaching Hospitals, Jessop Wing, Tree Root Walk, Sheffield S10 2SF, UK*

[2]*Department of Obstetrics and Gynecology, Bronx-Lebanon Hospital Center, Albert Einstein College of Medicine, The Bronx, NY 10457, USA*

[3]*Department of Obstetrics and Gynaecology, Chinese University of Hong Kong, Prince of Wales Hospital, Shatin, N.T., Hong Kong*

Correspondence should be addressed to Vidya A. Tamhankar; vidya.tamhankar@sth.nhs.uk

Academic Editor: Peter E. Schwartz

Objective. Women with infertility and recurrent miscarriages may have an overlapping etiology. The aim of this study was to compare the pregnancy loss in pregnancies after IVF treatment with spontaneous pregnancies in women with recurrent miscarriages and to assess differences related to cause of infertility. *Methods.* The outcome from 1220 IVF pregnancies (Group I) was compared with 611 spontaneous pregnancies (Group II) in women with recurrent miscarriages. Subgroup analysis was performed in Group I based on cause of infertility: tubal factor (392 pregnancies); male factor (610 pregnancies); and unexplained infertility (218 pregnancies). *Results.* The clinical pregnancy loss rate in Group I (14.3%) was significantly lower than that of Group II (25.8%, $p < 0.001$) and this was independent of the cause of infertility. However the timing of pregnancy loss was similar between Groups I and II. The clinical pregnancy loss rate in Group I was similar in different causes of infertility. *Conclusions.* The clinical pregnancy loss rate following IVF treatment is lower than that of women with unexplained recurrent miscarriages who conceived spontaneously. This difference persists whether the infertility is secondary to tubal factors, male factors, or unexplained cause.

1. Introduction

Infertility and miscarriage are two facets of reproductive failure that are said to have overlapping etiologies. A number of pathologies have been considered to be associated with both infertility and miscarriage, namely, polycystic ovarian disease [1], uterine septum, and uterine fibroid [2]. A higher prevalence of infertility has also been detected among patients with recurrent miscarriage [3].

The risk of miscarriage in women with infertility has been reported to range widely from 7% [4] to as high as 70% [5]. There are several explanations for these differences reported by various investigators. Firstly, the definition of miscarriage used by various investigators is quite different; some included biochemical losses while others reported only clinical pregnancy loss. Secondly, infertility itself is a rather heterogeneous condition with different underlying causes. It is possible that the miscarriage rate in women with different underlying causes of infertility may be different. Very few investigators have, however, examined the impact of infertility diagnosis on the miscarriage rate. Miscarriage rates are said to be the highest among PCOS as compared to other groups of infertility [6]. Thirdly, it is possible that infertility treatment itself may influence the likelihood of miscarriage. It has been reported that pregnancy following IVF treatment has a particularly high loss rate, with several reports on rates well over 30% [7], similar to that observed in women with a history of recurrent miscarriage.

Miscarriage may occur at different stages of the pregnancy, for example, biochemical loss prior to any ultrasound evidence of an intrauterine gestational sac, early clinical loss in which there is an ultrasound evidence of an intrauterine sac, fetal loss in first trimester after demonstration of fetal pole and heart beats, and second trimester loss. It is possible that various underlying pathology results in loss at different stages of the pregnancy. Patients with recurrent miscarriage and infertility are at a high risk of pregnancy loss. A similar pattern of miscarriage among these two cohorts of patients may indicate common pathogenesis of pregnancy loss in them. To the best of our knowledge, there has been no study that has compared the miscarriage rate between patients with recurrent miscarriage and infertility. Miscarriage rate among naturally conceived pregnancies is particularly difficult to measure and often underreported. As patients with recurrent miscarriage are closely monitored in our unit, this hurdle is easily overcome. The objective of our study is to compare the rate and pattern of miscarriage between spontaneous conceptions in women with history of recurrent miscarriage and IVF pregnancies in women with infertility.

2. Methods

The study was conducted at the Reproductive Medicine Unit, Jessop Wing, Sheffield. Women were included in the study from the recurrent miscarriage clinic and assisted conception unit. Data was retrospectively analyzed from a prospectively maintained database in the unit. Ethics approval was not required as patient identifying details were excluded from database.

2.1. Subjects. Two groups of subjects were included in the study.

Group I consisted of infertile women, who conceived following IVF ± ICSI treatment, for either tubal factor (Group IA), male factor (Group IB), or unexplained infertility (Group IC). Tubal factor (Group IA) was defined as patients who were unable to conceive due to tubal disease diagnosed by hysterosalpingogram (HSG) or laparoscopy. Male factor infertility (Group IB) was defined when there was abnormal semen analysis as per WHO 2010 criteria [8]. Unexplained infertility (Group IC) was defined when the basic infertility evaluation including midluteal progesterone, hysterosalpingogram, ultrasonography, and semen analysis all showed normal results. Out of 962 women in Group I who conceived with IVF, 144 women had at least one miscarriage previously and a quarter of these women had 2 miscarriages. None of these women had three or more miscarriages. The total number of previous miscarriages was 189 in this group giving a mean miscarriage rate (+SD) of 0.2 ± 0.4 per person.

Group II included women who conceived spontaneously with history of recurrent miscarriage of unknown etiology. Unexplained recurrent miscarriage was defined as subjects who had 3 or more consecutive miscarriages with no evidence of endocrine, immunological, anatomical, and genetic cause for their recurrent pregnancy loss following investigations according to an established protocol [9]. The investigations they had included karyotyping for both partners, antiphospholipid antibody (lupus anticoagulant, anticardiolipin antibody, and beta-2 glycoprotein) and thrombophilia screen,

thyroid function test, ultrasonography, and hysterosalpingogram. Unexplained recurrent miscarriage was a diagnosis of exclusion. The mean number of miscarriages in this group was 3.4 ± 0.6.

2.2. Exclusion Criteria. All patients above the age of 37 years were excluded from the study in order to reduce the confounding variable of age. IVF pregnancies involving donor gametes were also excluded from the study. Patients having IVF for etiologies other than tubal, male, or unexplained infertility were excluded. Biochemical pregnancy loss, multiple pregnancies, ectopic pregnancies, and pregnancies terminated for social reasons were excluded from analysis.

3. Treatment

Group I had in vitro fertilization (IVF) or intracytoplasmic sperm injection (ICSI) treatment depending on the clinical indication. As a default protocol, controlled ovarian stimulation with human recombinant FSH and GnRH antagonist was commenced in the follicular phase of the menstrual cycle. In some women, with poor ovarian reserve, GnRH agonist was used as a flare-up protocol. Serial ultrasound examinations and serum estradiol measurement were used to assess the ovarian response. When a minimum of 3 follicles reached a size of ≥ 17 mm, ovulation was triggered with human chorionic gonadotropin and oocyte retrieval was performed 36 hours later using standard ultrasound guided transvaginal approach. Collected oocytes were fertilized in vitro using IVF or ICSI as clinically appropriate. Progesterone was used for luteal phase support for 2 weeks in the form of vaginal pessaries and was discontinued on the day of pregnancy test as per the unit protocol. Embryo replacement was performed between days two and five. Pregnancy was diagnosed if plasma βHCG > 20 IU/L fourteen days after oocyte retrieval. Women with a positive pregnancy test were then followed up with serial Beta HCG assays and transvaginal scan at 6 weeks.

Group II women were seen in the recurrent miscarriage clinic within a week of positive home urine pregnancy test. They all received pregnancy support through the early pregnancy clinic. Follow-up was similar to Group I with serial Beta HCG assays and transvaginal scan at 6 weeks. None of these patients received any empirical treatment in the form of progesterone support or aspirin.

3.1. Pregnancy Outcome. Outcome was categorized into 6 groups as follows:

(i) Biochemical loss was defined when the Beta HCG values were higher than 20 IU/L with no ultrasound evidence of pregnancy.

(ii) Ectopic pregnancy was defined when ultrasound or laparoscopy confirmed the presence of ectopic gestation or when Beta HCG values were more than 1000 IU/L with no ultrasound evidence of intrauterine gestation.

TABLE 1: Demographic data of women with recurrent miscarriage and infertility.

	Infertility				(II) Unexplained recurrent miscarriage	p value
	(I) All infertility factors	(IA) Tubal infertility	(IB) Male infertility	(IC) Unexplained infertility		
Patients	962	304	473	185	368	
Conception cycles (n)	1220	392	610	218	611	
Body Mass Index, kg/m^2 (mean ± SD)	24.4 ± 3.8	24.7 ± 3.7	24.7 ± 4.1	23.8 ± 3.6	25.4 ± 4.9	$p = 0.092^*$
Age, years (mean ± SD)	32.5 ± 4.1	32.68 ± 4.1	32.2 ± 4.5	32.9 ± 3.1	32.1 ± 4.4	$p = 0.15^*$

*ANOVA used to compare means between different groups.

(iii) Clinical pregnancy was defined when there was positive pregnancy test accompanied by ultrasound evidence of intrauterine pregnancy.

(iv) Embryonic loss was defined as pregnancy loss after the presence of intrauterine gestational sac but prior to demonstration of fetal heart beats.

(v) Fetal loss was defined as pregnancy loss after fetal heart beats had been detected, but before 13 weeks of gestation.

(vi) Second trimester loss was defined as pregnancy loss beyond 13 weeks of gestation.

Conceptions without ultrasound evidence of intrauterine pregnancy (biochemical loss and ectopic) were excluded from the analysis.

Data in the two groups were compared with appropriate statistical test (Fisher's exact test, Student's t-test, and ANOVA one-way test) using GraphPad InStat version 3.10, GraphPad Software, San Diego, CA, USA, and SPSS for Windows, Rel. 20.0.0. 2011., SPSS Inc., Chicago.

4. Results

A total of 962 women who conceived after IVF treatment (Group I) and 368 women with unexplained recurrent miscarriage (Group II) were included in the study. Their demographic data is presented in Table 1. All groups were comparable with regard to mean age and BMI.

There were 1220 pregnancies in Group I. This was further divided into Groups IA, IB, and IC depending on the etiology (tubal, male, and unexplained). All women in these groups conceived with either IVF treatment ($n = 644$) or IVF + ICSI ($n = 576$). There were 611 pregnancies in Group II. These women had history of three of more previous miscarriages of unexplained etiology. In Figure 1, the rates of pregnancy loss between Group I and Group II are compared. The total clinical pregnancy loss in women with recurrent miscarriage (25.8%) was significantly higher than that of women with infertility who conceived following IVF treatment (14.3%). The embryonic loss rate, fetal loss rate, and second trimester loss rate were all significantly higher in women with recurrent miscarriage.

The pregnancy loss in subgroups IA, IB, and IC was individually compared to Group II yielding similar results,

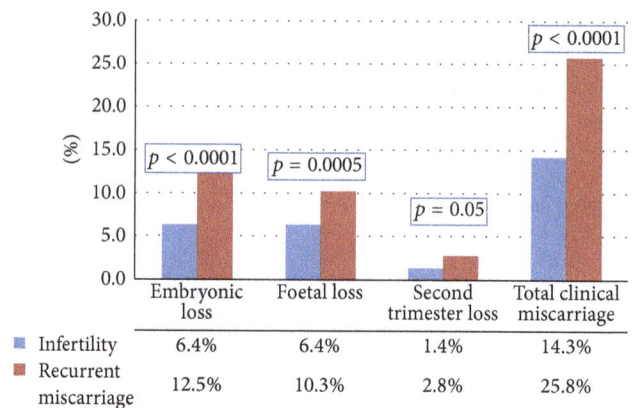

	Embryonic loss	Foetal loss	Second trimester loss	Total clinical miscarriage
■ Infertility	6.4%	6.4%	1.4%	14.3%
■ Recurrent miscarriage	12.5%	10.3%	2.8%	25.8%

Fisher's exact test used to compare the two groups

FIGURE 1: A comparison of the rates of pregnancy loss between women with infertility and recurrent miscarriage.

namely, Group IA (14.4% versus 25.8%; $p < 0.001$); Group IB (13.5% versus 25.8%; $p < 0.001$); and Group IC (15.9% versus 25.8%; $p < 0.002$).

In Figure 2, the pattern of pregnancy loss in both groups was compared. There was no difference between the two groups ($p = 0.7$).

In Figure 3, the pregnancy loss among the three subgroups of women with infertility (tubal, male, and unexplained) is compared. There was no difference in the rate of pregnancy loss among the three groups. In Figure 4, the pattern of pregnancy loss among the three groups was compared. Whilst embryonic loss in male infertility appeared highest among the three groups and fetal loss appeared highest in tubal infertility, the difference did not reach statistical significance ($p = 0.7$).

5. Discussion

In this study we compared the rate and pattern of miscarriage in two groups of women with reproductive failure, namely, women with recurrent miscarriage who conceived spontaneously and women with infertility who conceived following IVF treatment. We found significant differences between the pregnancy losses in these two groups. Studies

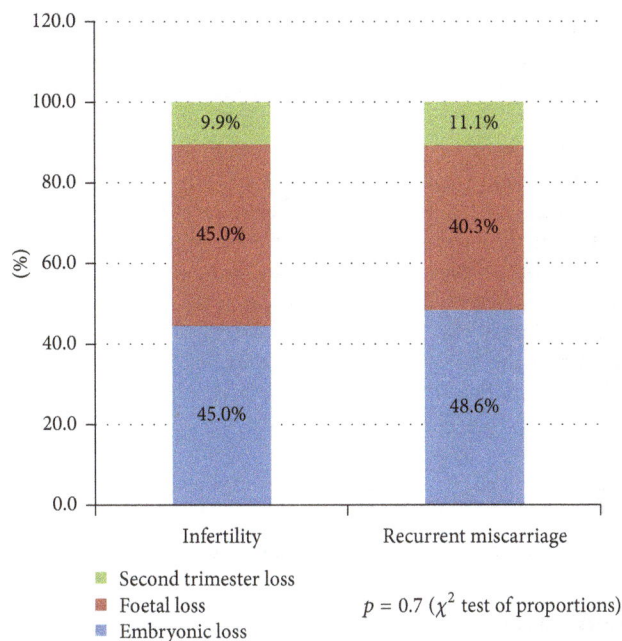

FIGURE 2: A comparison of the pattern of pregnancy loss between women with infertility and recurrent miscarriage.

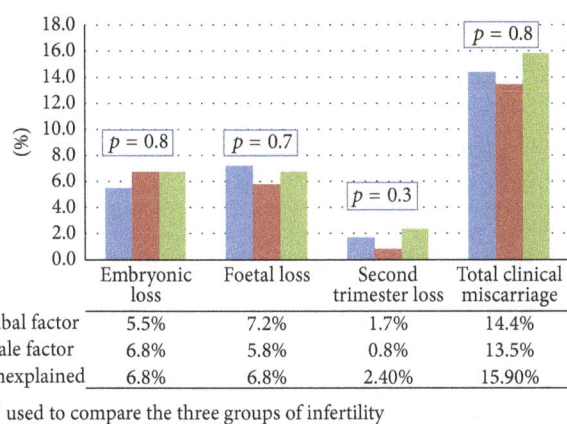

FIGURE 4: A comparison of the pattern of miscarriage in tubal, male, and unexplained infertility.

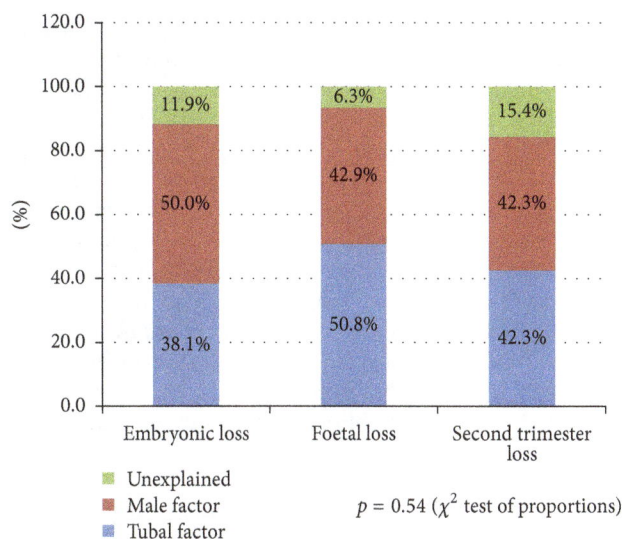

χ^2 used to compare the three groups of infertility

FIGURE 3: A comparison of the rates of pregnancy loss in tubal, male, and unexplained infertility.

have assessed pregnancy loss after IVF and in recurrent miscarriage patients, but no direct comparison has been made [10–13]. We performed this comparative study between these groups as common etiological factors exist for pregnancy loss in both of these groups [14].

5.1. Biochemical Loss. In our study, the biochemical loss rate was 22.5% among Group I who had IVF/ICSI treatment and 5% in Group II who conceived spontaneously. This is consistent with previous studies, where the biochemical loss rate has been reported to range from 22% to 31% [15–17] after IVF, which appears to be higher than the rate reported in women who conceive naturally which ranges from 8% to 22% [12, 18]. The apparently higher rate of biochemical loss in the former group could be a consequence of increased

surveillance of women undergoing IVF and hence this has been excluded from the study. In most IVF units, Beta HCG is measured 14 days after oocyte retrieval with the result that biochemical pregnancy is more likely to be detected. This is in contrast to women with recurrent miscarriage who wait until a few days after a missed period to do urine pregnancy test. By this time a significant proportion of biochemical pregnancy may have escaped detection. Hence to make a valid comparison of the biochemical loss rate between spontaneous conceptions in recurrent miscarriage and IVF pregnancies in infertility, the same method of surveillance is required for both groups, namely, measurement of serum BHCG 14 days after ovulation or oocyte retrieval. In this study, therefore, we have limited our comparison to clinical pregnancy loss which is after ultrasound confirmation of intrauterine pregnancy.

Biochemical pregnancies represent conceptions that have started to implant but fail to progress at a very early stage before clinical diagnosis of pregnancy is established. Endometrial factors, maternal age, stress, and sperm DNA fragmentation have been proposed as possible aetiological mechanisms for biochemical pregnancy [19]. Several studies have shown that biochemical pregnancies have positive prognosis on the outcome of subsequent IVF cycles [20–22]. Although we have not included biochemical pregnancies in our analysis due to methodological issues, they have prognostic significance for subsequent pregnancy outcome.

5.2. Clinical Miscarriages. We found that the overall clinical loss in the unexplained recurrent miscarriage group (25.8%) was significantly higher ($p = 0.001$) than the infertility group (14.3%). The rates observed in these two groups of subjects both appear to be higher than the rate observed in the general population (7.9% to 13.5%) [23, 24].

First Trimester Loss. Embryonic loss was significantly higher in recurrent miscarriage than that of the infertility group (12.5% versus 6.4%; $p < 0.0001$). The rate of fetal loss per clinical pregnancy in women with recurrent miscarriage (10.3%) was also significantly higher ($p = 0.03$) than that (6.4%) of the infertile group. A review of the literature has shown that pregnancy loss rate after documentation of fetal heart (fetal loss) was 3–6% in patients with no history of infertility and/or recurrent miscarriages [25–27]. In the infertile populations this ranges from 7 to 15% [28–30]. However, in women with a history of recurrent miscarriage, pregnancy loss after ultrasound documentation of fetal heart beats (fetal loss rate) has been shown to be higher, at 17–22% [31, 32]. Our observation in this study on fetal loss is consistent with earlier reports.

Second Trimester Loss. After the first trimester the pregnancy loss in the recurrent miscarriage group was 2.8% which represents a twofold increase in comparison with the infertility group (1.4%). This difference did not quite reach statistical significance ($p = 0.05$). This is almost certainly due to type 2 error. Verifying a significant difference between the two groups requires studies with larger sample sizes.

5.3. Spontaneous Conceptions versus IVF Treatment. One possible criticism of the study is that we compared the two groups of women who conceived with different methods, namely, spontaneous conception for women with recurrent miscarriage and IVF conception for women with infertility. Ideally comparison should be made when the method of conception is the same for two different groups of women. However women with recurrent pregnancy loss do not usually have a problem with conception and very few require assisted conception. Alternately one may compare only natural pregnancies in both groups, but women with infertility often require treatment to achieve conception. In our study the comparison between the two groups has been made on the assumption that IVF does not in itself alter the likelihood of clinical loss when compared with natural conception. Though limited information is available, the study by Schieve et al. has demonstrated that IVF does not increase the risk of clinical pregnancy loss when compared to natural conception [33].

5.4. Age as a Confounding Variable. It is well recognized that older women are more likely to have pregnancy loss. Hence to minimize the impact of age as a confounding variable we have excluded women over the age of 37 years in our study. Our data showed no significant difference in mean ages between women with recurrent miscarriage and different groups of infertility.

Comparison among Different Groups of Infertility. Our study has shown no significant differences in the rate of pregnancy loss among the three groups of infertility (Figure 3). The embryonic loss appeared highest in the male infertility and lowest in the tubal infertility. The pregnancy loss in the second trimester was highest in unexplained infertility and lowest in male infertility. These differences though did not reach statistical significance ($p = 0.54$). This is in contrast to the study by Omland et al. where the first trimester miscarriage rate and particularly those before 6 weeks of pregnancy were considerably lower in unexplained infertility in comparison with endometriosis and tubal factor [34].

To conclude, we found that women with unexplained recurrent miscarriage who conceived spontaneously have a higher risk of pregnancy loss than women who conceived after IVF treatment for tubal factor, male factor, or unexplained infertility. However the pattern of pregnancy loss remained the same. The rate and pattern of pregnancy loss following IVF were similar irrespective of the etiology of infertility.

Conflict of Interests

The authors report no conflict of interests.

References

[1] K. A. Cocksedge, T.-C. Li, S. H. Saravelos, and M. Metwally, "A reappraisal of the role of polycystic ovary syndrome in recurrent miscarriage," *Reproductive BioMedicine Online*, vol. 17, no. 1, pp. 151–160, 2008.

[2] A. S. D. Wold, N. Pham, and A. Arici, "Anatomic factors in recurrent pregnancy loss," *Seminars in Reproductive Medicine*, vol. 24, no. 1, pp. 25–32, 2006.

[3] C. B. Coulam, "Association between infertility and spontaneous abortion," *American Journal of Reproductive Immunology*, vol. 27, no. 3-4, pp. 128–129, 1992.

[4] M. W. Molo, M. Kelly, R. Balos, K. Mullaney, and E. Radwanska, "Incidence of fetal loss in infertility patients after detection of fetal heart activity with early transvaginal ultrasound," *Journal of Reproductive Medicine*, vol. 38, no. 10, pp. 804–806, 1993.

[5] R. B. Hakim, R. H. Gray, and H. Zacur, "Infertility and early-pregnancy loss," *American Journal of Obstetrics and Gynecology*, vol. 172, no. 5, pp. 1510–1517, 1995.

[6] M. Bahceci and U. Ulug, "Does underlying infertility aetiology impact on first trimester miscarriage rate following ICSI? A preliminary report from 1244 singleton gestations," *Human Reproduction*, vol. 20, no. 3, pp. 717–721, 2005.

[7] H.-C. Liu and Z. Rosenwaks, "Early pregnancy wastage in IVF (in vitro fertilization) patients," *Journal of In Vitro Fertilization and Embryo Transfer*, vol. 8, no. 2, pp. 65–72, 1991.

[8] T. G. Cooper, E. Noonan, S. von Eckardstein et al., "World Health Organization reference values for human semen characteristics," *Human Reproduction Update*, vol. 16, no. 3, pp. 231–245, 2010.

[9] T.-C. Li, T. Iqbal, B. Anstie et al., "An analysis of the pattern of pregnancy loss in women with recurrent miscarriage," *Fertility and Sterility*, vol. 78, no. 5, pp. 1100–1106, 2002.

[10] S. A. Brigham, C. Conlon, and R. G. Farquharson, "A longitudinal study of pregnancy outcome following idiopathic recurrent miscarriage," *Human Reproduction*, vol. 14, no. 11, pp. 2868–2871, 1999.

[11] J. S. Hyer, S. Fong, and W. H. Kutteh, "Predictive value of the presence of an embryonic heartbeat for live birth: comparison of women with and without recurrent pregnancy loss," *Fertility and Sterility*, vol. 82, no. 5, pp. 1369–1373, 2004.

[12] J. X. Wang, R. J. Norman, and A. J. Wilcox, "Incidence of spontaneous abortion among pregnancies produced by assisted reproductive technology," *Human Reproduction*, vol. 19, no. 2, pp. 272–277, 2004.

[13] E. Winter, J. Wang, M. J. Davies, and R. J. Norman, "Early pregnancy loss following assisted reproductive technology treatment," *Human Reproduction*, vol. 17, no. 12, pp. 3220–3223, 2002.

[14] O. B. Christiansen, H. S. Nielsen, and A. M. Kolte, "Future directions of failed implantation and recurrent miscarriage research," *Reproductive BioMedicine Online*, vol. 13, no. 1, pp. 71–83, 2006.

[15] H.-C. Liu, G. S. Jones, H. W. Jones Jr., and Z. Rosenwaks, "Mechanisms and factors of early pregnancy wastage in in vitro fertilization-embryo transfer patients," *Fertility and Sterility*, vol. 50, no. 1, pp. 95–101, 1988.

[16] S. Bjercke, T. Tanbo, P. O. Dale, L. Mørkrid, and T. Abyholm, "Human chorionic gonadotrophin concentrations in early pregnancy after in-vitro fertilization," *Human Reproduction*, vol. 14, no. 6, pp. 1642–1646, 1999.

[17] A. Hourvitz, L. Lerner-Geva, S. E. Elizur et al., "Role of embryo quality in predicting early pregnancy loss following assisted reproductive technology," *Reproductive BioMedicine Online*, vol. 13, no. 4, pp. 504–509, 2006.

[18] N. J. Ellish, K. Saboda, J. O'Connor, P. C. Nasca, E. J. Stanek, and C. Boyle, "A prospective study of early pregnancy loss," *Human Reproduction*, vol. 11, no. 2, pp. 406–412, 1996.

[19] J. J. K. Annan, A. Gudi, P. Bhide, A. Shah, and R. Homburg, "Biochemical pregnancy during assisted conception: a little bit pregnant," *Journal of Clinical Medicine Research*, vol. 5, no. 4, pp. 269–274, 2013.

[20] T. Levy, D. Dicker, J. Ashkenazi, D. Feldberg, M. Shelef, and J. A. Goldman, "The prognostic value and significance of preclinical abortions in in vitro fertilization-embryo transfer programs," *Fertility and Sterility*, vol. 56, no. 1, pp. 71–74, 1991.

[21] K. R. Pearson, R. Hauser, D. W. Cramer, and S. A. Missmer, "Point of failure as a predictor of in vitro fertilization treatment discontinuation," *Fertility and Sterility*, vol. 91, no. 4, pp. 1483–1485, 2009.

[22] G. W. Bates Jr. and E. S. Ginsburg, "Early pregnancy loss in in vitro fertilization (IVF) is a positive predictor of subsequent IVF success," *Fertility and Sterility*, vol. 77, no. 2, pp. 337–341, 2002.

[23] A.-M. Nybo Andersen, J. Wohlfahrt, P. Christens, J. Olsen, and M. Melbye, "Maternal age and fetal loss: population based register linkage study," *British Medical Journal*, vol. 320, no. 7251, pp. 1708–1712, 2000.

[24] X. B. Wang, C. Z. Chen, L. H. Wang et al., "Conception, early pregnancy loss, and time to clinical pregnancy: a population-based prospective study," *Fertility and Sterility*, vol. 79, no. 3, pp. 577–584, 2003.

[25] L. M. Hill, D. Guzick, J. Fries, and J. Hixson, "Fetal loss rate after ultrasonically documented cardiac activity between 6 and 14 weeks, menstrual age," *Journal of Clinical Ultrasound*, vol. 19, no. 4, pp. 221–223, 1991.

[26] S. R. Goldstein, M. Danon, and C. Watson, "An updated protocol for abortion surveillance with ultrasound and immediate pathology," *Obstetrics and Gynecology*, vol. 83, no. 1, pp. 55–58, 1994.

[27] M. R. Laufer, J. L. Ecker, and J. A. Hill, "Pregnancy outcome following ultrasound-detected fetal cardiac activity in women with a history of multiple spontaneous abortions," *Journal of the Society for Gynecologic Investigation*, vol. 1, no. 2, pp. 138–142, 1994.

[28] J. A. Keenan, S. Rizvi, and M. R. Caudle, "Fetal loss after early detection of heart motion in infertility patients. Prognostic factors," *The Journal of Reproductive Medicine*, vol. 43, no. 3, pp. 199–202, 1998.

[29] S. M. Qasim, R. Sachdev, A. Trias, K. Senkowski, and E. Kemmann, "The predictive value of first-trimester embryonic heart rates in infertility patients," *Obstetrics and Gynecology*, vol. 89, no. 6, pp. 934–936, 1997.

[30] K. E. Smith and R. P. Buyalos, "The profound impact of patient age on pregnancy outcome after early detection of fetal cardiac activity," *Fertility and Sterility*, vol. 65, no. 1, pp. 35–40, 1996.

[31] M. S. Opsahl and D. C. Pettit, "First trimester sonographic characteristics of patients with recurrent spontaneous abortion," *Journal of Ultrasound in Medicine*, vol. 12, no. 9, pp. 507–510, 1993.

[32] I. Van Leeuwen, D. W. Branch, and J. R. Scott, "First-trimester ultrasonography findings in women with a history of recurrent pregnancy loss," *American Journal of Obstetrics and Gynecology*, vol. 168, no. 1, pp. 111–114, 1993.

[33] L. A. Schieve, L. Tatham, H. B. Peterson, J. Toner, and G. Jeng, "Spontaneous abortion among pregnancies conceived using assisted reproductive technology in the United States," *Obstetrics & Gynecology*, vol. 101, no. 5, pp. 959–967, 2003.

[34] A. K. Omland, T. Åbyholm, P. Fedorcsák et al., "Pregnancy outcome after IVF and ICSI in unexplained, endometriosis-associated and tubal factor infertility," *Human Reproduction*, vol. 20, no. 3, pp. 722–727, 2005.

34

A Reappraisal of Women's Health Initiative Estrogen-Alone Trial: Long-Term Outcomes in Women 50–59 Years of Age

Eric Roehm

Volunteer Health Clinic, 4215 Medical Pkwy, Austin, TX 78756, USA

Correspondence should be addressed to Eric Roehm; ericfr3@gmail.com

Academic Editor: Marc J. N. C. Keirse

The Women's Health Initiative (WHI) Estrogen-Alone Trial randomized postmenopausal women, 50 to 79 years of age, with prior hysterectomy, to conjugated equine estrogens (CEE) or placebo with a 5.9-year median duration of CEE use. In 2013, the WHI published outcomes for additional extended follow-up. Reported here for the first time is an analysis of the number needed to treat with CEE rather than placebo for younger women (50–59 years) to prevent an adverse long-term outcome. For every 76 women randomized to CEE at 50–59 years, one less myocardial infarction occurred during the 13-year cumulative long-term follow-up. For every 37 women randomized to CEE at 50–59 years, one less woman experienced a global index endpoint (including coronary heart disease, invasive breast cancer, stroke, pulmonary embolism, colorectal cancer, hip fracture, and death) during the 13-year follow-up. Younger women (50–59 years), compared to older women, had more favorable cumulative long-term outcomes for MI and global index. Though a subgroup analysis is not an adequate basis for making primary prevention guideline recommendations, the WHI Estrogen-Alone Trial outcomes strongly suggest that a similar course of estrogen initiated at 50–59 years in postmenopausal women with prior hysterectomy results in significant long-term health benefit.

1. Introduction

The Women's Health Initiative (WHI) hormone trials are randomized, double blind, predominantly primary prevention trials, with long-term follow-up evaluating hormone therapy in postmenopausal women. The WHI Estrogen-Alone Trial randomized 10,739 postmenopausal women with prior hysterectomy to either 0.625 mg of conjugated equine estrogens (CEE) daily or placebo [1]. The WHI estrogen plus progestin trial randomized 16,608 postmenopausal women with a uterus to a combination of daily 0.625 mg of CEE and 2.5 mg of medroxyprogesterone acetate or placebo [2]. The strengths of these trials derive, in part, from their large size and long-term follow-up, with a 6.6-year median duration of follow-up in the WHI Estrogen-Alone Trial [3] after the completion of the intervention phase.

However, outcomes resulting from postmenopausal hormone therapy trials may be affected by multiple factors, including the specific estrogen or progestogen agent used, duration of therapy, and characteristics of the group of women treated [4–8]. The inclusion of older women in the WHI trial was recognized as potentially important before any outcomes were reported. The WHI researchers, in a trial design article when discussing the inclusion of older participants in the trial state, "…if the study interventions turn out to be equally efficacious in terms of relative risk reduction throughout the postmenopausal age range… [9]" indicating an awareness by the investigators prior to trial results being available that trial outcomes may vary with age.

The current report makes the case in which outcomes clearly differ by age at time of randomization to CEE in the WHI Estrogen-Alone Trial and that cumulative long-term outcomes for women 50–59 years of age show a net benefit with CEE. In contrast, the WHI trial authors did not take the position in which the evidence from the WHI Estrogen-Alone Trial showed an overall cumulative long-term benefit for younger women randomized to estrogen [3]. Outcome data is presented in detail in the current report to make the case for reinterpretation of the data and to provide a context for outcomes of younger women within the overall trial results for all participants.

TABLE 1: Women's Health Initiative Estrogen-Alone Trial, age of participants in estrogen/placebo (intervention) phase of trial.

Age at trial entry [3] Years (%, Number)	Age at end of CEE/placebo intervention phase[a]	Median age at randomization to CEE/placebo[b]	Median age of starting postmenopausal hormone replacement therapy in USA population [15–19]: <55 years of age
50–59 y (30.9%[c], 3313)	55–67	55	
60–69 y (45.2%, 4851)	65–77	64	
70–79 y (24.0%, 2575)	75–87	74	

[a]A minority of participants were older at the end of the intervention phase than those listed in the upper limits of the estimated age brackets. (Start of intervention phase: December 1993; end of enrollment for intervention phase: October 1998; end of intervention phase: February 29, 2004; median duration of intervention phase: 7.2 years; end of reported trial follow-up: September 30, 2010 [1, 3].)
[b]Estimates adjusted for age distribution of 50–59 y group (50–54 y/55–59 y = 1 : 1.37 ratio [14]) and for possible enrollment of participants at lower end of age bracket.
[c]Percentages do not add to 100% because of rounding anomaly.
CEE: conjugated equine estrogens; USA: United States of America.
Derived from data provided in [1, 3, 14–19].

2. Methods

For the analysis, in this paper, the number needed to treat (NNT) was assessed over the entire 13-year follow-up, including vboth the intervention and the postintervention phase, in order to help the clinician assess the overall impact of the effect of randomization to CEE in the WHI Estrogen-Alone Trial. The calculations were performed using SAS software (version 9.3) with an add-on module as per Bender [10, 11]. Calculations of the confidence intervals for NNT were calculated based on the Wilson score method as this appears to be the most reliable methodology [10]. The 22% of surviving participants in the WHI Estrogen-Alone Trial who did not consent to extended follow-up [12] are treated as lost to follow-up in the number needed to treat analysis. The number needed to treat provides additional information where the outcomes are initially reported as time to an event [13]. Other P values and confidence intervals for hazard ratios in this paper are as provided by the WHI investigators in prior reports.

3. WHI Estrogen-Alone Trial

At 40 clinical centers in the United States, the WHI Estrogen-Alone Trial enrolled 10,739 women 50–79 years of age with prior hysterectomy. Subgroup analysis by age was prespecified in the trial protocol [9]. For women at trial entry, 30.9% of participants were 50–59 years, 45.2% of participants were 60–69 years, and 24.0% of participants were 70–79 years of age [3].

The intervention phase lasted for a median duration of 7.2 years before the trial was stopped because of an elevated stroke rate in the CEE group (hazard ratio [HR]: 1.35; 95% nominal confidence interval [CI]: 1.07–1.70) [1, 3]. Median duration of CEE use was 5.9 years [12]. The median adherent time receiving CEE (ingestion of >80% pills) was 3.5 years [12]. The intervention phase plus the postintervention follow-up phase resulted in a cumulative long-term median follow-up of 13 years [3]. A total of 77.9% of surviving participants in the CEE group and 78.4% in the placebo group gave consent for the entire extended follow-up period [12]. The majority of women enrolled in the WHI Estrogen-Alone Trial were without preexisting cardiovascular disease, though, at trial entry, 4.1% had a history of prior myocardial infarction (MI) or coronary revascularization [1].

3.1. Age of Starting Estrogen/Placebo. The majority of WHI Estrogen-Alone Trial participants were randomized to CEE or placebo at a median age older than the typical age for starting postmenopausal therapy in clinical practice. The age for initiating CEE or placebo in the trial is shown in Table 1. The estimated median age for randomization to CEE or placebo is 55 years for the 50–59-year group, 64 years for the 60–69-year group, and 74 years of age for the 70–79-year group [1, 3, 14]. A managed care organization reporting on hormone replacement therapy for 1990–1995 showed a median age of 52 years for first time users of hormone replacement therapy [15]. In both the WHI Estrogen-Alone Trial and the WHI estrogen plus progestin trial, the majority of women with a prior history of hormone replacement therapy began at ≤55 years of age. (This can be determined by the previously reported mean age of menopause of trial participants [16, 17] in conjunction with published data on the number of years from menopause at time of starting initial prior course of hormone therapy [18].) Furthermore, a National Health and Nutrition Examination Survey in the United States from 1988 to 1994 reported that the majority of women using hormone replacement therapy started therapy within 1 year of menopause [19].

3.2. Outcomes for Women 50–79 Years of Age at Trial Entry. The only statistically significant outcome for all participants (50–79 years) in the WHI Estrogen-Alone Trial for the 13-year cumulative long-term follow-up was a reduction in invasive breast cancer with CEE (HR: 0.79; 95% CI: 0.65–0.97) [3]. There were no other statistically significant differences, including deep vein thrombosis (DVT), stroke, or hip fractures for cumulative long-term follow-up.

In the WHI Estrogen-Alone Trial, for 7.2-year median intervention phase, for all participants (50–79 years), there was no difference with CEE compared to placebo for CHD (coronary heart disease) defined as nonfatal MI or coronary death, the primary trial endpoint (HR: 0.94; 95% CI: 0.78–1.14) [3]. There was an increase in the CEE group CEE in the rate of stroke (HR: 1.35; 95% CI: 1.07–1.70), as well as

Intervention phase (7.2 years)

Outcome by age at trial entry (years of age)	Hazard ratio (95% CI)	P value for trend by age
Myocardial infarction		
50–59 y	0.55 (0.31–1.00)	
60–69 y	0.95 (0.69–1.30)	0.02
70–79 y	1.24 (0.88–1.75)	
Colorectal cancer		
50–59 y	0.71 (0.30–1.67)	
60–69 y	0.88 (0.53–1.47)	0.02
70–79 y	2.24 (1.16–4.30)	
All-cause mortality		
50–59 y	0.70 (0.46–1.09)	
60–69 y	1.01 (0.79–1.29)	0.04
70–79 y	1.21 (0.95–1.56)	
Global index		
50–59 y	0.84 (0.66–1.07)	
60–69 y	0.99 (0.85–1.15)	0.02
70–79 y	1.17 (0.99–1.39)	

Cumulative long term follow-up (13 years)
(intervention + postintervention phase)

Myocardial infarction		
50–59 y	0.60 (0.39–0.91)	
60–69 y	1.03 (0.82–1.31)	0.007
70–79 y	1.25 (0.95–1.65)	
Global index		
50–59 y	0.82 (0.68–0.98)	
60–69 y	1.03 (0.92–1.15)	0.01
70–79 y	1.10 (0.97–1.25)	

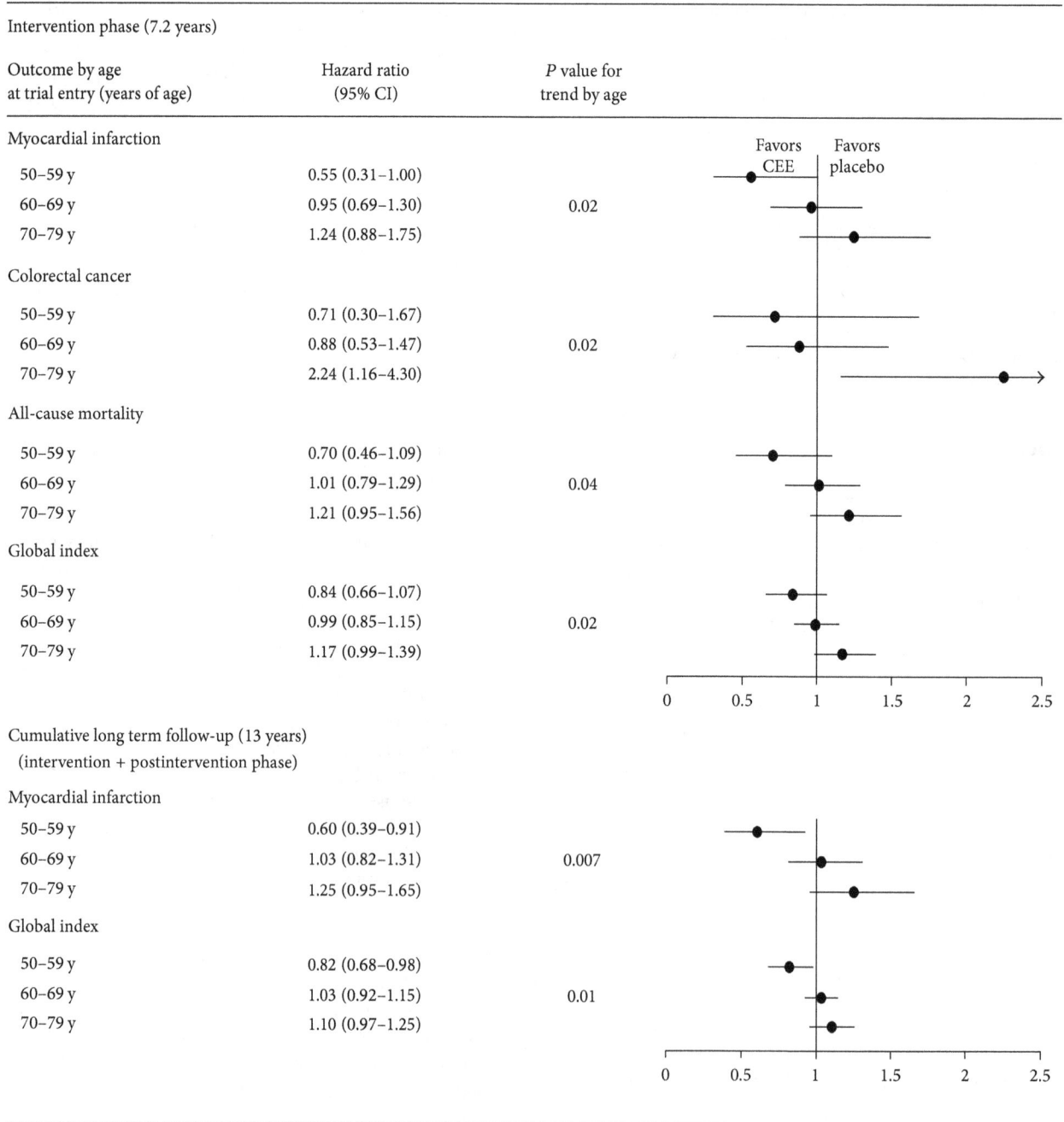

FIGURE 1: Primary and secondary trial outcomes with a significant trend by age (P for interaction) in Women's Health Initiative Estrogen-Alone Trial. CEE: conjugated equine estrogens; y: years of age. Source for outcomes: [3].

DVT (HR: 1.48; 95% CI: 1.06–2.07) [3]. Gall bladder disease occurred more frequently with CEE (HR: 1.55; 95% CI: 1.34–1.79) [3, 20]. Hip fractures (HR: 0.67; 95% CI: 0.46–0.96), all fractures (HR: 0.72; 95% CI: 0.64–0.80), and diabetes (HR: 0.86; 95% CI: 0.76–0.98) were less frequent in the CEE group [3]. Of note, the confidence intervals cited throughout this report are for nominal, unadjusted values.

3.3. Significant Trends by Age. Multiple trial outcomes in the WHI Estrogen-Alone Trial were more favorable in younger compared to older participants randomized to CEE. Hazard ratios by decade of age of participant for primary and secondary trial outcomes with a significant trend by age are shown in Figure 1. All outcomes with a statistically significant trend by age had a comparatively more favorable outcome for CEE initiation in younger women compared to older women: myocardial infarction (P = .02), total mortality (P = .04), colorectal cancer (P = .02), and global index (P = .02) for the intervention phase and myocardial infarction (P = .007) and global index (P = .01) for cumulative long-term follow-up [3].

TABLE 2: Women 50–59 years of age at trial entry: WHI Estrogen-Alone Trial outcomes, 13-year cumulative long-term follow-up (intervention phase + postintervention phase).

Outcome	Hazard ratio (95% CI) Women 50–59 years of age CEE versus placebo	P for interaction (trend by age) for all participants, 50–79 years
Coronary heart disease (primary trial endpoint)[a]	0.65 (95% CI, 0.44–0.96)[†]	0.12
Myocardial infarction	0.60 (95% CI, 0.39–0.91)[†]	0.007[‡]
Invasive breast cancer	0.76 (95% CI, 0.52–1.11)	0.70
All cancer types	0.80 (95% CI, 0.64–0.99)[†]	0.18
All-cause death	0.78 (95% CI, 0.59–1.03)	0.10
Global index[b]	0.82 (95% CI, 0.68–0.98)[†]	0.01[‡]

[a]Coronary heart disease: nonfatal myocardial infarction or coronary death.

[b]Global index represents the first event for each participant from among the following: coronary heart disease, stroke, pulmonary embolism, invasive breast cancer, colorectal cancer, hip fracture, or death due to other causes.

[†]95% confidence interval does not include 1.0.

[‡]Statistically significant (95% CI) P for interaction (trend by age).

CEE: conjugated equine estrogens; CI: confidence interval; WHI: Women's Health Initiative.

Source for outcomes: [3].

3.4. Intervention Phase Outcomes in Women 50–59 Years of Age. For the intervention phase (7.2 years), for women 50–59 years of age in the WHI Estrogen-Alone Trial, there was no statistically significant difference in CEE versus placebo for CHD (HR: 0.60; 95% CI: 0.35–1.04) [3]. There was no statistically significant reduction in MI (HR: 0.55; 95% CI: 0.31–1.00), invasive breast cancer (HR: 0.82; 95% CI: 0.50–1.34), and global index (HR: 0.84; 95% CI: 0.66–1.07) [3]. There was a reduced hazard ratio for CEE compared to placebo for coronary revascularization (HR: 0.56; 95% CI: 0.35–0.88), but the *P* for interaction by age was not statistically significant [3].

For adverse outcomes in the intervention phase, for CEE compared to placebo, in women 50–59 years of age, there was an increase in DVT (HR: 1.66; 95% CI: 0.75–3.67) which is consistent with the increase in DVT for all participants (50–79 years) [3]. Gall bladder disease increased for women 50–59 years of age with CEE (HR: 1.40; 95% CI: 1.10–1.78) [20, 21].

For women 50–59 years of age at trial entry, stroke rate for the intervention phase was similar for CEE and placebo groups (HR: 0.99; 95% CI: 0.53–1.85) [3]. (However, the *P* value (*P* = .77) for trend by age does not suggest that the hazard ratio for the younger age group (50–59 years) can reliably be considered different from the statistically significant elevated hazard ratio for stroke present in the entire group of women 50–79 years of age.)

A post hoc classification of stroke outcomes as ischemic or hemorrhagic showed a HR of 1.09 (95% CI, 0.54–2.21) for women 50–59 years of age randomized to CEE for ischemic strokes [22]. For women less than 10 years post menopause, the risk of ischemic stroke for CEE was increased (HR: 2.62; 95% CI: 1.01–6.81) during the intervention phase [22]. Another WHI report indicated that the increase in total stroke seen with women less than 10 years from menopause was attenuated when women with prior cardiovascular disease and >60 years were excluded (HR 1.23 versus 1.77) from an analysis of the combined WHI trials [23].

3.5. Long-Term Outcomes with a Hazard Ratio of Less than 1.0 in Women 50–59 Years of Age. With cumulative long-term follow-up of 13 years in the WHI Estrogen-Alone Trial, there were a number of outcomes with a reduced hazard ratio for CEE versus placebo in women 50–59 years of age at trial entry [3], Table 2. The hazard ratios comparing CEE to placebo were reduced for CHD (HR: 0.65; 95% CI: 0.44–0.96), myocardial infarction (MI) (HR: 0.60; 95% CI: 0.39–0.91), all cancer types (HR: 0.80; 95% CI: 0.64–0.99), and global index (HR: 0.82; 95% CI: 0.68–0.98) [3]. However, the outcomes of myocardial infarction and global index were the only outcomes with both a reduced hazard ratio and a statistically significant p for interaction for age for CEE versus placebo [3]. Invasive breast cancer was decreased with CEE for long-term follow-up in women 50–59 years of age (HR: 0.76; 95% CI: 0.52–1.11) similar to the statistically significant reduction in invasive breast cancer occurring for all participants 50–79 years of age randomized to CEE (HR: 0.79; 95% CI: 0.65–0.97) [3].

3.6. Magnitude of Favorable Long-Term Outcomes in Women 50–59 Years of Age. Annualized incidence rates allow direct comparison of the magnitude of the difference between CEE and placebo groups, while hazard ratios provide information on the relative difference in outcome, but not the absolute differences in outcome. In Figure 2, annualized incidence rates as well as hazard ratios [3] for the cumulative 13-year long-term follow-up in WHI Estrogen-Alone Trial are shown in graph form for the first time for the 50–59-year group with an adequate scale to allow a comparative assessment of the magnitude of the difference between CEE versus placebo for multiple outcomes.

3.7. Number Needed to Treat to Avoid Adverse Outcome in Women 50–59 Years of Age. The number of women needed to be randomized to CEE to prevent one woman from developing an adverse outcome during the cumulative 13-year follow-up in the WHI Estrogen-Alone Trial, for women 50–59 years of age, was calculated as noted in the Methods Section. This number-needed-to-treat analysis provides a measure of the summation effect of randomization to CEE versus placebo

Cumulative long-term FU (intervention + postintervention phase)
WHI Estrogen-Alone Trial, women 50–59 years of age, CEE versus placebo

Cases per 10,000 person-years (number of events)	CEE P 21 32 (42)(64)	CEE P 17 29 (35)(58)	CEE P 45 56 (90)(115)	CEE P 23 30 (46)(61)	CEE P 16 18 (33)(36)	CEE P 12 16 (25)(32)	CEE P 11 10 (22)(21)	CEE P 7 10 (15)(20)	CEE P 4 5 (9)(10)	CEE P 75 93 (147)(182)	CEE P 110 136 (214)(264)
Hazard ratio (95% CI)	0.65 (0.44–0.96)	0.60 (0.39–0.91)	0.78 (0.59–1.03)	0.76 (0.52–1.11)	0.96 (0.60–1.55)	0.79 (0.47–1.34)	1.06 (0.58–1.93)	0.76 (0.39–1.49)	0.88 (0.36–2.17)	0.80 (0.64–0.99)	0.82 (0.68–0.98)

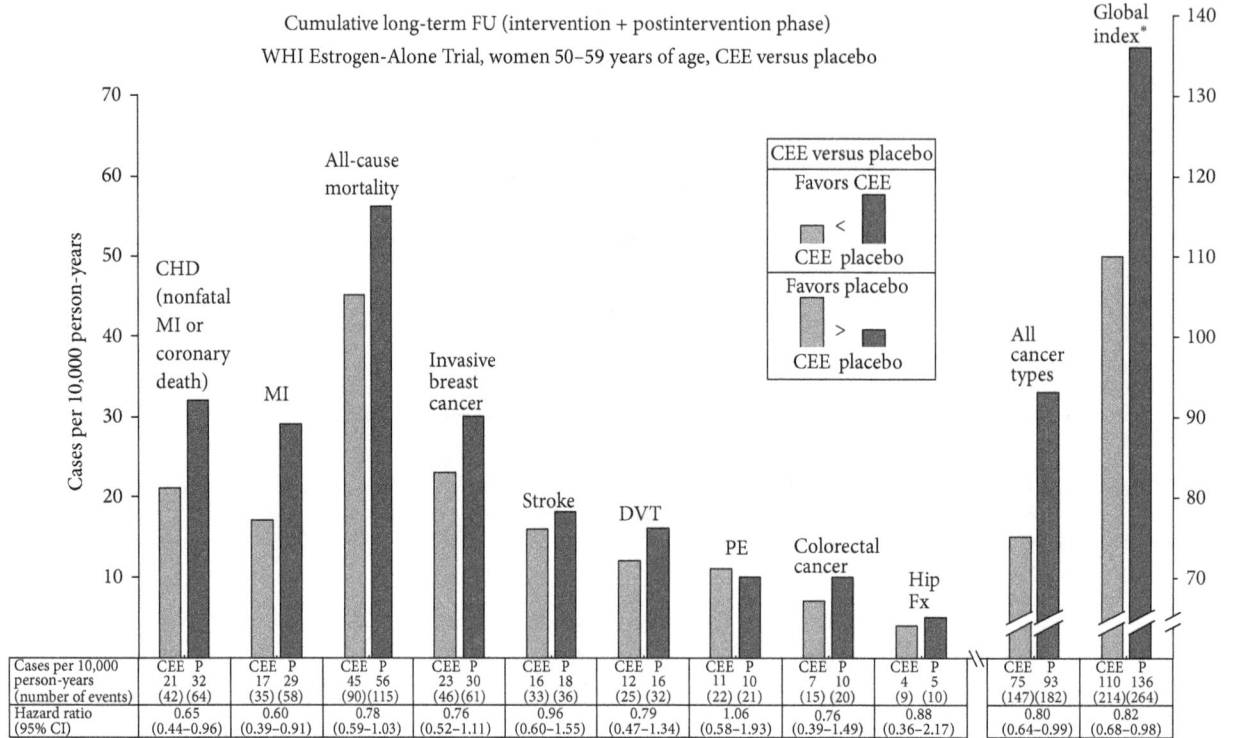

FIGURE 2: Outcomes for women 50-59 years of age at trial entry, conjugated equine estrogens (CEE) versus placebo, cumulative long-term follow-up (13 years), and WHI Estrogen-Alone Trial. * Global index represents the first event for each participant from among the following: coronary heart disease (nonfatal MI or coronary death), stroke, pulmonary embolism, breast cancer, colorectal cancer, hip fracture, or death due to other causes. CEE: conjugated equine estrogens; CHD: coronary heart disease; CI: confidence interval; DVT: deep vein thrombosis; FU: follow-up; Fx: fracture; MI: myocardial infarction; P: placebo; PE: pulmonary embolus; WHI: Women's Health Initiative. Source for outcomes: [3].

TABLE 3: Number of women needed to treat (randomized to CEE) to prevent one woman from developing a myocardial infarction or global index event, women aged 50–59 years at trial entry, Women's Health Initiative Estrogen-Alone Trial, and cumulative long-term outcomes.

Outcome	Cumulative long-term (13-year median duration) outcomes (intervention phase + postintervention phase) Number needed (95% CI) to treat	Effect
Myocardial infarction	76 (40.3–497.2)	1 less woman with a myocardial infarction
Global index[a]	37 (19.6–312.6)	1 less woman with a global index event

A number needed to treat analysis for MI and global index for the intervention phase for women aged 50–59 years did not show a statistically significant difference in outcomes for the CEE versus placebo group.

[a] A participant is counted as having a global index event if there is the diagnosis of one or more of the following occurring after randomization: coronary heart disease (nonfatal MI or coronary death), stroke, pulmonary embolism, invasive breast cancer, colorectal cancer, hip fracture, or death due to other causes.
CEE: conjugated equine estrogens; CI: confidence interval; MI: myocardial infarction; NS: not significant.
Derived (as per Methods Section) from data provided in [3].

for the entire 13-year cumulative follow-up period. For every 76 (95% CI, 40.3–497.2) women randomized to CEE rather than placebo at 50–59 years of age, there was one less woman having a myocardial infarction (MI) (Table 3). For every 37 (95% CI, 19.6–312.6) women randomized to CEE rather than placebo at 50–59 years of age, there was one less woman who developed a global index endpoint (coronary heart disease, invasive breast cancer, stroke, pulmonary embolus, colorectal cancer, hip fracture, and death from other causes).

A number-needed-to-treat analysis for MI and global index for the intervention phase for women 50–59 years of age

did not show a statistically significant difference in outcomes for the CEE versus placebo group.

3.8. WHI Estrogen-Alone Trial and Breast Cancer Reduction. In the WHI Estrogen-Alone Trial with cumulative long-term follow-up, CEE use for a 5.9-year median duration compared to placebo resulted in a statistically significant reduction in invasive breast cancer for women 50–79 years of age (HR: 0.79; 95% CI: 0.65–0.97) [3]. Breast cancer risk reduction was concentrated in women without benign breast disease or

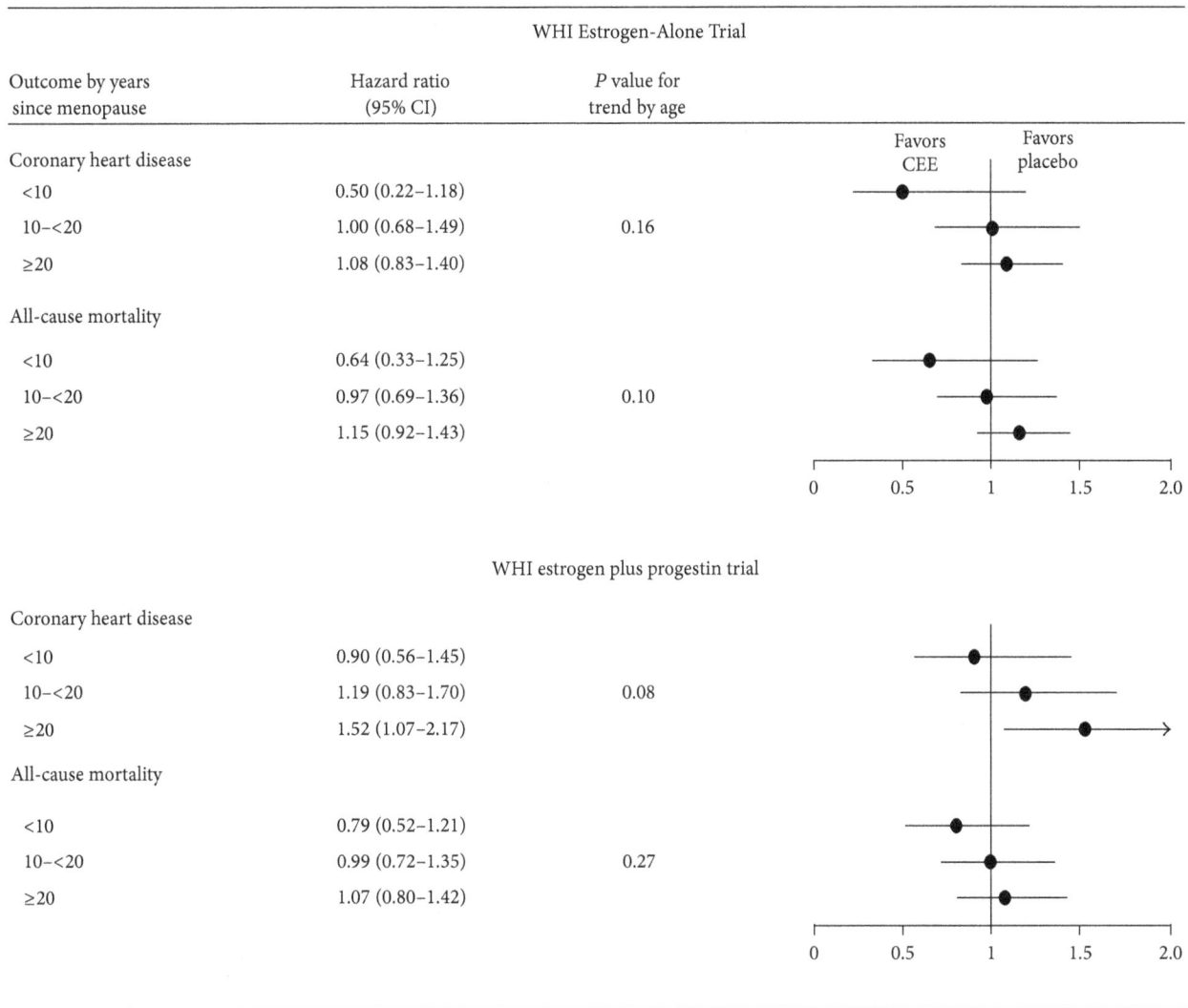

FIGURE 3: Intervention phase outcomes by years since menopause at trial entry of WHI Estrogen-Alone Trial and WHI estrogen plus progestin trial. CEE: conjugated equine estrogens; WHI: Women's Health Initiative. Sources for outcomes: [3, 23].

family history of breast cancer [24]. A sensitivity analysis showed that better adherence to estrogen use within the trial was associated with a lower risk of invasive breast cancer [24]. Women randomized to CEE compared to placebo were less likely to die of breast cancer (HR: 0.37; 95% CI: 0.13–0.91) and fewer women died from any cause after a breast cancer diagnosis (HR: 0.62; 95% CI: 0.39–0.97) [24]. In contrast, the WHI estrogen plus progestin trial for women 50–79 years of age showed an increase in invasive breast cancer with long-term follow-up (HR: 1.28; 95% CI: 1.11–1.48) [3], with the addition of 2.5 mg of medroxyprogesterone acetate daily to the same dose of CEE. The increased breast cancer risk was initially concentrated in women with prior postmenopausal hormone use [25]. The similar incidence rates of breast cancer for the placebo groups in the two trials suggest that the difference in outcome between the trials is primarily the result of the addition of medroxyprogesterone acetate to CEE [24].

3.9. WHI Trial Results Stratified by Years Since Menopause. Outcome data stratified by years since menopause [3, 23] has been published for the WHI Estrogen-Alone Trial and WHI estrogen plus progestin trial for the intervention phase (Figure 3). In both trials, there was a trend for better CHD and mortality outcomes with hormone therapy when comparing women closer to menopause with women farther from menopause.

There is a high degree of biologic plausibility that a woman's age and duration of time since menopause at initiation of hormone replacement therapy may affect clinical outcome [26]. The timing hypothesis, which is supported by primate work [27], proposes that hormone replacement therapy may have an adverse effect when begun late in menopause contrasting with beneficial effects on the more normal vessels typically present in younger women closer to time of menopause [26]. A WHI substudy of women 50–59 years of

TABLE 4: Women 50–59 years of age at trial entry, WHI Estrogen-Alone Trial Outcomes, intervention phase and postintervention phase, events, and relative risk.

Outcome	Intervention phase Events and relative risk (RR)[†]			Postintervention phase Events and relative risk (RR)[†]		
	CEE N = 1639	Placebo N = 1674	RR[†] (95% CI)	CEE N = 1223	Placebo N = 1232	RR[†] (95% CI)
	Events			Events		
CHD	21	35	0.61 (0.36–1.05)	21	29	0.73 (0.42–1.27)
MI	17	31	0.56 (0.31–1.01)	18	27	0.67 (0.37–1.21)
Death	35	50	0.71 (0.47–1.10)	55	65	0.85 (0.60–1.21)
Global index[a]	117	142	0.84 (0.67–1.06)	97	122	0.80 (0.62–1.03)

[†]Hazard ratios in WHI Hormone Trials apply a time to event analysis which can not be duplicated without full access to the data set. Relative risks in this table are calculated and shown (no time to event analysis) to allow comparison of the intervention phase and post intervention phase data.

[a]Global index represents the first event for each participant from among the following: coronary heart disease, stroke, pulmonary embolism, invasive breast cancer, colorectal cancer, hip fracture, or death due to other causes.

CEE, conjugated equine estrogens; CHD, coronary heart disease; CI, confidence interval; MI, myocardial infarction; RR, relative risk; WHI, Women's Health Initiative.

Source for the number of events and number of participants: [3, 12].

age showed significantly less coronary artery calcification, a quantitative marker for atherosclerotic plaque, in the CEE group compared to placebo [16]. The Kronos early estrogen prevention study (KEEPS) involved a younger, healthier group of newly menopausal women who developed minimal disease over the treatment period of 4 years [28]. KEEPS showed no statistically significant difference in coronary calcification or carotid artery intima-media thickness scores for women treated with estrogen and progesterone compared to the placebo group [28].

4. Long-Term Follow-Up for Clinical Outcomes Is Optimal

The WHI Estrogen-Alone Trial results indicate that long-term follow-up is required to fully assess the effects of estrogen in postmenopausal women. For all participants (50–79 years) in the WHI Estrogen-Alone Trial, a reduction in invasive breast cancer only became statistically significant with approximately an additional 5 years of follow-up after the completion of the CEE intervention phase [1, 12]. Similarly, in women 50 to 59 years of age, there were nonsignificant trends for a reduction in MI and global index in the CEE group at the completion of the 7.2-year intervention phase that only became statistically significant after years of additional follow-up subsequent to the completion of the CEE intervention phase [3, 12].

The single published Kaplan-Meier estimate for women 50–59 years of age (known to the author) from the WHI Estrogen-Alone Trial is for the outcome of CHD for the intervention phase of the trial [29]. The Kaplan-Meier curves of cumulative hazard for CHD in regard to CEE versus placebo for the intervention phase showed a divergence developing with time over the median of 7.2 years of follow-up [29]. In

Table 4, outcome events and relative risk for both the intervention and postintervention phase of the trial are shown for CHD, MI, death, and global index using data derived from prior WHI publications [3, 12]. Given the data as shown in Table 4, diverging curves for CHD for the intervention phase would persist and maintain a pattern of diverging curves when followed beyond the end of the intervention phase. The data for MI, death, and global index for women 50–59 years of age would also show diverging curves extending beyond the intervention phase if presented as a Kaplan-Meier estimate of cumulative hazard.

The only published Kaplan-Meier estimate extending at least 10 years for hormone replacement therapy for women less than 60 years of age in a primary prevention trial is from the Danish osteoporosis prevention study (DOPS) [30]. Diverging outcomes extending past the 10-year drug intervention were shown in DOPS, comparing hormone therapy (estradiol plus or minus norethisterone acetate, started within 2 years of menopause) to no medication, for the combined endpoint of death or hospital admission for heart failure or MI in this randomized, unblinded study [30] (Figure 4).

If Kaplan-Meier cumulative hazard estimates extending through 10 years had been published for the WHI Estrogen-Alone Trial for CHD, death, MI, or global index endpoints for women 50–59 years of age, similar diverging outcome curves to the DOPS data would be shown. Long-term follow-up of cardiovascular, cancer, and mortality outcomes through 10 years, including at least 5 years of follow-up after completion of hormone therapy, is advisable to adequately assess the effects of hormone replacement therapy.

Of note, in DOPS, where 81% of the women received both estrogen and progestin, participants had predominantly favorable outcomes [30], while women 50–59 years of age in the WHI estrogen plus progestin trial had negative outcomes or trends for coronary artery disease, stroke, deep venous

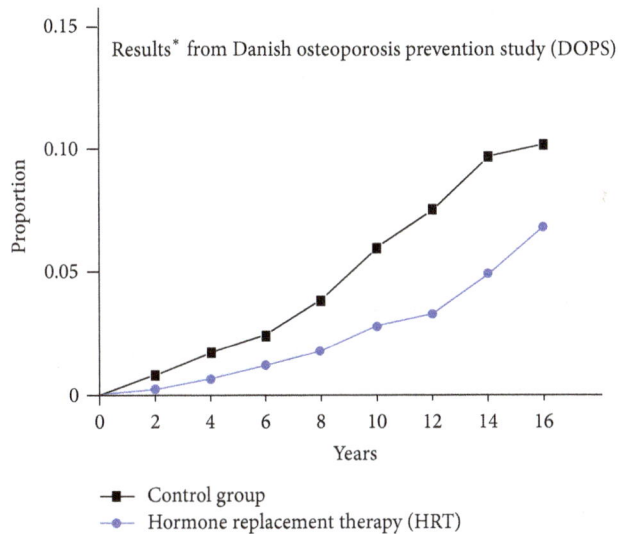

FIGURE 4: Cumulative hazard of developing death or hospitalization due to heart failure or myocardial infarction. *Modified from Schierbeck [30].

thrombosis, and pulmonary embolism [3]. The difference between the trials may be due in part to the very different populations in the trials (younger women, ≤2 years from menopause and with lower cardiovascular risk profiles in DOPS), as well as the particular hormone therapy and duration of therapy used in the trials, though this remains conjecture.

4.1. Factors Affecting Long-Term Outcomes. The long duration of the follow-up of the WHI Estrogen-Alone Trial may have influenced outcomes. The 13-year median cumulative follow-up included the intervention phase and the 6.6-year median duration postintervention phase of the trial. The WHI trial study's authors reported on that time duration for their most recent comprehensive article on outcomes [3] and, hence, that time duration was used in this paper.

The initial adverse effect of CEE on stroke and DVT documented during the intervention phase that diminished in the postintervention phase may have been simply the waning of the adverse effect that occurred after CEE was discontinued. The similarity of the relative risks in the intervention and postintervention phase for myocardial infarction, CHD, death, invasive breast cancer, and global index suggests a possible perseverance of a beneficial effect of CEE that lasted beyond cessation of the medication. If vascular beneficial effects occurred during the intervention phase, the ramification of these effects would tend to continue to manifest beyond the point in time when CEE was discontinued. The mechanism of the persistent effects of hormone therapy after cessation in regard to invasive breast cancer is beyond the scope of this paper.

The unblinding occurred when the trial was stopped because of an increased risk of stroke in the CEE group [1]. This would not tend to lead to preferential reporting of adverse events in the placebo group participants during the

postintervention follow-up. Hence, the unblinding of the trial in the post intervention phase is unlikely to bias the reporting of adverse outcomes in favor of the CEE group.

5. Age as an Important Subgroup

Age was prespecified in the WHI trial protocol as a subgroup for analysis. A limited number of subgroup analyses in the WHI hormone trial reports were thought to be important enough to warrant stratifying primary outcomes in the presentation of the initial WHI trial results [1, 2]. In the WHI estrogen plus progestin trial 2002 publication, there were four such subgroups: clinical center, age, prior to disease, and randomization status in the low-fat diet trial [2]. Similarly, in the WHI Estrogen-Alone Trial initial 2004 publication, primary outcome comparisons were presented as hazard ratios from Cox proportional hazard analyses stratified by only three subgroups: age, prior disease, and randomization status in the low-fat diet trial [1]. Age was an important consideration in the trial, with the protocol defining specific target age enrollment percentages [9]. Though a subgroup analysis of multiple biomarkers obtained from blood draw analysis in a nested case control study was also prespecified by protocol, this analysis was reported only after initial publication of trial results [29, 31, 32]. The biomarker subgroup analysis was performed for a comparatively limited number of outcomes [3, 12, 29, 31, 32].

6. Limitations of This Analysis

This paper concerns a subgroup analysis of women 50–59 years of age at trial entry in the WHI Estrogen-Alone Trial. Subgroup analyses are subject to statistical problems: limiting conclusions for subgroup analyses to those with a statistically significant p for interaction is helpful. A limitation of this analysis is that CHD, the primary trial outcome, did not have a statistically significant P for interaction ($P = .08$ for intervention phase [3]). This trial also reflects the outcomes for only a single formulation of estrogen: CEE.

Multiple primary and secondary endpoints underwent evaluation for trend by age (P for interaction). Four primary or secondary endpoints in the intervention phase and two in the cumulative long-term follow-up had a significant trend by age at the .05 significance level. For the 20 primary and secondary trial endpoints [3] in the WHI Estrogen-Alone Trial undergoing analysis by age, one significant P for interaction would be expected by chance alone in the intervention phase and one by chance alone for cumulative long-term follow-up at the .05 level of significance.

The number-needed-to-treat analysis includes the extended follow-up phase which is unblinded and with incomplete participant follow-up. These same limitations are present for all WHI reported annualized incidence percentages and rates for postintervention and cumulative long-term follow-up [3, 12, 24, 33, 34].

Nominal 95% confidence intervals are reported without adjustment for multiple outcomes, sequential repeated data analysis, multiple subgroup analyses, and extension of trial follow-up with incomplete participation. This is true for this report and for the majority of the published WHI trial outcome results [3, 12, 20, 24, 32–34]. There has been no publication from the WHI Estrogen-Alone Trial of a primary or secondary trial endpoint fully adjusted for these factors (except for a benefit with CEE for all fractures [1]) which achieves statistical significance for any follow-up interval, including stroke or DVT in women 50–79 years of age [1, 3, 12, 23, 24, 29, 32].

7. Conclusions

Women 50–59 years of age at time of randomization to CEE or placebo in the WHI Estrogen-Alone Trial were similar in median age to women initiating hormone replacement therapy in clinical practice. In the intervention phase, for women 50–59 years of age with CEE, there was an increased risk of DVT, gall bladder disease, and stroke, while the reduction in MI, invasive breast cancer, and global index of events was not statistically significant. With cumulative 13-year long-term follow-up, women 50–59 years of age with CEE showed a reduction in MI, as well as a reduced global index of events. The increased risk of stroke and DVT in the intervention phase for women 50–79 years of age, which did not show significant trends with age, declined with cessation of CEE. Long-term follow-up including at least 5 years of follow-up after completion of hormone therapy is necessary to optimally evaluate effects of hormone replacement therapy on cardiovascular, cancer, and mortality outcomes. Though a subgroup analysis does not provide an adequate basis for making guideline recommendations for primary prevention, the preponderance of evidence in the WHI Estrogen-Alone Trial strongly suggests an overall benefit with CEE with cumulative long-term follow-up in women 50–59 years of age. These potential benefits only apply to women with prior hysterectomy and for duration of CEE use similar to what was used in the trial. The WHI Estrogen-Alone Trial data does not provide information on longer durations of use and strongly suggests that initiation of hormone therapy at significantly later ages is harmful.

Conflict of Interests

The author declares that there is no conflict of interests regarding the publication of this paper.

References

[1] G. L. Anderson and M. Limacher, "Effects of conjugated equine estrogen in postmenopausal women with hysterectomy: the Women's Health Initiative randomized controlled trial," *The Journal of the American Medical Association*, vol. 291, no. 14, pp. 1701–1712, 2004.

[2] Writing Group for the Women's Health Initiative Investigators, "Risks and benefits of estrogen plus progestin in healthy postmenopausal women: principal results from the Women's health initiative randomized controlled trial," *The Journal of the American Medical Association*, vol. 288, no. 3, pp. 321–333, 2002.

[3] J. E. Manson, R. T. Chlebowski, M. L. Stefanick et al., "Menopausal hormone therapy and health outcomes during the intervention and extended poststopping phases of the women's health initiative randomized trials," *The Journal of the American Medical Association*, vol. 310, no. 13, pp. 1353–1368, 2013.

[4] F. Grodstein, J. E. Manson, M. J. Stampfer, and K. Rexrode, "Postmenopausal hormone therapy and stroke: role of time since menopause and age at initiation of hormone therapy," *Archives of Internal Medicine*, vol. 168, no. 8, pp. 861–866, 2008.

[5] M. Canonico, E. Oger, G. Plu-Bureau et al., "Hormone therapy and venous thromboembolism among postmenopausal women: impact of the route of estrogen administration and progestogens: the ESTHER study," *Circulation*, vol. 115, no. 7, pp. 840–845, 2007.

[6] B. Liu, V. Beral, A. Balkwill, J. Green, S. Sweetland, and G. Reeves, "Gallbladder disease and use of transdermal versus oral hormone replacement therapy in postmenopausal women: prospective cohort study," *British Medical Journal*, vol. 337, article a386, 2008.

[7] N. L. Smith, M. Blondon, K. L. Wiggins et al., "Lower risk of cardiovascular events in postmenopausal women taking oral estradiol compared with oral conjugated equine estrogens," *The Journal of the American Medical Association Internal Medicine*, vol. 174, no. 1, pp. 25–31, 2014.

[8] C. L. Shufelt, C. N. B. Merz, R. L. Prentice et al., "Hormone therapy dose, formulation, route of delivery, and risk of cardiovascular events in women: findings from the Women's Health Initiative Observational Study," *Menopause*, vol. 21, no. 3, pp. 260–266, 2014.

[9] The Women's Health Initiative Study Group, "Design of the women's health initiative clinical trial and observational study," *Controlled Clinical Trials*, vol. 19, no. 1, pp. 61–109, 1998.

[10] R. Bender, "Calculating confidence intervals for the number needed to treat," *Controlled Clinical Trials*, vol. 22, no. 2, pp. 102–110, 2001.

[11] R. Bender, "Calculation of Confidence Intervals for NNT," http://www.rbsd.de/SOFTWARE/nnt_ci.sas.

[12] A. Z. LaCroix, R. T. Chlebowski, J. E. Manson et al., "Health outcomes after stopping conjugated equine estrogens among postmenopausal women with prior hysterectomy: a randomized controlled trial," *The Journal of the American Medical Association*, vol. 305, no. 13, pp. 1305–1314, 2011.

[13] D. G. Altman and P. K. Andersen, "Calculating the number needed to treat for trials where the outcome is time to an event," *British Medical Journal*, vol. 319, no. 7223, pp. 1492–1495, 1999.

[14] R. L. Prentice, M. Pettinger, and G. L. Anderson, "Statistical issues arising in the women's health initiative," *Biometrics*, vol. 61, no. 4, pp. 899–911, 2005.

[15] M. T. Connelly, M. Richardson, and R. Platt, "Prevalence and duration of postmenopausal hormone replacement therapy use in a managed care organization, 1990–1995," *Journal of General Internal Medicine*, vol. 15, no. 8, pp. 542–550, 2000.

[16] J. E. Manson, M. A. Allison, J. E. Rossouw et al., "Estrogen therapy and coronary-artery calcification," *The New England Journal of Medicine*, vol. 356, no. 25, pp. 2591–2602, 2007.

[17] R. L. Prentice, R. Langer, M. L. Stefanick et al., "Combined postmenopausal hormone therapy and cardiovascular disease: toward resolving the discrepancy between observational studies and the Women's Health Initiative clinical trial," *American Journal of Epidemiology*, vol. 162, no. 5, pp. 404–414, 2005.

[18] R. L. Prentice, J. E. Manson, and R. D. Langer, "Benefits and risks of postmenopausal hormone therapy when it is initiated soon

after menopause," *American Journal of Epidemiology*, vol. 170, no. 1, pp. 12–23, 2009.

[19] Department of Health and Human Services and National Center for Health Statistics, "National Health and Nutrition Examination Survey. Use of Hormone Replacement Therapy among Postmenopausal Women in the United States, 1988–94," http://www.cdc.gov/nchs/data/nhanes/databriefs/hrtinwomen .pdf.

[20] D. J. Cirillo, R. B. Wallace, R. J. Rodabough et al., "Effect of estrogen therapy on gallbladder disease," *The Journal of the American Medical Association*, vol. 293, no. 3, pp. 330–339, 2005.

[21] J. E. Manson, R. T. Chlebowski, and A. K. Aragaki, "Hormone therapy use and outcomes in the women's health initiative trials—reply," *The Journal of the American Medical Association*, vol. 311, no. 4, pp. 417–418, 2014.

[22] S. L. Hendrix, S. Wassertheil-Smoller, K. C. Johnson et al., "Effects of conjugated equine estrogen on stroke in the Women's Health Initiative," *Circulation*, vol. 113, no. 20, pp. 2425–2434, 2006.

[23] J. E. Rossouw, R. L. Prentice, J. E. Manson et al., "Postmenopausal hormone therapy and risk of cardiovascular disease by age and years since menopause," *The Journal of the American Medical Association*, vol. 297, no. 13, pp. 1465–1477, 2007.

[24] G. L. Anderson, R. T. Chlebowski, A. K. Aragaki et al., "Conjugated equine oestrogen and breast cancer incidence and mortality in postmenopausal women with hysterectomy: extended follow-up of the Women's Health Initiative randomised placebo-controlled trial," *The Lancet Oncology*, vol. 13, no. 5, pp. 476–486, 2012.

[25] G. L. Anderson, R. T. Chlebowski, J. E. Rossouw et al., "Prior hormone therapy and breast cancer risk in the women's health initiative randomized trial of estrogen plus progestin," *Maturitas*, vol. 55, no. 2, pp. 103–115, 2006.

[26] M. E. Mendelsohn and R. H. Karas, "HRT and the young at heart," *The New England Journal of Medicine*, vol. 356, no. 25, pp. 2639–2641, 2007.

[27] T. B. Clarkson and S. E. Appt, "Controversies about HRT—lessons from monkey models," *Maturitas*, vol. 51, no. 1, pp. 64–74, 2005.

[28] S. M. Harman, D. M. Black, F. Naftolin et al., "Arterial imaging outcomes and cardiovascular risk factors in recently menopausal women: a randomized trial," *Annals of Internal Medicine*, vol. 161, no. 4, pp. 249–260, 2014.

[29] J. Hsia, R. D. Langer, J. E. Manson, Women's Health Initiative Investigators et al., "Conjugated equine estrogens and coronary heart disease: the women's health initiative," *Archives of Internal Medicine*, vol. 166, no. 3, pp. 357–365, 2006.

[30] L. L. Schierbeck, L. Rejnmark, C. L. Tofteng et al., "Effect of hormone replacement therapy on cardiovascular events in recently postmenopausal women: randomised trial," *British Medical Journal*, vol. 345, no. 7881, Article ID e6409, 2012.

[31] J. E. Manson, J. Hsia, K. C. Johnson et al., "Estrogen plus progestin and the risk of coronary heart disease," *The New England Journal of Medicine*, vol. 349, no. 6, pp. 523–534, 2003.

[32] J. D. Curb, R. L. Prentice, P. F. Bray et al., "Venous thrombosis and conjugated equine estrogen in women without a uterus," *Archives of Internal Medicine*, vol. 166, no. 7, pp. 772–780, 2006.

[33] G. Heiss, R. Wallace, G. L. Anderson et al., "Health risks and benefits 3 years after stopping randomized treatment with estrogen and progestin," *The Journal of the American Medical Association*, vol. 299, no. 9, pp. 1036–1045, 2008.

[34] R. T. Chlebowski, G. L. Anderson, M. Gass et al., "Estrogen plus progestin and breast cancer incidence and mortality in postmenopausal women," *The Journal of the American Medical Association*, vol. 304, no. 15, pp. 1684–1692, 2010.

35

Mode of Vaginal Delivery: A Modifiable Intrapartum Risk Factor for Obstetric Anal Sphincter Injury

Marta Simó González,[1] **Oriol Porta Roda,**[1] **Josep Perelló Capó,**[1]
Ignasi Gich Saladich,[2] **and Joaquim Calaf Alsina**[1]

[1]*Department of Gynecology and Obstetrics, Hospital de la Santa Creu i Sant Pau, Universidad Autónoma de Barcelona,*
 C/Mas Casanovas 90, 08025 Barcelona, Spain
[2]*Clinical Epidemiology Unit, Hospital de la Santa Creu i Sant Pau, Universidad Autónoma de Barcelona,*
 C/Mas Casanovas 90, 08025 Barcelona, Spain

Correspondence should be addressed to Marta Simó González; msimo@santpau.cat

Academic Editor: Marc J. N. C. Keirse

The aim of this study was to analyze the comparative risks of this anal sphincter injury in relation to the type of intervention in vaginal delivery. We performed an observational, retrospective study of all vaginal deliveries attended at a tertiary university hospital between January 2006 and December 2009. We analyzed the incidence of obstetric anal sphincter injury for each mode of vaginal delivery: spontaneous delivery, vacuum, Thierry spatulas, and forceps. We determined the proportional incidence between methods taking spontaneous delivery as the reference. Ninety-seven of 4526 (2.14%) women included in the study presented obstetric anal sphincter injury. Instrumental deliveries showed a significantly higher risk of anal sphincter injury (2.7 to 4.9%) than spontaneous deliveries (1.1%). The highest incidence was for Thierry spatulas (OR 4.804), followed by forceps (OR 4.089) and vacuum extraction (OR 2.509). The type of intervention in a vaginal delivery is a modifiable intrapartum risk factor for obstetric anal sphincter injury. Tearing can occur in any type of delivery but proportions vary significantly. All healthcare professionals attending childbirth should be aware of the risk for each type of intervention and consider these together with the obstetric factors in each case.

1. Introduction

Obstetric anal sphincter injury encompasses third and fourth degree perineal tearing that occurs during delivery, according to Sultan's classification. This classification considers perineal injuries as a 3rd degree tear when there is any involvement of the anal sphincter and 4th degree tear when the anal epithelium is involved. This classification is incorporated in the RCOG guidelines and included in the Green Top Guidelines for the Management of Third and Fourth-Degree Perineal Tears Following Vaginal Delivery. Third degree tears are further classified into three subgroups according to the extent of damage to the external anal sphincter and internal anal sphincter [1, 2]. This classification is summarized in Table 1.

The incidence of obstetric anal sphincter injury varies between 0.5 and 5% of vaginal deliveries and it is the most common cause of anal incontinence in healthy women [3].

Obstetric anal sphincter injury is a serious complication of childbirth due to its notable maternal morbidity, its serious physical and emotional effects, and its impact on quality of life. Awareness of the factors most frequently associated with this injury is essential and can help obstetricians perform safer deliveries for both mother and child.

Many authors have studied the risk factors for obstetric anal sphincter injury and there is unanimity that its incidence is higher in occiput posterior and in instrumental deliveries with forceps [4]. Instruments used in the delivery room, however, can vary greatly between centers and countries. Most trials concerning instrumental deliveries considered forceps and vacuum in their analysis [5].

Spatulas are unarticulated instruments used mainly in French-speaking countries and a few other countries in Europe, Africa, and Latin American. The two most commonly used types of spatulas are Thierry and Teissier. Both

TABLE 1: Sultan's classification of perineal trauma.

1st degree	Laceration of vaginal epithelium or perineal skin only	
2nd degree	Involvement of the perineal muscles but not the anal sphincter	
3rd degree	Disruption of the anal sphincter muscles	3a: <50% thickness of external sphincter torn
		3b: >50% thickness of external sphincter torn
		3c: internal sphincter torn
4th degree	Third degree tear with disruption of the anal epithelium as well	

TABLE 2: Types of vaginal delivery.

Type of delivery		Total (%)	ACC %
Spontaneous		3109 (68.69%)	68.69%
Vacuum		149 (3.29%)	31.31%
Forceps	553 (12.21%)	207 Kjelland (37.43%)	
		346 Naegele (62.57%)	
Thierry spatulas		715 (15.79%)	
Total		**4526 (100%)**	**100%**

types consist of two independent symmetric levers that are used to propel the fetal head forward, avoiding squeezing between the two branches. Teissier spatulas are shorter and less commonly used than the Thierry type [6]. Spatulas have classically been considered less aggressive than forceps on the basis of neonatal morbidity, and literature concerning their use and their maternal morbidity is scarce [7]. In daily clinical practice in our hospital, we use vacuum, forceps, and Thierry spatulas for instrumental deliveries. To our knowledge, no studies to date have compared all three interventions. The aim of this study was to analyze the comparative risk of obstetric anal sphincter injury in relation to the method used in instrumental deliveries.

2. Materials and Methods

We carried out an observational, retrospective study by analyzing data from the computerized database of all deliveries at Hospital de la Santa Creu i Sant Pau from January 1, 2006, until December 31, 2009. Our institution is a tertiary referral hospital in Barcelona, Spain. Personal identification details were omitted in all cases to ensure anonymity. The study was approved by the local Clinical Research Ethics Committee.

We included all vaginal deliveries of a singleton fetus in vertex presentation that occurred in our center during the study period. Exclusion criteria were birth by caesarean section, multiple births, and births with noncephalic presentations.

Our hospital is a training center for specialist physicians and midwives. Spontaneous deliveries can be attended by either physicians or midwives following a common protocol. The mother chooses the position in which she wants to give birth, but the perineum should always be visible to the attendant to permit "hands-on" perineal protection. Mediolateral episiotomy is only used when the attendant considers this necessary. Trainee physicians and midwives are closely overseen by a specialist in their field at all times. Instrumental vaginal deliveries are only performed by physicians. We perform and teach instrumental vaginal interventions using forceps, Thierry spatulas, and vacuum. The type of instrument is selected at the discretion of the attending physician, depending on the obstetric situation. When obstetric anal sphincter injury is diagnosed, primary repair is carried out in accordance with established guidelines.

The main outcome, obstetric anal sphincter injury, was classified according to the Sultan's classification [2]. Variables analyzed were type of delivery (spontaneous, vacuum, forceps, or Thierry spatulas), age, parity, anesthesia (epidural or local), type of labor onset (spontaneous or induction), duration of labor (hours from the beginning of the active phase of the first stage of labor until delivery), attendant (OBGYN trainee, OBGYN specialist, midwife, and midwife trainee), neonatal weight, and umbilical cord pH values.

The incidence of obstetric anal sphincter injury was analyzed according to the attendant and the type of vaginal delivery. Spontaneous vaginal birth was taken as the reference as it has the lowest incidence of this injury. We compared this with the other types of vaginal delivery (vacuum, forceps, and spatulas) rather than comparing the different types of instrumental delivery with each other.

2.1. Statistical Analysis. All variables were assessed in relation to the main outcome: obstetric anal sphincter injury. For categorical variables, the bivariate relationship was determined using contingency tables and inference with the corresponding chi-square or Fisher's exact test. For quantitative variables, the t-test for independent measurements was used. Multivariate analysis (logistic regression) was carried out. This analysis included all variables with a trend in the bivariate approach ($P \leq 0.10$) or with clinical relevance. In all cases, the significance level used was the 5% ($\alpha = 0.05$) with a bilateral approach. Analysis was performed using the SPSS Statistics V19.0.

3. Results

A total of 4526 vaginal births were recorded during the study period. Obstetric anal sphincter injury occurred in 97 cases, giving an incidence of 2.14% (CI 95% = 1.72–2.57).

Table 2 summarizes the different types of vaginal delivery. Our instrumentation rate was 31.31% for vaginal deliveries and 23.31% for all deliveries (including cesarean deliveries). According to the Sultan's classification, there were 93 3rd degree injuries (spontaneous 33, vacuum 3, forceps 22, and Thierry spatulas 35) and four 4th degree injuries (forceps 3 and Thierry spatulas 1).

Table 3 summarizes the results of the bivariate analysis. No significant differences were found between the obstetric anal sphincter injury and nonobstetric anal sphincter injury groups regarding maternal age, mode of onset of labor, duration of labor, or umbilical cord pH values at birth. We

TABLE 3: Summary of bivariate analysis results.

Variable	Categories	OASI	NO OASI	P value
Maternal age**	Years	31.33 (4.95)	31.02 (5.50)	P = 0.541
Parity*	Primipara	**70 (2.9%)**	**2324 (97%)**	**P < 0.001**
	Multipara	**27 (1.3%)**	**2104 (98.7)**	
Labor onset*	Spontaneous	75 (2%)	3622 (98%)	P = 0.287
	Induction	22 (2.7%)	807 (97.3%)	
Delivery duration	Hours	6.15 (3.64)	6.15 (5.04)	P = 0.995
Anesthesia*	Without	**8 (1.1%)**	**736 (98.9%)**	**P = 0.026**
	With	**89 (2.4%)**	**3693 (97.6%)**	
Type of delivery*	Spontaneous	**33 (1.1%)**	**3076 (98.9%)**	**P < 0.001**
	Vacuum extraction	**4 (2.7%)**	**145 (97.3)**	
	Forceps	**25 (4.5%)**	**528 (95.5%)**	
	Thierry's spatulas	**35 (4.9%)**	**680 (95.1%)**	
Assistant*	OBGYN	**18 (5.7%)**	**298 (94.3%)**	**P < 0.001**
	OBGYN trainee	**63 (2.3%)**	**2943 (97.7%)**	
	Midwife	**4 (1.1%)**	**349 (98.9%)**	
	Midwife trainee	**6 (0.7%)**	**822 (99.3%)**	
Neonatal weight**	Grams	3438.35 (408.40)	3263.89 (508.93)	**P < 0.001**
Umbilical cord pH**	Umbilical artery	7.22 (0.074)	7.23 (0.001)	P = 0.181

*Categorical variables: number and percentageof cases.
**Quantitative variables: mean and standard deviation.

TABLE 4: Summary of multivariate analysis results.

Variable			Coeff.	P	OR	CI 95% Lower OR	CI 95% Upper OR
Neonatal weight (grams)			0.001	0.002	1.001	1.000	1.001
Mode of delivery	Spontaneous delivery			P < 0.001	1*		
	Instrumental delivery	Vacuum	0.920	0.087	2.509	0.876	7.189
		Forceps	1.408	**<0.001**	**4.089**	2.406	6.949
		Thierry spatulas	1.569	**<0.001**	**4.804**	2.962	7.792

*Reference group.

found that differences were statistically significant in the bivariate analysis for parity ($P < 0.01$), anesthesia ($P = 0.026$), attendant ($P < 0.01$), type of vaginal delivery ($P < 0.01$), and birth weight ($P < 0.01$). Neither parity nor anesthesia, however, was significant in the multivariate analysis, and both were excluded from the final model. Table 4 shows the results obtained in the multivariate analysis.

The type of vaginal delivery ($P < 0.01$), the attendant ($P < 0.01$), and neonate birth weight ($P < 0.01$) showed statistically significant differences in the multivariate analysis. As neonatal weight is a nonmodifiable factor, we focused on the two factors in which we can intervene, the attendant and the type of vaginal delivery.

We analyzed the incidence of obstetric anal sphincter injury for each type of vaginal intervention. Women who had a spontaneous delivery had the lowest incidence of injury (1.1%), followed by vacuum extraction (2.7%) and forceps (4.5%). The use of Thierry's spatulas showed the highest incidence (4.9%). When comparing the differences in incidence of obstetric anal sphincter injury between spontaneous and instrumental delivery, we found significant results ($P < 0.01$).

Vacuum extraction showed no significant differences (OR = 2.50). Forceps (OR = 4.08) and Thierry spatulas (OR = 4.80) showed statistically significant differences ($P < 0.01$). The risk of obstetric anal sphincter injury during delivery was fourfold higher using forceps and almost fivefold higher using Thierry spatulas than for spontaneous delivery.

The incidence of obstetric anal sphincter injury differed significantly in relation to the attendant ($P < 0.01$). OBGYN specialists showed a high incidence of injury (5.7%) compared to trainee physicians (2.3%), midwives (1.1%), and resident midwives (0.7%). It should be taken into account, however, that only physicians (both specialists and trainees) perform instrumental deliveries at our centre.

In terms of evaluation of the model, the Hosmer-Lemeshow test for goodness of fit showed no significant results ($P = 0.548$). The discrimination index (AUC-ROC) showed a value of 0.72, indicating good discrimination. We also calculated the ROC curve in the final model using 2 variables (neonatal weight and type of delivery) and 3 variables (adding attendant). The results showed similar values: 0.720 and 0.725.

4. Discussion

The main finding in this study was that the risk of obstetric anal sphincter injury differed in relation to the type of intervention in a vaginal delivery. Spatulas and forceps showed a significantly higher incidence of injury than spontaneous delivery and the incidence of injury was highest for Thierry spatulas.

Multivariate analysis identified the variables type of vaginal intervention, attendant, and neonatal weight as risk factors for obstetric anal sphincter injury in our group of patients. These results show special care should be taken when reviewing for tears so as to rule out obstetric anal sphincter injury in cases of high neonatal weight and in cases of instrumental delivery.

As neonatal weight is a nonmodifiable factor, we focus from here on the types of vaginal intervention during delivery and the attendant. In relation to vaginal intervention, we did not find many studies about the rate of instrumental delivery. In a multicentric study including data from 49 university hospitals in France in 2007, Mangin et al. published an interesting article about the rates of instrumental delivery. They concluded that the rate of operative delivery differed from one center to the other, ranging from 5.3 to 34.1% of all births [7]. In our setting of a university tertiary department where we perform and teach all types of instrumentation our rate of instrumentation (31.3% for vaginal deliveries and 23.31% for all deliveries) could be considered within a common range.

Our results agree with earlier publications which found that several variables that were initially considered as risk factors for obstetric anal sphincter injury, such as primiparity, were later associated with instrumental extraction [8]. Episiotomy was not considered a variable due to the difficulty in credibly and objectively assessing this from the available data. Nevertheless, we do not consider our results were influenced by episiotomy because there is no consensus about the effect of this intervention with respect to tearing [9, 10].

The decision regarding the indication for instrumental delivery and the choice of instrument depended on the criteria of the attending physician. The fact that our analysis included all types of vaginal delivery gave us a wide view. Most studies to date have compared rates of obstetric anal sphincter injury for vacuum with rates for forceps. However, we compared the incidence of such injury in spontaneous vaginal delivery between three types of vaginal instrumentation: vacuum, spatulas, and forceps. We considered that this approach provided a new and more complete and objective picture of the real risk of each intervention.

Spontaneous delivery should be prioritized over other methods as an elective approach whenever feasible because of its lowest risk for this complication. The risk should be thoroughly evaluated when a delivery attendant considers a vaginal intervention is needed. The relative risk of obstetric anal sphincter injury for each type of intervention and its potential impact on the quality of life of the mother should be taken into account when selecting the instrument.

Our results support other studies showing that vacuum extraction has the lowest risk of obstetric anal sphincter injury among instrumental deliveries and should be considered, when obstetrically indicated, before other types of intervention. The higher risk of obstetric anal sphincter injury associated with the use of Thierry's spatula and forceps should be kept in mind when assessing their indication. Although spatulas may be considered less aggressive than forceps for neonatal morbidity, the risk for the mother must also be taken into account.

A final point worthy of consideration is the statistically significant difference found in relation to the attendant. OBGYN had the highest incidence of obstetric anal sphincter injury, but we did not consider this in the final statistical model. In our setting as a teaching hospital, OBGYN specialists intervene directly only in difficult deliveries. They supervise medical trainees and midwives but rarely intervene in spontaneous deliveries. Furthermore, midwives and midwife trainees never perform instrumental deliveries. For these reasons, we considered the results related to the variable "attendant" were biased. Nevertheless, we calculated the ROC curve using two models: with and without the attendant variable. The similar results support our argument that including attendant in the final model would not improve our results regarding the other two significant variables: neonatal weight and type of delivery.

In conclusion, all professionals attending a delivery of any type must be aware of the risks of obstetric anal sphincter injury. When an instrumental delivery is indicated, the most adequate approach should be carefully assessed, considering its potential impact. Such considerations could play a key role in reducing the incidence of obstetric anal sphincter injury and improving the maternal outcomes of childbirth.

5. Limitations and Strengths

Our study has several limitations. First, it was an observational, retrospective study of the register of our normal clinical practice, and occiput position or episiotomy was not systematically recorded in our database. Second, when intervention in a vaginal delivery was considered necessary, the decision concerning the type of intervention was left up to the specialist and, as in many operative and surgical techniques, this variable is difficult to standardize. The strengths of our paper are, however, the wide number of patients included and the comparison of the different modes of vaginal intervention. To our knowledge, these three interventions have not been compared together previously.

Ethical Approval

The Ethics Committee at Hospital de la Santa Creu i Sant Pau approved this trial on July 13, 2010 (Code number: 46/2010).

Conflict of Interests

The authors declare no conflict of interests.

Acknowledgment

The authors thank Carolyn Newey for editing assistance.

References

[1] A. H. Sultan and R. Takar, "Lower genital tract and anal sphincter trauma," *Best Practice & Research Clinical Obstetrics & Gynaecology*, vol. 16, pp. 99–116, 2002.

[2] A. H. Sultan and C. Kettle, "Diagnosis of perineal trauma," in *Perineal and Anal Sphincter Trauma Diagnosis and Clinical Management*, A. H. Sultan, R. Thakar, and D. E. Fenner, Eds., vol. 2, pp. 13–19, SpringerScience+Business Media, London, UK, 2007.

[3] M.-C. Marchand, H. Corriveau, M.-F. Dubois, and A. Watier, "Effect of dyssynergic defecation during pregnancy on third- and fourth-degree tear during a first vaginal delivery: a case-control study," *American Journal of Obstetrics & Gynecology*, vol. 201, no. 2, pp. 183.e1–183.e6, 2009.

[4] T. C. Dudding, C. J. Vaizey, and M. A. Kamm, "Obstetric anal sphincter injury: incidence, risk factors, and management," *Annals of Surgery*, vol. 247, no. 2, pp. 224–237, 2008.

[5] C. O'Herlihy, "Obstetric perineal injury: risk factors and strategies for prevention," *Seminars in Perinatology*, vol. 27, no. 1, pp. 13–19, 2003.

[6] I. Boucoiran, L. Valerio, A. Bafghi, J. Delotte, and A. Bongain, "Spatula-assisted deliveries: a large cohort of 1065 cases," *European Journal of Obstetrics Gynecology and Reproductive Biology*, vol. 151, no. 1, pp. 46–51, 2010.

[7] R. Mangin, Z. Ramanah, L. Aouar et al., "Données 2007 de l'extraction instrumentale en France: résultats d'une enquête nationale auprès de l'ensemble des centres hospitalo-universitaires," *Journal de Gynécologie Obstétrique et Biologie de la Reproduction*, vol. 39, no. 2, pp. 121–132, 2007.

[8] J.-P. Menard, M. Provansal, H. Heckenroth, M. Gamerre, F. Bretelle, and C. Mazouni, "Maternal morbidity after Thierry's spatulas and vacuum deliveries," *Gynecologie Obstetrique Fertilite*, vol. 36, no. 6, pp. 623–627, 2008.

[9] E. Twidale, K. Cornell, N. Litzow, and A. Hotchin, "Obstetric anal sphincter injury risk factors and the role of the mediolateral episiotomy," *Australian and New Zealand Journal of Obstetrics and Gynaecology*, vol. 53, no. 1, pp. 17–20, 2013.

[10] S. Alouini, L. Rossard, B. Lemaire, P. Mégier, and L. Mesnard, "Anal sphincter tears after vaginal delivery: risk factors and means of prevention," *Revue Medicale de Liege*, vol. 66, no. 10, pp. 545–549, 2011.

Permissions

List of Contributors

Sharda Brata Ghosh
Saudi German Hospital, Dubai, UAE

Y. M. Mala
Department of Obstetrics & Gynaecology, Lok Nayak Hospital, Maulana Azad Medical College, Delhi 110002, India

Habtamu Demelash
Department of Public Health, College of Medicine and Health Sciences, Madawalabu University, Goba, Bale, Ethiopia

Dabere Nigatu and Ketema Gashaw
Department of Nursing, College of Medicine and Health Sciences, Madawalabu University, Goba, Bale, Ethiopia

A. J. van der Ven, J. M. Schaaf and E. Pajkrt
Department of Obstetrics and Gynaecology, Academic Medical Center, P.O. Box 22700, 1100 DE Amsterdam, Netherlands

J. M. Schaaf
Department of Medical Informatics, Academic Medical Center, Amsterdam, Netherlands

M. A. van Os and C. J. M. de Groot
Department of Obstetrics and Gynaecology, VU University Medical Center, Amsterdam, Netherlands

M. C. Haak
Department of Obstetrics and Gynaecology, Leiden University Medical Center, Leiden, Netherlands

B. W. J. Mol
School of Paediatrics and Reproductive Health, University of Adelaide, SA 5000, Australia

Selda Uysal
Gynecology and Obstetrics Department, Ataturk Training and Research Hospital, Basin Sitesi, Yesilyurt, 35360 İzmir, Turkey

Ahmet Zeki Isik
Gynecology and Obstetrics Department, Izmir University Hospital, 35360 İzmir, Turkey

Serenat Eris
Gynecology and Obstetrics Department, Isparta Obstetrics and Pediatrics Hospital, 32000 Isparta, Turkey

Seyran Yigit
Pathology Department, Ataturk Training and Research Hospital, Basin Sitesi, Yesilyurt, 35360 İzmir, Turkey

Yakup Yalcin
Gynecologic Oncology Department, Suleyman Demirel University Hospital, 32000 Isparta, Turkey

Pelin Ozun Ozbay
Gynecology and Obstetrics Department, Aydın Obstetrics and Pediatrics Hospital, 09100 Aydın, Turkey

Jayasri Basu, Bolek Bendek, Enyonam Agamasu, Carolyn M. Salafia, Aruna Mishra, Nerys Benfield, Ronak Patel and Magdy Mikhail
Department of Obstetrics & Gynecology, Bronx Lebanon Hospital Center, 1650 Grand Concourse, Bronx, NY 10457, USA

Yibeltal Tebekaw, Yohana James Mashalla and Gloria Thupayagale-Tshweneagae
Department of Health Studies, University of South Africa, Pretoria, South Africa

Simon J. Hogg
Peter MacCallum Cancer Centre, St Andrews Place, East Melbourne, Melbourne, VIC 3002, Australia

Kenny Chitcholtan and Peter H. Sykes
Department of Obstetrics and Gynaecology, University of Otago, Christchurch, 2 Riccarton Avenue, Christchurch 8011, New Zealand

Wafaa Hassan and Ashley Garrill
School of Biological Sciences, University of Canterbury, Private Bag 4800, Christchurch 8140, New Zealand

Qian Meng, Xiucui Luo, Yingping Mu and Wen Xu
Department of Obstetrics, Lianyungang Maternity and Child Health Care Hospital, Lianyungang 222000, China

Qian Meng, Li Shao, Chao Gao, Li Gao, Jiayin Liu and Yugui Cui
The State Key Laboratory of Reproductive Medicine, Center of Clinical Reproductive Medicine, First Affiliated Hospital of Nanjing Medical University, 300 Guangzhou Road, Nanjing 210029, China

Kevin C. Ching and Jules H. Sumkin
Department of Radiology, University of Pittsburgh, 200 Lothrop Street, Suite 3950, Presby South Tower, Pittsburgh, PA 15213, USA

Natsuko Kobayashi, Shigeru Aoki and Tsuneo Takahashi
Perinatal Center for Maternity and Neonates, Yokohama City University Medical Center, 4-57 Urafunecyou, Minami-ku, Yokohama, Kanagawa 232-0024, Japan

Mari S. Oba
Department of Biostatistics and Epidemiology, Yokohama City University Graduate School of Medicine and University Medical Center, Yokohama, Japan

Fumiki Hirahara
Department of Obstetrics and Gynecology, Yokohama City University Hospital, Yokohama, Japan

Andreia Matos, Alda Pereira da Silva, Maria Clara Bicho and Conceição Afonso
Genetics Laboratory, Lisbon Medical School, University of Lisbon, 1649-028 Lisbon, Portugal

Maria José Areias
Júlio Diniz Maternity, Maria Pia Hospital, 4050-371 Porto, Portugal

Irene Rebelo
Department of Biochemistry, Faculty of Pharmacy and Institute for Molecular and Cell Biology, University of Porto, 4050-313 Porto, Portugal

Manuel Bicho
Genetics Laboratory, Lisbon Medical School, University of Lisbon, 1649-028 Lisbon, Portugal
Rocha Cabral Institute, 1250-047 Lisbon, Portugal

C. E. Shehu
Department of Obstetrics and Gynaecology, Usmanu Danfodiyo University Teaching Hospital, PMB 2370, Sokoto 840001, Sokoto State, Nigeria

M. A. Yunusa
Department of Psychiatry, Usmanu Danfodiyo University Teaching Hospital, PMB 2370, Sokoto 840001, Sokoto State, Nigeria

Leona C. Poon and Kypros H. Nicolaides
Harris Birthright Research Centre of Fetal Medicine, King's College Hospital, Denmark Hill, London SE5 9RS, UK

Shoji Kaku, Fuminori Kimura and Takashi Murakami
Department of Obstetrics and Gynecology, Shiga University of Medical Science, Shiga 520-2192, Japan

Seishi Furukawa and Hiroshi Sameshima
Department of Obstetrics & Gynecology, Faculty of Medicine, University of Miyazaki, Miyazaki 889-1692, Japan

Marianne J. Rutten, Gemma G. Kenter and Marrije R. Buist
Centre for Gynaecologic Oncology Amsterdam, Academic Medical Centre, Amsterdam, Netherlands

Gabe S. Sonke
Department of Medical Oncology, Netherlands Cancer Institute, P.O. Box 22700, 1100 DE Amsterdam, Netherlands

Anneke M. Westermann
Department of Medical Oncology, Academic Medical Centre, Amsterdam, Netherlands

Willemien J. van Driel
Centre for Gynaecologic Oncology Amsterdam, Netherlands Cancer Institute, Netherlands

Johannes W. Trum
Centre for Gynaecologic Oncology Amsterdam, Netherlands Cancer Institute, Netherlands
Centre for Gynaecologic Oncology Amsterdam, Free University Medical Centre, Amsterdam, Netherlands

Vinayak Smith
Alice Springs Hospital, Department of Obstetrics and Gynaecology, Alice Springs, NT 0870, Australia

Tiki Osianlis
Monash IVF, 252 Clayton Road, Clayton, VIC 3168, Australia

Beverley Vollenhoven
Monash IVF, 252 Clayton Road, Clayton, VIC 3168, Australia
Monash Health, Women's and Children's Program, Monash Medical Centre, Clayton Road, Clayton, VIC 3168, Australia
Department of Obstetrics and Gynaecology, Monash University, Clayton, VIC 3168, Australia

Stephen J. Genuis
Faculty of Medicine, University of Calgary and University of Alberta, 2935-66 Street, Edmonton, AB, Canada T6K 4C1

Dorette J. Noorhasan
Division of Reproductive Endocrinology and Infertility, Department of Obstetrics, Gynecology and Women's Health, New Jersey Medical School, UMDNJ, Newark, NJ 07103, USA
University Reproductive Associates, Hasbrouck Heights, NJ 07604, USA
Fertility Specialists of Texas, 5757 Warren Parkway, Suite No. 300, Frisco, TX 75034, USA

Michael Cho and Aimee Seungdamrong
Division of Reproductive Endocrinology and Infertility, Department of Obstetrics, Gynecology and Women's Health, New Jersey Medical School, UMDNJ, Newark, NJ 07103, USA
University Reproductive Associates, Hasbrouck Heights, NJ 07604, USA

Khaliq Ahmad
University Reproductive Associates, Hasbrouck Heights, NJ 07604, USA
Department of Obstetrics and Gynecology, Texas Tech University Health Sciences Center School of Medicine, Lubbock, TX 79430, USA

David H. McCulloh
Division of Reproductive Endocrinology and Infertility, Department of Obstetrics, Gynecology and Women's Health, New Jersey Medical School, UMDNJ, Newark, NJ 07103, USA
University Reproductive Associates, Hasbrouck Heights, NJ 07604, USA
NYU Fertility Center, New York University Langone Medical Center, New York, NY 10016, USA

Peter G. McGovern
Division of Reproductive Endocrinology and Infertility, Department of Obstetrics, Gynecology and Women's Health, New Jersey Medical School, UMDNJ, Newark, NJ 07103, USA
University Reproductive Associates, Hasbrouck Heights, NJ 07604, USA
Department of Obstetrics and Gynecology, Saint Luke's Roosevelt Hospital, New York, NY 10019, USA

Norman D. Goldstuck
Department of Obstetrics and Gynaecology, Faculty of Medicine and Health Sciences, Stellenbosch University and Tygerberg Hospital, Western Cape, South Africa

Dirk Wildemeersch
Gynecological Outpatient Clinic and IUD Training Center, Rooseveltlaan 43/44, 9000 Ghent, Belgium

Ayman A. A. Ewies and Zahid R. Khan
Department of Obstetrics and Gynaecology, Birmingham City Hospital, Birmingham, West Midlands B18 7QH, UK

Michael C. Pitter
Department of Obstetrics & Gynecology, Columbia University Medical Center, New York, NY 10032, USA

Serene S. Srouji and Antonio R. Gargiulo
Department of Obstetrics and Gynecology, Center for Infertility and Reproductive Surgery, Brigham and Women's Hospital, Harvard Medical School, 75 Francis Street, Boston, MA 02115, USA

Leslie Kardos
Department of Obstetrics and Gynecology, California Pacific Medical Center, 475 Brannan Street, San Francisco, CA 94107, USA

Usha Seshadri-Kreaden
Department of Clinical Affairs, Intuitive Surgical Inc., 1266 Kifer Road, Building 101, Sunnyvale, CA 94086, USA

Helen B. Hubert
Stanford University School of Medicine Emerita, 1043 Oakland Avenue, Menlo Park, CA 94025, USA

Glenn A. Weitzman
Nashville Fertility Center, 345 23rd Avenue, Nashville, TN 37203, USA

Aliya B. Aziz and Nida Najmi
Department of Obstetrics and Gynaecology, Aga Khan University Hospital, Karachi 74800, Pakistan

Feras Sendy
Obstetrics and Gynecology Department, King Fahad Medical City, Riyadh, Saudi Arabia

Eman AlShehri and Amani AlAjmi
King Khalid University Hospital, King Saud University, Riyadh, Saudi Arabia

Elham Bamanie and Surekha Appani
Obstetrics and Gynecology Department, King Abdulaziz Medical City, King Saud Bin Abdualziz University for Health Science (KSAU-HS), Riyadh, Saudi Arabia

Taghreed Shams
Obstetrics and Gynecology Department, King Abdulaziz Medical City, King Saud Bin Abdulaziz University for Health Science (KSAU-HS), P.O. Box 9515, Jeddah 21423, Saudi Arabia

F. J. Valenzuela, J. Vera, C. Venegas, F. Pino and C. Lagunas
Department of Basic Sciences, Universidad del Bío-Bío, Campus Fernando May, Avenida Andres Bello s/n, Chillán, Chile
Grupo de Ciencias Biotecnológicas, Basic Sciences Department, Universidad del Bío-Bío, Avenida Andres Bello s/n, Chillán, Chile

Divyesh Thakker
Department of Pharmacology, SAL Institute of Pharmacy, Ahmadabad, Gujarat 380060, India

Amit Raval
Department of Pharmaceutical Systems and Policy, School of Pharmacy, West Virginia University, Morgantown, WV 26506, USA

Isha Patel
Department of Biopharmaceutical Sciences, Bernard J. Dunn School of Pharmacy, Shenandoah University, Winchester, VA 22601, USA

Rama Walia
Department of Endocrinology, Post-Graduate Medical Education and Research Institute (PGIMER), Chandigarh 160012, India

Apollinaire G. Horo, Abdoul Koffi, Konan Seni, Kacou Edèle Aka and Mamourou Kone
Department of Gynaecology and Obstetrics, Teaching Hospital of Yopougon, Félix Houphoüet Boigny (FHB) University, Abidjan, Côte d'Ivoire

Judith Didi-Kouko Coulibaly
Oncology Department, Félix Houphoüet Boigny (FHB) University, Teaching Hospital of Treichville, Abidjan, Côte d'Ivoire

Boris Tchounga
PACCI Program, IeDEAWest Africa Collaboration, Abidjan, Côte d'Ivoire

Phyllis C. Leppert and Friederike L. Jayes
Duke University School of Medicine, Durham, NC 27710, USA

James H. Segars
Unit on Reproductive Endocrinology and Infertility, Program on Pediatric and Adult Endocrinology, NICHD, NIH, Bethesda, MD 20892-1109, USA

Niharika Khanna and Stephanie Arnold
Department of Family & Community Medicine, University of Maryland, MD, USA

Aparna Ramaseshan
Department of Obstetrics and Gynecology, University of Maryland School of Medicine, Baltimore, MD 21201, USA

Kalpana Panigrahi
Department of Epidemiology, Center for Global Health & Development, College of Public Health, University of Nebraska Medical Center, Omaha, NE, USA

Mark D. Macek
Department of Dental Public Health, University of Maryland School of Dentistry, Baltimore, MD, USA

Bijaya K. Padhi
Asian Institute of Public Health, Bhubaneswar, Odisha, India

Diptirani Samanta
Department of Medical Oncology, Acharya Harihar Regional Cancer Center, Cuttack, Odisha, India

Surendra N. Senapati
Department of Radiation Oncology, Acharya Harihar Regional Cancer Center, Cuttack, Odisha, India

Pinaki Panigrahi
Department of Epidemiology, Center for Global Health & Development, College of Public Health, University of Nebraska Medical Center, Omaha, NE, USA
Department of Pediatrics, University of Nebraska Medical Center, Omaha, NE, USA

Bart Jan Voskamp, Brenda M. Kazemier, Eva Pajkrt and Wessel Ganzevoort
Department of Obstetrics and Gynecology, Room H4-232, Meibergdreef 9, Academic Medical Center, 1105 AZ Amsterdam, The Netherlands
Julius Center for Health Sciences and Primary Care, University Medical Center Utrecht, Universiteitsweg 100, 3584 CG Utrecht, The Netherlands

Ben Willem J. Mol
The Robinson Institute, School of Paediatrics and Reproductive Health, University of Adelaide, Adelaide, SA 5005, Australia

Maarten Buimer
Department of Obstetrics and Gynecology, Skaraborgs Sjukhus, Skövde, 541 85 Västra Götaland, Sweden

Ewoud Schuit
Department of Obstetrics and Gynecology, Room H4-232, Meibergdreef 9, Academic Medical Center, 1105 AZ Amsterdam, The Netherlands
Julius Center for Health Sciences and Primary Care, University Medical Center Utrecht, Universiteitsweg 100, 3584 CG Utrecht, The Netherlands

Anouk Pels and Wessel Ganzevoort
Department of Obstetrics and Gynecology, Academisch Medisch Centrum, Meibergdreef 9, 1105 AZ Amsterdam, Netherlands

Vidya A. Tamhankar and Junhao Yan
Department of Reproductive Medicine, University of Sheffield, Sheffield Teaching Hospitals, Jessop Wing, Tree Root Walk, Sheffield S10 2SF, UK

Beiyu Liu
Department of Obstetrics and Gynecology, Bronx-Lebanon Hospital Center, Albert Einstein College of Medicine, The Bronx, NY 10457, USA

Tin-Chiu Li
Department of Obstetrics and Gynaecology, Chinese University of Hong Kong, Prince of Wales Hospital, Shatin, N.T., Hong Kong

Eric Roehm
Volunteer Health Clinic, 4215 Medical Pkwy, Austin, TX 78756, USA

Marta Simó González, Oriol Porta Roda, Josep Perelló Capó and Joaquim Calaf Alsina
Department of Gynecology and Obstetrics, Hospital de la Santa Creu i Sant Pau, Universidad Autónoma de Barcelona, C/Mas Casanovas 90, 08025 Barcelona, Spain

Ignasi Gich Saladich
Clinical Epidemiology Unit, Hospital de la Santa Creu i Sant Pau, Universidad Autónoma de Barcelona, C/Mas Casanovas 90, 08025 Barcelona, Spain

www.ingramcontent.com/pod-product-compliance
Lightning Source LLC
Chambersburg PA
CBHW080458200326
41458CB00012B/4009